The Palgrave Handbook of Gender and Healthcare

The Palgrave Handbook of Gender and Healthcare

Second Edition

Edited by

Ellen Kuhlmann
University Campus Suffolk, UK and University of Aarhus, Denmark

and

Ellen Annandale
University of Leicester, UK

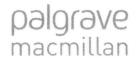

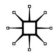
First published in hardback in 2010 and second edition as paperback 2012 by PALGRAVE MACMILLAN

Palgrave Macmillan in the UK is an imprint of Macmillan Publishers Limited, registered in England, company number 785998, of Houndmills, Basingstoke, Hampshire RG21 6XS.

Palgrave Macmillan in the US is a division of St Martin's Press LLC, 175 Fifth Avenue, New York, NY 10010.

Palgrave Macmillan is the global academic imprint of the above companies and has companies and representatives throughout the world.

Palgrave® and Macmillan® are registered trademarks in the United States, the United Kingdom, Europe and other countries.

ISBN 978–1–137–01514–3   paperback

This book is printed on paper suitable for recycling and made from fully managed and sustained forest sources. Logging, pulping and manufacturing processes are expected to conform to the environmental regulations of the country of origin.

A catalogue record for this book is available from the British Library.

A catalog record for this book is available from the Library of Congress.

Contents

Figures

Tables

Boxes

Contributors

Shelly N. Abdool holds an MA in Political Science (Gender and Development) from the University of Western Ontario, Canada. She is currently a technical officer in the Department of Gender, Women and Health at the World Health Organization. Her work focuses on developing practical tools to build capacities of national partners to mainstream gender analysis methods in health sector activities and support country partners in their efforts to improve the health of women and men through gender-responsive plans, policies and actions. Her publications also date back to work on women's health in rural India (*Journal of International Women's Studies*, 2005).

Joy Adamson holds a PhD in Social Medicine from Bristol University, UK. She has a background in both qualitative research methods and epidemiology and is currently Senior Lecturer in the Department of Health Sciences, University of York, UK. Key areas of research are health and healthcare of older people and macro and micro determinants of healthcare consultation. Recent publications include two articles in the *British Journal of General Practice*: 'Exploring the Impact of Patient Views on "Appropriate" Use of Services and Help-seeking: Mixed Method Study' (2009) and 'Age and Gender Interaction in Reported Help Seeking in Response to Chest Pain' (2008).

Avni Amin holds a PhD in International Health from Johns Hopkins University, Bloomberg School of Hygiene and Public Health, Baltimore, USA. She is currently a technical officer in the Department of Gender, Women and Health at the World Health Organization. Her work focuses on evidence generation on gender and health, and supporting gender mainstreaming in technical programmes such as HIV/AIDS. Her most recent publication dates back to work on gender and rights-based approaches to addressing HIV/AIDS among sex workers in India including a paper *Risk, Morality, and Blame* (Washington DC: Center for Health and Gender Equity, 2004).

Ellen Annandale holds a PhD in Sociology from Brown University, USA. She is Professor of Sociology at the University of Leicester, UK, and the Editor-in-Chief of *Social Science & Medicine*. Her work focuses on the relationship between feminist and gender theories and the way that questions about the health of women and men are framed and studied. Her most recent publications are *Women's Health and Social Change* (Routledge, 2009) and the co-edited (with Elianne Riska) edition of *Current Sociology, New Connections: Towards a Gender-inclusive Approach to Women's and Men's Health* (Sage, 2009).

Pat Armstrong holds a PhD in Sociology from Carleton University, Ottawa, and is a Professor in Sociology at York University, Canada. She holds a Canadian Health Services Research Foundation/Canadian Institutes of Health Research Chair in Health Services and chairs Women and Health Care Reform. Her research focuses on gender and health services, using a political economy perspective. Most recently, she has co-authored *Critical to Care: The Invisible Women in Health Services* (University of Toronto Press, 2008), *About Canada: Health Care* (Fernwood, 2008); '*They Deserve Better': The Long Term Care Experience in Canada and Scandinavia* (CCPA, 2009) and co-edited *Women's Health: Intersections of Policy, Research, and Practice* (Women's Press, 2008).

Jim Barry holds a PhD in Sociology with Politics from Birkbeck College, University of London, UK. He is Professor of Gender and Organization Studies at the University of East London. Research interests include gender, new public management and social movements. He is co-author (with Mike Dent and Maggie O'Neill) of *Gender and the Public Sector* (Routledge, 2003), was Guest Editor of the special issue of *Equal Opportunities International*, 'Gender, Management and Governance in the Public Sector' in 2007 and co-author (with Elisabeth Berg and John Chandler) of 'Essentially Political: Gender and the Politics of Care in Mumbai' in the *International Feminist Journal of Politics* (2010). He is Associate Editor of *Gender, Work & Organization* and member of the Editorial Advisory Board of *Equal Opportunities International*.

Susan E. Bell holds a PhD in Sociology from Brandeis University, USA. She is currently Professor of Sociology and A. Myrick Freeman Professor of Social Sciences at Bowdoin College in Maine, USA. Her scholarship investigates the experience of illness, women's health, and visual and performative representations of the politics of cancer, medicine and women's bodies. Her most recent publications are 'Artworks, Collective Experience, and Claims for Social Justice' (with Alan Radley, *Sociology of Health and Illness*, 2007), and *DES Daughters: Embodied Knowledge and the Transformation of Women's Health Politics* (Temple, 2009).

Cecilia Benoit holds a PhD in Sociology from the University of Toronto, Canada. She is currently a Scientist at the Centre for Addictions Research of British Columbia and Professor in the Department of Sociology at the University of Victoria. Apart from ongoing research focused on the occupation of midwifery and the organization of maternity care in Canada and internationally, she is involved in a variety of projects that employ mixed methodologies to investigate the health of different vulnerable populations. Her most recent publication is a co-edited edition of *Current Sociology*, 'Comparative Perspectives on the Professions' (2009, with Ivy Lynn Bourgeault).

Elisabeth Berg holds a PhD and is a Professor of Sociology in the Department of Human Work Science, Luleå University of Technology, Sweden, and Visiting

Professor at the University of East London, UK. She is a member of the Editorial Advisory Board of the journal *Equal Opportunities International*. Her work focuses on the relationship between gender, management and professionals. She has published on 'Women's Positioning in a Bureaucratic Environment: Combining Employment and Mothering' (2003) and 'New Public Management and Social Work in Sweden and England', *International Journal of Sociology and Social Policy* (2008, with John Chandler and Jim Barry).

Chloe E. Bird holds a PhD from the University of Illinois, Urbana, USA. She is Senior Sociologist at the RAND Corporation, Professor of Sociology at Pardee RAND Graduate School, USA, and Associate Editor of the journal *Women's Health Issues*. Her work focuses on gender differences in health and healthcare. Her recent publications include a co-authored article on 'Neighbourhood Socioeconomic Status and Biological "Wear & Tear" in a Nationally Representative Sample of US Adults', in the *Journal of Epidemiology and Community Health* (2010), and the *Handbook of Medical Sociology*, 6th edition (co-edited with Peter Conrad, Allen Fremont and Stefan Timmermans, Vanderbilt University Press, 2010).

Robert H. Blank holds a PhD in Political Science from the University of Maryland, USA. He is currently a Research Scholar at the New College of Florida, USA, and Professor at the University of Canterbury, Christchurch, New Zealand. He has published numerous articles and more than 35 books on health and biomedical policy including *End of Life Decision Making* (MIT, 2007, edited with Janna C. Merrick), *Comparative Health Policy*, third edition (Palgrave Macmillan, 2010, with Viola Burau) and *Condition Critical* (Fulcrum, 2007, with Richard D. Lamm). Current areas of interest include health priority setting, medical technology assessment and neuroscience policy.

Ivy Lynn Bourgeault holds a PhD in Community Health from the University of Toronto, Canada. She is currently Professor of Health Sciences at the University of Ottawa, CIHR/Health Canada Research Chair in Health Human Resource Policy, and Scientific Director of the Population Health Improvement and Ontario Health Human Resources Research Networks. She has edited (with Robert Dingwall and Raymond De Vries) *The Sage Handbook of Qualitative Methods in Health Research* (Sage, 2010).

Alex Broom holds a PhD in Sociology from La Trobe University, Melbourne, Australia. He is Associate Professor of Sociology and Australia Research Council Future Fellow at the School of Social Science, the University of Queensland, Australia. He is a Visiting Professor at Jawaharlal Nehru University, India and Brunel University, London, UK and Director of Social Science Research for the Network of Researchers in the Public Health of Complementary and Alternative Medicine. Recent books include: *Traditional, Complementary and Alternative*

Medicine and Cancer Care (Routledge, 2007), *Men's Health: Body, Identity and Social Context* (Wiley-Blackwell, 2009), and *Health, Culture and Religion in South Asia* (Routledge, 2011).

Viola Burau holds a PhD from the University of Edinburgh, Scotland. She is Associate Professor of Public Policy in the Department of Political Science, University of Aarhus, Denmark. Her work analyses, mostly from a cross-country comparative perspective, the policies and politics of welfare services and the governance of professions. Her most recent publications include the co-authored (with Hildegard Theobald and Robert H. Blank) research monograph *Governing Home Care* (Edward Elgar, 2007), 'Governing Medical Performance' (special issue of *Health Economics, Policy and Law*, 2009) and the co-authored (with Robert H. Blank) third edition of *Comparative Health Policy* (Palgrave Macmillan, 2010).

Joan Busfield, who initially trained as a clinical psychologist at the Tavistock Clinic, London, has a PhD from the University of Essex, UK, where she is a Professor of Sociology. Her books include *Men, Women and Madness: Understanding Gender and Mental Disorder* (Macmillan, 1996), *Health and Health Care in Modern Britain* (Oxford University Press, 2000) and *Rethinking the Sociology of Mental Illness* (ed., Blackwell, 2001). Her recent research has focused on the pharmaceutical industry; for instance, 'Pills, Power, People: Sociological Understandings of the Pharmaceutical Industry' (*Sociology*, 2006).

Sarah Cant holds an Msc (Econ) in Sociology as Applied to Medicine and is a Principal Lecturer in Sociology and Social Science at Canterbury Christ Church University, UK. Her research has focused on healthcare that stands outside state provision, namely the private sector and complementary and alternative medicine (CAM). In particular, she has developed an interest in the processes of professionalization, focusing on questions of power, legitimacy and trust. Her most recent funded research in this area has centred on the use of CAM by nurses and midwives and is published in *Social Science & Medicine* (2011).

John Chandler holds a PhD from Luleå University of Technology, Sweden. He is a Reader in Organization Studies in the Business School, University of East London, UK. His work currently focuses on public services management and the social consequences of managerialism in various contexts, particularly higher education, health and social care. Recent publications include an article in *Qualitative Research in Accounting and Management* (2008) entitled 'Academics as Professionals or Managers?' and another (with Jim Barry and Elisabeth Berg) in *Public Administration* (2007), 'Women's Movements and New Public Management: Higher Education in Sweden and England'.

Anoshua Chaudhuri holds a PhD in Economics from the University of Washington, USA, and an MA in Economics from the Delhi School of

Economics, India. She is currently Associate Professor in the Department of Economics, San Francisco State University. Her research is in health economics with a focus on global health. Recent work includes disparities in health outcomes, health payments and health services utilization among children and the elderly as a result of health programmes and policies in South and South-east Asian countries. She is also working on issues around intergenerational support for the elderly in South Asia and among the South Asian Diaspora.

Ling-fang Cheng holds a PhD from the University of Essex, UK. Currently she is Associate Professor in the Graduate Institute of Gender Studies, Kaohsiung Medical University, Taiwan and the Editor-in-Chief of *Gender Equality Quarterly* (Ministry of Education, Taiwan). Her work focuses on gender relations in the medical profession, professional–user relations, and gender and health issues. As a member of the Advisory Committee for Gender Equity at the Ministry of Education, Taiwan, she is actively involved in integrating gender into medical and nursing education. Her most recent publication is *A Dialogue between Medicine and Society* (Qunxue, 2008).

Raymond De Vries holds a PhD in Sociology from the University of California, Davis, and is Professor in the Bioethics Program and the Departments of Obstetrics and Gynaecology and Medical Education at the University of Michigan Medical School, USA. He is currently studying the history of bioethics; regulation of science; international research ethics; difficulties of informed consent; bioethics and the problem of suffering; and ethics of non-medically indicated surgical birth. He is author of *A Pleasing Birth: Midwifery and Maternity Care in the Netherlands* (Temple University Press, 2005), and co-editor of *The View from Here: Bioethics and the Social Sciences* (Blackwell, 2007).

Eugene Declercq holds a PhD in Political Science from Florida State University, USA. He is a Professor of Community Health Sciences and Assistant Dean for Doctoral Education at the Boston University School of Public Health and Professor in the Department of Obstetrics and Gynaecology of the Boston University School of Medicine.

Lesley Doyal holds an MSc (Econ) from the London School of Economics. She is Emeritus Professor in the School for Policy Studies, University of Bristol, UK, and Visiting Professor, University of Cape Town, South Africa. She is especially interested in gender and health issues from international and comparative perspectives, and has recently completed a series of studies of HIV-positive African migrants in London which were set within a paradigm of intersectionality. Publications from this work have appeared in *Culture, Health and Sexuality, Social Science & Medicine* and *Sexualities*. She is currently finishing a book, *Living with HIV and Dying from AIDS*.

Jane Edwards holds a PhD in the Sociology of Health and Illness from the University of Adelaide, Australia. She has a long-standing interest in the relationship between gender, sexuality and health and between 2004 and 2008 was a member of the South Australian Ministerial Advisory Committee on Gay and Lesbian Health. Currently, she is with the Centre for Work and Life at the University of South Australia undertaking research on the impact of work–life issues on sustainable lifestyles.

Elizabeth Ettorre holds a PhD in Sociology from the London School of Economics. She is currently Professor of Sociology in the School of Sociology and Social Policy, University of Liverpool, UK. Her work focuses on women and health. In this area, she has developed specific interests in reproduction, drugs, embodiment and depression. Her most recent publications are *Culture Bodies and the Sociology of Health* (Ashgate, 2010), *Revisioning Women and Drugs: Gender Power and the Body* (Palgrave Macmillan, 2007) and *Reproductive Genetics, Gender and the Body* (Routledge, 2002).

Anne E. Figert holds a PhD in Sociology from Indiana University, USA. She is currently Associate Professor in the Department of Sociology, Loyola University, Chicago, USA. Her work focuses on expertise, medicalization and HIV/AIDS service provision. Her recent publications include articles on medicalization, HIV/AIDS housing policy and on the relationship between scientific and religious authority.

Paul Galdas holds a PhD in Nursing from the University of Leeds, UK. He is currently Senior Lecturer in the Department of Health Sciences at the University of York, UK. His scholarly work focuses on the intersections of gender and ethnicity with men's health-related behaviours and experiences, with a particular focus on cardiovascular health and the South Asian community.

Claudia García-Moreno is a physician from Mexico with a Masters in Community Medicine from the London School of Hygiene and Tropical Medicine, UK. She was involved in the negotiations for the Plan of Action of the ICPD in 1994 and the Beijing Declaration and Platform of Action in 1995 and has led WHO's work on gender and health and on violence against women. She coordinated the WHO Multi-Country Study on Women's Health and Domestic Violence, initiated and chaired the Sexual Violence Research Initiative and is on the editorial board of several public health journals, including *Development in Practice* and *Reproductive Health Matters*.

Leah Gilbert holds a PhD as well as an MPH. She is Professor of Health Sociology in the Department of Sociology, University of the Witwatersrand, Johannesburg, South Africa. She has published widely on social aspects of dentistry, the role of pharmacy in primary healthcare, and medical and healthcare pluralism. Her current research focuses on health professionals in the context of HIV/AIDS, and the social complexity of anti-retroviral therapy. She is one of the authors (with Terry-Ann Selikow and Liz Walker) of *Society, Health and Disease in a Time of HIV/ AIDS: An Introductory Reader for Health Professionals* (Macmillan, 2010).

Kate Hunt holds a PhD from Glasgow University, UK, and is an Honorary Professor in the Division of Community-based Sciences there. She is also a Professorial Fellow at Stirling University, UK. For many years she has conducted research on social and gender inequalities in health and on understandings of health and illness. She currently leads a research programme on Gender and Health at the UK Medical Research Council's Social and Public Health Sciences Unit at Glasgow University. She co-edited (with Ellen Annandale) *Gender and Health Inequalities* (Open University Press, 2000).

Carol Kingdon holds a PhD in Sociology and is currently a Senior Research Fellow at the Faculty of Health, University of Central Lancashire, UK. Her research areas are midwifery and women's health. She has published widely on aspects of caesarean delivery for maternal request and is the author of *Sociology for Midwives* (Quay Books, 2009).

Ineke Klinge holds a PhD in Biomedicine. She is currently Associate Professor of Gender/Diversity Medicine at School Caphri, Maastricht University, the Netherlands, and was previously Visiting Professor in Gender Medicine at Göttingen University, Germany. Her research focuses on innovation of biomedical and health research methodologies through integration of sex and gender. Since 2000 she has executed successive projects in the field for the European Commission of which the GenderBasic project was selected as a 'success story' of the 6th Framework Programme. She edited a special volume of *Gender Medicine* (2007) on 'Bringing Gender Expertise to Biomedical and Health Research'.

Petra Kolip holds a PhD in Psychology. She is Professor of Prevention and Health Promotion at Bielefeld University, Germany. Her research interests pertain to the interaction between the medical system and patients, focusing especially on women's health issues; gender mainstreaming in healthcare systems; and gender-adequate healthcare and prevention. Her most prominent books are (with Ellen Kuhlmann) *Gender und Public Health* (2005); and (edited with Klaus Hurrelmann) *Geschlecht, Gesundheit und Krankheit* (2002). She published a Gender Health Report for Germany in 2005 and a Gender Health Report for Switzerland in 2006 (both with Julia Lademann).

Ellen Kuhlmann holds a PhD in Sociology and an MA in Public Health. She is currently Visiting Professor of Sociology, University Campus Suffolk, UK and University of Aarhus, Denmark. Trained as a nurse, she also has extensive clinical experience. Key areas of research are health policy, healthcare organization and management, and the professions, including cross-country comparison and gender-sensitive approaches. Recent publications include *Modernising Health*

Care (Policy Press, 2006) and *Rethinking Professional Governance: International Directions in Healthcare* (co-edited with Mike Saks, Policy Press, 2008).

Toine Lagro-Janssen holds a PhD in Medicine, is a registered and practising GP and holds a Professorship in Women's Health. She is a Principal Lecturer and Head of the Unit of Women's Health at the Medical Centre, Radboud University Nijmegen, the Netherlands. Her key areas of research are: gender in medical education and professional development; intimate partner violence and sexual abuse; pelvic floor problems; reproductive health issues, especially home delivery; and female students/doctors, careers and leadership.

Martha E. Lang holds a PhD in Sociology from Brown University, USA. She is currently Visiting Assistant Professor in Sociology/Anthropology and Coordinator of Gay, Lesbian, Bisexual and Transgendered Resources at Guilford College, North Carolina, USA. Her work focuses on the interrelationships of gender, race, class and sexual orientation on health outcomes. Her most recent publication, co-authored with Patricia Rieker and Chloe Bird, is 'Understanding Gender and Health: Old Patterns, New Trends and Future Directions', in the *Handbook of Medical Sociology*, 6th edition (Vanderbilt University Press, 2010).

Christa Larsen holds a PhD from the University of Essen in Germany and studied sociology, political sciences and economics in Germany and the United States. She is currently the Managing Director of the Institute for Economics, Labour and Culture (IWAK) at Goethe-University Frankfurt, Germany. Her research focuses on regional labour market and skills monitoring, including health human resource planning and management. She is the coordinator of the European Network of Regional Labour Market Monitoring (RLMM) and has developed a monitoring system for nurses in the region of Hesse, Germany. She has also led several European projects on illegal employment in home care.

Vivian Lin holds a MPH and DrPH from the University of California Berkeley, USA. She is Professor of Public Health at La Trobe University in Melbourne, Australia, and has worked previously in health policy for various Australian state governments. She is also Vice President for Scientific Affairs for the International Union for Health Promotion and Education (IUHPE) and a board member of the Cooperative Research Centre on Aboriginal Health. She works closely with the World Health Organization (Western Pacific Regional Office) on health promotion and health systems issues. Her most recent book *China Health Policy in Transition,* was published bilingually by Peking University Medical Press in 2010.

Helen L'Orange is an Honorary Associate, School of Public Health, La Trobe University, Melbourne, Australia. She has been instrumental in policy development and programme implementation in government at local, national and international levels. This includes consultancies with the WHO on women and health and several years as Head of the Australian Office for the Status of Women. Her most recent publication is the *Western Pacific Region Baseline Assessment Report* prepared as part of a WHO-wide 2008 baseline assessment of the WHO Strategy on Integrating Gender Analysis and Actions into the work of WHO (2009).

Tulsi Patel is Professor of Sociology and teaches in the Department of Sociology, Delhi School of Economics, Delhi University, India. Her research interests include gender and society, anthropology of reproduction and childbirth knowledge systems, medical sociology, sociology of kinship and family, and old age. She has authored *Fertility Behaviour: Population and Society in a Rajasthan Village* (Oxford University Press, 2006), and edited *The Family in India: Structure and Practice* (Sage, 2005) and *Sex Selective Abortion in India: Gender, Society and New Reproductive Technologies* (Sage, 2007).

Sarah Payne holds a PhD in Social Policy from Bristol University, UK, where she is currently a Professor in Health Policy and Gender in the School for Policy Studies. Her research focuses on gender inequalities in health and gender equity in health policy. Recent studies have explored differences in mental health, suicidal behaviour, colorectal cancer, access to healthcare, as well as gender equity and gender mainstreaming. Her latest publications include *The Health of Men and Women* (Polity, 2006), and *How Can Gender Equity Be Improved through Health Systems?* (World Health Organization, 2009).

Patricia P. Rieker holds a PhD in Sociology from the University of Pittsburgh, USA. She is an adjunct Professor of Sociology, Boston University and Associate Professor of Psychiatry at Harvard Medical School. Her current work is focused on cross-national comparisons of gender and health, evaluation of public health interventions and the gender gap in child health. Recent publications include a co-authored book (with Chloe E. Bird), *Gender and Health: The Effects of Constrained Choices and Social Policies* (Cambridge University Press, 2008), and she is a main author of *Introduction to Process Evaluation in Tobacco Use, Prevention and Control* (US Centers for Disease Control, 2008).

Elianne Riska holds a PhD from Stony Brook University, New York State, USA. She is currently Professor of Sociology at the Swedish School of Social Science, University of Helsinki, Finland. Her recent articles examine gender and medical education in the *Handbook of the Sociology of Medical Education* (Routledge, 2009) and women physicians in Lithuania in the journal *Gender Issues* (2008). She has examined men's health in her book *Masculinity and Men's Health* (Rowman and Littlefield, 2004), and in a chapter on men's mental health in *Men's Health* (Wiley-Blackwell, 2009), and co-edited a monograph issue (with Ellen Annandale) on gender and health for *Current Sociology* (2009).

Kakoli Roy holds both a PhD and MA in Economics. She is currently a Senior Economist at the Centers for Disease Control of Prevention (CDC), United States Department of Health and Human Services. Her current research interests include integrating economic methods in assessing the burden of disease and health inequalities in the USA, public health systems and workforce research, and analysing inequities in health outcomes and healthcare access in low-income countries. Before joining CDC, she was a Senior Fellow at the Center for Development Research (ZEF), University of Bonn, Germany.

Jane Sandall holds a PhD in Sociology from Surrey University, UK, and initially worked as a midwife. She is currently Professor of Social Sciences and Women's Health in the Department of Public Health, King's College, London, UK. She is leading a programme of work in the King's Patient Safety Research Centre on clinical innovation and new health technologies and the implementation of patient safety strategies in acute medicine and maternity care. She has interests in how the social and cultural shaping of maternal health policy influences the organization and delivery of services, and exploring safety and quality initiatives in healthcare.

Toni Schofield holds a PhD in Government and Public Administration from the University of Sydney, Australia. She is currently Associate Professor in the Faculty of Health Sciences at the University of Sydney. Her research focuses on sociological and policy dimensions of a range of topics in health, especially gender, health and healthcare, maternity services, class and health inequalities, workplace health, and harm minimization in young people's alcohol use. The principal objective of her work is to analyse and understand the social dynamics involved in the distribution and embodiment of health and illness in order to identify barriers and opportunities for public interventions to redress them.

Terry-Ann Selikow holds a Masters in Sociology from the University of the Witwatersrand, Johannesburg, South Africa, and a PhD in the Sociology of Education from the University of Alberta, Canada. She is a Lecturer in the Department of Sociology, University of the Witwatersrand, Johannesburg, where she teaches courses in Health Sociology. Her research and publications are in the area of youth sexuality and HIV/AIDS with a particular focus on gendered dynamics in South Africa. She is one of the authors (with Leah Gilbert and Liz Walker) of *Society, Health and Disease in a Time of HIV/AIDS: An Introductory Reader for Health Professionals* (Macmillan, 2010)

Hilary Standing holds a PhD in Social Anthropology from London University. She was a professorial fellow at the Institute of Development Studies, University of Sussex, and is now Emeritus Professor at the University of Sussex, UK. Her key areas of research are health systems development in the context of rapid transitions and conceptual and policy issues in gender and health equity. A specialist on South Asia, her recent publications include co-editing (with Gerald Bloom) a special issue of *Social Science & Medicine* (66, 2008) on 'Future Health Systems' and editing (with Andrea Cornwall and Andrea Lynch) *IDS Bulletin*, 39 (2008) on 'Unsafe Abortion: A Development Issue?'.

Rebecca Sutherns holds a PhD in Rural Studies from the University of Guelph, Canada, which focused on rural maternity care. She now specializes in researching and creating sustainable, accessible models of healthcare for marginalized populations. She also maintains a facilitation, strategic planning and policy analysis consulting business called Sage Solutions.

Hildegard Theobald holds a PhD in Political Science from the Free University of Berlin, Germany. She is Professor at the Research Centre on Ageing and Society, Vechta University, Germany. Her research focuses on care policies – development and outcomes – and care work and professionalization in an international comparative and transnational perspective. Conceptually, she combines approaches in international comparative welfare state research, public policy research and theories on inequality and intersectionality. Recent publications include a co-authored book (with Viola Burau and Robert H. Blank), *Governing Home Care: A Cross-national Comparison* (Edward Elgar, 2007).

Edwin van Teijlingen holds a PhD in Sociology from the University of Aberdeen, UK. He is Professor of Maternal and Perinatal Health at Bournemouth University, UK. His key areas of research include public health and the relationship between culture and the organization of maternity care. He has published on a wide variety of topics, including qualitative research methods. His co-edited books include *Birth by Design: Pregnancy, Maternity Care and Midwifery in North America and Europe* (with Raymond De Vries, Cecilia Benoit and Sirpa Wrede; Routledge, 2001) and *Midwifery and the Medicalization of Childbirth* (with George Lowis, Peter McCaffery and Maureen Porter; Nova Science, 2004).

Peter Watts holds a PhD in Sociology from Brunel University, UK. He is currently a Senior Lecturer in Sociology in the Department of Applied Social Sciences at Canterbury Christ Church University, UK. His academic interests include complementary and alternative medicine, sexuality and medicine and governmentality. His most recent publication, co-authored with Sarah Cant and Annmarie Ruston, is 'Negotiating Competency, Professionalism and Risk: The Integration of Complementary and Alternative Medicine by Nurses and Midwives in NHS Hospitals', *Social Science & Medicine* (2011).

Sirpa Wrede holds a PhD in Sociology from Åbo Akademi University, Finland. She is Research Fellow at the Collegium for Advanced Studies and University Lecturer and Adjunct Professor in Sociology at the University of Helsinki. Her key areas of research are the historical as well as contemporary reconfigurations of professionalism and professional power. She currently conducts research on professional expertise and welfare professionalism in 'glocalizing' welfare systems and leads a four-year research project on the shaping of occupational subjectivities of migrant care workers.

Preface to the Second Edition

Since the first edition of the *Palgrave Handbook of Gender and Healthcare* was published in 2010, interest in the gender dimensions of healthcare has continued to grow worldwide. As the 29 chapters in this expanded and updated edition of the *Handbook* show, the social and health sciences have much to offer to anyone seeking to understand how and why gender matters to the delivery of healthcare and, consequently, to the health of men and women in societies and to healthcare systems worldwide. They help us to see that gender differences, which may easily turn into inequalities in access to care and the provision of care, are often socially created and politically motivated. Hence, gendered health inequalities are pliable and open to change, should political will be found at the level of national and local governments, healthcare organization and professional associations.

Increased global connectivity directs our attention to the shared vulnerability and precariousness of lives and health around the world. As social relations of gender change and become more complex, so too do the health experiences of men and women. Health systems are also undergoing significant change as they respond to the international marketization of care, adopt neoliberal policies which lay emphasis on private-sector management models, and adapt to the increased mobility of patients, citizens and healthcare providers as well as to changing demands for healthcare services. The need to bring a gender lens to bear on these matters has never been greater.

It is therefore an opportune time to take stock and form a platform for future research and practice. This second edition includes new chapters on health human resource management and policy; end-of-life care; and complementary and alternative medicine; and also revised Introduction and Conclusion chapters. Covering health issues from early life to the end of life, this revised edition charts why a gender lens is important to patient care and to the work of healthcare practitioners and policy-makers in various parts of the world. As well as summarizing and evaluating existing research knowledge, it provides practical insights and poses questions for future research.

In developing the Handbook we have greatly benefited from constructive comments and valuable feedback that we received from colleagues and reviewers and at various conferences. The Handbook would not have been possible without enthusiastic support from our colleagues from across the world; they have authored a unique collection of chapters covering a wide range of topics from a range of geopolitical perspectives. We are thankful to all of the authors and to our publisher at Palgrave, Philippa Grand, for their continuing collaboration over the past couple of years since the publication of the first edition and for their enthusiasm and support for bringing gender onto the agenda of healthcare and policy-makers.

Ellen Annandale and Ellen Kuhlmann

March 2012

Introduction

Bringing Gender to the Heart of Health Policy, Practice and Research

Ellen Kuhlmann and Ellen Annandale

Gender is known to be strongly associated with health status and to exert a significant influence upon help-seeking and the delivery of healthcare, but it has been a relatively low policy priority for many governments and also within the health professions until very recently. Heightened awareness of gender equity issues and the introduction of gender mainstreaming policies have increased interest in gender in relation to health around the world. Yet the current evidence base is scattered and fragmentary. Attempts to mainstream gender into healthcare often turn out to be simplified reports of sex differences without taking account of the complex life conditions of men and women and the gendered dimensions of the organization and delivery of healthcare. Added to this, changing health policies, together with globalization and ageing societies, accelerate dynamics in healthcare systems that may affect women and men in different ways. New emerging social inequalities may create new demands on health policy-makers and health professionals that need further empirical investigation.

This is an optimum time to draw state-of-the-art thinking on gender and healthcare together into one compilation. Consequently, this edited Handbook brings together international experts from different countries and academic disciplines. The collection takes a critical and reflective approach and explores the challenges and opportunities of bringing gender to the heart of health policy, practice and research. Starting with more general issues of gendering health policy, healthcare and human resources and exploring the social patterning of health and illness, key themes in the debates over health reform are then addressed, such as access to services, the organization of care and professional development and education in healthcare.

A particular strength of this edited Handbook is a more integrated and context-sensitive approach to changing healthcare and gender relations than is currently available. This includes attention to men's and women's health, actor-centred and institutional approaches to healthcare, as well as to the

1

needs of service users and professionals. Another innovative feature of the book is the use of case studies from Anglo-American, continental European and developing countries. And yet another advance is its focus on the intersections between gender and a wide range of social inequalities, such as, for instance, 'race', age, sexual orientation and place.

In our Introduction we begin by locating the sex–gender debate in the context of 21st-century healthcare and outline key definitions and concepts that recur across the various chapters and topics of this Handbook. Here, the gender mainstreaming approach is indicative and provides a springboard for flagging the field of contemporary healthcare through the lens of gender. This is the theme of the following section which highlights the opportunities and risks of gender being mainstreamed into the policy and practice of healthcare as well as the blind spots that it generates. Finally, we introduce the structure of the Handbook and highlight key issues discussed in the chapters.

Locating gender

Gender-sensitive healthcare and women's healthcare issues are increasingly moving from the margins of feminist activism to the mainstream of health policy; and men's health and well-being has also emerged as a new field over the past decade. A growing body of public statistics and epidemiological research reveals differences between the health of men and women – mainly studied in relation to illnesses and rarely in relation to health and well-being – that are usually discussed as disadvantages for women, and increasingly also for men (Annandale, 2009a). Reliable databases and evidence-based policies are the backbone of gender-sensitive research, but they do not tell us much about the reasons *why and how* disadvantages come about. All too often research focuses only on a cluster of proximate causes, be they quantitatively or qualitatively defined, and the relationship between gender and health loses its structural moorings. Without these moorings we are left with similarities and differences in women's and men's health status and similarities and differences in their experience of health and illness for which we have no real explanation beyond a generalized sense that they are related to women's and men's positioning within society (Annandale, 2009b). But health research rarely takes a system – or healthcare – approach that would help to explore opportunities for more systematic policy interventions towards gender-sensitive healthcare.

Furthermore, the concepts of sex and gender are often re-merged into one single concept of 'gender'. To give only some examples, in medicine and clinical research gender is increasingly debated but underpinned by a new emergent biologism – that is, using the language of gender while actually talking about sex differences and subsequently offering medical solutions. Similarly, within the discourse of changing gender relations in the health workforce, the sex category (numbers of males and females in occupations and professions) is utilized as a means of explaining or predicting changes in the content of healthcare or the power of a professional group (gender category). This is embodied in the discourse of the so-called feminization of medicine and occurs where, for instance, trends towards more gender-sensitive clinical decision-making or patient-centred medicine are read off from growing numbers of women doctors; much the same is true for the assumption that women may bring about a decline of medical power. Yet another version of the problematic conflation of sex–gender is the implicit but widely shared assumption that 'women will do things right' due to their 'caring nature' which has led to an overall neglect of gender policies and gender-sensitive research in the mainly female health professional workforce, from nursing to complementary and alternative therapists.

In summary, gender mainstreaming policies and the new discourses of 'gender medicine' or 'sex-specific medicine' are shadowed by unsolved gender troubles. So the new gender policies are becoming more easily digestible for a wide range of policy-makers and health professionals – practitioners as well as researchers – and gender-sensitive healthcare is torn from its original feminist linkages, including the problems with the sex–gender distinction and social relations of power. In this Handbook we do not attempt to debate the theoretical and epistemological queries raised by the sex and gender categories (see, for example, Clarke and Olesen, 1999), but we do call for greater caution and suggest ways to unpack the sex–gender dimensions and relocate the gender category more systematically in its social context, including structural, cultural and action dimensions and how they intersect.

Here we would like to recall that the sex–gender distinction originated in psychiatry about half a century ago and was taken up by feminist scholars as an attempt to counteract biologism and the devaluation of women. Within this binary framework, 'sex' marks the biological and 'gender' the social category. For many years, this distinction has served health activists in their bid to challenge biological explanations for social inequalities and bring the social constructions and configurations of inequality into sight (for an overview, see Annandale and Hunt, 2000); it has fuelled the hopes of many women (and some men) that what is socially constructed can be rearranged. At the same time, the 'gender binary' has always been a matter of controversy in feminist theory. Numerous attempts to cross the sex–gender divide and/or expand the binary framework give proof of the demands for more fluid and flexible gender concepts that are better able to integrate structural, biological and social constructionist dimensions of gender and health (see, for example, Connell, 2011; Lorber, 2005).

Two approaches have been particularly important in healthcare, namely the concept of 'doing gender' (West and Zimmerman, 1987) that highlights action and process dimensions, and the concept of diversity that attempts to link gender and other categories of social inequality, like race, class or sexual orientation (Sen and Iyer, 2012). More recently, the concept of intersectionality is gaining currency. The intersectional approach also attempts to incorporate diversity and multiple differences but brings a more dynamic dimension to the (un-)making of inequalities, that may even question the master status of the gender category itself (for an overview, see Bates et al., 2012).

Taken together, these concepts are enabling us to better understand the processes and micro-politics of social inequalities, but they often fail to adequately explore the institutional contexts. While the role of women and men as active players and the differences within them are brought into view, this does not necessarily empower people to change the unhealthy gender relations in society. Thus a major shortcoming of the 'doing gender' and the 'diversity' approaches is a neglect of the institutional conditions that either constrain or enable choices for health (Bird and Rieker, 2008), and intersectionality may even reinforce the need for an institutional embeddedness, because gender may easily get lost in the jungle of diversity and differences.

Here, the concept of gender mainstreaming marks a new era that places gender-sensitive healthcare in the context of public policy and the respective institutional and organizational architecture, thereby opening up new chances for interventions towards gender equality (Council of Europe, 1998; United Nations, 1999; see also Bacchi and Eveline, 2010; Kuhlmann and Annandale, 2012). However, before we turn our attention to the new gender mainstreaming policies, it is important to keep in mind that the unsolved problems of the sex–gender binary and universal categories of 'woman' and 'man' are also embedded in the mainstream of healthcare.

The concept of gender mainstreaming

The concept of gender mainstreaming is part of new governance approaches in public sector services. As such it also applies to the health sector where it is supported by international organizations, such as the United Nations (1999), the World Bank (2011) and the World Health Organization (WHO Euro, 2001, 2011a) as well as the European Union (Council of Europe, 1998). Gender mainstreaming is an umbrella term for new approaches to both gender equality and policy-making; it is open to various definitions and political strategies, including redefinitions of the relationship between difference/equality and nature/culture that is embodied in the sex–gender distinction. We draw on the definition of gender mainstreaming adapted by WHO:

> ... the process of assessing the implications for women and men of any planned action, including legislation, policies or programmes, in any area and at all levels. It is a strategy for making women's as well as men's con-

cerns and experiences an integral dimension in the design, implementation, monitoring and evaluation of policies and programmes in all political, economic and social spheres, such that inequality between men and women is not perpetuated. The ultimate goal is to achieve gender equality. (WHO, 2007: n.p.)

Based on the 1995 Beijing platform of the fourth International World Conference of Women, gender mainstreaming is itself a result of both feminist critiques of essentialist approaches to women and a response to the changing governance of the public sector. Woodward (2008: 290) characterizes these two dimensions of gender mainstreaming as 'a tool to transform gender relations through public policy' and 'a reflection of the equality/difference debate in feminist theory'. When it comes to healthcare, gender mainstreaming is assigned a double role: as an approach to reduce social inequalities in health which, at the same time, improves the quality and efficiency of the provision and delivery of healthcare. This linkage calls for new mechanisms of accountability and the removal of the 'organisational plaque', as a report from the Karolinska Institute dubbed the male bias embedded in healthcare services and reform strategies (Sen et al., 2007: 17). Accordingly, gender mainstreaming provides a new opportunity for more diverse and contextualized approaches on gender relations, and for closer links with health policy processes, medical governance and the organizational restructuring of healthcare.

This approach expands previous feminist research and theorizing on welfare states that has mainly looked at institutionalized masculinities (Connell, 1987) and how women as 'outsiders' are becoming 'insiders' and players in the policy process. Existing research highlights that political opportunity structures for gender-sensitive healthcare are not only arising from feminist and women's healthcare activism but also from – seemingly gender-neutral – new demands for tighter regulation of healthcare providers and an overall changing governance of public sector services. For instance, new models of governing and monitoring services, in particular target-setting, standardization and evidence-based health policies, provide new opportunities for the development of gender-sensitive performance indicators, as for instance explored in the US healthcare system (McKinley et al., 2001). However, the new managerial regimes also create incentives towards prioritizing indicators that are financially inexpensive and easy to measure, quantifiable and comparable across organizations and countries. As a consequence, gender analysis may easily turn out as a statistical exercise of counting men and women – that is, using the sex category as a proxy for gender issues.

One key conclusion drawn from the literature is that opportunity structures have expanded from the macro-level of institutional regulation and policies to the meso-level of healthcare providers, organizations and service users

(Kuhlmann and Bourgeault, 2008). As already noted, another important trend is the growing body of research into men's health that expands the concept of gender beyond women's issues (Broom and Tovey, 2009; Courtenay, 2011). Negotiations around gender-sensitive care are thereby becoming more complex, including decentralized models of governance and a broader range of players and interests. And to make things even more complicated, driving forces may also operate beyond formal institutions, for instance the creation of more gender-sensitive expert knowledge in the context of international and European research agendas and the development of clinical guidelines (for example, HEN, 2005; Payne, 2009; Sen et al., 2007).

Taken together, gender mainstreaming opens up new opportunities but also entails new forms of governance in healthcare which are based on managerialist regimes and markets which embody the logics of neutral organizations and unmarked subjects acting rationally in order to maximize their benefit (Kuhlmann, 2006; Sandall et al., 2009). Mainstreaming therefore does not necessarily transform the gendered substructure of the organization and content of healthcare shaped by hegemonic masculinities; mainstreaming policies may also reproduce the colonizing mindset of the western world (Debusscher, 2011).

With respect to the health professional workforce, mainstreaming policies may have some positive effects within the medical profession but gender equality is not (yet) a yardstick of performance in the entire professional workforce and usually no matter of concern in predominantly female professional groups, like nursing (Davies, 2002) and complementary and alternative medicine (Cant et al., 2011). Added to this, an emergent field of health human resource planning and policy largely ignores the complex gendered nature of the health workforce and reduces this to sex-disaggregated data analysis (Standing, 2000; WHO, 2011b). Consequently, organizations as well as professions do not necessarily concern themselves with equality issues. While new mainstreaming policies may provide some incentives towards equality, there may also be other rationalities of organizations and professional groups that counteract gender policies, including ignorance as well as overt conflict of interest with powerful male actors (Bourgeault, 2005; Sandall et al., 2009). These conditions and possibly divergent trends call for new approaches to the analysis of policy processes and further empirical investigation.

Why gender-sensitive healthcare and how to move beyond uniform categories?

The persistence of unequal gender relations in society and their negative impact on the quality and efficiency of healthcare is based on two mechanisms: first, gender differences are ignored as far as the needs for and demands on healthcare are concerned; and second, gender bias is deeply embedded in the institutions and organizations that provide healthcare services. It is important to understand the different analytical dimensions of gender and how their connectedness plays out differently in the various fields of healthcare. To name only some of the most prominent examples, gender shows up as male bias in the field of coronary health that leads to poor quality healthcare for women and stereotypical 'masculinities' that may also effect men's health negatively (Emslie and Hunt, 2009; Riska, 2004); as medicalization of women's reproductive capacities and life course changes, like caesarean section and hormone replacement therapy (De Vries et al., 2001; WHI, 2002); as neglect of women-specific healthcare needs like breast cancer treatment, and male-specific care needs such as for prostate cancer; or as an overprescription of psychotropic drugs due to stereotyped images of women as the mentally weak sex – and conversely, a lack of services for men with mental illness.

Yet the call for tighter regulation of care providers and performance measurements do offer new opportunities to negotiate both quality and gender equality. These opportunities arise above all in the increasing necessity for the standardization and transparency of treatment via clinical guidelines, as well as the definition of performance indicators for quality and efficiency. In this situation, mainstreaming gender into research and evaluation can uncover unwarranted variations in the treatment of men and women. It turns the spotlight on structural deficits of healthcare systems and the lack of evidence and guidelines for gender-sensitive and patient-centred treatments (Kuhlmann, 2009).

However, it does not tell us *how* to define the healthcare needs of different groups of women and men and set the targets and standards for 'good' care with respect to both quality and efficiency. The key questions, 'Who serves as the standard and why?' and 'What counts as evidence?', go largely unanswered. This also brings new challenges and the demand for moving beyond gender mainstreaming into perspective. One conclusion drawn from the blind spots of contemporary mainstreaming policies is a need for context-sensitive approaches that take account of the many differences within men and women as groups. Other important issues that need further investigation are globalization and transnationalism and the new challenges of overcoming nationalism in health policy-making; this includes bringing a gender approach into the healthcare needs of a diverse user population as well as into the governance of an increasingly international health professional workforce (Bourgeault and Wrede, 2011; Yeates, 2008).

Flagging the field: the structure of the Handbook

This Handbook draws state-of-the-art debates and research into gender and into healthcare together. At the same time it extends existing research by putting forward both critical debate and practical guidance on how to make healthcare more sensitive to the needs of various different groups of men and women. It draws appreciably upon critical feminist analyses as a thorn in the side of mainstream healthcare as it has challenged the masculinist tradition of healing and sex segregation and maldistribution of care work.

The two motivations for developing this Handbook were: first, to bring politics and power more firmly to the heart of the analysis of health and healthcare and therefore to highlight their interconnections; and second, to breach the boundaries between professionals and users and to take into account the inter-sections of both perspectives. This also helps to overcome an illness-centred approach – and the related dominance of biomedicine and doctors – and to bring the resources for health and well-being into sight. These goals recall and re-establish the aims and experiences of the women's health movement of the 1970s onwards (BWHBC, 1973; Ehrenreich and English, 1974; Fee and Krieger, 1994; for an overview see Kuhlmann, 2009). At the same time, collectively, the chapters in this Handbook take into account the ever expanding scope of gen-der research in healthcare, for example towards greater recognition of men's healthcare needs and the global dimensions of health inequalities (Annandale and Riska, 2009; Sen et al., 2002; WHO, 2009).

The Handbook is divided into five parts and 29 chapters that follow topical issues in contemporary debates around changing health policy and healthcare governance. The structure mirrors the different dimensions of policy (Part I), society (Part II), users (Part III), the organization of care (Part IV) and the pro-fessions (Part V). Each chapter concludes by highlighting key messages in a summary and provides suggestions for key reading.

Gendering healthcare and policy: Part I

Part I of the Handbook provides an introduction and overview of current debates on gender and healthcare, including policies, governance, manage-ment and assessment and the evaluation of research in an international context. It addresses classic topics, such as equity and equality, and medicali-zation that often affect women and men in different ways, as well as gendered dimensions of new health policies and the demands of globalization and transnational policy-making. The collection of chapters also takes the different conditions of gender-sensitive healthcare in developing and developed coun-tries into account.

In Chapter 1, *Re-visiting Gender Justice in Health and Healthcare,* Sarah Payne and Lesley Doyal clarify the key terms of gender equality and gender equity and outline their practical implications for healthcare. This includes a discus-sion of some of the obstacles to the achievement of equality and equity in health policy and the difficulties involved in gender mainstreaming in health-care. They highlight that the health gap between women and men reflects biological as well as gender influences.

Gender equity issues are also taken up in Chapter 2, *Gender Equality and International Health Policy Planning*, by Shelly N. Abdool, Claudia García-Moreno and Avni Amin, who continue the focus on policy planning. They highlight two essential conditions of gender-sensitive health policy planning; namely, political commitment and technical expertise. The authors emphasize the significance of politicizing gender-sensitive healthcare and review a number of different approaches. Useful tools for improving technical expertise are also introduced. Finally, they highlight the benefits of a gender approach in health policy planning that leads to more equal and effective healthcare services.

Hilary Standing also addresses health policy issues in Chapter 3, *Gender Equity and Health Sector Reforms in Low and Middle-income Countries,* but with a focus on equity and the situation of low and middle-income countries. She argues for the need to move beyond universalism in order to address the ways in which specific groups and individuals are disadvantaged. Specifically, this calls for comprehensive national-level databases that include gender-disaggregated data as well as an adequate institutional infrastructure and – national and local – advocacy and capacity to monitor the implementation and progress of gender equity.

Chapter 4, *Gendering Health Human Resource Policy and Management,* by Ellen Kuhlmann, Ivy Lynn Bourgeault, Christa Larsen and Toni Schofield, complements the attention to health policy and management issues by setting focus on health human resources and on high-income countries. The authors highlight how the technocratic nature of this emergent field may fuel a revival of the sex category as a proxy for complex gendered health workforce dynamics. Such dynamics are furthermore explored by drawing on case study material into skill-mix and task-shifting in Canada, Australia and Germany.

In Chapter 5, *Gender-sensitive Indicators for Healthcare,* Vivian Lin and Helen L'Orange move our attention towards policy implementation. The authors explore how gender-sensitive indicators can alert governments and the public to policy and programme successes and failures. They highlight a need to develop gender-sensitive health indicators which go beyond the reproductive health of women, and call for more attention to be paid to men's health. Some illustrative cases of how gender-sensitive indicators can be linked to policy-making are also provided.

Chapter 6, *Gender Assessment: European Health Research Policies,* by Ineke Klinge, is also concerned with issues of policy implementation, but shifts the focus from the international level towards the European Union (EU) and biomedical research. Klinge gives illustrative examples of how contemporary research programmes are assessed and how this may further an overall sensitivity towards sex and gender differences in medical research. She argues for an intersectional approach to differences that can effectively reduce any potential risk of biological or racial essentialism.

Chapter 7, by Susan E. Bell and Anne E. Figert, reviews a classic issue of feminist critique in the context of changing healthcare in 21st-century societies;

namely, *Gender and the Medicalization of Healthcare.* In their analysis the authors show that medicalization theory has significantly expanded in various ways as it has shifted away from the initial focus on professional dominance to include active participation of patients/consumers, and also takes account of globalization processes and new developments, such as geneticization and pharmaceuticalization.

The social patterning of health by gender: Part II

Part II of the Handbook highlights the intersections between biological and social dimensions of health and gender. It introduces theoretical and methodological concerns and tackles gender and social inequalities in health. The chapters show how biological conditions intersect with male and female stereotypes, social constructions of health and illness and the institutional conditions of healthcare systems. Particular attention is given to the key areas of reproductive health, coronary heart disease, mental health, HIV/AIDS, and end-of-life care. This selection of areas directs our attention towards major challenges facing public health policy, including chronic illness of high incidence and prevalence, mental health, and new infectious diseases as well as death and dying. The authors consider how male and female stereotypes may have an impact on care in the form of either neglect of women's or of men's healthcare needs, as well as the intersections between gender, race and culture.

In Chapter 8, Chloe E. Bird, Martha E. Lang and Patricia P. Rieker explore *Changing Gendered Patterns of Morbidity and Mortality.* They introduce the 'constrained choices' approach to understand the complex antecedents of the morbidity and mortality differences between men and women and the ways their choices are constrained. They highlight that policy decisions can shape factors far beyond the control of individuals which directly affect health, including the safety and quality of the food supply, exposure to cigarette smoke in public spaces, and even the prevalence of HIV in high-risk populations in the local community.

In Chapter 9, *Reproductive Regimes: Governing Gendered Bodies,* Elizabeth Ettorre and Carol Kingdon examine the intersections between biological and social dimensions of gender and health with special reference to reproduction. In so doing the authors draw attention to a key issue of long-standing importance to women's health and highlight the new connections between the governance of pregnant bodies and medicalization, like physicians' appropriation of choice discourses that may serve to extend pregnant women's support for medicalization and contribute to the rise in caesarean section rates.

Elianne Riska, in Chapter 10, *Coronary Heart Disease: Gendered Public Health Discourses,* takes us to a major challenge of public policy across the globe, namely the prevention of coronary heart disease. She spotlights the benefits of gender analysis in a field of healthcare that is of high significance for men and women but fundamentally dominated by a masculinist discourse. This discourse not only causes significant disadvantages and poor quality of care for women with coronary heart disease but also neglects the needs of other than white middle-class men.

Chapter 11, *Gender and Mental Health,* by Joan Busfield, reviews definitions and measurements through the lens of gender but directs our attention to a field of healthcare that is, unlike coronary heart disease, harnessed more tightly to female stereotypes. The analysis shows that the way in which the concepts of mental health and illness are defined and measured affects the observed gender balance in overall levels of mental health. Busfield critically discusses individualized approaches and highlights the significance of social circumstances and practical social support.

In Chapter 12, Leah Gilbert and Terry-Ann Selikow explore *HIV/AIDS and Gender.* They bring into focus the ongoing challenges of infectious diseases that not only affect men and women differently but also vary significantly between different regions of the globe. Focusing on sub-Saharan Africa, the authors highlight the urgent need to develop a broader conception of HIV/AIDS that is located within the socio-economic and cultural environment, rather than focusing on individualized approaches. This is especially important for women, whose economic dependence on men increases their vulnerability to HIV/AIDS.

Finally in this Part, Alex Broom, in Chapter 13, *Gendering End-of-life Care,* seeks to unpack some of the moral, ideological and political underpinnings of 'modern dying' and examines intersections of gender and end-of-life care. The author primarily refers to the western world and reveals how the forms of care that people pursue in the context of terminal diagnoses can be heavily influenced by gendered ideas about agency, self-responsibility and self-help. A better understanding of the gendered demands and expectations may help to improve end-of-life care for both men and women.

Equity and access to healthcare: Part III

Part III brings the service user into perspective, focusing on equity and access to healthcare through the lens of gender. The chapters make clear that influences on access and equity stem from institutional barriers and from the impact of gender expectations on perceptions of health and help-seeking. Differences in the social conditions of life often create different healthcare needs, demands and desires, not only between men and women but also within the two groups. However, healthcare systems typically fail to respond adequately to these differences, thus creating and even reinforcing inequalities. This may affect not only women but also men's well-being and the health of older people, as well as services for particularly vulnerable groups, such as gay and lesbian people, and young mothers and children; it may also cause negative effects for women living in rural areas.

Chapter 14, *Gender and Help-seeking: Towards Gender-comparative Studies*, by Kate Hunt, Joy Adamson and Paul Galdas, highlights the need to review existing research on help-seeking that has often over-generalized that women consult primary care more than men. The authors apply a gender-comparative approach and thereby provide a more nuanced picture. For example, their analysis shows that men do not delay longer in seeking help for colorectal cancer – a major contributor to premature mortality – and that men and women commonly present to healthcare use as a 'last resort'.

Kakoli Roy and Anoshua Chaudhuri, in Chapter 15, *Gender Differences in Healthcare Utilization in Later Life*, bring older people into perspective, a group that is rapidly gaining significance in ageing societies. Besides certain universal commonalities of older people's use of healthcare, their analysis reveals significant variation. In developed countries, older women generally report better self-assessed health than men or levels of health that are comparable to men, but greater utilization of healthcare services. In developing countries, however, women tend to report worse health than men alongside lower utilization of services.

In Chapter 16, *Men's Health and Well-being*, Toni Schofield focuses on men as gendered service users. She highlights that men's health is constructed by a contrast with women's health, and this construction mainly relies on binary categories and statistical fabrication. She shows that men's health discourse does not provide evidence for an overall disadvantage of men as a group, but some groups of men are in real health trouble that stems basically from dynamics of class and ethnicity, combined with the practices of enacting masculinities.

Jane Edwards, in Chapter 17, *The Healthcare Needs of Gay and Lesbian Patients*, directs our attention to a group of service users whose healthcare needs have broadly been neglected. She discusses the problematic effects of heteronormative and heterosexist cultures and society that makes the healthcare needs of non-heterosexual people invisible. She points out that access to care is insufficient to address these needs; services themselves must also be appropriate and acceptable if the complex healthcare needs of the diverse group of non-heterosexual people are satisfactorily to be addressed.

Chapter 18, *Mothers and Children: What Does Their Health Tell Us about Gender?*, by Tulsi Patel, makes gender differences in two of the most vulnerable groups visible. Focusing on Asia, and specifically on India, she reveals significant differences in the health of girls and boys; for example, of the two-fifths proportion of malnourished children in South Asia, more girls than boys are malnourished. However, women's and girls' ill-health is not simply correlated with poverty and availability of healthcare facilities, it is also shaped by familial politics, such as daughter dislike and sex-selective abortion technologies.

In Chapter 19, *Gender, Health, Care and Place: Living in Rural and Remote Communities*, Ivy Lynn Bourgeault and Rebecca Sutherns challenge common assumptions of there being a more healthy life in rural areas. Their analysis shows that, contrary to the common stereotype of small communities having strong social ties, women's social networks may be more limited in rural areas resulting in fewer sources of support. Policy development must therefore address broader social determinants of health, including better employment opportunities, transportation and childcare resources.

The organization and delivery of healthcare: Part IV

Part IV brings the significance of healthcare organizations into view. It unpacks the gendered nature of the organization and delivery of care and counteracts seemingly gender-neutral, although often gender-stereotyped, policy and management discourses. The case studies address topical issues, such as health promotion and the new management of professional performance and also direct attention towards new emerging areas of care, such as home care. By contrast, the overall gender-neutral discourse of healthcare organization and delivery is complemented with a specific focus on healthcare for women, namely the Centres for Women's Health as an alternative to the mainstreaming of healthcare services.

Chapter 20, *The New Management of Healthcare: 'Rational' Performance and Gendered Actors,* by Jim Barry, Elisabeth Berg and John Chandler, reviews key issues of health reform from a gender perspective. The authors explore a gendered subtext of the new public management (NPM) practices that are characterized by masculine performativity. However, NPM embodies both opportunities and challenges. For example, it offers new career opportunities for women prepared to take managerial roles with high income and power but raises the question of whether there are alternatives to masculinist managerialism.

Viola Burau, Hildegard Theobald and Robert H. Blank consider *Old Age Care Policies: Gendering Institutional Arrangements across Countries* in Chapter 21. This leads us back to healthcare for older people, but by exploring opportunities and challenges from an institutionalist perspective. The authors use cross-country comparison – Sweden and Japan – and are able to identify the gendered selectivity of institutions and the gendered power relations embedded in them. At the same time, they show that institutions do not tell the full story since power relations and informal care must also be considered.

In Chapter 22, *Primary Prevention and Health Promotion: Towards Gender-sensitive Interventions,* Petra Kolip introduces an approach that links the Public Health Action Cycle model with the concept of gender mainstreaming. Arguing from a public health perspective, she uses research into smoking prevention, drink-driving and workplace health to highlight that intervention planning and implementation informed by gender theories may improve the quality and efficacy of health promotion and primary prevention.

Chapter 23, *Gender and Maternal Healthcare,* by Jane Sandall, Cecilia Benoit, Edwin van Teijlingen, Sirpa Wrede, Eugene Declercq and Raymond De Vries, addresses key issues in maternal healthcare which have resonance in the international arena. Using Canada, the USA, Finland and the UK as comparative case studies, the analysis shows that, in all four countries, inequalities in maternal and infant healthcare have risen up the policy agenda but solutions being put forward to reduce inequalities vary among countries, including institutional changes as well as changing health behaviour and family culture.

Pat Armstrong concludes this part of the Handbook in Chapter 24, *Women's Health Centres: Creating Spaces and Institutional Support,* by evoking a key goal – and dream – of the women's health movement. She critically reviews support for Women's Health Centres in 21st-century society and highlights new challenges and negative effects of neoliberal policy agendas. The illustrative case of Canada makes clear that gender-based analysis itself embodies challenges: it can strengthen health planning and service delivery for governments, but broadening the mandate towards gender issues may also provoke tensions with women's healthcare.

The professions as 'catalyst' of gender-sensitive healthcare: Part V

Part V focuses on the health professions as mediators between institutions and service users that may either encourage or discourage gender-sensitive care. Recent changes in health policy, together with professionalization and new demands from service users, have provided the conditions for various new dynamics in the health professional workforce. Thus the chapters discuss general international trends of growing numbers of women in medicine, often labelled as 'feminization', the advancement of gender issues in medical research, and new strategies to include gender sensitivity in training and professional development. These matters are complemented by a consideration of gender issues in typically female-gendered professions, like nursing and complementary and alternative medicine.

In Chapter 25, *Women in the Medical Profession: International Trends,* Elianne Riska sheds light on a topical issue in health policy and medical debate. Drawing on empirical evidence from various health systems, the analysis reveals that gender segregation of specialties is a universal pattern in healthcare; accordingly, this pattern refutes the homogenization argument of the 'feminization of medicine' view. She shows that while women doctors can have a more empathic practice style, little or no gender differences have actually been found in clinical decision-making to date.

Chapter 26, *Sex, Gender and Health: Developments in Medical Research,* by Toine Lagro-Janssen, directs our attention to medical education as a switchboard for gender-sensitive healthcare and explores opportunities for integrating gender. She reveals three persistent principles in medicine that act as barriers towards the introduction of gender in scientific medical research; namely, gender blindness, andronormativity and the predominantly biomedical concept of illness.

However, examples of best practices and the successful integration of gender into medical curricula are also discussed.

In Chapter 27, *Gender Mainstreaming at the Cross-roads of Eastern-Western Healthcare*, Ling-fang Cheng, Ellen Kuhlmann and Ellen Annandale argue the need for context-sensitive approaches that help to unpack the structure and content of healthcare as well as the sex and gender categories. The illustrative case of Taiwan reveals that the composition of the workforce by sex does not predict opportunities for gender mainstreaming, while performance indicators and measurements can be a highly efficient strategy of implementation.

Sirpa Wrede, in Chapter 28, *Nursing: Globalization of a Female-gendered Profession,* directs our attention towards the nursing profession. She places the gendered professionalization processes in a global context and explores how the globalization of nursing along national pathways produces new, complex orderings of nurses within the wider profession, and how references to professionalism and skill are utilized in these processes. She calls for a gender-sensitive analysis that considers the intersections of gendered injustice with other local and global forms of inequality.

Finally, in Chapter 29, *Complementary and Alternative Medicine: Gender and Marginality*, Sarah Cant and Peter Watts conclude by exploring the apparent affinity between complementary and alternative medicine (CAM), women's health concerns and feminist agendas, and the extent to which CAM has the potential to create spaces for gender-sensitive healthcare. They show that although CAM provides some opportunities for female practitioners, it is more generally connected with marginality, as is shown by the usage patterns by men and women from minority ethnic groups.

The future outlook

Bringing gender to the heart of health policy, practice and research is increasingly recognized as an urgent need and an essential condition for improved healthcare for women and men (WHO, 2011b). At the same time, attempts to mainstream gender into healthcare, policy and research are challenging. Gender policies place various new demands on the agenda and this often causes resistance from policy-makers, researchers and practitioners alike, ranging from mere ignorance to overt conflict. Above all claims for gender-sensitive healthcare and the new mainstreaming policies cause uncertainty; this includes questions about what gender actually means when applied to healthcare and how the new gender policies can be implemented effectively.

Here, this Handbook fills the gaps by providing more critical and theoretically informed analysis alongside a rich source of case study material. There is no easy answer or 'standard approach' to how to get gender mainstreaming right in healthcare, but a number of helpful tools and 'best practices' exist, such as the identification of gender-sensitive indicators for policy planning and evaluation, and the implementation of gender assessment in research programmes and funding schemes. There are also worst case scenarios of persistent inequalities and devaluation of women and their healthcare needs that call for urgent action; one such example is the statistical phenomenon of 'missing women' due to sex-selective abortion and neglect of girls in some south Asian regions but also in countries like the United Kingdom (Gill and Mitra-Kahn, 2009). Another shocking example is the gendered nature of HIV/AIDS in sub-Saharan Africa that causes high risks for women and a growing incidence of AIDS. Both examples underscore the need for context-sensitive gender approaches that take account of intersecting inequalities as well as globalization and transnational processes in healthcare. These examples, amongst others, also recall that women's health is an essential dimension of gender-sensitive healthcare and gender mainstreaming policies (see also Weisman et al., 2010; WHO, 2009).

In our concluding chapter to the Handbook we highlight key issues that emerged from the selection of chapters in this book of how and why gender can be brought to the heart of healthcare. We will argue the need for making connections between sex and gender on the macro, meso and micro-levels of healthcare. We will also open up some of the black boxes of gender and healthcare, such as the lack of gender-sensitive approaches in complementary and alternative medicine (Cant et al., 2011; Flesch, 2007) and the intersections between ethnicity, gender and healthcare (Bourgeault and Wrede, 2011; Ahmad and Bradby, 2008). We believe this Handbook will be a valuable resource for a wide range of academics, including health practitioners such as doctors, nurses and alternative therapists, managers, policy-makers and researchers.

References

Ahmad, W. I. U. and H. Bradby (eds) (2008) *Ethnicity, Health and Health Care: Understanding Diversity, Tackling Inequality* (Oxford: Blackwell).

Annandale, E. (2009a) 'Health and Gender', in W. Cockerham (ed.), *The New Companion to Medical Sociology* (New York: Wiley-Blackwell), 97–112.

Annandale, E. (2009b) *Women's Health and Social Change* (London: Routledge).

Annandale, E. and K. Hunt (2000) (eds) *Gender Inequalities in Health* (Buckingham: Open University Press).

Annandale, E. and E. Riska (2009) 'New Connections: Towards a Gender-inclusive Approach to Women's and Men's Health', *Current Sociology*, 57 (2), 123–33.

Bacchi, C. and J. Eveline (eds) (2010) *Mainstreaming Politics: Gendering Practices and Feminist Theory* (Adelaide: University of Adelaide Press), at: www.adelaide.edu.au/press/titles/mainstreaming/, accessed 3 October 2011.

Bates, L., K. Springer and O. Hankivsky (2012: forthcoming) 'Gender and Health: Relational, Biosocial and Intersectoral Approaches', *Social Science & Medicine*, Special Issue.

Bird, C. and P. Rieker (2008) *Gender and Health. The Effects of Constrained Choices and Social Policies* (New York: Cambridge University Press).

Bourgeault, I. L. (2005) 'Rationalization of Health Care and Female Professional Projects', *Knowledge, Work and Society,* 3 (1), 25–52.

Bourgeault, I. L. and S. Wrede (2011) 'Caring across Borders: Contrasting the Contexts of Nurse Migration in Canada and Finland', in C. Benoit and H. Hallgrimsdottir (eds), *Finding Dignity in Health Care and Health Care Work* (Toronto: University of Toronto Press), 65–86.

Broom, A. and P. Tovey (eds) (2009) *Men's Health: Body, Identity and Social Context* (London, Wiley-Blackwell).

BWHBC – The Boston Women's Health Book Collective (1973) *Our Bodies, Ourselves* (New York: Simon and Schuster).

Cant, S., P. Watts and A. Ruston (2011) 'Negotiating Competency, Professionalism and Risk: The Integration of Complementary and Alternative Medicine by Nurses and Midwives in NHS Hospitals', *Social Science & Medicine,* 72, 529–36.

Clarke, A. E. and V. L. Olesen (eds) (1999) *Revisioning Women, Health, and Healing* (New York: Routledge).

Connell, R. W. (1987) *Gender and Power* (Sydney: Allen and Unwin).

Connell, R. (2011) *Confronting Equality: Gender, Knowledge and Global Change* (Oxford: Polity Press).

Council of Europe (1998) *Gender Mainstreaming. Conceptual Framework, Methodology and Presentation of Good Practice,* Final Report (EG-S-MS), Strasbourg.

Courtenay, W. (2011) *Dying To Be Men* (London: Routledge).

Davies, C. (2002) 'What about the Girl Next Door? Gender and the Politics of Self-Regulation', in G. Bendelow, M. Carpenter, C. Vautier and S. Williams (eds), *Gender, Health and Healing: The Public/Private Divide* (London: Routledge), 91–107.

Debusscher, P. (2011) 'Mainstreaming Gender in European Commission Development Policy: Conservative Europeanness?', *Women's Studies International Forum,* 34 (1), 39–49.

De Vries, R., C. Benoit, E. van Teijlingen and S. Wrede (2001) *Birth by Design* (New York: Routledge).

Ehrenreich, B. and D. English (1974) *Complaints and Disorders. The Sexual Politics of Sickness* (London: Compendium).

Emslie, C. and K. Hunt (2009) 'Men, Masculinities and Heart Disease: A Systematic Review of the Qualitative Literature', *Current Sociology,* 57, 155–91.

Fee, E. and N. Krieger (eds) (1994) *Women's Health, Politics, and Power* (New York: Baywood).

Flesch, H. (2007) 'Silent Voices: Women, Complementary Medicine, and the Co-optation of Change', *Complementary Therapies in Clinical Practice,* 13 (3), 166–73.

Gill, A. and T. Mitra-Kahn (2009) 'Explaining Daughter Devaluation and the Issue of Missing Women in South Asia and the UK', *Current Sociology,* 57 (5), 684–703.

HEN – Health Evidence Network – WHO Regional Office Europe (2005) *What Evidence Is There about the Effects of Health Care Reforms on Equity, Particularly in Health?*, at: www.euro.who.int/Document/E87674.pdf, accessed 19 October 2009.

Kuhlmann, E. (2006) *Modernising Health Care. Rethinking Professions, the State and the Public* (Bristol: Policy Press).

Kuhlmann, E. (2009) 'From Women's Health to Gender Mainstreaming and Back Again: Linking Feminist Agendas and Health Policy', *Current Sociology,* 57 (2), 135–54.

Kuhlmann, E. and E. Annandale (2012) 'Researching Transformations in Health Services and Policy in International Perspective', *Current Sociology,* Special Issue, 60 (4).

Kuhlmann, E. and I. L. Bourgeault (2008) 'Gender, Professions and Public Policy: New Directions', *Equal Opportunities International,* 27 (1), 5–18.

Lorber, J. (2005) *Breaking the Bowls: Degendering and Feminist Change* (New York: W. W. Norton & Co).

McKinley, E. D., J. W. Thompson, J. Briefer-French, L. S. Wilcox, C. S. Weisman and W. C. Andrews (2001) 'Performance Indicators in Women's Health: Incorporating Women's Health in the Health Plan Employer Data and Information Set' (HEDIS), *Women's Health Issues*, 12 (1), 46–58.

Payne, S. (2009) *How Can Gender Equity Be Addressed through Health Systems?*, Joint Policy Brief 12, World Health Organization, on behalf of the European Observatory on Health Systems and Policies, at: www.euro.who.int/document/E92846.pdf, accessed 11 October 2009.

Riska, E. (2004) *Masculinities and Men's Health: Coronary Heart Disease in Medical and Public Discourse* (Lanham: Rowman & Littlefield).

Sandall, J., C. Benoit, S. Wrede, S. F. Murray, E. R. van Teijlingen and R. Westfall (2009) 'Social Service Professional or Market Expert: Maternity Care Relations under Neoliberal Healthcare Reform', *Current Sociology*, 57 (4), 529–53.

Sen, G., A. George and P. Östlin (2002) (eds) *Engendering International Health: The Challenge of Equity* (Cambridge, MA: MIT Press).

Sen, G., P. Östlin and A. George (2007) *Unequal, Unfair, Ineffective and Inefficient. Gender Inequality in Health Care: Why It Exists and How We Can Change It*, Final report to the WHO Commission on Social Determinants of Health, at: www.eurohealth.ie/pdf/WGEKN_FINAL_REPORT.pdf, accessed 19 October 2009.

Sen, G. and A. Iyer (2012: forthcoming) 'Who Gains, Who Loses and How: Leveraging Gender and Class Intersections to Secure Health Entitlements', *Social Science & Medicine*, Special Issue.

Standing, H. (2000) 'Gender: A Missing Dimension in Human Resource Policy and Planning for Health Reforms', *Human Resources for Health Development Journal*, 4 (1), 27–42.

United Nations (1999) *Women and Health. Mainstreaming the Gender Perspective into the Health Sector* (New York: UN Publication Sales No 99.IV.4).

Weisman, C. S., C. H. Chuang and S. Hutson Scholle (2010) 'Still Piecing It Together: Women's Primary Care', *Women's Health Issues*, 20, 228–30.

West, C. and D. Zimmerman (1987) 'Doing Gender', *Gender & Society*, 1, 125–51.

WHI – Righting Group for the Women's Health Initiative Investigators (2002) 'Risks and Benefits of Estrogen Plus Progesterone in Healthy Post-menopausal Women', *Journal of the American Medical Association*, 288, 321–33.

WHO (2007) *Glossary*, at: www.euro.who.int/GEM/strategy/20070426_7, accessed 19 October 2009.

WHO (2009) *Women and Health. Today's Evidence, Tomorrow's Agendas* (Geneva: WHO).

WHO (2011a) *Gender Mainstreaming in EWHO: Where Are We Now?* Report of the Baseline Assessment of the WHO Gender Strategy (Geneva: WHO).

WHO (2011b) *Human Rights and Gender Equality in Health Sector Strategies: How To Assess Policy Coherence* (Geneva: WHO).

WHO Euro (2001) *Mainstreaming Gender Equity in Health*, Madrid Statement (Copenhagen: WHO Euro).

Woodward, A. E. (2008) 'Too Late for Gender Mainstreaming? Taking Stock in Brussels', *Journal of European Social Policy*, 18 (3), 289–302.

World Bank (2011) *World Development Report 2012: Gender Equality and Development* (New York: World Bank).

Yeates, N. (2008) *Globalizing Care Economies and Migrant Workers* (Basingstoke: Palgrave Macmillan).

Part I
Gendering Healthcare and Policy

1
Re-visiting Gender Justice in Health and Healthcare

Sarah Payne and Lesley Doyal

Introduction

Debates about gender justice are now common in public policy in general and in the health sector in particular. The promotion of greater equality between women and men has become a key theme in both national and international policy debates. However there has often been confusion about what 'equality' means in this context and how it might be achieved. The terms 'gender equality' and 'gender equity' are both in widespread use but there has sometimes been a lack of clarity about the distinctions between them as well as their practical implications.

Most discussions of gender justice begin with the argument that women and men should be regarded as being of equal moral value. Where there are no relevant differences between them, then fairness and justice dictate that they should be treated equally. That is to say, men and women should both have equal access to the same goods and services which are required in order to flourish in all spheres of economic and social life. But where there are biological or social differences between the two groups that affect the capacity of either to optimize their potential for health, then it will be unjust to treat them as though they were the same and to do so may well lead to further inequalities. When women and men have different needs then the planning of services should reflect this. In these circumstances, equity as well as equality should be a guiding principle.

This chapter will begin by reviewing recent debates on the significance of these issues in the context of healthcare. This is followed by discussion of some of the obstacles to the achievement of equality and equity in health policy and the difficulties involved in gender mainstreaming in healthcare. The chapter also examines some of the internal challenges found in many policy settings and the ways in which the moral case for gender justice is affected by the wider global environment.

The emergence of gender equality strategies

During the 1970s and 1980s women's organizations around the world became increasingly active on a number of issues of global importance. This is usually referred to as second wave feminism, and reflected a growth in feminist movements in richer countries, especially in Europe and the USA. But it was also a period of increasing activism among women's groups in poorer countries of the South. At the same time the United Nations and other international organizations began a series of conferences and other policy initiatives (see also Chapter 2 by Abdool et al. and Chapter 3 by Standing).

This early period of activism was based on a recognition of biological and (some) social differences between women and men and highlighted the evident failure of many societies to meet the particular needs of women. Thus campaigns argued for the universal right of all women to control their fertility through safe and affordable contraception and abortion as well as effective and appropriate care during pregnancy and labour. Other health-related issues that came into focus included the social condoning (and sometimes encouragement) of gender-based violence in general and the practice of female genital mutilation (FGM) in particular (Doyal, 2002; Petchesky, 2003).

Both activists and academics also emphasized that the health of many women was profoundly shaped by their relative poverty. Hence any attempts to promote their reproductive or sexual well-being would have to be located within a strategy which also addressed their economic and social lives. That is to say, women's need for healthcare might be common across the world but there were major inequalities in their access to services and other means of support. Hence it was argued that concern about gender issues need to be at the heart of development policies and funding.

These arguments contributed to a shift in broader development debates away from the more traditional framework of 'women in development' (WID) which highlighted the greater burden of women in relation to paid and unpaid work, as well as their relative lack of access to a wide range of resources. Instead a new 'gender and development' (GAD) perspective was constructed (Hafner-Burton and Pollack, 2002). This new approach emphasized the relational nature of women's position, and brought inequalities between women and men into a broader structural context (Barton, 2004; Razavi and Miller, 1995). The GAD perspective was in line with a growing critique of the failures of international efforts to relieve poverty, and an appreciation of the adverse effects of global restructuring on many women.

Changing patterns of employment, for example, were shown to have had a major impact on women's health. This reflected their increasing participation in paid labour alongside their continuing responsibility for domestic work and the care of dependents. Many women do gain both material and social benefits from work outside the home. However, these trends have also generated new risks that affect women in particular as they take up insecure jobs in what are often unhealthy and unregulated conditions (Doyal, 2002; Pearson, 2000).

These conceptual developments were accompanied by the collection of a growing volume of evidence on gender inequalities in the global context. Together they provided the basis for a more complex and holistic understanding of the connections between women's health and well-being, their reproductive potential and their social and economic status. This in turn made possible the emergence of new formulations of political objectives in terms of both gender equality and gender equity. However, the meaning of these terms themselves and their implications for policy still needed further clarification.

Gender equality or gender equity?

From the 1990s the terms gender equality and gender equity became increasingly visible in policy documents and position statements from national, international and supranational organizations. But too often there was a lack of clarity about how these terms should be used in referencing political as well as practical differences between the position of women and men. What did each term imply in relation to desired outcomes and what strategies should be deployed to bring them about?

The rise of the discourse of gender equality

The objectives of the 1994 Cairo Conference on Population and Development (ICPD) were broadly drawn to include the promotion of gender equality as well gender equity and the empowerment of women. However, the use of these terms was not well thought through, and their meanings were strongly contested among participants at the conference (Petchesky, 2003). It was argued by faith-based organizations in particular that women were 'natural' homemakers and hence were not in need of equal rights at work. Similarly the domestic relations between women and men were said to be divinely ordained, making the notion of female sexual rights inappropriate. This led to the principle of gender equity being used to justify treating women differently to men in ways that other participants and commentators perceived to be unfair and inappropriate (Barton, 2004).

Given these debates, the UN adopted gender equality in preference to gender equity in developing the objectives for the Beijing Platform for Action of 1995. This decision was based on a growing recognition that in certain situations the use of the term gender equity could be predicated on perceptions of 'difference' and concepts of social justice which were not in themselves value-free or objective. Hence the notion of gender equality was deemed to be preferable in order to avoid perpetuating what could be seen as gender-based discrimination (UN, 2001). Gender equality continues to be the preferred term for the majority of organizations and institutions charged with reducing the inequalities between men and women. Within the United Nations for example, responsibility for gender mainstreaming is held by the Office of the Special Advisor on Gender Issues and the Advancement of Women (OSAGI). Their aim is to achieve gender equality between women and men which is defined as:

> ... the equal rights, responsibilities and opportunities of women and men and girls and boys. Equality does not mean that women and men will become the same but that women's and men's rights, responsibilities and opportunities will not depend on whether they are born male or female. (OSAGI, 2001: 1)

Similarly the World Bank and the International Monetary Fund both use the concept of gender equality in defining their approach to development work and funding, and in the working of their own internal organization (World Bank, 2007). In the European Union discourses around gender also use the concept of equality rather than equity, and the UK and Norway, for example, have both recently passed legislation which requires the public sector actively to promote gender equality throughout all their activities (EHRC, 2009).

The goal of gender equity in the context of health policy

But despite this growing preference for the term gender equality, some international organizations are continuing to use the notion of gender equity. This is found mostly in debates about health policy and, as we shall see, it reflects the importance of biological as well as social differences in shaping the morbidity and mortality of women and men. The United Nations Population Fund (UNFPA), for example, does talk in the *State of the World's Population* (2005) about the achievements realized by the promotion of gender equality. However, reproductive rights are described in the same document as 'a measure of equity' (UNFPA, 2005: 2). Similarly, the *Global Monitoring Report 2007* (World Bank, 2007) refers to gender equality in its overall assessment of gender differences in the impact of development, but talks of gender equity when looking at health differences between women and men.

The Millennium Development Strategy now stands as the broadest consensus statement on global policy initiatives. And here again the language of gender equality and empowerment is paramount (if somewhat rhetorical) with the third Millennium Development Goal (MDG3) calling for actions to address the economic, political and citizenship rights of women (Barton and Prendergast, 2004). MDG5, on maternal mortality, is also aimed specifically at women (see also Chapter 18 by Patel and Chapter 23 by Sandall et al.). But here the focus is not on gender equality per se but on the healthcare needs of women resulting directly from their biological potential to bear children. The clearest argument for the importance of combining both concepts in a health setting is found in documents from the World Health Organization. Here both gender equality and gender equity are used in coherent and systematic ways for analysis and policy development (WHO, 2002; 2008a; see also Chapter 2 by Abdool et al.). The differences in the meaning and implications of the two concepts are described as follows:

> Gender equality means the absence of discrimination on the basis of a person's sex in opportunities, allocation of resources or benefits, and access to services. [...] Gender equity means fairness and justice in the distribution of benefits, power, resources and responsibilities between women and men. The concept recognizes that women and men have different needs, power and access to resources, and that these differences should be identified and addressed in a manner that rectifies the imbalance between the sexes. (WHO, 2002: 3)

So why are these issues of terminology different in the context of health? Why should equity be a central concept alongside equality when this option has been rejected in other policy arenas? The key reason for this lies in the biological sex differences between women and men. In the context of education or employment, for example, it is social obstacles alone which prevent gender equality in outcomes. However, the same cannot sensibly be argued in the context of health. While gender inequalities and differences are clearly important, biology itself is also a major determinant of health and a failure to recognize this can create further inequalities between women and men. Biological differences cannot be removed but their potentially harmful effects can be mitigated through social policies which take them properly into account.

Sex, gender and health

Differences between women and men in their experiences of health and illness are well known (Payne, 2006). Male and female patterns of mortality and morbidity show significant variation. Moreover, the nature of these differences varies between countries and regions, and between different social groups. Life expectancy is one of the most commonly used indicators of differences in health and it is now higher for women in virtually every country in the world (Payne, 2006). However, the size of this female advantage in longevity varies considerably. In 2006, for example, male life expectancy at birth in Iraq was 19 years lower than female life expectancy, while in the Russian Federation it was 13 years lower (WHO, 2008b). The narrowest gaps are usually found in the poorest countries where life expectancy in general is low (Payne, 2006; WHO, 2008b).

Male and female patterns of morbidity or ill-health also vary around the world. These are more complex than mortality differences, since they depend on what kinds of illness are taken into account and how ill-health is measured. However, it is clear that women are at greater risk of some communicable diseases such as malaria, sexually transmitted infections and HIV infection as well as non-communicable conditions such as depression, anxiety and arthritis. They also experience a much higher burden of reproductive ill-health. Men on the other hand, have a higher risk of intentional and non-intentional injuries and alcohol-related problems.

Sex and health

These variations in morbidity and mortality can be explained in part by the underlying biological differences between women and men. It is now accepted, for example, that women's potential for greater longevity than men has a genetic element (Wizemann and Pardue, 2000). On the other hand, women's reproductive capacities generate certain risks and these will cancel out their potential for greater longevity if they are not met in effective and appropriate ways. Similarly, men's inherently greater vulnerability to early heart disease will be exacerbated if wider public health policies do not deal effectively with their greater exposure to related risk factors.

Whatever policies are put in place, these biological factors make it impossible to achieve 'equal' health for women and men. Instead, the only realizable goal will be to ensure that both men and women are able to maximize their potential for health within the constraints of their biological sex (Anand and Sen, 1995). And it is here that strategies for gender equity should come into play to meet the inherently different needs of the two sexes.

Gender inequalities and differences in health

But despite the importance of biology, many of the health variations between women and men are also social in origin. Environmental factors interact with biological influences in shaping gender differences in exposure to potential risks, in access to health-promoting resources and in health and illness behaviour. They also affect the ways in which health workers and carers respond to the different needs of males and females (Payne, 2006). Thus far these issues have been explored mainly through a female lens. This is reflected in an extensive literature on the links between women's health problems and their relative poverty, their heavy burden of both waged and domestic labour, their low social status and their vulnerability to gendered violence and other forms of abuse (Doyal, 1995; Payne, 2006). This concentration on women is not surprising given the structural disadvantage so many face in accessing the resources needed to optimize their health. However, the focus is now beginning to open up as the links between 'maleness' and health are increasingly explored (Courtenay, 2000; Robertson, 2007; see also Chapter 16 by Schofield).

We know, for example, that men are more likely than women to be in the most dangerous jobs. But there is also an association between masculinities and risk-taking with men being more likely than women to be involved in alcohol-related accidents (Payne, 2006). Similarly, many cultures sanction (or even 'require') hazardous behaviours such as cigarette smoking and tobacco use as a demonstration of masculinity. This is reinforced by the fact that in most societies men are likely to have more resources than women to spend on such habits. An emphasis on stoicism and 'soldiering on' may also require men to dismiss symptoms of ill-health and this can be a contributing factor in a number of serious health problems (Payne, 2006).

Men are no different from women in that they also experience health problems that are gender-based. Both the psychological and the structural dimensions of masculinities play a significant role in the creation of avoidable health problems in men as well as generating inequitable health policies through placing obstacles in the way of appropriate care. However, it is important to note that these gendered aspects of male health cannot be fitted easily into the framework of gender inequalities used to analyse the potential health hazards facing women. Though men may be damaged by the social construction of masculinities they are rarely harmed in any direct way by gender inequalities themselves. This is not of course surprising in the context of male-dominated societies where men have socially sanctioned advantages in the allocation of both responsibilities and rewards. Hence 'difference' rather than 'inequality' is the key concept here.

We can conclude from this review that both gender equity and gender equality are important principles in addressing avoidable unfairness in health outcomes between women and men. However, as Annandale (2009) points out, the gap between conceptual models and empirical analysis means that there is still little agreement on how these principles can best be put into practice. The next section will illustrate this through an exploration of some of the challenges of gender mainstreaming in healthcare.

Gender mainstreaming in healthcare: internal problems and contradictions

Gender mainstreaming has developed as the key strategy in the pursuit of gender justice across a range of private and public policy settings. The UN defines this approach as follows:

Mainstreaming a gender perspective is the process of assessing the implications for women and men of any planned action, including legislation, policies or programmes, in all areas and at all levels. It is a strategy for making women's as well as men's concerns and experiences an integral dimension of the design, implementation, monitoring and evaluation of policies and programmes in all political, economic and societal spheres so that women and men benefit equally and inequality is not perpetuated. The ultimate aim is to achieve gender equality. (UN, 1997: 27)

These ideas have been widely adopted, with international organizations often taking the lead. However, documented evidence of successes has so far been limited, especially in the health sector. As Elsey and colleagues point out:

Despite the work of gender advocates over many years, achieving a fully gender mainstreamed health sector has proved to be an elusive goal, with often seemingly insurmountable obstacles. (Elsey et al., 2002: 8)

These limitations stem in large part from the fact that initiatives have focused mainly on service delivery rather than the wider social determinants of health. But even within the limits of this relatively narrow approach, the available evidence has highlighted three key problems in most initiatives: confusion of aims and objectives; lack of an appropriate evidence base at individual and organizational levels; and wider social and political constraints on the underlying processes of gender transformation.

Lack of clarity in aims and objectives

Confusion about the differences between equity and equality is still evident in gender mainstreaming strategies in the health sector. Rigorous debates about the desired outcomes of interventions are rarely held; indeed it seems that in some cases the initiation of a policy is seen as enough in itself. There is often little clarity about what gender equity in health would look like in practice. Instead initiatives have tended to focus on more easily measurable outputs relating to equality issues in the health labour force and in the distribution of services (Elsey et al., 2005). Following the model of mainstreaming adopted in other sectors, attempts have been made to promote greater equality among healthcare workers. This has been especially evident in medicine where women were traditionally in the minority. Though this has now been transformed with female doctors in the majority in many countries, medicine remains male-dominated, with women still occupying less senior positions in the profession and being in a tiny minority in prestigious specialties such as surgery (see Chapter 25 by Riska on women in the medical profession).

The implementation of gender mainstreaming in the context of service delivery is more complex and hence more difficult to evaluate. Attempts have so far focused on a relatively narrow range of equality issues including changes in patterns of delivery and the targeting of services at specific groups, especially in the fields of reproductive health and HIV/AIDS (Hardee, 2005). Some attempts have been made to capture qualitative data on the particular ways in which women (and more rarely men) experience the services provided (Hardee, 2005). However, there have been very few attempts to operationalize or to measure the impact of gender-sensitive initiatives on male and female differences in health outcomes themselves. Hence the notion of gender equity has rarely been taken seriously in the practice of mainstreaming in healthcare.

Lack of an appropriate evidence base

It has long been recognized that one of the major problems in promoting gender sensitivity in health services is the lack of an adequate evidence base. In response to this, women's health activists have been calling for the collection and analysis of more 'disaggregated' national and local health data. Some progress has been made with the development by WHO of a set of reproductive health indicators to be used in global monitoring (WHO, 2001). This was followed by the creation of a wider set of gender-sensitive indicators incorporating measures for both men and women, including maternal mortality ratios, rates of self-reported depression, individual autonomy in decision-making on household budgeting and on health behaviours, and the performance of health systems, including gender differences in the use of various services, in waiting times and in expenditures (Ben-Abdelaziz, 2007). However, these are not clearly linked in conceptual terms to the pursuit of gender equality and/or equity.

Effective gender mainstreaming is also limited by the lack of an extensive and accurate knowledge base on the ways in which social and biological influences interact to shape the health of women and men. This is obviously important in relation to health problems that are biologically specific to one sex or the other. It has been argued by men's health advocates, for example, that not enough work has been done on prostate cancer compared with cancer of the breast. But it is also essential that gender analysis is applied to the many health problems which affect both men and women, but are experienced differently in terms of symptoms, treatment and prognosis. One of the most frequently cited examples of such problems is that of coronary heart disease. There is now growing evidence of gender differences in how symptoms are experienced and presented. For example, women more often experience 'silent' myocardial infarction without the acute pain reported by men. Some tests used to diagnose heart disease seem to be less accurate for women than for men, while women sometimes receive less treatment then men and are also more likely to die in the first year after diagnosis (Wilkins et al., 2008).

Behind this lack of knowledge is continuing bias in the choice of topics and the design of many medical studies. The lack of research on the biology of sex differences in coronary heart disease has been a long-standing concern

(Sen and Östlin, 2007). Many critics have highlighted the white male bias in the selection of study samples and some countries have attempted to remedy this inequity. However, there is little evidence that such strategies have been successful. In the USA, for example, despite the requirement that all biomedical research funded by the National Institutes of Health (NIH) should include gender disaggregated analysis and data, recent reviews suggest that changes have been very limited (Geller et al., 2006).

In sum, more interdisciplinary research is needed using both social science and biomedical perspectives if the implications of gender on patterns of heart disease (and similar health problems) in women and men are to be properly understood. Unless and until it is clear how particular patterns of health and illness are related to sex and gender it will be impossible to promote either equality or equity in mainstreaming strategies (see also Chapter 6 by Klinge).

Complex politics of gender mainstreaming

But even if this knowledge base were to be improved there would still be significant political challenges inherent in any attempt to promote either equity or equality in mainstreaming. This reflects the reality that interventions of this kind are not simply technical exercises that can be achieved by following a textbook. Nor can they be done through a single specialist unit. Rather, responsibility needs to be clearly allocated within the relevant organization and power distributed in ways that enable potentially radical changes to be carried out. Similarly, commitment to the underlying values must be widely shared. Existing evidence and anecdotal accounts suggest, however, this is rarely the case.

The need for shared values is particularly difficult to ensure given the fact that gender equality initiatives may be embedded in very different ethical frameworks. The arguments used by gender activists are usually based on the idea of social justice and health as a human right. Most women's organizations involved in gender equality and gender equity work from a women's rights perspective as embodied in international declarations. WHO's own gender mainstreaming strategy is built on the principle articulated in their constitution that:

> The enjoyment of the highest attainable standard of health is one of the fundamental human rights of every human being without distinction of race, religion, political belief, economic or social condition. (WHO, 2002: 2)

There is also a 'business case' for gender equality and equity based on the argument that health outcomes will be improved, and resources used more efficiently, if bias is not allowed to distort rational decision-making. The 'business case' focuses on the need for efficiency and 'good stewardship' in the planning and provision of health services. The World Bank (2007), for example, argues that economies grow more quickly in countries where women and men are relatively equal, due to increased productivity and greater efficiency in the allocation of labour both in the wider economy and in private households. Buvinic and King (2007), in a report for the International Monetary Fund, argue that gender equality is smart economics, not only because women's increased participation in the labour market increases economic growth, but also because the health of households is improved when women have more control over the use of resources. Sometimes these policy justifications are used simultaneously, as described by the UN Office of the Special Advisor on Gender Issues and the Advancement of Women: 'Equality between women and men is seen both as a human rights issue and as a precondition for, and indicator of, sustainable people-centered development' (OSAGI, 2001: 1).

Thus participants in a single organization may be working toward what appear to be the same goals but are doing so with a different set of values. The implications of these different foundations for the effective implementation of gender mainstreaming have so far received little attention.

When the two approaches lead to the same policies then clearly there will not be a problem. Indeed it is this apparent convergence of interests that has made possible much of the progress achieved thus far. However, problems may arise when resources are scarce and when efficiency gains are not immediately obvious to those holding the power. Under these circumstances gender justice issues may well be seen as an optional add-on (Bremen and Shelton, 2007; Sen and Östlin, 2007). These contradictions are likely to become increasingly apparent in the current economic climate where social justice is rarely high on the list of priorities in the health sector.

Obstacles to the promotion of gender mainstreaming in healthcare: the global context

In recent years health policy at both national and international levels has been shaped by neoliberal economic policies and associated ideological shifts. The main manifestation of this has been broadly characterised as Health Sector Reform (HSR). Different versions of HSR have been carried out in both rich and poor countries, and in the latter case it has often been accompanied by structural adjustment policies of various kinds. There is considerable evidence that these policies have reinforced gender inequities in a number of ways – usually to the detriment of women (Standing, 2002; see also Chapter 3 by Standing).

The focus on decentralization in the Americas, for example, with strong systems of state governance, can be compared with the very different situation in sub-Saharan Africa. Here the context is one of public health sector crisis, with weak state governance and an increasing role for the private sector. Standing (2002) points out that the private sector is not uniformly bad for women, and that private care can include services from non-profit providers such as women's health organizations. However, some not-for-profit services, especially those provided by faith-based organizations, may seek to reinforce traditional, patriarchal values and thus increase gender inequity.

Private sector care may also limit the extent to which national or international organizations can promote gender equality and equity (Standing, 2002). Similarly, HSR has often led to the introduction or extension of fees for services followed by a greater reduction in use of healthcare by women than men (Mackintosh and Tibandebage, 2006; Standing, 2002). In a number of countries user fees for reproductive health services have contributed to increased rates of maternal and infant mortality, while fees for treatment for sexually transmitted infections have led to a greater fall in service use among women than among men (Mackintosh and Tibandebage, 2006). Women are also disadvantaged by health insurance schemes, as fewer women work in jobs which qualify for health insurance and fewer earn enough to pay insurance premiums (Mackintosh and Tibandebage, 2006). In addition, women are often unable to access money in their own right, and household decisions on the allocation of resources are likely to mean that women's healthcare needs are unmet (Doyal, 2002).

This bias will frequently go unnoticed due to the unavailability of gender-sensitive indicators to measure the efficiency and effectiveness of policies. Disability-adjusted life years (DALYs) are widely used for this purpose but fail to measure the full impact of some illnesses on quality of life.

HSR and related economic and social trends have further damaged many women's health through increasing the scale of their domestic responsibilities. Reductions in public expenditure in the health sector have limited the availability of care, especially for those living with chronic illness. In many parts of the world this has meant that women have little choice but to provide unpaid care in the home, often to the detriment of their own health (Mackintosh and Tibandebage, 2006; Standing, 2002). This trend has of course been greatly exacerbated by the global HIV pandemic which has consumed vast quantities of scarce healthcare resources while hugely increasing the burden of domestic caring, especially among older women (see also Chapter 12 by Gilbert and Selikow). Together the effect of these various developments has often been to increase gender equality with little sign of corresponding policies to promote gender equity.

Conclusion

We have seen that any strategy for enabling women and men to optimize their health will necessitate the use of both gender equity and gender equality as underpinning principles. For this to have happened, the following are crucial: the development of equitable policies based on sex differences in health needs, and their implications for appropriate care. In many ways this will be the easiest part of the process, provided that the appropriate knowledge base is available. The challenges of promoting gender equality in health and healthcare will be much greater. Differences between the social constructions of maleness and femaleness are deeply embedded in all aspects of the individual psyche and in the wider social order. Any shift towards 'healthier' models of gender will be a complex and difficult process and will involve changes far beyond the health sector. These issues have been at the heart of many feminist debates over the years and are beginning to emerge in the literature on men's health. But there are no easy solutions.

Even more challenging will be the achievement of gender justice. As we have seen, gender inequalities are much more pervasive and more damaging to women than they are to men. If this unfairness is to be tackled it will require a radical transformation of gender relations. A major restructuring will be needed in the divisions of labour, of resources and of status between women and men across a range of social and economic settings. These changes would be complex and difficult to achieve and, as we have seen, they are likely to be resisted at both individual and institutional levels. It is always difficult to persuade those with status and power to relinquish them. But without such changes, improvements achieved from mainstreaming gender will only be partial and neither women nor men will be able to fully realize their biological potential for health.

Summary

- The promotion of gender equality and gender equity between women and men has become a key theme in national and international policy debates since the 1990s.
- Gender equality refers to an absence of discrimination in relation to opportunities, resources, benefits and access to services.
- Gender equity refers to justice in the distribution of power, resources and responsibilities.
- Policies to promote health need to address both equality and equity. In particular, the health gap between women and men reflects biological as well as gender influences, which means that equality in health outcomes is an unrealistic policy objective.

Key reading

Doyal, L. (2002) 'Putting Gender into Health and Globalisation Debates: New Perspectives and Old Challenges', *Third World Quarterly*, 23 (2), 233–50.
OSAGI – Office of the Special Advisor on Gender Issues and the Advancement of Women (2001) *Gender Mainstreaming: Strategy for Promoting Gender Equality* (New York: OSAGI, United Nations Department of Economic and Social Affairs).

Payne, S. (2006) *The Health of Men and Women* (Cambridge: Polity).
Sen, G., A. George and P. Östlin (eds) (2002) *Engendering International Health: The Challenge of Equity* (Cambridge, MA: MIT Press).

Acknowledgement

The authors thank Len Doyal for his great help with the philosophical underpinnings of this paper.

References

Anand, S. and A. Sen (1995) *Gender Inequality in Human Development: Theories and Measurement* (New York: UNDP).

Annandale, E. (2009) *Women's Health and Social Change* (Abingdon: Routledge).

Barton, C. (2004) 'Global Women's Movements at a Crossroads: Seeking Definition, New Alliances and Greater Impact', *Socialism and Democracy*, 18 (1), 151–84.

Barton. C. and L. Prendergast (eds) (2004) *Seeking Accountability on Women's Human Rights: Women Debate the Millennium Development Goals* (Mumbai: Women's International Coalition for Economic Justice).

Ben-Abdelaziz, F. (2007) 'Women's Health and Equity Indicators', *International Journal of Public Health*, 52, S1–2.

Breman, A. and C. Shelton (2007) 'Structural Adjustment Programs and Health', in I. Kawachi and S. Wamala (eds), *Globalization and Health* (Oxford: Oxford University Press), 219–33.

Buvinic, M. and E. M. King (2007) 'Smart Economics', *Finance and Development*, 44 (2), at: www.imf.org/external/pubs/ft/fandd/2007/06/king.htm, accessed 19 May 2009.

Courtenay, W. (2000) 'Constructions of Masculinity and Their Influence on Men's Well-being: A Theory of Gender and Health', *Social Science & Medicine*, 50, 1385–1401.

Doyal, L. (1995) *What Makes Women Sick? Gender and the Political Economy of Health* (Basingstoke: Macmillan).

Doyal, L. (2002) 'Putting Gender into Health and Globalisation Debates: New Perspectives and Old Challenges', *Third World Quarterly*, 23 (2), 233–50.

EHRC – Equalities and Human Rights Commission (2009) *Gender Equality Duty*, at: www. equalityhumanrights.com/advice-and-guidance/public-sector-duties/introduction-to-the-public-sector-duties/gender-equality-duty/, accessed 21 September 2009.

Elsey, H., R. Tolhurst and S. Theobald (2002) *Gender Mainstreaming in Sector Wide Approaches, Policy Briefing* (Liverpool: Liverpool School of Tropical Medicine).

Elsey, H., R. Tolhurst and S. Theobald (2005) 'Mainstreaming HIV/AIDS in Development Sectors: Have We Learnt the Lessons from Gender Mainstreaming?', *AIDS Care*, 17 (8), 988–98.

Geller, S. E., M. G. Adams and M. Carnes (2006) 'Adherence to Federal Guidelines for Reporting of Sex and Race/Ethnicity in Clinical Trials', *Journal of Women's Health*, 15 (10), 1123–31.

Hafner-Burton, E and M. A. Pollack (2002) 'Gender Mainstreaming and Global Governance', *Feminist Legal Studies*, 10 (3), 285–98.

Hardee, K. (2005) *The Intersection of Gender, Access, and Quality of Care in Reproductive Services: Examples from Kenya, India, and Guatemala* (Washington, DC: USAID).

Mackintosh, M. and P. Tibandebage (2006) 'Gender and Health Sector Reform', in S. Razavi and S. Hassim (eds), *Gender and Social Policy in a Global Context* (Basingstoke: Palgrave Macmillan and UNRISD), 237–57.

OSAGI – Office of the Special Advisor on Gender Issues and the Advancement of Women (2001) *Gender Mainstreaming: Strategy for Promoting Gender Equality* (New York: OSAGI, United Nations Department of Economic and Social Affairs).

Payne, S. (2006) *The Health of Men and Women* (Cambridge: Polity).

Pearson. R. (2000) 'Moving the Goalposts: Gender and Globalisation in the Twenty-First Century', *Gender and Development,* 8 (1), 10–19.

Petchesky, R. (2003) *Global Prescriptions: Gendering Health and Human Rights* (London: Zed Books).

Razavi, S. and C. Miller (1995) *From WID to GAD: Conceptual Shifts in the Women and Development Discourse* (Geneva: UNRISD).

Robertson, S. (2007) *Understanding Men and Health: Masculinities, Identity and Well-being* (Maidenhead: Open University Press).

Sen, G., A. George and P. Östlin (eds) (2002) *Engendering International Health: The Challenge of Equity* (Cambridge, MA: MIT Press).

Sen, G. and P. Östlin (2007) *Unequal, Unfair, Ineffective and Inefficient. Gender Inequity in Health: Why It Exists and How We Can Change It,* Final Report to the WHO Commission on Social Determinants of Health, at: www.eurohealth.ie/pdf/WGEKN_FINAL_REPORT. pdf, accessed 19 October 2009.

Standing, H. (2002) 'Frameworks for Understanding Health Sector Reform', in G. Sen, A. George and P. Östlin (eds), *Engendering International Health: The Challenge of Equity* (Cambridge, MA: MIT Press), 347–71.

UN – United Nations (1997) *Mainstreaming the Gender Perspective into all Policies and Programmes in the United Nations* (New York: ECOSOC, United Nations).

UN – United Nations (2001) *Important Concepts Underlying Gender Mainstreaming* (New York: United Nations Office of the Special Advisor on Gender Issues and the Advancement of Women).

UNFPA – United Nations Population Fund (2005) *State of the World's Population 2005: The Promise of Equality: Gender Equity, Reproductive Health and the Millennium Development Goals* (New York: United Nations Population Fund).

WHO – World Health Organization (2001) *Reproductive Health Indicators for Global Monitoring: Report of Second Interagency Meeting* (Geneva: WHO).

WHO – World Health Organization (2002) *Mainstreaming Gender Equity in Health: The Need to Move Forward – Madrid Statement* (Geneva: WHO).

WHO – World Health Organization (2008a) *Strategy for Integrating Gender Analysis and Actions into the Work of WHO* (Geneva: WHO).

WHO – World Health Organization (2008b) *World Health Statistics 2008* (Geneva: WHO).

Wilkins, D., S. Payne, G. Granville and P. Branney (2008) *The Gender and Access to Health Services Study Final Report* (London: Department of Health), at: www.dh.gov.uk/en/ Publicationsandstatistics/Publications/PublicationsPolicyAndGuidance/DH_092042, accessed 24 August 2009.

Wizemann, T. and M. Pardue (2000) *Exploring the Biological Contributions to Human Health: Does Sex Matter?* (Washington, DC: National Academy Press).

World Bank (2007) *Global Monitoring Report 2007: Confronting the Challenges of Gender Equality and Fragile States* (New York: World Bank).

2
Gender Equality and International Health Policy Planning*

Shelly N. Abdool, Claudia García-Moreno and Avni Amin

Introduction

The 1995 Fourth World Conference on Women, held in Beijing, led to increased international efforts to scale up gender mainstreaming across sectors, including in health (UN, 1995). In the health sector gender mainstreaming has multiple objectives. First and foremost, as in other sectors, its goal is to achieve gender equality. Second, its methods and tools aim to identify and address both the harmful ways that gender inequality damages the health of women and girls as well as the ways that the socialization of gender norms, roles and relations influence health behaviours and outcomes of different groups of women and men (Sen et al., 2007). A final objective is to address institutional conditions of the health system and wider society, such as unequal distribution of decision-making authority, that can reinforce patterns of inequality (Ravindran and Kelkar-Khambete, 2008; Walby, 2005). Enabling policy environments or mechanisms for equal participation of women and men can also contribute to health equity and sustainability in the health sector (Theobald et al., 2002) and to agenda-setting. All of these objectives require both technical expertise and political commitment in order to achieve the ultimate goal of gender equality.

In international health the blending of technical expertise and political commitment has implied different efforts and strategies. As authors have shown (see Chibber et al., 2008; Donner, 2003; Fathalla, 2008; Ribeiro et al., 2008; Sen et al., 2007; Standing, 2000; Theobald et al., 2002), applying various gender mainstreaming tools and methods, gender and women's health advocates have worked to:

1. Further develop a women's health agenda that encompasses determinants of women's health including and beyond reproductive health;
2. Increase attention and develop methodologies to uncover how and why gender norms/behaviours and gender inequality operate as a determinant of health for different groups of women and men; and

3. Ensure that health policy planning involves women and men as equal partners and beneficiaries in line with human rights principles of equality, non-discrimination and participation.

Progress has been steady in some areas, notably the first area. The second area has seen promising progress with issues such as sexual and other forms of gender-based violence (SGBV), early marriage, masculinities and commercial sex work increasingly posited as important influences on health behaviours and outcomes for women and men (García-Moreno et al., 2005; WHO, 2001; WHO, 2007). Progress has been patchy, however, with respect to the third area, which requires sustained political commitment and systemic changes in the ways health policies are planned and implemented (Donner, 2003; Sen et al., 2007).

This chapter focuses on international health policy planning, and discusses challenges and successes in promoting gender equality. It first identifies four minimum elements for the integration of gender equality in health policy planning. As international health policy planning is influenced by the broader gender and development policy paradigms, a brief overview of policy approaches is provided to underscore that if the framework used for health policy planning is not based on principles of social justice and an explicit attention to gender equality, it is difficult for the resulting policies to promote it in meaningful, sustainable ways. The chapter then discusses progress in integrating gender equality in health policy planning, identifies challenges and proposes some ways forward. Examples demonstrating ways that gender equality has been a core element of policy planning in the areas of violence against women and HIV/AIDS are used throughout. Both of these areas are a reflection of some of the stark manifestations of gender inequality, related to stigma and unequal power relations, particularly in the area of sexual negotiation and decision-making. The chapter concludes by reiterating what international feminist practice has taught us for years: commitment to gender equality requires technical expertise, human resources, budgetary allocations and multiple stakeholder involvement to translate health policies into action-able outcomes.

Minimum elements for gender mainstreaming in health policy planning

As strategies to achieve gender equality are inherently context-specific, there are many tools and methods for addressing gender equality, or to mainstream gender, in health policy planning. A set of minimum elements, however, can be identified from the various efforts to guide health policy planning processes. As discussed by authors such as Bloom and Standing (2008),

Gwatkin et al. (2004), Siddiqi et al. (2009) and Sen et al. (2002; 2007), minimum elements could include:

1. Use of gender analysis methods and tools when generating evidence to inform health policy planning and development;
2. Establishing mechanisms for meaningful participation of female and male stakeholders, including civil society organizations such as patient advocate groups, health professional associations and representative groups of marginalized populations;
3. Developing and implementing strategic legislative and policy frameworks based on human rights and gender equality principles to explicitly protect the most vulnerable groups in society; and
4. Creating and/or strengthening existing oversight functions/mechanisms to ensure that existing forms of discrimination against men or women from any social group are neither reinforced nor upheld through health policy.

Violence against women: a case study for minimum standards to integrate gender in health policy planning

Globally, at least one out of every three women has been beaten, coerced into sex or otherwise abused in her lifetime. Violence against women (VAW) tends to be more common in settings where power relationships between men and women are unequal, with violence used as a tool to force or maintain women into subservient positions or to 'discipline' them; husbands and male partners are often the perpetrators (Heise and García-Moreno, 2002). It is used to maintain gender inequalities and social hierarchies, often perpetuated by a culture of silence and denial. Thus, violence against women is sustained by and helps to sustain women's unequal status in society. It has a major impact on women's health and well-being and that of their children, and thus is a major public health issue and a human rights concern which occurs across the life-span (García-Moreno et al., 2005). This case study illustrates how the four elements above have contributed to the recognition and policy development on violence against women in the international public health agenda.

Minimum element 1: Using gender analysis when reviewing evidence for health policies

Violence ranks among the leading causes of death for people aged 15 to 44 years, accounting for about 14 per cent of deaths among males and seven per cent of deaths among females worldwide; and for every person who dies as a result of violence, many more are injured or traumatized (Krug et al., 2002). At face value these statistics point to violence as a major cause of death and disability for young men and less so for young women. When gender analysis is applied, the evidence highlights important differences in the forms and consequences of violence that women and men experience, with clear implications for health and other policies. For example, in some countries half to two-thirds of female deaths from violence are by a partner, whereas intimate partners account for only four per cent of male homicides (Heise and García-Moreno, 2002). For women, most violence happens behind closed doors and from family members, whereas men are more exposed to violence outside of the home, by strangers. The focus on physical injury also reflects a common outcome of violence for men, whereas for women violence more often leads to a range of physical, sexual, reproductive and mental health problems. For years violence against women, particularly by intimate partners, was seen as a private matter rather than a crime or a public health problem to be dealt with. The production and analysis of data on violence have informed the international health policy agenda, positing violence against women as a public health issue for urgent policy and programmatic action.

Minimum element 2: The equal involvement of various types of male and female stakeholders in policy development

Years of activism by women's organizations coupled with gender analysis of health and violence have contributed to a greater recognition of violence against women in public policy agendas at global, regional and national levels. A public health and human rights approach recognizes addressing gender inequality as a key element to violence prevention and response. More recently, men have joined forces with women's groups and taken a more active role in challenging gender norms that perpetuate or condone violence generally and against women in particular (WHO, 2007). A high-level panel of men against violence against women has recently been appointed by the UN Secretary General as part of his campaign for the elimination of violence against women. Professional associations such as the World Federation of Obstetricians and Gynaecologists are developing policies and guidelines to educate and raise awareness among their constituencies about violence.

Minimum element 3: Developing and implementing strategic legislative and policy frameworks based on human-rights and gender equality principles

Following 1995 Fourth World Conference on Women in Beijing, many countries implemented legal reforms or introduced new laws to address 'family' or 'domestic violence' and, in some countries, sexual violence. Other countries have revised laws which, by discriminating against women, can increase their vulnerability to violence (and HIV infection), such as those related to property and inheritance rights. Health policies in many countries are beginning to address intimate partner violence and sexual violence in health services. However, challenges remain. In some countries violence against women still lacks priority in policy-making, continues to be shrouded in silence, and is considered a personal or private matter. Services for victims are often inadequate and where they exist may be limited to urban areas, with providers lacking the understanding and knowledge required. There is limited or no investment in prevention, which requires attention to important structural and other determinants, including those related to gender equality and women's empowerment. Many of these challenges are closely related to a low level of political commitment to address gender-based violence, despite the evidence that it is a public health issue of significant concern.

Minimum element 4: Establishing oversight mechanisms to ensure that the principles of gender equality are upheld and to monitor progress

Women's groups remain watchful and are constantly lobbying for policy change, resources and implementation of policies and plans. Changes to the law, to public health norms and to service provision provide at times for oversight mechanisms, but in most places institutional mechanisms still are lacking or need strengthening.

Overview of approaches to gender equality in health policy planning

Approaches to addressing women in development and gender planning have evolved over the years. International health policy planning has mirrored these approaches (see, for example, March et al., 1999; PAHO, 1997; Sen et al., 2002; 2007). Discussions on international health policy planning should therefore begin from an understanding of the characteristics and assumptions of these approaches in order to assess their impact on health policies and gender equality goals.

The welfare approach

The welfare approach to development policy planning stems from the 'women in development' (WID) philosophy (Moser, 1993; Taylor, 1999). Utilitarian arguments are used: women should be involved because they will contribute to better development outcomes. Concerns about social justice or gender equality are of lesser priority as it is assumed that robust economic progress will contribute to such objectives. This lack of priority means that the minimum elements for gender equality are unlikely to occur within this policy approach. The welfare approach is based on the assumption that motherhood is the most important and valued role for women (Moser, 1993; PAHO, 1997; Taylor, 1999), inferring that a comprehensive gender analysis (minimum element 1) is not likely to happen when assessing health needs. In health policies, this translates into an emphasis on women's reproductive roles, particularly motherhood.

The emphasis on girls' education *only* as it relates to later fertility and child health outcomes is another example. With respect to the four minimum elements, the welfare approach falls short.

The equity approach

The equity approach is also based on the assumption that involving women is good for economic progress. Its assumptions shift however, to acknowledge that women's roles and responsibilities are three-fold: reproductive, productive and community service (Moser, 1993). The recognition of women's roles beyond motherhood is a significant shift – and, in health, accommodates minimum element 1 of using gender analysis methods to examine health needs beyond those related to motherhood. The recognition of women's multiple roles has contributed to analyses of the gender-based division of labour which have found that the distribution of power and benefits within the health workforce is still skewed in many contexts – with more men in decision-making positions and in higher-paid positions than women (George, 2008). The equity approach assumes that only state interventions can eliminate gender inequality (Taylor, 1999; Williams et al., 1994). This implies an opportunity to put in place minimum elements 2 and 3 – both related to political mechanisms to support gender equality. However, the continued focus on economic progress means that gender equality is not always a guiding principle, which could lead to limitations in establishing oversight mechanisms (minimum element 4).

The anti-poverty approach

The anti-poverty approach continues to be popular among NGOs and women's groups from the developing world and emerged to counterbalance top-down planning and policy approaches (Moser, 1993; Taylor, 1999). In considering both poverty and women's inequality, this approach provides space for looking at differential allocation (access to and control over) of resources for women and men, which infers the application of broader gender analysis methods as a tool for evidence-based policy (minimum element 1). As this approach was born from political movements and grassroots organizations, it can more easily accommodate the creation of oversight mechanisms to ensure principles of equality are upheld (minimum element 4).

Examples of anti-poverty approaches in international health and development policy planning include the recognition that women's lesser access to and control over resources such as income, education and health information has an impact on their health. These resources represent determinants of health that must be addressed to improve health outcomes. Another example is the push towards community-based initiatives (CBI) to foster bottom-up approaches to health planning. This approach promotes a 'determinants of health' approach and the principle that health is central to development (WHO EMRO, 2009).

It promotes addressing basic economic needs such as vocational training for women or men, and sponsoring micro-credit initiatives or other income-generating activities. CBI can be considered both as a vehicle (or mechanism) for meaningful participation of women and men and a strategic policy framework (minimum elements 2 and 3), indicating that this approach may be conducive to promoting gender equality in health policy. At the same time, some approaches have tended to marginalize women from mainstream policies with these economic development activities (Grown et al., 2005).

The efficiency approach

The efficiency approach became popular following the debt crisis in the 1980s. Similar to the welfare approach, it is not explicitly committed to the principles of social justice and gender equality. Addressing gender inequality in this approach is important because inequality obstructs economic progress, not because equality is a valid goal in and of itself (Moser, 1993; Taylor, 1999; Williams et al., 1994). This, on its own, excludes this approach from fulfilling minimum elements 2 to 4 as political will is likely to be weak as a result. The efficiency approach is reflected in the now-replaced Structural Adjustment Programmes (SAPs) which focused on increasing efficiency and productivity, including in the health sector (see also Chapter 3 by Standing). These policies tend to downplay harmful gender norms, roles and relations that lead to inequitable health outcomes or ignore their impact altogether. This indicates a failure to fulfil minimum element 1; that is, using gender analysis methods to inform policies. Without a solid evidence base on gender equality and health, this approach cannot meet the remaining minimum elements set out for addressing gender equality in health policy planning.

The equality approach

The equality approach targets women due to their burden of inequality. It promotes activities such as legislative review, policy revision and/or development designed to promote gender equality. It further supports the establishment of mechanisms for gender equality and women's autonomy (Moser, 1993; PAHO, 1997; Williams et al., 1994). All four minimum elements can be accommodated within this policy approach: understanding women in their broader gendered context allows the use of gender analysis methods (minimum element 1), attention to facilitating women's entry into the workforce includes ensuring mechanisms for equal participation of women and men (minimum element 2), the promotion of legislative review and policy development speaks directly to minimum element 3 and the introduction of mechanisms to sustain gender equality accommodates minimum element 4 on the creation of oversight functions for gender equality.

Box 2.1 includes an example of health policy planning based on the equality approach. The example fulfils all four minimum elements for ensuring gender

Box 2.1 Involving people living with HIV in delivery of HIV/AIDS services in Kenya

The Family Planning Association of Kenya (FPAK) implemented a project to integrate comprehensive HIV/AIDS care into its existing network of sexual and reproductive health services, with support from *Deutsche Gesellschaft für Technische Zusammenarbeit* (GTZ). The project involved building the capacity of FPAK staff, enhancing delivery and demand through the active participation of people living with and affected by HIV/AIDS. The delivery of expanded services involved the provision of anti-retrovirals using voluntary counselling and treatment programmes and the prevention of mother-to-child transmission of HIV as entry points in selected FPAK clinics. Action research was conducted to better understand the use of anti-retrovirals by women, including potential interactions with oral contraceptives. This has led to participatory capacity building of community-based outreach staff and peer educators, including people living with HIV, who can support women with adherence and in accessing psychosocial care through mentoring and based on their own experiences.

To ensure active participation of people living with HIV and the implementation of the Greater Involvement of People Living with HIV/AIDS (GIPA) declaration, the programme ensured that people living with HIV were employed as paid staff, included on the site advisory committees, and integrated into the management and advisory board for FPAK. This has led to people living with HIV having a stronger sense of commitment to this long-term work, with possibilities for career development, and it has reduced stigma and discrimination against people living with HIV from other staff. It has also increased the credibility of the HIV/AIDS services within the communities served, among other HIV/AIDS service organizations, and among men and women living with HIV.

Sources: IPPF, 2005; UNAIDS, 2006.

equality in health policy planning. While the equality approach tends to highlight women's equality, the initiative described here encompasses both women and men to reduce inequalities for people living with HIV. In so doing, this also facilitates their equal involvement in planning interventions of direct relevance to their lives. The project is based on a human rights framework for programming designed to protect the most marginalized – corresponding to minimum element 3. The target population could not have been defined without the application of gender analysis methods to HIV data and services in Kenya (minimum element 1). In creating space for the equal and meaningful participation of women and men living with HIV (through paid service) and establishing oversight functions such as the advisory committee that led to decreased stigma, it fulfils the final two minimum elements for promoting gender equality in health policy planning.

The empowerment approach

The empowerment approach emerged as a response to welfare, equity, anti-poverty and efficiency approaches, which tend to treat women as a homogenous group (Moser, 1993; Taylor, 1999; Williams et al., 1994). This allows use of gender analysis (minimum element 1) when examining women's (or men's) health needs and status as it acknowledges more than sex differences and assumes multiple roles and identities for men and women. This approach aims to empower women and men to be self-reliant, and emphasizes diversity and broader socio-political factors as important influences on women's and men's lives (Moser, 1993; Williams et al., 1994). This approach therefore creates space for fostering meaningful and equal participation of women and men in health policy planning (minimum element 2).

The emphasis on broader socio-political influences implies the need for legislative and policy frameworks (minimum element 3) as well as oversight functions based on human rights and gender equality principles (minimum element 4). Like the equality approach, the empowerment approach allows for all four minimum elements for promoting gender equality in international health policy planning. Box 2.2 highlights this through an example dealing with health workers in various settings. All four minimum elements for promoting gender equality in international health policy planning are reflected in this project. The development of workshop materials to sensitize health workers on gender and health requires the application of gender analysis methods (minimum element 1). The focus on engaging with health workers (male and female) to create space for them to learn, share experiences and express needs can be considered as mechanisms to foster equal participation of different groups (minimum element 2).

In summary, it appears that the first minimum element – of using gender analysis to generate evidence to inform health policy planning – is possible in several of the policy approaches. Gender analysis requires technical expertise and political commitment to ensure this analysis is used for evidence-based policy-making. However, the second, third and fourth minimum elements – all requiring political commitment and technical expertise in institutional aspects of gender mainstreaming – are harder to achieve and more likely to be implemented in the anti-poverty, equality and empowerment approaches. These three policy approaches are therefore the most conducive frameworks

Box 2.2 Health Workers for Change: Gender-sensitive interventions for health infrastructure and quality of care

The Health Workers for Change (HFWC) intervention was developed by the Women's Health Project at the University of Witswatersrand in South Africa to provide high quality, gender-sensitive health services. Through a series of workshops, it engaged and empowered healthcare workers to critically analyse interpersonal aspects (for example, provider–client relations) of quality, sensitized them to how gender relations affect health, and helped them take action to improve other aspects of quality of care (for example, inadequate physical infrastructure, lack of human resources). The intervention was subsequently adapted and used in seven sites in Argentina, Ghana, Kenya, Nigeria and the United Republic of Tanzania.

An impact evaluation of HFWC showed that health workers were able to integrate their heightened understanding of gender issues into their daily practices. In HFWC acceptability studies, health workers described many situations in which they had blamed women (for example, for coming late for treatment), although they recognized that gendered power relations often prevented women from coming earlier. After the intervention, positive measurable changes in health workers' relationships with their clients were noted, along with improved service. These included increased privacy for female patients, greater promptness in services, improved availability of drugs and supplies, greater cleanliness and improved communication. Health workers also took more initiative in problem-solving, including in relation to the supply of drugs and equipment. For example, in Nigeria the primary health care staff requested and received supplies and equipment from the community, including a delivery couch, a urine analysis facility and blood pressure apparatus. In Kenya, after the intervention, the facility staff consulted administrators about the lack of water and electricity and a decision was made to use the facility-held proportion of user fees to fence the facility and install electricity.

Sources: Onyano-Ouma et al., 2001; Vlassof and Fonn, 2001.

to advance gender equality in health policy planning. This further indicates that when both technical expertise on the application of gender analysis methods and gender politics (or the creation of political infrastructure based on the principles of gender equality) is combined with political commitment, efforts to address gender equality in health policy planning are more likely to succeed.

Where are we today?

The good news: Progress exists to promote gender equality in health policy planning

The simple, straightforward answer to ever-persistent questions about the added value of gender mainstreaming in health is that it contributes to good public health practice. As health is defined beyond the absence of illness, it is imperative to explore all factors that influence health behaviours and outcomes (Chibber et al., 2008; Sen et al., 2002; 2007). Despite reticence and apparent stagnation, commitments to gender equality remain prominent in international instruments and frameworks such as the Millennium Development Goals (see also Chapter 3 by Standing and Chapter 18 by Patel). This is seen as a means to achieve social justice and enhance the effectiveness of health sector actions. Health policy planners have been using evidence from various sources to pinpoint and address root causes of disease and illness that stem from socio-cultural norms at household and community levels.

For example, in HIV/AIDS health policy planning and programmatic responses globally, addressing gender inequalities as a determinant of the epidemic is now widely recognized (Ehrhardt et al., 2009; see also Chapter 12 by Gilbert and Selikow). This progress can be attributed to multiple factors including global advocacy efforts by civil society groups (HIV-positive groups, women's groups and other advocates) who have successfully lobbied to place gender inequalities, including gender-based violence, at the centre of HIV/AIDS policy planning and response. There has also been increased effort and emphasis placed on gathering evidence on gender inequalities to inform HIV/AIDS policy and programming. Such evidence has driven much of the work that the international community is currently undertaking in this area.

As a result of these factors, the broader international community, including inter-governmental agencies and bilateral and multilateral donors, have increasingly recognized the intersections between gender inequality and HIV infection and have contributed to ensuring that addressing this is on the international health agenda. Several international commitments to addressing gender inequalities in HIV/AIDS response exist, including the UNGASS Declaration of Commitments in 2001 and 2006. In 2007, the Policy and Coordinating Board (PCB) of UNAIDS specifically requested UNAIDS to address gender substantially in HIV/AIDS programming. Such a call to action will surely influence national health policy planning, technical cooperation between countries, and support from UNAIDS and other international organizations. At the Replenishment Conference of the Global Fund for AIDS, Tuberculosis and Malaria (GFATM) in Berlin and the Sixteenth GFATM Board meeting in 2007 an explicit commitment was made to integrate gender into GFATM infrastructure and to ensure that national responses consider the role of gender across the three diseases. In 2008 the Global Fund invested in the development and approval of their Gender Equality Strategy and its implementation plan (WHO, 2009). Other donor programmes, including the US President's Emergency Plan for AIDS Relief (PEPFAR) and the World Bank's Multi-country HIV/AIDS Programme (MAP), have also committed to ensuring that their responses to HIV/AIDS programmes incorporate gender (Ashburn et al., 2009).

This type of high-level commitment creates an enabling environment for health policy planning to systematically address gender inequality. Within such an environment, with a range of different stakeholders involved, the minimum elements are more likely to be fulfilled: gender analysis methods become central to evidence generation, political mechanisms are established to ensure equal and meaningful participation, and legal and policy frameworks and oversight mechanisms (such as the GFATM's Gender Equality Strategy) are developed. Box 2.3 includes a case study on experiences with gender mainstreaming in national HIV/AIDS policy-making in Kenya. The case study is illustrative of the ways that blending technical expertise on gender and HIV/AIDS and political commitment to address gender equality in HIV/AIDS policies and programmes make a difference to the policy planning process.

The bad news: Despite an international framework and commitment, reticence is predominant

In spite of decades of attention to gender equality, questions still arise within the health sector about the added value of gender mainstreaming. Reticence towards addressing gender equality in the health sector can be attributed to multiple factors. First, the predominant biomedical approach – despite increasing attention to determinants of health over the past decade – leads to general conclusions that physiological factors are what matter most for health and illness (Fathalla, 2008; Ravindran and Kelkar-Khambete, 2008). This approach feeds the continued misconception that gender refers simply to biological differences between women and men. Furthermore, the biomedical model itself has been biased towards a male norm. Measures of the burden of disease, while important tools for health policy planners, do not provide the full story of facilitating and inhibiting causes of ill-health for women and men (Chibber et al., 2008; Sen et al., 2007).

Second, like other determinants of health, those related to gender equality, such as education, income-generation opportunities and legal protections are outside of the health sector and therefore often seen as outside of health policy planners' mandate. The lack of consultation across sectors, and of valuing expertise from multiple sources within the health sector, means that the health policy planning process risks remaining in stagnant, biomedical waters.

Third, developments in international health policy, and the global health and aid architecture generally, continue to be gender-blind or even worse, opposed to promoting gender equality in international health policy and planning. These

Box 2.3 Mainstreaming gender into the Kenya national HIV/AIDS strategic plan: Gender and HIV/AIDS Technical Subcommittee and the POLICY Project, Kenya

In Kenya, despite overwhelming evidence that the incidence of HIV/AIDS among women was rising at a high rate and women were being infected at an earlier age than men, there were no explicit strategies to address this. In 2001 the Kenya National AIDS Control Council formed a technical subcommittee on gender and an HIV/AIDS task force. It was agreed that the best approach would be to 'engender' the existing Kenya national HIV/AIDS strategic plan – a key document that guided and coordinated all responses to HIV/AIDS in Kenya.

The technical subcommittee's mandate was to formulate guidelines and create a strategic framework through which gender concerns could be integrated into the analyses, formulation and monitoring of policies and programmes relating to the five priority areas of the Kenya national HIV/AIDS strategic plan, so as to ensure that the beneficial outcomes are shared equally by all – women, men, boys and girls.

The gender and HIV/AIDS technical subcommittee included government representatives, as well as a broad cross-section of more than 36 organizations and sectors such as the Society for Women against AIDS in Kenya, Women Fighting AIDS in Kenya and the Kenya AIDS NGOs Consortium. This was the first time that HIV/AIDS groups and gender advocacy organizations had come together in an official forum to inform policy-making at the national level.

In 2002, the subcommittee completed a detailed analysis of Kenya's national plan, highlighted the gender considerations in each part of the plan and provided recommendations for how to address these in the strategy. The findings of the analysis are contained in the document *Mainstreaming Gender into the Kenya National HIV/AIDS Strategic Plan: 2000–2005*, which was adopted by the National AIDS Control Council in 2002. The document also contains comprehensive guidelines and strategies for mainstreaming gender in HIV/AIDS plans and a tool kit for assessing how far gender has been mainstreamed within policies and projects. Kenya's approach could serve as a model for other countries seeking to integrate gender-sensitive approaches into national strategies. While the document continues to inform the current Kenya national HIV/AIDS strategic plan, which is valid until 2009–10, there remain gaps in operationalizing and implementing concrete gender-responsive actions in the HIV/AIDS response, including explicit budgetary allocations, targets and indicators to measure progress on gender-responsive strategies.

Source: Gender and HIV/AIDS Technical Subcommittee, National AIDS Control Council Kenya, 2002.

include health-sector reforms initiated in the 1990s, health workforce crises affecting primarily countries in Asia and Africa resulting in a critical shortage of skilled health workers, and the debt and financial crises which, by reducing donor and government allocations to health and other areas of social protection, can undermine the health of the most vulnerable groups, including women and children (Nanda, 2002; WHO, 2006; 2009). For example, the imposition of user fees, related to the health-sector reforms, has a particular effect on women's access to health services as they are the primary users of public-sector services and least likely to have access to or control over financial resources (Nanda, 2002). Similarly, a shortage of nurses and doctors and the migration of skilled health workers from low-income to high-income countries has, in several countries, resulted in transfer of responsibilities for healthcare provision to communities and households where, given gender norms and roles, women bear the burden of caring for families and communities.

Fourth, gender equality has been progressively de-politicized over the years. A sense of *gender fatigue* has crept into health offices as some get caught up in counting the number of times that the word gender is used and others only address gender as a process of socialization, without addressing the unequal power relations between and among women and men that result. The dissociation of gender equality from feminist (and other forms of social) activism has led to a multiplicity of tools and methods across sectors thereby diluting harmonized attempts to put right unequal structures rooted in gender inequality (Ravindran and Kelkar-Khambete, 2008; Sen et al., 2007).

This de-politicization contributes in two other ways to resistance to gender equality in health policy planning. First, institutional gender mainstreaming has often been limited to aspects of human resources rather than the need for broader systemic reforms aimed at positioning gender equality as a guiding principle for the way an institution does business. Institutional reforms have tended to be framed around issues of sex parity, pay equity and work-life balance – contributing to resistance and criticisms of 'positive discrimination' in favour of women. While these are important issues, the lack of attention to systemic changes in the ways that institutional decisions are made or in the distribution of power among men and women often remains unchallenged (George, 2008). International commitments to human rights and gender equality underscore the importance of principles such as participation, non-discrimination and equality. Institutional responses to gender equality should therefore reflect these principles by enabling women and men to participate on equal terms in the way an institution delivers on its mandate for its staff, partners and beneficiaries. Areas such as education or training opportunities to facilitate access to senior management positions – or political office, as set out in the targets for Millennium Development Goal 3 (Grown et al., 2005) – need to become part of institutional reforms. When these are ignored, attention is concentrated on goal-setting within human resource policies alone; when this is complete, the 'work' to mainstream gender within an institution is erroneously assumed to be have been completed (Daly, 2005).

Finally, gender equality has been watered down by the very process set in place to achieve it: gender mainstreaming. In mainstreaming gender across health programmes (or line ministries), the tendency has been to de-specialize gender units and expertise, thereby weakening sound technical oversight and guidance. Health policy planners may not have the technical expertise to adequately undertake gender analysis. When there is no central unit to guide and spearhead such technical inputs, substantive attention to gender equality wanes (Daly, 2005; Mukhopadhyay, 2006). This is paradoxical: an objective of gender mainstreaming is to achieve and promote gender equality in all programmes and avoid creating parallel, vertical programmes on gender. The historic recent announcement of the creation of a new UN agency for women illustrates the necessity of having such a central unit despite the UN-wide mandate for gender mainstreaming, bringing some of these discussions to a full circle. Yet, this very process has led to decreased specialization and an assumption that 'anyone can do gender'; an assumption that would not be put forth in other technical health areas. Where they exist, gender or women's units (or focal points) often lack the resources and the political support to do their work effectively. The lack of attention given to creating sustainable mechanisms for technical expertise on gender equality in health policy planning can be interpreted as part of the resistance to change and the de-politicization of gender work, ultimately weakening the power earned by women, and men, after decades of activism to ensure that women's health and gender equality become standing agenda items in international health policy.

The recognition of the importance of gender equality and women's empowerment as a determinant of health has undoubtedly grown in the past 15 years and some examples of global and national policies that have integrated gender issues demonstrate that (see also Chapter 5 by Lin and L'Orange, Chapter 6 by Klinge and Chapter 24 by Armstrong). While progress has been made, particularly at policy level, enormous challenges remain and the recognition and commitment in policies needs to be translated into concrete investments and actions.

Conclusion

Despite several gender and health policy planning tools (Donner, 2003; Gender and Health Group, 2008; Horne et al., 1999; PAHO, 2008; Williams et al., 1994), there continues to be a gap between policies for gender equality in health and actual implementation. The emphasis, thus far, has been on getting gender equality on the policy agenda and less so on developing sustainable mechanisms – including political and financial commitment – required to put these policies into action through effective implementation once they are on the agenda. Monitoring and evaluation processes rarely reflect a gender perspective. There is a predominant focus on incorporating gender considerations into the situation analysis phase of health planning (or country profiles for policy development) while scaling up specific activities to address the problems has tended to be piecemeal. As mentioned at the outset, addressing gender equality in health policy planning requires both technical expertise and political commitment. This is a particular challenge as often one or both of these are missing. Some proposals which could help move things forwards include the following:

- *Increase capacity of policy planners to carry out gender analysis and develop appropriate interventions to respond to the issues identified in ways that are sustainable*

Understanding how gender socialization and gender inequality impact on women and men's vulnerability to different risks, access to heath information and services, ability to protect themselves from ill-health and to exercise their rights fully, and on health outcomes, is a necessary step to addressing these issues in policy. It is therefore critical to build capacity for this among health policy-makers and planners. This includes strategies to integrate this into the basic education of public health professionals, and into in-service training and continuing-education programmes. This will enable minimum element 1 – using gender analysis when reviewing evidence for health policies – to be undertaken more systematically.

- *Establish mechanisms for meaningful participation of women and men in health planning and programme implementation*

As shown by the example in Box 2.3 from Kenya it is possible to engage multiple stakeholders in policy design in a meaningful way when the conditions are there. The Gender and Health Equity Network (GHEN) supported some interesting experiences that sought to involve women in decisions related to the organization and delivery of services. One of them in China (Jing et al., 2008) explored approaches to increasing women's participation in local health planning so as to enhance the responsiveness and accountability of health facilities to women's needs and thus lead to the improvement of gender equality and health equity. It found that while there was potential to increase women's participation in local health planning this would require substantial institutional transformation of the All-China Women's Federation. George (2003) documented how for participatory processes for improving sexual and reproductive health service delivery to lead to change requires the broad participation of users, taking into account the social contexts and policy and delivery systems, addressing power relations, and improving the representation of marginalized groups within communities and service delivery systems.

• *Adequately resource implementation frameworks*

Commitments to gender equality must trickle down to policy implementation frameworks (such as strategies or plans), monitoring and evaluation activities in order to address the multiple objectives of gender mainstreaming. For this to occur, political will and commitments to posit gender equality at the centre of international health policy agendas are required. However, this is not enough. In order to reduce gender-based health inequities, resources (human, technical and financial) are required to ensure proper implementation. Budgetary allocations should ensure provision for capacity-building, implementation activities and dedicated, trained human resources, at least in the initial stages, to identify the specific actions required and ensure monitoring and follow-up.

• *Establish monitoring and evaluation mechanisms for institutional oversight*

In very basic terms, what gets measured gets done. If gender equality is not woven into policy monitoring and evaluation systems, it is likely to be downgraded to a lower priority. Indicators used for monitoring must go beyond mere counting where women and men are in policy planning and outcomes to capture measures of substantive equality. When monitoring is limited to formal measures of equality alone, the challenges raised above ensue.

• *Initiate operations research to assess different modes of implementation and integration of gender equality into specific health programmes*

It is necessary to build up a convincing body of evidence of how best to ensure the gains from gender equality programming in health. This should contribute to lowering the resistance encountered and to making the case for more budget allocation.

The integration of gender equality perspectives into health policies and programmes should ultimately lead to better outcomes for women and men of different groups as a first priority – as well as towards more equitable, effective health programmes, services and policies.

Summary

• Addressing gender equality in health policy planning requires both technical expertise and political commitment.
• Broader policy frameworks can either enable or hinder the promotion of gender equality. Anti-poverty, equality and empowerment policy approaches are those best suited for work on gender equality in health policy planning.

- If gender equality is absent from policy monitoring and evaluation systems, it is likely to be downgraded to second-degree priority and have less tangible outcomes on health status and policy-planning processes.
- It is necessary to build up a convincing body of evidence of how best to ensure the gains from gender equality programming in health.
- Gender mainstreaming, if rendered apolitical (or de-politicized), remains limited in its scope to promote and achieve gender equality.
- The integration of gender equality perspectives into health policies and programmes should ultimately lead to better outcomes for women and men as well as towards more equitable, effective health programmes, services and policies.

Key reading

AIDS Support and Technical Assistance Resources Project, USAID (2009) *Integrating Gender Strategies to Improve HIV and AIDS Interventions: A Compendium of Programs in Africa* (Washington, DC: International Centre for Research on Women).

Sen, G., A. George and P. Östlin (eds) (2002) *Engendering International Health: The Challenge of Equity* (Cambridge, MA: MIT Press).

Sen, G., A. George and P. Östlin (2007) *Unequal, Unfair, Ineffective and Inefficient: Gender Inequity in Health. Why It Exists and How We Can Change It,* Final report to the WHO Commission on Social Determinants of Health, at: www.who.int/social_determinants/ resources/csdh_media/wgekn_final_report_07.pdf, accessed 6 March 2009.

Note

*These are the views of the authors and do not reflect official policy of the World Health Organization.

References

Ashburn, K., N. Oomman, D. Wendt and S. Rozenzweig (2009) *Moving beyond Gender as Usual* (Washington, DC: Center for Global Development).

Bloom, G. and H. Standing (2008) 'Introduction – Future Health Systems: Why Future? Why Now?', *Social Science & Medicine,* 66, 2067–75.

Chibber, K. S., R. L. Kaplan, N. S. Padian, S. J. Anderson, P. M. Ling, N. Acharya, C. Van Dyke and S. Krishnan (2008) 'A Common Pathway toward Women's Health', *Global Public Health,* 3 (1), 26–38.

Daly, M. (2005) 'Gender Mainstreaming in Theory and Practice', *Social Politics, International Studies in Gender, State & Society,* 12 (3), 433–50.

Donner, L. (2003) *Including Gender in Health Planning: A Guide for Regional Health Authorities* (Winnipeg: Prairie Women's Health Centre of Excellence).

Ehrhardt, A. A., S. Sawires, T. McGovern, D. Peacock and M. Weston (2009) 'Gender, Empowerment and Health: What Is It? How Does It Work?', *Journal of Acquired Immune Deficiency Syndrome,* 51 (Suppl 3), S96–S105.

Fathalla, M. (2008) *Issues in Women's Health and Rights: International, Arab Regional and Egyptian Perspectives* (Cairo: International Planned Parenthood Federation, Arab World Region).

García-Moreno, C., H. Jansen, M. Ellsberg, L. Heise and C. Watts (2005) *WHO Multi-country Study on Women's Health and Domestic Violence against Women* (Geneva: World Health Organization).

Gender and Health Group, Liverpool School of Tropical Medicine (2008) *Gender and Health Guidelines*, at: www.liv.ac.uk/lstm/groups/gender_health/index.htm, accessed 14 January 2009.

Gender and HIV/AIDS Technical Sub Committee, National AIDS Control Council, Kenya (2002) *Mainstreaming Gender into the Kenya National HIV/AIDS Strategic Plan: 2000–2005* (Kenya: National AIDS Control Council).

George, A. (2003) 'Using Accountability to Improve Reproductive Health Care', *Reproductive Health Matters*, 11 (21), 161–70

George, A. (2008) 'Nurses, Community Health Workers, and Home Carers: Gendered Human Resources Compensating for Skewed Health Systems', *Global Public Health*, 3 (S1), 75–89.

Grown, C., G. R. Gupta and A. Kes (2005) *Taking Action: Achieving Gender Equality and Empowering Women*, UN Millennium Project, Task Force on Education and Gender Equality (London: Earthscan).

Gwatkin, D. R., A. Bhuiya and C. G. Victora (2004) 'Making Health Systems More Equitable', *The Lancet*, 364, 1273–80.

Heise, L. and C. García-Moreno (2002) 'Violence against Intimate Partners', in E. Krug, L. Dahlberg, J. Mercy, A. B. Zwi and R. Lozano (eds), *World Report on Violence and Health* (Geneva: World Health Organization), 89–121.

Horne, T., L. Donner and W. E. Thurston (1999) *Invisible Women: Gender and Health Planning in Manitoba and Saskatchewan and Models for Progress* (Winnipeg: Prairie Women's Health Centre of Excellence).

IPPF – International Planned Parenthood Federation (2005) *Models of Care Project: Linking HIV/AIDS Treatment, Care and Support in Sexual and Reproductive Health Care Settings* (London: IPPF).

Jing, F., J. Kaufman and L. Yunguo (2008) *Health Service Planning and Women's Organisations in Poor Rural China: The Case of Dafang County, Guizhou Province*, GHEN Working Paper No. 1 (Sussex: IDS).

Krug, E., L. Dahlberg, J. Mercy, A. B. Zwi and R. Lozano (eds) *World Report on Violence and Health* (Geneva: World Health Organization).

March, C., I. Smyth and M. Mukhopadhyay (1999) *A Guide to Gender-Analysis Frameworks* (London: Oxfam GB).

Moser, C. (1993) *Gender Planning and Development: Theory, Practice and Training* (London: Routledge).

Mukhopadhyay, M. (2006) 'Mainstreaming Gender or "Streaming" Gender Away: Feminists Marooned in the Development Business', *IDS Bulletin*, 35 (4), 95–103.

Nanda, P. (2002) 'Gender Dimensions of User Fees: Implications for Women's Utilization of Health Care', *Reproductive Health Matters*, 10 (20), 127–34.

Onyango-Ouma, W., R. Laisser, M. Mbilima, M. Araoye, P. Pittman, I. Agyepong, M. Zakari, S. Fonn et al. (2001) 'An Evaluation of "Health Workers For Change" in Seven Settings: A Useful Management and Health System Development Tool', *Health Policy and Planning*, 16 (Suppl. 1), 24–32.

PAHO – Pan American Health Organization (1997) *Workshop on Gender, Health and Development: Facilitator's Guide* (Washington, DC: PAHO).

PAHO – Pan American Health Organization (2008) *Guide for Analysis and Monitoring of Gender Equity in Health Policies* (Washington, DC: PAHO).

Ravindran, T. K. S. and A. Kelkar-Khambete (2008) 'Gender Mainstreaming in Health: Looking Back, Looking Forward', *Global Public Health*, 3 (S1), 121–42.

Ribeiro, P. S., K. Jacobsen, C. D. Mathers and C. García-Moreno (2008) 'Priorities for Women's Health from the Global Burden of Disease Study', *International Journal of Gynecology and Obstetrics*, 102 (1), 82–90.

Sen, G., A. George and P. Östlin (eds) (2002) *Engendering International Health: The Challenge of Equity* (Cambridge, MA: MIT Press).

Sen, G., A. George and P. Östlin (2007) *Unequal, Unfair, Ineffective and Inefficient: Gender Inequity in Health. Why It Exists and How We Can Change It*, Final Report to the WHO Commission on Social Determinants of Health, at: www.who.int/social_determinants/resources/csdh_media/wgekn_final_report_07.pdf, accessed 6 March 2009.

Siddiqi, S., T. I. Masud, S. Nishtar, D. H. Peters, B. Sabri, K. M. Bile and M. A. Jama (2009) 'Framework for Assessing Governance of the Health System In Developing Countries: Gateway to Good Governance', *Health Policy*, 90 (1), 13–25.

Standing, H. (2000) 'Gender – A Missing Dimension in Human Resource Policy and Planning for Health Reforms', *Human Resources for Health Development Journal*, 4 (1), 27–42.

Taylor, V. (1999) *Gender Mainstreaming in Development Planning: A Reference Manual for Governments and Other Stakeholders* (London: Commonwealth Secretariat).

Theobald, S., R. Tolhurst and H. Elsey (2002) 'Introductory Comments: The Background and Structure of the Resource Pack', in S. Theobald, R. Tolhurst and H. Elsey (eds), *Papers Presented at 'Sector Wide Approaches: Opportunities and Challenges for Gender Equity in Health* (London: Gender and Health Group, Liverpool School of Tropical Medicine), 1–9.

UNAIDS (2006) *Greater Involvement of People Living with or Affected by HIV/AIDS (GIPA)* (Geneva: UNAIDS).

UN – United Nations (1995) *Beijing Declaration and Platform for Action*, A/CONF.177/20, at: www.un.org/esa/gopher-data/conf/fwcw/off/a-20.en, accessed 9 May 2009.

Vlassof, C. and S. Fonn (2001) 'Health Workers for Change as a Health Systems Management and Development Tool', *Health Policy and Planning*, 16 (Supplement 1), 47–52.

Walby, S. (2005) 'Gender Mainstreaming: Productive Tensions in Theory and Practice', *Social Politics: International Studies in Gender, State & Society*, 12 (3), 321–43.

Williams, S., J. Seed and A. Mwau (1994) *The Oxfam Gender Training Manual* (Oxford: Oxfam UK and Ireland).

Wilson, M. and M. Daly (1994) 'Spousal Homicide', *Juristat Service Bulletin*, 14, 1–15.

WHO – World Health Organization (2001) *Transforming Health Systems: Gender and Rights in Reproductive Health* (Geneva: World Health Organization).

WHO – World Health Organization (2006) *The Global Shortage of Health Workers and Its Impact*, Fact Sheet No. 302 (Geneva: World Health Organization).

WHO – World Health Organization (2007) *Engaging Men and Boys to End Gender Inequity in Health* (Geneva: World Health Organization).

WHO – World Health Organization (2009) *Integrating Gender into HIV/AIDS Programmes in the Health Sector: Tool to Improve Responsiveness to Women's Needs* (Geneva: World Health Organization), at: www.who.int/gender/documents/gender_hiv_guidelines_en.pdf, accessed 24 September 2009.

WHO EMRO – WHO Regional Office for the Eastern Mediterranean (2009) *Community Based Initiatives*, at: www.emro.who.int/cbi/cbi_introduction.htm, accessed 23 August 2009.

3
Gender Equity and Health Sector Reforms in Low and Middle-income Countries

Hilary Standing

Introduction

Health sector reforms have been taking place in rich and poor countries alike at an accelerating pace over the last two decades. While some common themes can be discerned, such as responding to changing population needs and managing the rising costs of healthcare, a range of drivers underlies health sector reform (HSR) policies and approaches in different places and times. The gender implications of HSR did not, however, receive much attention until relatively recently. This chapter discusses some key narratives of HSR in low and middle-income countries, where the pressures to reform and the challenges faced have been particularly intense. After considering definitions and concepts, it outlines major strands of HSR, contextualizing them in relation to different regional experiences. It then discusses the gender issues that they have raised, using illustrations from different country settings. It concludes by reflecting on the gaps and omissions in HSR programmes from a gender perspective and notes other international development initiatives that have come to the fore in the past decade and influenced thinking about healthcare, bringing more aware-ness of gender issues and implications and contributing to changing the terms of the debate about gender and health systems development.

Definitions and concepts: gender equity and health sector reform

The ubiquitousness of gender inequities in health has been highlighted by a large body of research (Doyal, 1995; Sen et al., 2002; 2007). Gender is one of the profound markers of difference in epidemiology, health status, health behaviours, health risks and vulnerabilities and access to and use of health resources. First, biological and genetic endowments and social relations come together to create gendered health needs from health conditions which may be specific to women and men, or affect women and men differently. Second, the social relations of gender create cultural and societal biases such as unequal access to treatment and care. They underlie structural biases, such as unequal entitlements stemming from disadvantages in the labour market. Third, health-care production has a strong gender aspect. The health workforce is very gender-differentiated, with segments, such as nursing, often specific to one gender, and high levels of gender stratification by occupational category (see Chapter 28 by Wrede). Women tend to be the unpaid care workforce in households. Gender also interacts with other economic and social determinants such as poverty, class, age, sexual orientation and race in creating and maintaining inequities across these dimensions (Doyal, 1998; see also Chapter 1 by Payne and Doyal).

Biases and inequities affecting women and girls are located at the level of households and family relationships, communities, health facilities and also in the processes and institutions which determine policies, resource allocations and decision-making. While the precise nature of these is contextually variable, their existence is pervasive and rooted in the ideologies and power relations of gendered social systems (Sen et al., 2007). These social relations can also produce and replicate inequities which adversely affect men. For example, male-specific occupational health risks and socially approved and encouraged forms of masculinity producing greater risk-taking behaviours can lead to higher levels of avoidable morbidity and mortality (Greig et al., 2000; Meryn, 2007).

The health sectors of most countries have been undergoing change, particularly over the past few decades, so trying to define HSR can be like hitting a moving target (Standing, 2002a). One generic definition is provided by Berman and Bossert:

> Health sector reform can be defined as 'strategic, purposeful change' – strategic in the sense of addressing significant, fundamental dimensions of health systems; purposeful in the sense of having a rational, planned basis – to improve health system performance in terms of well-defined outcomes. (2000: 2)

This definition is used to distinguish between what they describe as purposive attempts to improve health sector functioning, whether through large or small policy changes; and broader health systems change stemming from larger economic and political pressures on a particular country or region. However, this is not a sustainable distinction. In practice, it is impossible to abstract reforms from their context: most of the impetus towards HSR in low and middle-income countries – and the ensuing debate about outcomes – has come precisely from these larger pressures.

This is particularly clear from the way the language of health sector reform, as expressed by international agencies and some governments, changed over the decade from the early 1990s when the 'first generation' of reforms began. These were overwhelmingly supply-side driven in the sense that reform agendas focused on a set of technical and institutional changes to the architecture of the health sector. These included improving management systems, more efficient human resources use, reforming financing mechanisms, introducing cost control measures and cost effectiveness approaches and working more closely with private actors (Cassels, 2006).

Various forms of decentralization of management, resources and financing were also a prominent policy prescription during this decade. These reform attempts had mixed results. For example, during the period 1994 to 1998, a consortium of ten international donors, including the World Bank, United Nations (UN) agencies and several bilateral (country) donors, financed a major health sector reform programme by the Government of Zambia using a blueprint approach of introduction of user fees, decentralization of management and introduction of an essential service package. The period over which this took place saw a *worsening* in a number of key health indicators such as the Infant Mortality Rate (IMR), yet so great was the commitment to the blueprint that most of these donors regarded the programme as successful until very late in the process (Simms, 2000). Clearly, 'success' depended on what was being measured. In this era, change was focused on technical and managerial reforms to improve the functions of government bureaucracies. The impact on and outcomes of service delivery were neglected and the voices of users were silent (Standing, 2000).

By the end of the 1990s, language and approaches had shifted somewhat as the failure of reforms in a number of poor countries to deliver any obvious improvements to health sector performance was becoming apparent. Other international initiatives, such as the health-focused Millennium Development Goals (MDGs) which have clear targets for improvements in maternal and child health and priority diseases, as well as in gender equality (UNDP, n.d.) gained prominence in policy and financing (see also Chapter 2 by Abdool et al.). From another perspective, widening gaps between rich and poor in health status and healthcare access (for example in China and other Asian countries) also raised serious questions about the content and direction of reforms. A more nuanced approach to the complexities of reforming health systems began to emerge, with greater emphasis on linking reforms to broader national anti-poverty and social protection strategies, involvement of a wider range of actors, particularly from civil society, in planning, delivery and monitoring of services, and renewed debate about the role and capacities of governments in safeguarding the health of their citizens. At the same time, there was a further shift towards vertical approaches to programmes, with the movement of large amounts of funding into HIV and AIDS prevention and treatment and other disease-specific programmes. Neither approach necessarily took gender equity issues into consideration.

In this chapter, HSR is understood not just as a technocratic planning activity but as a social process that is embedded in the larger macroeconomic and political shifts which have taken place over the past two decades. This way of conceptualizing HSR encompasses the effect of health sector reforms on gender equity (Standing, 2002a). As will be noted, despite the changing discourses on HSR and a substantial body of evidence on the significance of gender in the production of health inequities, gender issues have often struggled to surface in the various manifestations of reforms in different times and places.

What are the links between health sector reforms and gender equity?

The concept of health sector reform (HSR) has different meanings in different national and regional contexts. Many of the financial and political drivers for HSR are the same but the degree of national ownership varies and the reform options adopted differ from country to country and region to region. For instance, HSR has a different 'flavour' in Latin America than in sub-Saharan Africa. This reflects partly the objectively different conditions in the two continents, and partly the extent to which HSR has been driven by international donor agencies such as the World Bank and European bilateral aid agencies seeking to finance reforms according to often predetermined scripts about cost-effective and efficient health systems (Gómez Gómez, 2000). This means that the issues raised for gender equity are not the same in all contexts.

Three perspectives provide useful and complementary ways of linking gender and health issues to HSR. In an early attempt to characterize the links, Standing (1997) distinguished between a *women's health needs approach* and a *gender equity approach*. The former focuses on women-specific health needs, particularly reproductive healthcare needs. In the context of HSR, this approach allows us to ask questions such as: 'How well do health systems respond to women's health needs?'; or 'Does HSR improve or worsen the responsiveness of health systems to these needs?' A gender equity approach is concerned more centrally with gendered power relations and the processes by which they produce and reproduce inequalities in access to health status, outcomes and resources (see, for example, Sen et al., 2002). This approach allows us to ask questions about whether health status, outcomes and resources are distributed differentially between women and men, how and why they are distributed in those ways and how HSR affects these relations of distribution.

Mackintosh and Tibandebage (2006) add a third perspective which they characterize as *applying a gender lens to institutions and institutional processes*. This prompts questions about the assumptions underlying institutional policy and practice. For instance, what assumptions are made about women's position as dependents or as earners in households and how do these get reflected in financing policy? Is there an unstated assumption that women are available to care for sick people in the household and that this care capacity has infinite flexibility? As they note, health systems are not neutral to gender but express the gender hierarchies and historical biases of the societies within which they have developed. Attempts to reform them may therefore reflect or reinforce them as well as challenge them.

These three perspectives are all helpful in examining HSR gender impacts. In the following sections, they are used to explore how examples and experiences of HSR from different regions and times raise different issues for gender and health equity.

Sub-Saharan African countries under 'first generation' HSR

The term health sector reform (HSR) is perhaps most associated with a set of policy prescriptions that were concentrated in low and middle-income countries during the late 1980s to the early 1990s and focused on the institutional and financial reforms described earlier as 'first generation' HSR. In low-income countries of sub-Saharan Africa and South Asia, HSR has been strongly driven by external agencies, particularly multilateral agencies such as the World Bank and the European Union and bilateral donors such as the UK that have provided substantial aid to the health sectors of developing countries. The 1980s were a crisis decade for the social sectors in these countries. Their economies were experiencing severe turbulence and governments were increasingly unable to deliver on their commitments to maintain or expand the basic services that had been built up. In many countries, public services came close to collapse, resulting in health facilities emptied of drugs and equipment and health workers unable to live on their devalued wages and increasingly selling their services in a developing informalized healthcare market.

During this period, countries needing loans from the International Monetary Fund (IMF) to address their fiscal crises and stabilize their economies and currencies were required to adopt structural adjustment programmes (SAPs) as a condition of support. The SAPs of this period reflected the prevailing neoliberal orthodoxy in global macroeconomic policy. This was based on implementing free-market solutions to the fiscal crises engulfing countries, particularly privatization, deregulation and the removal of trade barriers, and the reining in of government expenditure to reduce the size of government. In some cases, this entailed reductions in social sector expenditure (Stewart, 1995). Structural adjustment processes are one of the important drivers of HSR programmes in these countries.

The other major driver of HSR was a set of policy prescriptions for institutional reforms to what were seen as generic failures in public sector performance in many countries (see, for example, Berman, 1993; Cassels, 1995). As Standing (2002a) notes, the need for institutional reform was addressed to a different but related agenda that was also donor-driven, namely improving governance by creating more efficient, accountable bodies and redefining the relationships between the state, service providers and users. Increasingly during this decade the institutional reform agenda came to be addressed through a different aid instrument: the Sector Wide Approach (SWAp). This sought to break away from the proliferation of often poorly coordinated donor-funded projects and harmonize external resources to a collaborative financing framework negotiated with national ministries of health and finance, with agreed institutional reforms to health sector functioning (Cassels, 1997).

Concern about gender impacts arose in the context of a lack of acknowledgement of the gendered dimensions of HSR prescriptions and strategies, for instance, the fact that poor women are major users of publicly provided services, that the health sector workforce is highly gendered in terms of occupations and levels of seniority, and that women provide the main informal care work in households. This led to a body of work that particularly explored the gender equity aspects of policy and programme approaches to HSR (Doyal, 2003; Evers and Juarez, 2003; Mackintosh and Tibandebage, 2006; Standing, 1997; 2000; 2002a; 2002b).

Mackintosh and Tibandebage (2006) characterize the approach to HSR during the 1990s as a shift to greater commodification of healthcare, where services became increasingly provided through market payment mechanisms, particularly private out-of-pocket expenditure, with government-subsidized packages of essential care based on cost-effectiveness criteria. It also signalled the shift at that time in dominant views of the role of government (World Development Report, 1993) manifest, for instance, in an emphasis on the contracting-out of services to independent providers. What is striking about this period of HSR is how profound the gender impacts may have been and yet how inadequate is the evidence base for understanding them. Both Standing (1997) and Mackintosh and Tibandebage (2006) hypothesize a range of likely impacts but lament the lack of research on many of them. For instance, we have only very patchy information on the gender-differentiated effects of any changes to health worker terms and conditions and job grading, so it is difficult to reach any conclusions about whether and in what ways HSR either adversely affected women health workers or improved their situation.

The actual impacts, both immediate and long-term, of first generation HSR programmes in sub-Saharan Africa have been most documented in relation to changes in health financing options, particularly the introduction of user charges for government health services, diagnostic tests and drugs, which still remain in place in many of these countries. Women and children are by far the largest users of basic healthcare (PHC) services in poor countries. This is because these services are heavily weighted towards provision of preventive and curative services for maternal and child health. Informal payments have been increasingly a feature of public sector provision as health staff try to make up for inadequate wages, or request users to buy drugs and equipment in the market as there are none in the facilities. It is therefore possible that introducing transparent charges would decrease costs for these services – although there is no indication that gender was taken into account when user charges were introduced. However, it is also possible that they would disadvantage women due to women's often greater struggle to obtain cash for personal expenses, including medical purposes.

Some evidence suggests that user charges have had a disproportionate impact on women since their introduction from the mid-1980s to the early 1990s. In particular, they were associated with reduced use of maternal health services (Ekwempu et al., 1990; Kutzin, 1995; Standing, 2002a; see Box 3.1).

Other forms of financing encouraged under HSR during this period of first generation reforms, and subsequently, included community-based financing mechanisms such as local risk-pooling for social insurance, and private insurance for formal-sector workers. Again, the evidence on their gender impacts is limited. But, as Mackintosh and Tibandebage (2006) note, attempts to change financing mechanisms tended to rely on assumptions about capacity to access income within or outside the household that did not differentiate between women and men. Yet there is considerable evidence that women are often disadvantaged in terms of access. For instance, they are less likely to hold formal-sector jobs, or they may need to gain access to cash or income through

Box 3.1 Gender impact of user charges under HSR in sub-Saharan Africa

A study in Nigeria found that between 1983 and 1988, when fees were introduced, maternal deaths in the Zaria region increased by 56 per cent. This was associated with a decline of 46 per cent in the number of deliveries in the main hospital and a threefold increase in obstetric complications. The interval between admission and surgery increased significantly as relatives had to go and search for money (Ekwempu et al., 1990).

There were similar findings from Zimbabwe (Kutzin, 1995) where the greater enforcement of user charges in the early 1990s was followed by a decline of 30 per cent in the use of maternal and child health (MCH) services, and the number of babies born before their mothers reached hospital increased by four per cent. In Nairobi, the introduction of user fees at a Nairobi sexually transmitted infections clinic resulted in a fall, over nine months, of 56 per cent in attendance by women and a 40 per cent decrease for men (results for 2004, quoted in Mackintosh and Tibandabage, 2006).

husbands or other household members. These constraints limit full participation in such schemes.

In conclusion, accounts of the impacts of first generation HSR on gender equity in sub-Saharan Africa generally emphasize their actual or likely negative effects in a context of almost no attention given by policy-makers to possible gender impacts and little information on outcomes. This is now compared with the experience of HSR in Latin America.

Latin America: a stronger focus on gender equity?

From the early 1990s onwards, most countries in the Latin American region had started reforms of their health and social security systems. Some of the drivers are similar in that the 1990s was a period of considerable economic instability in this region and responses to macroeconomic crisis were governed by the prevailing neoliberal economic consensus of the multilateral agencies described above. Several commentators also note that the similarities in trends in HSR across regions reflect a globalized approach to restructuring social policy (Ewig, 2006; Flores, 2006; Gómez Gómez, 2000), as economic liberalization and privatization were extended to areas such as health. In this region, health sector reforms have been concentrated in three areas of institutional change: decentralization to subnational governments and entities; reform of social security systems, particularly through private financing arrangements to expand health insurance; and improving service delivery through diversification of providers and, in some places, development of essential-services packages (Gómez Gómez, 2000). However, while critical of neoliberalism and its general consequences for gender equity, commentary and debate about HSR have also noted HSR's potential for improving access to healthcare. Latin America has historically very high levels of social, economic, gender and other inequalities, which are reflected in serious health inequalities. Reforms have been seen as central to addressing these inequalities (see Box 3.2).

There are other important differences from the situation in many countries of sub-Saharan Africa. National ownership of reforms has been stronger as – although influenced by them – they have not been driven mainly by external agencies. They have been taking place in the context of relatively strong states and with a higher level of national debate and involvement of civil society. Various political traditions of solidarity in some countries such as Costa Rica and Brazil have produced more emphasis on negotiating citizen participation. Most importantly, the women's movement has been an extremely strong advocate for health and gender equity across the region. Women have fought for progressive legislation and programmes on women's health, particularly in the area of sexual and reproductive health, and have taken on controversial issues such as access to safe abortion services (see for example, Jaquette, 1994; Soares and Sardenberg, 2008). The Pan American Health Organization (PAHO)

Box 3.2 Latin America: Opening up spaces for integrating gender into HSR

In relation to gender equity, women's advocacy organizations and health activists have influenced and monitored reforms in a number of key reforming countries over the last decade, including Chile, Mexico and Peru (Ewig, 2008; Langer and Catino, 2006). Despite this history of engagement, the evidence base on the extent to which gender equity measures have been incorporated into reform programmes and adverse impacts have been avoided is uneven. However, studies undertaken so far indicate a range of outcomes. In the context of a discussion of HSR in Peru, Ewig (2008) considers the general impact in Latin America of HSR based on neoliberal reforms. She notes that these have been seen to be detrimental to women's interests as they have had both negative distributional effects and have particularly ignored women's role in social reproduction. But she argues that in Peru they nevertheless opened up space for more positive outcomes through a decentralization process that recognized some of women's specific health needs and leadership roles.

For Mexico, Langer and Catino (2006) give an upbeat assessment of the progress of recent reforms. Mexico's HSR programme, including a restructured health insurance scheme (*Seguro Popular*) is specifically addressing women's health needs and increasing coverage to poor women. It is also, and unusually, seeking to address the more hidden forms of discrimination and exclusion through integrating a gender perspective into all aspects of the reforms, using a national centre focused on gender equity.

includes social participation as one of its guiding criteria for technical support and its Women, Health and Development Program has been very influential in raising the profile of gender equity in the region in the context of HSR (Gómez Gómez, 2000). These differences have contributed to greater public engagement in the enactment of reforms than in countries where they have been imposed externally.

The gender impacts of HSR in Colombia have been analysed by Ewig and Bello (2009), using secondary data from different national surveys at different time periods. They ask three key questions about gender equity in the context of HSR. Have the reforms increased financial equity in healthcare costs between women and men? Does the health system respond to women's health needs? Do the new policies create or reinforce inequalities in the benefits offered to women and men?

Colombia's health reforms, which began in the early 1990s, have generally been considered progressive, and resulted in Colombia receiving a high ranking in a quality assessment of the world's health systems (WHO, 2000) for increasing universal coverage and equity. The reforms took place in the context of a new, inclusionary Constitution in 1991 which laid down a universal right to social security. It also followed a decade of women's activism which had made considerable gains in the sphere of family and workplace rights, in institutionalizing gender mainstreaming in the policy arena, and in getting women's reproductive health needs addressed in policy and planning (Beall, 1998).

The health reforms replaced a segmented system in which the richest 10 per cent were served by the private sector, less than half of the formal sector workforce were covered by national social security, and public services were in practice expensive and inaccessible to the poor and those living in remote areas (Ewig and Bello, 2009). In its place, a universal coverage system for health social security was created. This provided a package of guaranteed services through individual insurance in a managed market where consumers could choose between different providers. It provided subsidized benefits for the poor. It was thus a 'mixed' system combining a state-regulated system committed to universal principles with elements of market-based provision. Nonetheless, universality has remained a commitment rather than a reality, as continuing economic weakness constrained the state's capacity to accomplish the full transformation. A degree of segmentation continued after the reforms, with two different sets of insurers and insurance regimes serving contributory and state-subsidized beneficiaries respectively and with a hierarchy of benefits among the subsidized groups depending on their socio-economic status. Some of the poor still remain outside the insurance system and depend on existing public provision.

Returning to the questions posed by Ewig and Bello (2009), have the reforms increased financial equity in healthcare costs between women and men? They suggest that the reforms had potential to improve financial gender equity in Colombia in three ways. First, dependents were provided with complete health insurance. This is beneficial to the large number of women working in the informal sector who do not have access to the contributory regime in their own right. The reforms significantly increased coverage for both men and women but even more for women. In 2003, 66 per cent of men and 71 per cent of women were covered by either the contributory or the subsidized scheme. Second, the system is a risk-pooling one where all workers pay the same salary percentage. For women this mitigates their reproductive health risk which very importantly becomes a shared societal responsibility. Third, the subsidized scheme for those unable to pay into the contributory scheme gives priority to vulnerable groups, including pregnant women and women-headed households who, in 2003, constituted over 30 per cent of households. In terms of the value of healthcare benefits, the reforms have most benefited those in the subsidized scheme. Despite these gender gains, out-of-pocket health expenditure for non-subsidized services – though much reduced – remains a greater burden for women due to their higher use of services.

The next question posed by Ewig and Bello (2009) related to whether the reformed health system responds to women's health needs. Despite the principle of universality, there are significant differences between what is covered under the contributory and subsidized schemes and in the quality of care offered. These have emerged as a result of the unequal capitalization of the insurance funds. This has opened up a gap between better-off and poorer women, particularly in reproductive healthcare. One important indicator is that, between 1998 to 2006, maternal mortality among women under the subsidized scheme was twice as high as among those under the contributory scheme.

The final question posed by Ewig and Bello (2009) was whether the new policies create or reinforce inequalities between women and men in the benefits offered. Here, they note that women are concentrated more in the subsidized scheme with its inferior coverage and quality and that some groups of women, such as Afro-descendents and displaced women, are particularly likely to lack coverage. This points to a more complex stratification than gender on its own. Running through the narrative of continuing inequalities in Colombia is the stratification of poverty and its complex linkages with gender and race. A more nuanced analysis remains to be done which would include how the reforms have affected inequalities between poor men and non-poor women.

Conclusion

This section reflects on lessons from the regional experiences of HSR and considers the gaps and disconnections in the changing relationship between HSR and gender equity. The experiences of sub-Saharan Africa and Latin America show both similarities and differences in the forces driving the reforms and in the way the reforms have played out in relation to gender equity concerns. The experience of much of sub-Saharan Africa under the first generation externally driven reforms of the mid-1980s to the early 1990s is generally one of complete gender invisibility. Except in South Africa, where a new political dispensation facilitated an explicitly rights-based concept of reform in all sectors, the question was simply not raised. This has meant that information on gender impacts has been generally hard to find, but such data that exist, such as on financial regimes, have led to negative assessments of impact. In Latin America, a more complex picture emerges. Despite similarities in the macroeconomic drivers and general direction of reforms, there are positive narratives. Salient here is the role of strong women's movements in driving demands for programmes addressing women's health needs. In both sub-Saharan Africa and Latin America the intersections between poverty, gender and other markers of inequality emerge starkly and are a reminder of the importance of not seeing women and men as homogeneous groups in terms of policy impacts.

From a gender perspective, looking back at the reforms of the late 1980s to early 1990s, a striking feature has been the disconnection between the dominant discourses and practices of HSR and those of rights and gender mainstreaming that dominated gender and health advocacy (Standing, 2002b). Yet this is also the decade of the Cairo agenda – the commitments from the International Conference on Population and Development (1994) which many governments signed up to and which laid out a comprehensive agenda on reproductive health and gender equity. These commitments were further underscored by the 'Platform for Action' of the Fourth World Conference on Women in Beijing in 1995. This also called for UN commitment to gender mainstreaming to institutionalize analysis of the gender impacts of policies, a call which was formally ratified by UN member states (Hafner-Burton and Pollack, 2002; see also Chapter 2 by Abdool et al.). Rights-based approaches underlay most of the health activism and were increasingly adopted by agencies working in health programming at the time. However, there has been little reflection of these in national reforms until recently (Ijeoma, 2006; Langer and Catino, 2006).

Common across regions was the way in which these progressive initiatives seemingly went on either above or below the radar of HSR. Arguing that health sector reform programmes largely marginalized the Cairo agenda, Standing (2002b) suggests that part of the reason lay in the weak links between reproductive health advocates and national and international actors in HSR. From an operational perspective, Berer (2002) argues that HSR undermined reproductive healthcare through disease-based prioritizing of public funding and disregard of evidence on the effectiveness of reproductive health interventions. More generally, even in Latin America, where women's health advocacy has been very strong, it did not necessarily influence the overall HSR process. Ewig and Bello (2009) note that, despite the high level of public engagement in the development of constitutional reform and a decade of gender activism in relation to healthcare, this activism did not connect with the HSR process in Colombia. However, one of the lessons of the reform experience is that universalism, though an essential basis for health equity, needs supplementing with measures to ensure that specific needs stemming from social and economic inequalities are addressed, and that indirect gender and other biases do not create further inequalities.

Nonetheless, some of the major international development initiatives of the past decade have brought greater prominence to gender and health equity issues and opened a larger space for local and international gender and health advocacy to influence debates and policies. Renewed effort to meet the health-related MDGs in poor countries, particularly Goal 5 to reduce maternal mortality, has refocused attention on maternal health (see also Chapter 23 by Sandall et al.). This in turn has led to an understanding that healthcare delivery systems have to be radically improved, if maternal mortality is to fall substantially (Freedman, 2003).

Gender and health equity has also figured prominently as the theme of one of the component reports of the World Health Organization's Social Determinants of Health Commission (Sen et al., 2007), providing a comprehensive analysis of the embeddedness of gender and power relations in the production, consumption and distribution of healthcare. Recent concern over the state of the world's health sector workforce, including lack of qualified staff and maldistribution of the workforce in poor countries, has brought recognition of the critical importance of gender in shaping all aspects of healthcare work (Joint Learning Initiative, 2004; Reichenbach, 2007; WHO, 2006). As with many aspects of gender and health equity, Reichenbach (2007) stresses how inadequate data availability limits the improvement of gender analysis in this area. Many countries do not have human resources data disaggregated by sex. Data insufficiency has been a recurring theme in the literature on gender and HSR. A number of initiatives have begun to address this gap (Standing, 2006). These include the extension of gender budgets to the health sector and the development of gender-sensitive health indicators (WHO Kobe Centre, 2003; see also Chapter 5 by Lin and L'Orange).

Summary

Major international development initiatives have facilitated a richer, more substantive debate about gender and health sector reforms over the past few years. In particular, both national and international gender advocacy is connecting more effectively to reform processes. There is also greater recognition of the complexity of gender-linked inequalities and the need to go beyond universalism to address the ways in which specific groups and individuals are disadvantaged. However, operationalizing insights from gender equity analysis at national and programme level remains a challenge. Key requirements for this include the following:

- strengthened national capacity to collect, analyse and use gender disaggregated data;
- adequately resourced institutional infrastructure for gender analysis, policy development and monitoring, such as gender units at national and subnational level;
- independent national and local 'informed advocacy' capacity to monitor gender impacts of reforms and encourage wider political debate about health inequalities.

Key reading

Doyal, L. (2003) *Gender and Health Sector Reform: A Literature Review and Report from a Workshop at Forum 7* (Geneva: Global Forum for Health Research), at: www.isn.ethz.ch/ isn/Digital-Library/Publications/Detail/?ots591=0C54E3B3-1E9C-BE1E-2C24-A6A8C70 60233&lng=en&id=47972, accessed 15 May 2009.

Evers, B. and M. Juárez (2003) *Understanding the Links: Globalization, Health Sector Reform, Gender and Reproductive Health* (New York: Ford Foundation).

Ewig, C. and A. H. Bello (2009) 'Gender Equity and Health Sector Reform in Colombia: Mixed State-Market Model Yields Mixed Results', *Social Science & Medicine*, 68 (6), 1145–52.

Standing, H. (2002) 'Frameworks for Understanding Health Sector Reform', in G. Sen, A. George and P. Östlin (eds), *Engendering International Health: The Challenge of Equity* (Cambridge, MA: MIT Press), 347–71.

Acknowledgement

I would like to thank Peroline Ainsworth for her assistance in locating references and materials for this article.

References

Beall, J. (1998) 'Trickle-down or Rising Tide? Lessons on Mainstreaming Gender Policy from Colombia and South Africa', *Social Policy and Administration*, 32 (5), 513–34.

Berer, M. (2002) 'Editorial. Health Sector Reforms: Implications for Sexual and Reproductive Health Services', *Reproductive Health Matters*, 10 (20), 6–15.

Berman, P. (1995) 'Health Sector Reform in Developing Countries: Making Health Development Sustainable', *Health Policy*, 32 (1–3), 13–28.

Berman, P. and T. Bossert (2000) *A Decade of Health Sector Reform in Developing Countries: What Have We Learned?* Paper prepared for the DDM Symposium 'Appraising a Decade of Health Sector Reform in Developing Countries', Washington, DC, 15 March 2000, International Health Systems Group, Harvard School of Public Health, at: http:// hsphsun3.harvard.edu/ihsg/publications/pdf/closeout.PDF, accessed 14 May 2009.

Cassels, A. (1995) *Health Sector Reform: Key Issues in Less Developed Countries*, WHO Forum on Health Sector Reform, Discussion Paper No. 1, SHS/NHP/95.4 (Geneva: World Health Organization).

Cassels, A. (1997) *A Guide to Sector-wide Approaches for Health Development. Concepts, Issues and Working Arrangements*, WHOIARAI97.12 (Geneva: World Health Organization).

Cassels, A. (2006) 'Health Sector Reform: Key Issues in Less Developed Countries', *Journal of International Development*, 7 (3), 329–47.

Doyal, L. (1995) *What Makes Women Sick – Gender and the Political Economy of Health* (Basingstoke: Macmillan).

Doyal, L. (1998) *Gender and Health: A Technical Document* (Geneva: World Health Organization).

Doyal, L. (2003) *Gender and Health Sector Reform: A Literature Review and Report from a Workshop at Forum 7* (Geneva: Global Forum for Health Research), at: www.isn.ethz. ch/isn/Digital-Library/Publications/Detail/?ots591=0C54E3B3-1E9C-BE1E-2C24-A6A8 C7060233&lng=en&id=47972, accessed 15 May 2009.

Ekwempu, C. C., D. Maine, M. B. Oloruka, E. S. Essien and M. N. Kisseka (1990) 'Structural Adjustment and Health in Africa, Letter to *The Lancet*', *The Lancet*, 336, 56–7.

Evers, B. and M. Juárez (2003) *Understanding the Links: Globalization, Health Sector Reform, Gender and Reproductive Health* (New York: Ford Foundation).

Ewig, C. (2006) 'Global Processes, Local Consequences: Gender Equity and Health Sector Reform in Peru', *Social Politics*, 13 (3), 427–55.

Freedman, L. (2003) 'Strategic Advocacy and Maternal Mortality: Moving Targets and the Millennium Development Goals', *Gender and Development*, 11 (1), 97–108.

Flores, W. (2006) *Equity and Health Sector Reform in Latin America and the Caribbean from 1995 to 2005: Approaches and Limitations*, Report commissioned by the International Society for Equity in Health, Chapter of the Americas, at: www.iseqh.org/docs/HSR_equity_report2006_en.pdf, accessed 22 October 2009.

Gómez Gómez, Elsa (2000) *Equity, Gender and Health Policy Reform in Latin America and the Caribbean Economic Commission for Latin America and the Caribbean*, paper presented at the VIII Regional Conference on Women in Latin America and the Caribbean, Lima, Peru, 8–10 February 2000 (Washington, DC: Pan American Health Organization, Women, Health and Development Program).

Greig, A., M. Kimmel and J. Lang (2000) 'Men, Masculinities and Development: Broadening Our Work Towards Gender Equality', *Gender in Development Monograph Series*, No. 10, United Nations Gender and Development Programme, at: www.health.columbia.edu/pdfs/men_masculinities.pdf, accessed 14 May 2009.

Hafner-Burton, E. and M. A. Pollack (2002) 'Mainstreaming Gender in Global Governance', *European Journal of International Relations*, 8 (3), 339–73.

Ijeoma, A. N. (2006) 'Viewpoint: Health Sector Reform in Nigeria: A Perspective on Human Rights and Gender Issues', *Local Environment*, 11 (1), 127–40.

Jaquette, J. (ed.) (1994) *The Women's Movement in Latin America: Participation and Democracy* (Boulder: Westview Press).

Joint Learning Initiative (2004) *Human Resources for Health. Overcoming the Crisis*, Global Health Equity Initiative (Cambridge, MA: Harvard University Press).

Kutzin, J. (1995) 'Experience with Organizational and Financing Reform of the Health Sector', *Current Concerns SHS Paper No. 8*, SHS/CC/94.3 (Geneva: World Health Organization).

Langer, A. and J. Catino (2006) 'A Gendered Look at Mexico's Health Sector Reform', *The Lancet*, 368 (9549), 1753–5.

Mackintosh, M. and P. Tibandebage (2006) 'Gender and Health Sector Reform: Analytical Perspectives on African Experience', in S. Razavi and S. Hassim (eds), *Gender and Social Policy in a Global Context: Uncovering the Gendered Structure of 'the Social'* (Basingstoke: Palgrave), 237–57.

Meryn, S. (2007) 'Editorial. Growing Global Focus on Men's Health', *Journal of Men's Health & Gender*, 4 (4), 382–5.

Reichenbach, L. (ed.) (2007) *Exploring the Gender Dimensions of the Global Health Workforce*, Global Equity Initiative (Cambridge, MA: Harvard University Press).

Soares, G. and C. Sardenberg (2008) 'Campaigning for the Right to Legal and Safe Abortion in Brazil', *IDS Bulletin*, 39 (3), 55–61.

Sen, G., A. George and P. Östlin (2002) *Engendering International Health: The Challenge of Equity* (Cambridge, MA: MIT Press).

Sen, G., P. Östlin and A. George (2007) *Unequal, Unfair, Ineffective and Inefficient. Gender Inequality in Health Care: Why It Exists and How We Can Change It*, Final report to the WHO Commission on Social Determinants of Health, at: www.eurohealth.ie/pdf/WGEKN_FINAL_REPORT.pdf, accessed 15 May 2009.

Simms, C. (2000) 'Health Reformers' Response to Zambia's Childhood Mortality Crisis', IDS Working Paper No. 121 (Brighton: Institute of Development Studies).

Standing, H. (1997) 'Gender and Equity in Health Sector Reform Programmes: A Review', *Health Policy and Planning*, 12 (1), 1–18.

Standing, H. (2000) *Gender Impacts of Health Sector Reforms: The Current State of Policy and Implementation*, Paper presented at the ALAMES (Latin American Association of Social Medicine) meeting, Havana, Cuba, 3–7 July 2000.

Standing, H. (2002a) 'Frameworks for Understanding Health Sector Reform', in G. Sen, A. George and P. Östlin (eds), *Engendering International Health: The Challenge of Equity* (Cambridge, MA: MIT Press), 347–71.

Standing, H. (2002b) 'An Overview of Changing Agendas in Health Sector Reforms', *Reproductive Health Matters*, 10 (20), 19–28.

Standing, H. (2006) 'Gender Equity and Health Indicators in the Context of Health Reforms', *International Journal of Public Health*, 51, 3–4.

Stewart, F. (1995) *Adjustment and Poverty: Options and Choices* (New York: Routledge).

UNDP (n.d.) *About the MDGs: Basics – What are the Millennium Development Goals?*, United Nations Development Programme, at: www.undp.org/mdg/basics.shtml, accessed 15 May 2009.

World Development Report (1993) *Investing in Health* (Washington, DC: World Bank and Oxford University Press).

WHO Kobe Centre (2003) *Report of the Expert Working Group on Gender-sensitive Leading Health Indicators* (Kobe: WHO Centre for Health and Development), at: www.who.or.jp/library/cm_report.pdf, accessed 15 May 2009.

WHO (2000) *The World Health Report 2000: Health Systems: Improving Performance* (Geneva: World Health Organization).

WHO (2006) *The World Health Report 2006: Working Together for Health* (Geneva: World Health Organization).

4
Gendering Health Human Resource Policy and Management

Ellen Kuhlmann, Ivy Lynn Bourgeault, Christa Larsen and Toni Schofield

Introduction

Over recent years, health human resources (HHR) have rapidly moved up on the policy agenda in most countries. International organizations like the World Health Organization, the United Nations and the European Union have all drawn attention to a dramatic future shortage of health human resources in all areas of the world and called for urgent action (Commission of the European Communities, 2008; Kampala Declaration, 2008; WHO, 2006). Shortages and inefficient use of existing skills together with changes in the composition of the health professional workforce by age, gender and citizenship have created a need for more systematic policy interventions and new forms of health human resource management. Yet health policy reforms and scholarly debate over how to manage health human resources more effectively have largely ignored the fact that the healthcare division of labour is structured by gender, and that any change in the sector is imbued with complex gender dynamics.

In this chapter we bring a gender lens to HHR policy, planning and management. We are specifically interested in healthcare systems in high-income countries that have public responsibility for healthcare, that assure health services for their citizens and also have a strong legal commitment to gender equality. This is intended to complement existing research into gender and HHR that is primarily related to low and middle-income countries (George, 2007; Standing, 2000; WHO, 2011; see also Chapter 3 by Standing). We also focus primarily, although not exclusively, on doctors and nurses as the cornerstones of healthcare systems, and on the new demands for managing skills and shifting tasks (for example, skill-mix) within and between these health professional groups. We employ a context-sensitive approach that takes the institutional characteristics and the actors of healthcare systems into account (Wrede, 2010), drawing on case studies from Canada, Australia and Germany using material from a number of studies carried out by the authors together with secondary sources.

The chapter begins with an overview of the contemporary debates into HHR, taking into account different dimensions of planning, managing and governing the health workforce and how these dimensions are gendered. This is followed by the illustrative country case studies into the implementation of skill-mix approaches that are currently in the focus of health policy-makers across the globe and that are expected to use existing skills more efficiently. Finally, we will highlight key issues in bringing a gender lens to contemporary health human resource policy, planning and management.

Mapping the field of HHR through a gender lens

Increasing recognition of human resources as the core of healthcare systems has created an emergent field of HHR research and policy that cuts across disciplines and is transnational in nature. Indeed, HHR hosts various different approaches that include the dimensions of planning, policy and management. One of the more established strands of HHR research dates back to 1970s models of 'manpower planning'. These experienced a revival in the 1990s onwards and the concurrent translation into more complex models and non-sexist terms, like for instance, 'workforce planning' or 'health human resource planning' (Dal Poz et al., 2009; Health Canada, 2007). Other strands have emerged more recently and address complex issues involved in managing HHR and implementing innovative HHR policy (for an overview, see Birch and Bourgeault, 2007).

The topics covered under the umbrella of HHR are also diverse, spanning from classic HR themes – like work hours, skills, coordination of tasks – towards more recent issues of workforce governance (Dieleman et al., 2011) and the migration and mobility of health professionals (Bourgeault and Wrede, 2011; Buchan, 2008; Wismar et al., 2011). In addition, there are connections between HHR and approaches within the realm of the sociology of professions, of organizations and of work (for instance, Bourgeault and Mulvale, 2006; Dubois et al., 2006; Kuhlmann, 2006; Schofield, 2009). These approaches are especially useful in *deepening* the field of HHR policy and management; we will come back to this further down when discussing the policy dimensions of HHR.

WHO and European organizations have been especially influential in *broadening* the field and putting the relevance of HHR onto the policy agenda of national states (Commission of the European Communities, 2008; OECD, 2010a; WHO, 2006; see also Dussault et al., 2010; Rechel et al., 2006; Wismar et al., 2011). In parallel with these international efforts, concepts of HHR policy have also emerged nationally. Here, Canada has an internationally recognized pioneering role (Birch et al., 2009; Dubois and Singh, 2009; Health Canada, 2007) but Australia has also a tradition of HHR management (Palmer and Short, 2010; Schofield, 2009); and there are examples in the European context, such as in the Netherlands (RGO, 2008).

A gender lens can inform different topics related to HHR, some of which are discussed in greater detail in this Handbook (see Parts IV and V, especially Chapter 20 by Barry et al.; Chapter 25 by Riska; and Chapter 28 by Wrede). In this chapter we focus on core dimensions in contemporary HHR debates, namely policy, planning and management, that have thus far received only minimal recognition from a gender perspective. Clearly, these dimensions overlap but the analytical distinction helps us to better highlight the different ways gender matters in an emergent field of HHR.

Health human resource planning

The planning of the health workforce increasingly enjoys currency in health policy but no coherent approach exists. A recent Policy Brief of the European Observatory on Health Systems and Policies identifies four main approaches, including: health worker to population ratio; the utilization and demand approach; the service–target approach; and the health and service needs approach (Dussault et al., 2010: 9). Many of these approaches have been applied most often in a uni-professional manner despite a growing awareness of the complexity of health workforce issues. Even before the reinvigorated interest in HHR management due to contemporary and future predicted work-force crises, scholars identified that interventions focused on a single issue or a single profession in isolation have never been adequate; a change in one aspect of the system often intersects with other aspects and creates complex dynamics (Bourgeault et al., 2008; see also Chapter 3 by Standing).

Efforts towards developing more comprehensive and systematic models for HHR planning have been reinforced more recently (Birch et al., 2009; Dal Poz et al., 2009). Yet arguments for more complex HHR planning models are in stark contrast to the actual policies. Dussault and colleagues, in their European assessment, revealed that HHR policy typically focuses on 'establishing training numbers and related costs, rather than developing a comprehensive strategy covering compensation, working conditions, recruitment and retention issues' (2010: 6).

From a gender point of view, typical approaches are problematic in two ways. First, despite calls for more complex planning models and an increasing awareness of gender issues in mainstream policy, none of these models fully incorporates critically important gender dimensions – such as for instance skill-mix, working time, occupation, and earning – as for instance recommended by WHO (2011). Where gender is mentioned, it is mostly reduced to sex-based analysis (for example, Lavallee et al., 2009). So the 'gendering' of HHR is at risk of becoming a mere statistical exercise, like for example counting the numbers of men and women in different professional groups or lamenting the 'feminization' of the health workforce (Wismar et al., 2011). Second, the risk of limiting gender to sex-disaggregated data is problematically reinforced by existing planning policies that primarily focus on 'training numbers' or the 'health worker to population approach', as described by Dussault and colleagues (2010). In this situation, HHR planning exercises tend to reduce the challenging complexity of gendered workforce dynamics to sex category, which is more easily digestible for the forecasting models (see also Kazanjian, 1993).

In summary, contemporary HHR planning no longer totally ignores gender issues; instead, it creates new forms of 'limited inclusion' by reducing gender to sex category. A growing body of sex-disaggregated workforce data is without doubt useful and necessary, but this does not automatically bring about greater gender-sensitivity to HHR planning. Currently, neither of the existing models and policies shows any signs of giving consideration to the complexity of gendered dynamics.

Health human resource management

The management of human resources is one of the most complex strands of the HHR debates that includes managing the work of health professionals and managing organizations that deliver the services. Within this context, a number of issues are relevant that are traditionally influenced by gender. First and foremost, it is well known that social-cultural gender arrangements shape the structural location of men and women in the health workforce as well as the classification of caring and curing, formal and informal work, skilled and unskilled work, and so on (Armstrong and Armstrong, 1996; George, 2007). The horizontal and vertical segregation by sex is also linked to issues of part-time work, career chances and work-life balance (Jong et al., 2006; Özbilgin et al., 2011; Van den Brink, 2011). All of these issues have gendered implications for HHR that may release complex dynamics in the health workforce.

The most dynamic area of HHR management relates to contemporary skill-mix and task-shifting concepts to which we now turn our attention. In line with the transnational nature of the wider concept of HHR, skill-mix and task-shifting are gaining currency in otherwise different healthcare systems (Bourgeault et al., 2008; Delamaire and Lafortune, 2010; Dubois and Singh, 2009). Indeed, changing the skill-mix is an essential element of the transformations in health policy across the globe (for an overview, see Kuhlmann and Annandale, 2012) that fuels many different hopes for making healthcare systems more efficient and responsive to the changing needs of the population.

This prominent role of skill-mix is underscored by a recent WHO report (2011) suggesting skill-mix as one out of four areas where gender equality should be assessed. Here, it is important to keep in mind that every attempt to negotiate the balance of skills and the distribution of tasks is inevitably linked with a need to re-negotiate the gender order of the healthcare system and the gendered division of care work. This is especially obvious when looking at the two core groups of doctors and nurses: the former linked with a masculinist image of biomedical 'cure' work and the gender-exclusive strategies of the medical profession, and the latter with a 'female' image of care work. A large body of scholarly work has highlighted the various different dimensions of gender and the ways of making and unmaking gender inequality in the health professional workforce (Kuhlmann and Bourgeault, 2008; see also the chapters in Part V of this volume). Yet the different strands of scholarly work are poorly connected and the relevance of gender is in stark contrast to the debates in the field of HHR that largely ignore gender dimensions or reduce them to the sex category in similar ways as described with respect to HHR planning.

Dubois and Singh (2009) have recently suggested an expansion from looking at the *distribution* of skills towards the *management* of skills. From a gender perspective this expansion may be useful because it moves beyond sex-disaggregated data and the mere counting of numbers. Yet there are little, if any, attempts by HHR to include the gender dimension more systematically.

George, in her review for the 'Women and Gender Equity Knowledge Network and the Health Systems Knowledge Network' of the WHO Commission on Social Determinants of Health has highlighted the risks of deskilling and how this may create gender inequalities:

> [. . .] measures like substitution and delegation, which affect the professional ordering of health systems, cannot be seen as technical interventions alone. The gender dynamics of these measures need to be considered on a contextual basis, with an assessment of how gender hierarchies among health occupations are formally and informally sustained or subverted, in order to eliminate rather than exacerbate current inequalities across health occupations. It is essential that delegation be seen as part of long term planning and investment efforts that skilfully restructures health systems to do more in different ways, rather than as a means to stretch farther on a cheaper basis, often falling back on unsupported female labour. (George, 2007: 6; see also Chapter 28 by Wrede)

In the current climate of cost-efficiency and budget cuts, skill-mix policies clearly bear the risk of reinforcing the 'unhealthy' connections between 'female–care–deskilling'. At the same time, there may be new opportunities for shifting gendered hierarchies between nurses and doctors, for example through re-negotiation prescribing tasks and developing new roles for highly qualified nurses (Kroezen et al., 2011); but here may also be adverse effects or no impact in the hierarchical order of the health professional workforce. There is an overall need for empirical research into the dynamics that new health policies release in the gendered division of labour in order to avoid simplistic, stereotyped connections between 'female' and 'deskilling' (Heitlinger, 2003; see also Chapter 28 by Wrede) as well as high-flying expectations that skill-mix may bring about greater equality.

Health human resource policy

Just as the management of HHR has been gender-blind, so too has HHR policy. A recent review of the HHR literature has assessed equity and equality issues and revealed a number of more general limitations of contemporary policy interventions. The authors conclude:

> The articles show that although improved equity and/or equality was, in a number of interventions, a goal (mostly as an eventual objective or implicit in the values underlying policies and in the language used to articulate them), inclusiveness in policy development, and fairness and transparency in policy implementation, were often not adequate to guarantee the corresponding desired health workforce scenario (i.e. one that expresses and embodies the values of equity and equality to the extent intended prior to implementation). (Dieleman et al., 2011: 8)

In their review, Dieleman and colleagues (2011) are not particularly concerned with gender equity and equality but the results point towards more general problems of HHR that indeed have gendered implications. Most importantly, the findings raise questions about how and why the values of equity and equality have been 'lost' in the policy development and implementation processes (see also Sen et al., 2007). Here, sociological approaches come in that may help deepening our understanding of policy processes and the management of health human resources, as mentioned previously.

One key problem is that contemporary policy interventions are shaped by the new governance and new public management approaches established in western countries, that embody the mindset of 'rational knowledge' and bureaucratic management and consequently, deny their connections with power and the wider social contexts (Kuhlmann, 2006; see also Chapter 20 by Barry et al. and Chapter 21 by Burau et al.). From a feminist point of view, the problems of knowledge claims to universal truth and neutrality have especially been highlighted by the work of Donna Haraway (1988; see also Chapter 26 by Lagro-Janssen).

The emergent field of HHR may be described as *technocratic* in character, insofar as the organization, management and distribution of the resources involved in public governance are heavily influenced by the knowledge and understanding of professional 'experts' committed to 'rational choices' and the power of 'objective' and (gender) neutral knowledge (Kuhlmann, 2006; Schofield, 2009). So why is this kind of HHR a problem, and how is it gendered?

Basically the application of the dominant HHR approaches does not permit policy-makers and planners to identify and understand the *gendered social dynamics* responsible for producing the problem of shortages of human resources and maldistribution of skills (see, for example, Jeon and Hurley, 2007, with reference to the impact of gender on medical human resource planning in Canada). For example, responding to measurable decreases in workforce participation by health professional groups by creating and funding increased health student places leaves unaddressed why graduates of health education and training programmes do not stay in the health workforce and are reluctant to work outside urban and regional centres. It is an approach that relies on assumptions about workforce motivations rather than empirical evidence on precisely who its members are, what they do, and the relations and conditions under which they work (Schofield, 2009). This is particularly apparent in relation to the 'leakage' of the health workforces, or the problem of retention. One prominent example is the implication that a workforce characterized as 'relatively young and predominantly female' poses retention problems because young women are expected to leave full-time, paid employment to establish and prioritize family life. By contrast, research has revealed much more complex conditions, including a growing wish and demand of male doctors to reduce their work hours (Jong et al., 2006; Kuhlmann, 2006).

There is basically no large-scale, systematic social scientific research that could provide policy-makers and planners with a basis for understanding how and why health workforce participation assumes the patterns that it does. And to make things even worse, an existing body of 'small scale' and more focused research into the health workforce (mainly developed in the realm of feminist research and gender studies) is largely ignored. In short, HHR and gender research are obviously oceans apart and there are few signs that knoweldge can flow between them.

How gender matters

The WHO has recently published a useful manual on how to assess gender equality in health sector strategies; this includes detailed indicators and categories for the health workforce. The authors suggest assessing:

> [. . .] four key areas of education of health workers: recruitment and retention, skill mix and deployment. It should also address the three main employment dimensions in the labour force: occupation, working time and earnings. (WHO, 2011: 115)

While these suggestions are very helpful, they need further investigation directed towards the role of the organization. Organizations release dynamics in the health workforce that either reduce or reinforce gendered inequality within and between the health professions (see also Chapter 20 by Barry et al.). Schofield (2012) has explored the relevance of these dynamics in the Australian health workforce. She argues that the protection and contestation of professional territory and power is a process that is intrinsic to the establishment and reproduction of occupational boundaries in healthcare and that gender is central to it. Nevertheless, little is known and understood about how gender dynamics are played out in this process. Also, Bourgeault and Mulvale (2006), drawing on research in Canada, have highlighted that the gendered dominance of medicine is structurally embedded in the organizations of healthcare and the ways services are provided.

In Germany, analysis of hospital statistics suggests that women doctors in hospitals with private ownership may have better career chances compared to their colleagues in public or voluntary-sector hospitals (unpublished data, Larsen and Kuhlmann). Consequently, health policy changes towards privatization and public–private partnerships impact on the horizontal and vertical gendered division of labour. Taken together, these examples bring the relevance of *intersecting dynamics* of policy, organization, profession and gender into perspective, which are ignored in scholarly HHR debates.

Similarly to the planning policies, this shortcoming of HHR cannot simply be explained by a lack of more complex analytical models. For instance, more than a decade ago Standing (2000) introduced a comprehensive framework and suggested ways of exploring the gendered dynamics of HHR. This includes a number of indicators that are related to four major dimensions of health policy reform, namely reduction of costs and increasing efficiency; improving staff performance; improving equity in the distribution of services; and development of health resource planning and policy (HRPP) capacity (Standing, 2000: 38–40). This kind of approach requires excavating and embellishing. Without it, we will be led back to the problematic nature of contemporary HHR that lacks of a deeper understanding of its social moorings and institutional contexts. In what follows we provide an illustrative example on how to bring gender back into HHR.

Contextualizing HHR in Canada, Australia and Germany

Healthcare systems are all under pressure to manage human resources more effectively. While the reform concepts are broadly similar in western countries, HHR policy is shaped by national regulatory contexts and therefore often turns out differently. The three countries selected for our analysis represent nationally coordinated systems of health insurance systems in different regions of the world – Canada and Australia – that have established more complex HHR policies and management procedures (Australian Health Workforce Advisory Committee 2006; Birch and Bourgeault, 2007), and Germany as an EU member state with the longest tradition of a Statutory Health Insurance (SHI) system but poorly developed HHR management (SVR, 2009). All have introduced gender equality laws and have guidelines and monitoring systems on the level of organizations and professions in place. Table 4.1 provides an overview of major

Table 4.1   Governance of HHR in Canada, Australia and Germany

Indicators	Canada	Australia	Germany
Workforce governance	Federalist; decentralized planning, implementation of HHR policy with national advice and coordination	Federalist; centralized national planning and implementation of HHR policy with collaboration of States/Territory health agencies	Federalist; decentralized, network-based, corporatist SHI regulatory structure; collaboration between state agencies and medical profession
Legal framework	Structural embeddedness of medical dominance through historical statutes; some recent shifts for professional regulation	Government support for medical dominance; some changes since 2005 towards 'substitution' of 'medical' services	Strong regulation and protection of medical tasks and markets; protection of titles of doctors and nurses
Regulatory bodies	Although not consistent across all provinces/territories, a shift towards self-regulation for (nearly) all health professions	Co-regulation between national government/health bureaucracy and boards of all health professions	Part of SHI system with doctors representing the provider side; few attempts towards more plural regulatory bodies
Models of HHR planning	Emphasis on medicine and nursing with an increasing focus on needs-based rather than supply-based modelling	Technocratic approach with a focus on demand and supply factors affecting health workforce policy and planning	Emphasis on regulating influx in medical schools; supply-based modelling focusing on doctors, mainly nationally trained
Recruitment policies	Primarily national but a significant proportion of medical (24%) and nursing staff (8%) are from abroad	Combination of national and international; high proportions of doctors (48%) and nurses (30%) born overseas	Primarily national with low international recruitment (doctors: 6%; nurses: 3%) but some change, especially EU mobility

Source: authors

Table 4.2 Health workforce patterns in Canada, Australia and Germany

Indicators	Canada (2009)	Australia (2006)	Germany
Doctors:			
% women	36%^^^	37%^	42%*** (2009)
% with foreign nationality	24%^^^	48%^	5.7%** (2008)
Ratio: doctors to 1000 population	2.4*	2.75^	3.6* (2009)
Registered nurses:			
% women	94%^^	91%^	86%**** (2006)
% with foreign nationality	8%^^	30%^	3.4%** (2008)
Ratio: nurses to 1000 population	9.4*	9.8^	10.7* (2009)
Ratio: nurses to doctors	4:1*	3.5:1^	3:1* (2009)

Sources:
* OECD (2010b)
** Ognyanova and Busse (2011)
*** KBV (2011)
**** GBE (2011)
^ Australian Institute of Health and Welfare (2009)
^^ CIHI (2010a)
^^^ CIHI (2010b)

HHR governance arrangements and Table 4.2 of key indicators of the health workforce in comparative perspective.

Canada, and similarly Australia, show more advanced regulation and integration of a wider range of health professional groups, more extensive use of international recruitment and better recognition of needs-based and demand-side factors affecting HHR policy and modelling. Germany, by contrast, shows a narrow approach of supply-side planning that is focused on doctors and a nationally trained health workforce (Table 4.1). Interestingly, though, sex-segregation is significantly stronger in Canada and Australia when compared to Germany; this pattern holds true for both medicine and nursing (Table 4.2). With these institutional characteristics and workforce patterns as a backdrop we now explore in more detail the gendered dimensions of skill-mix and task-shifting in our three countries.

Skill-mix and task-shifting: dismantling gendered HHR dynamics

Skill-mix and task-shifting are 'core' dimensions of HHR that are largely about decisions of *who* does *what* to whom, when and for how much. A Policy Brief for the European Observatory of Health Systems and Policies has highlighted some key recommendations:

- Skill-mix initiatives can focus on changing professional roles directly – through role or skill extension, delegation and introducing a new type of worker – and those that change roles indirectly via modifications in the interface between services (i.e. where care is provided).

- Skill-mix initiatives may be motivated by both qualitative objectives or concerns (quality improvement, professional development and quality of work life concerns) and by quantitative considerations (shortages, mal-distribution and cost-effectiveness).
- Policy instruments to support the effective implementation of skill-mix initiatives can include:
  - modifying or introducing new professional roles through the development of different organizational and regulatory arrangements;
  - supporting new or enhanced professional roles through collective financing (i.e. involving them in public provision) and changing financial incentive structures; and
  - ensuring the educational foundations (competencies and capacity) for the new and expanded professional roles.
- Across all initiatives it is also essential to have the support of new professional roles by the affected professional organizations and by government.
- Skill-mix initiatives must be driven by need and be sensitive to the health system and health professional climate; one-size-fits-all approaches are not helpful. (Bourgeault et al., 2008)

Crucially, all of these dimensions and the decisions about 'who does what' are influenced by gender both historically and in the contemporary period, and shaped by institutional contexts of healthcare systems. The case study material which follows dismantles some of the gendered dimensions without claiming to draw a comprehensive picture of the gendered dimensions of HHR.

Canada

Health human resources in Canada have waxed and waned from shortages to surpluses for both the medical and nursing profession. With the advent of provincial/territorial public health insurance schemes (otherwise known as Medicare) in the late 1960s and early 1970s, there was a shortage of physicians and nurses to meet the needs of Canadian citizens now universally covered for healthcare. By the 1980s and 1990s, concerns over rising healthcare costs caused both federal and provincial governments to implement substantial cuts to healthcare spending.

In the early 1990s, a report prepared for the Conference of Deputy Ministers (CDM) of Health addressed issues regarding physician supply and demand in Canada – known as the Barer-Stoddart Report (1991). The context for this report was a perceived surplus of physicians but also the broader context of healthcare cost constraints. The scope of the report was far-reaching, addressing issues of the selection, training, supply, distribution and support of future physicians. One of the key task-shifting recommendations of the report was to rapidly expand the utilization of nurse practitioners, nurses who have an expanded scope of practice to diagnose, prescribe and order tests for a limited range of conditions. Although the report made a range of recommendations, few, other than reduced opportunities for international medical graduates (IMGs) and a ten per cent decrease in the number of undergraduate medical school positions, were implemented (Birch and Bourgeault, 2007).

But before the end of the decade, the pendulum seemed to shift back when medical professional associations, working groups and other politically active organizations started to discuss shortages of physicians, calling for a reversal of the reduction in enrolment in medical schools; indeed they proposed an increase of 27 per cent. Part of the problem with the projections made in the Barer-Stoddart report of 1991 was that they did not take into account the impact of the 'feminization' of the medical profession on volume of services. Many female physicians, but increasingly younger cohorts of male physicians, were simply not working the same hours or at the same capacity as older, largely male practitioners (Jeon and Hurley, 2007).

So as to help prevent HHR policy swings, the federal/provincial/territory Advisory Committee on Health Delivery and Human Resources (ACHDHR) was established in 2002 to provide a national forum for discussion and information-sharing. It developed a Pan Canadian HHR Framework to facilitate the enhancement of partnerships between governments and other stakeholders so as to build a more collaborative approach to HHR planning. One of its key recommendations was to enhance the capacity to achieve the appropriate mix of health providers and deploy then in service delivery models that make full use of their skills. To this end, Health Canada made significant investments through the provinces and territories to support interprofessional, collaborative care initiatives. In the province of Ontario, these funds were used to foster the development of interprofessional family health teams, including among others family physicians, nurses and nurse practitioners, social workers, pharmacists and physiotherapists. Such task-shifting was enabled by the Regulated Health Professions Act of 1993. Initially, these interprofessional initiatives were led by family physicians, but more recently a series of nurse-practitioner-led family health clinics have been established, though not without some criticism from organized medical interest groups.

Thus, although there have been concerted efforts to shift the provision of who does what across Canada, with some success, these have resulted in some 'pushback' from organized medicine even in the face of support and participation in these initiatives by a growing number of physicians intent on working differently than their predecessors. But just as some medical tasks are shifted to nurses/nurse practitioners, more and more direct care nursing tasks are also being shifted down to practical nurses, personal support workers and family members in an overall attempt to rationalize care (Birch and Bourgeault, 2007; Bourgeault and Mulvale, 2006). These decisions are made based on gendered assumptions that someone will be available at home to provide this care, which increasingly is less likely with the predominance of dual-income families (Armstrong and Armstrong, 1996). Although such reforms may be gender-blind, their implications most certainly are not.

Australia

In Australia, impending health workforce shortages have raised policy concerns about skill-mix and the division of tasks within healthcare institutions. These concerns were addressed most directly and explicitly in 2005 when a major national policy advisory body, the Australian Productivity Commission, conducted an extensive investigation of the health workforce. In commenting on shortages of medical professionals, especially in regional, rural and remote areas, the Commission reported at length on the limited utilization of the skills of the health workforce as a whole. It proposed to policy-makers the establishment of what it called professional substitution – an intervention whereby a range of health professionals other than doctors would, at government expense, be able to provide certain medical services and to prescribe medications, both the exclusive preserve of doctors.

With the restructuring of education for nurses and allied health professionals since the 1970s that saw a major shift to university-based training, the Productivity Commission noted the wider dissemination of complex skills and competencies in the health workforce. Such a development, it reasoned, meant that human health resources were required to address anticipated increases in demand for health services in the coming decades were by no means in short supply. It was evident that professional and organizational dynamics imposed barriers to health services' access to these resources (Schofield, 2009).

Significantly, however, Australian governments (national, State and Territory) rejected the Commission's proposal, adopting and implementing the recommendations submitted by the Australian Medical Association (AMA) to the Commission's review. The AMA openly opposed professional substitution, favouring delegation by doctors to appropriately trained nursing and allied health colleagues. The implementation of this recommendation has seen some significant relinquishment by medicine in performing some tasks, assigning them to nurses and allied health professionals. This has been particularly evident in community-based clinics or 'medical centres'. Yet doctors robustly maintain control and supervision in the process. Accordingly, medicine continues to exert considerable power and authority with respect to boundaries between health occupations and the pattern of skill-mix that accompanies them.

Given that nursing and the allied health professions are heavily female-dominated, while medicine continues to be male-dominated (Table 4.2), it is evident that medical dominance of healthcare and the distribution of human health resources is profoundly gendered. Clearly, there are significant consequences of this for the organization and management of HHR, particularly in responding to projected health workforce shortages. But health policy-makers and workforce planners have been consistently gender-blind in their responses (Schofield, 2009). The discourse of health workforce policy and planning in Australia has been overwhelmingly technocratic, eschewing any acknowledgement of the role of organizational dynamics such as those related to professional territory maintenance and gendered work in health service institutions.

Germany

The German system provides little flexibility for changing professional roles or creating new ones that touch on the tasks of doctors. For many years doctors have been very successful in protecting medical skills and markets. The other side of the coin is 'slow motion' in the professionalization of nursing, including blockades against academic education as well as against full recognition and state protection as a self-governing profession. Yet the role of doctors as the 'palace guard' of the health workforce has come under scrutiny and issues of skill-mix and task-shifting are gaining currency in the health policy discourse (SVR, 2009). Change is driven by financial pressures and by professionalization claims of nurses and other groups and, in addition, by an increasing shortage of doctors in some regions, especially in the eastern parts; there are also bottom-up-driven changes by emergent forms of a more inclusive medical professionalism (Kuhlmann, 2006). The notions of quality assurance and patient-centred care and safety, by contrast, serve the medical profession as demarcation against the claims of nurses and are therefore more conservative elements. Added to this, there are also no signs of the users loudly calling for shifting tasks (Bourgeault et al., 2008; Kuhlmann, 2006).

There is a lack of policy instruments that could help to systematically modify roles and create new ones. A few pilot projects have been introduced, primarily related to community nursing and physician assistants. Yet 'delegation of work' – from doctors to nurses and from qualified nurses to less qualified staff – is the dominant pattern. Substitution of doctors and prescribing tasks of nurses are highly contested areas; besides legal barriers, the power of the medical profession currently prevents more substantive changes in the distribution of tasks. Compared to this, changes in the educational foundations are more successful than transformation in the organization of work, including developing an academically trained nursing profession. But neither the legal framework nor the educational system are adequately prepared for shifting tasks (SVR, 2009).

Viewed through the lens of gender the lack of more complex HHR policies seems to act as a conservative force and 'stabiliser' of the gendered division of labour; growing economic pressures may even reinforce the unequal relationships between doctors and nurses. For example, regional health labour market analysis reveals divergent HHR management patterns in hospital doctors and nurses: while overall staffing levels increased (from 2004–08) eight per cent in the group of doctors, nurses faced a loss of one per cent.

In contrast to the gendered hierarchy of professions, the educational system is (slightly) more dynamic and has opened up some career pathways for nurses that better equip them for re-negotiating skills and tasks. Here, the main driving forces are broader changes in the educational system due to European laws and guidelines. So Europeanization, in this case, furthers an upgrading of nursing and might thereby help to reduce gendered inequality in HHR.

Another more dynamic element is the organization. The balance between doctors and nurses and within the nursing profession varies according to the organizational settings. For instance, public hospitals have shown the most radical cuts in qualified nursing staff, but have invested in nursing aides; by contrast, private hospitals have expanded all levels of nursing staff, but to a lesser degree in low-qualified segments of nursing (data: authors' calculations, based on Hospital Statistics Hesse, 2010).

In summary, the findings suggest that conservative forces preserving or even reinforcing gendered hierarchies are strongest on the level of the professions, while dynamics may come in 'sideways' through changing organizational settings and educational foundations that may further less hierarchical relationships. This underlines the significance of intersecting dynamics and the need for gendering HHR beyond the sex segregation of the health workforce.

Conclusions

This chapter has set out to bring a gender lens to the field of HHR policy and management in western healthcare systems. We have argued that all areas of healthcare are deeply structured by gender and, consequently, HHR is in need of a more systematic inclusion of gendered dynamics in management, planning and policy.

Our mapping exercise now brings more general problems of an emergent field of HHR into view. Next to a lack of gender sensitivity, the wider goals of equity and equality and the complex social dimensions of human resources get lost in contemporary HHR policy and management. Despite the availability of complex HHR models, priority is given to numbers and also to the medical profession. In this situation, we can observe new forms of 'limited inclusion' of gender as a sex category that sits more easily with the 'technocratic' approach of contemporary HHR and the demand for 'rational knowledge' to inform health policy-makers. So the major problem is not just to develop more complex and gender-sensitive models, but to understand the processes of *translation* into practice and the role of policy. Our analysis furthermore highlights a lack of connection between HHR research and a large body of (mainly feminist) more complex research into the gendered nature of healthcare work, organizations and professions. Thus, existing knowledge is not used efficiently in HHR.

Our case study material reveals that changes in the institutional governance arrangements, in the health professions and the organizations together with the educational system, intersect and shape the specific outcome of gendered workforce dynamics. At the same time, the comparative approach clearly highlights that there is no uniform pattern and easy explanation of *how* policy changes are linked to gender equality. For instance, more integrated and needs-based HHR approaches in Canada, and similarly in Australia, do not necessarily challenge an existing strong (horizontal) sex-segregation of the health professional workforce.

Assessing HHR through the lens of gender raises more general questions on how contexts matter in HHR management and challenges universal assumptions about the nature of health human resources and how they should be managed more effectively. This includes challenging a revival of sex category as a substitute for complex gendered dynamics in the health workforce.

Summary

- Healthcare is deeply structured by gender but HHR management and policy largely ignore the complexity of gendered dynamics.
- An emergent field of HHR does not fully ignore gender issues, but creates new forms of 'limited inclusion' of gender as sex category that sits more easily with the technocratic nature of HHR and wider public sector management.
- The revival of sex category in HHR as a substitute for complex gendered dynamics is reinforced by an overall disconnection between feminist research and HHR debates.
- Context-sensitive analysis of the implementation of skill-mix and task-shifting highlights intersecting gendered dynamics between governance, professions, organization and the educational foundations that need to be unpacked in order to understand the making and unmaking of inequality.

Key reading

Bourgeault, I. L., E. Kuhlmann, E. Neiterman and S. Wrede (2008) 'How to Effectively Implement Optimal Skill-mix and Why', *Health Evidence Network – European Observatory on Health Systems and Policies, Policy Brief Series*, at: www.euro.who.int/document/hsm/8_hsc08_ePB_11.pdf, accessed 10 August 2011.

Schofield, T. (2009) 'Gendered Organizational Dynamics: The Elephant in the Room for Australian Allied Health Workforce Policy and Planning', *Journal of Sociology*, 45 (4), 383–400.

Standing, H. (2000) 'Gender: A Missing Dimension in Human Resource Policy and Planning for Health Reforms', *Human Resources for Health Development Journal*, 4 (1), 27–42.

WHO (2011) *Human Rights and Gender Equality in Health Sector Strategies: How to Assess Policy Coherence* (Geneva: World Health Organization).

References

Armstrong, P. and H. Armstrong (1996) *Wasting Away: The Undermining of Canadian Health Care* (Toronto: Oxford University Press).

Australian Health Workforce Advisory Committee (2006) *The Australian Allied Health Workforce: An Overview of Workforce Planning Issues*, AHWAC Report 2006.1 (Sydney: AHWAK).

Australian Institute of Health and Welfare (2009) *Health and Community Services Labour Force 2006*, National Health Labour Force Series No. 42, Cat. No. HWL 43 (Canberra: AIHW).

Barer-Stoddart Report – Barer, M. L. and G. L. Stoddart (1991) *Toward Integrated Medical Resource Policies for Canada*, Report prepared for the Federal/Provincial and Territorial Conference of Deputy Ministers of Health (Vancouver: University of British Columbia).

Birch, S. and I. L. Bourgeault (eds) (2007) 'Health Human Resources Research in Canada', *Canadian Public Policy*, 33 (Supplement), S1–S99.

Birch, S., G. Kephart, G. T. Murphy, L. O'Brien-Pallas, R. Alder and A. MacKenzie (2009) 'Health Human Resource Planning and the Production of Health: Development of an Extended Analytical Framework for Needs-based Health Human Resources Planning', *Journal of Public Health Management Practice*, November (Supplement), S56–S61.

Bourgeault, I. L., E. Kuhlmann, E. Neiterman and S. Wrede (2008) 'How To Effectively Implement Optimal Skill-mix and Why', *Health Evidence Network – European Observatory on Health Systems and Policies, Policy Brief Series*, at: www.euro.who, accessed 10 August 2011.

Bourgeault, I. L. and G. Mulvale (2006) 'Collaborative Health Care Teams in Canada and the US: Confronting the Structural Embeddedness of Medical Dominance', *Health Sociology Review*, 15 (5), 481–95.

Bourgeault, I. L. and S. Wrede (2011) 'Caring across Borders: Contrasting the Contexts of Nurse Migration in Canada and Finland', in C. Benoit and H. Hallgrimsdottir (eds), *Finding Dignity in Health Care and Health Care Work* (Toronto: University of Toronto Press), 65–86.

Buchan, J. (2008) 'How Can the Migration of Health Professionals Be Managed so as To Reduce Any Negative Effects on Supply', *Health Evidence Network – European Observatory on Health Systems and Policies*, Policy Brief Series, at: www.euro.who, accessed 10 August 2011.

CIHI – Canadian Institutes of Health Information (2010a) *Regulated Nurses: Canadian Trends, 2005 to 2009*, at: https://secure.cihi.ca/estore/productFamily.htm?pf=PFC1565 &locale=en&lang=EN&mediatype=0, accessed 2 October 2011.

CIHI – Canadian Institutes of Health Information (2010b) *Supply, Distribution and Migration of Canadian Physicians, 2009*, at: https://secure.cihi.ca/estore/productSeries. htm?pc=PCC34, accessed 2 October 2011.

Commission of the European Communities (2008) *Green Paper on the European Workforce for Health*, Brussels, 10.12.2008, COM(2008) 725 final, at: http://ec.europa.eu/health/ph_systems/workforce_en.htm, accessed 10 August 2011.

Dal Poz, M. R., N. Gupta, E. Quain and A. L. B. Soucat (eds) (2009) *Handbook on Monitoring and Evaluation of Human Resources for Health* (Geneva: World Health Organization).

Delamaire, M. L. and G. Lafortune (2010) 'Nurses in Advanced Roles: A Description and Evaluation of Experiences in 12 Developed Countries', *OECD Working Papers*, No. 54 (Paris: OECD).

Dieleman, M., D. M. P. Shaw and P. Zwanikken (2011) 'Improving the Implementation of Health Workforce Policies through Governance: A Review of Case Studies', *BMC Human Resources for Health*, 9:10, at: www.human-resources-health.com/content/9/1/10, accessed 10 August 2011.

Dubois, C.-A. and D. Singh (2009) 'From Staff-mix to Skill-mix and Beyond: Towards a Systemic Approach to Health Workforce Management', *BMC Human Resources for Health*, 7:87, at: www.human-resources-health.com/content/7/1/87, accessed 10 August 2011.

Dubois, C.-A., M. McKee and E. Nolte (2006) *Human Resources for Health in Europe* (Maidenhead: Open University Press).

Dussault, G., J. Buchan, W. Sermeus and Z. Padaiga (2010) *Assessing Future Health Workforce Needs, Policy Summary 2*, WHO, on behalf of European Observatory on Health Systems and Policies.

GBE – Gesundheitsberichterstattung des Bundes und der Länder (2011) *Beschäftigte ausgewählter Berufe nach Geschlecht*, at: www.gbe-bund.de, accessed 23 September 2011.

George, A. (2007) 'Human Resources for Health: A Gender Analysis', paper prepared for the Women and Gender Equity Knowledge Network and the Health Systems Knowledge Network of the WHO Commission on Social Determinants of Health, at: www.who.int/social_determinants/resources/human_resources_for_health_wgkn_2007.pdf, accessed 10 August 2011.

Haraway, D. (1988) 'Situated Knowledges: The Science Question in Feminism and the Privilege of a Partial Perspective', *Feminist Studies*, 14 (2), 583–90.

Health Canada (2007) *A Framework for Collaborative Pan-Canadian Health Human Resources Planning* (Ottawa: Health Canada).

Heitlinger, A. (2003) 'The Paradoxical Impact of Health Care Restructuring in Canada on Nursing as a Profession', *International Journal of Health Services*, 33 (1), 37–54.

Jeon, S. and J. Hurley (2007) 'The Relationship between Physician Hours of Work, Service Volume and Service Intensity', *Canadian Public Policy*, 33 (Supplement), 17–30.

Jong, J. de, P. Heiligers, P. P. Groenewegen and L. Hingstman (2006) 'Why Are Some Medical Specialists Working Part-time, While Others Work Full-time?', *Health Policy*, 78, 235–48.

Kampala Declaration (2008) *Health Workers for All and All for Health Workers*, Global Health Workforce Alliance.

KBV – Kassenärztliche Bundesvereinigung (2011) *Arztzahlstudie 2010: Daten, Fakten, Trends*, at: www.kbv.de/publikationen/36943.html, accessed to August 2011.

Kazanjian, A. (1993) 'Health-manpower Planning or Gender Relations? The Obvious and the Oblique', in E. Riska and K. Wegar (eds), *Gender, Work and Medicine: Women and the Medical Division of Labour* (London: Sage), 147–71.

Kroezen, M., L. van Dijk, P. P. Groenewegen and A. L. Francke (2011) 'Nurse Prescribing of Medicines in Western European and Anglo-Saxon Countries: A Systematic Review of the Literature', *BMC Health Services Research*, 11:127, at: www.biomedcentral.com/1472-6963/11/127, accessed 10 August 2011.

Kuhlmann, E. (2006) *Modernising Health Care. Reinventing Professions, the State and the Public* (Bristol: Policy Press).

Kuhlmann, E. and E. Annandale (2012) 'Researching Transformations in Health Services and Policy in International Perspective', *Current Sociology*, Special Issue, 60 (4).

Kuhlmann, E. and I. L. Bourgeault (2008) 'Gender, Professions and Public Policy: New Directions', *Equal Opportunities International*, 27 (1), 5–18.

Lavallee, R., P. Hanvoravongchai and N. Gupta (2009) 'Use of Population Census Data for Gender Analysis of the Health Workforce', in M. R. Dal Poz, N. Gupta, E. Quain and A. L. B. Soucat (eds), *Handbook on Monitoring and Evaluation of Human Resources for Health* (Geneva: World Health Organization), 103–11.

OECD (2010a) *International Migration of Health Workers*, Policy Brief (Paris: OECD).

OECD (2010b) *Health at a Glance* (Paris: OECD).

Ognyanova, D. and R. Busse (2011) 'A Destination and a Source Country: Germany', *Euro Observer*, 13 (2), 5.

Özbilgin, M. F., M. Tsouroufli and M. Smith (2011) 'Understanding the Interplay of Time, Gender and Professionalism in Hospital Medicine in the UK', *Social Science & Medicine*, DOI:10.1016/j.socscimed.2011.03.030, accessed 10 August 2011.

Palmer, G. and S. Short (2010) *Health Care and Public Policy: An Australian Analysis*, 4th edition (Melbourne: Palgrave Macmillan).

Rechel, B., C.-A. Dubois and M. McKee (eds) (2006) *The Health Care Workforce in Europe. Learning from Experience* (Copenhagen: WHO Regional Office for Europe), at: www.euro.who.int/Document/E89156.pdf, accessed 10 August 2011.

RGO – Advisory Council on Health Research (2008) *Health Services Research: The Future of Health Services Research in the Netherlands*, RGO 59E (The Hague: Health Council of the Netherlands), at: www.rgo.nl, accessed 31 July 2011.

Schofield, T. (2009) 'Gendered Organizational Dynamics: The Elephant in the Room for Australian Allied Health Workforce Policy and Planning', *Journal of Sociology*, 45 (4), 383–400.

Schofield, T. (2012: forthcoming) 'The Global Health Workforce "Crisis" and Inequities in Health Care Access: Advancing a Gender and Organisations Approach to Policy, Research and Practice', in S. Short and F. McDonald (eds), *The Health Workforce Global Continuum* (London: Ashgate).

Sen, G., P. Östlin and A. George (2007) *Unequal, Unfair, Ineffective and Inefficient. Gender Inequality in Health Care: Why It Exists and How We Can Change It*, Final report to the WHO Commission on Social Determinants of Health, at: www.eurohealth.ie/pdf/WGEKN_FINAL_REPORT.pdf, accessed 12 August 2011.

Standing, H. (2000) 'Gender: A Missing Dimension in Human Resource Policy and Planning for Health Reforms', *Human Resources for Health Development Journal*, 4 (1), 27–42.

SVR – Advisory Council on the Assessment of Developments in the Health Care System (2009) *Cooperation and Responsibility. Prerequisites for Target-oriented Health Care*, Advisory Report, English summary, at: www.svr-gesundheit.de, accessed 15 August 2011.

Van den Brink, M. (2011) 'Scouting for Talent: Appointment Practices of Women Professors in Academic Medicine', *Social Science & Medicine*, 72 (12), 2033–40.

WHO (2006) *The World Health Report 2006. Working Together for Health* (Geneva: World Health Organization).

WHO (2011) *Human Rights and Gender Equality in Health Sector Strategies: How To Assess Policy Coherence* (Geneva: World Health Organization).

Wismar, M., I. A. Glinos, C. B. Maier, G. Dussault, W. Palm, J. Bremner and J. Figueras (2011) 'Health Professional Mobility and Health Systems: Evidence from 17 European Countries', *Euro Observer*, 13 (2), 1–4.

Wrede, S. (2010) 'How Country Matters: Studying Health Policy in a Comparative Perspective', in: I. Bourgeault, R. Dingwall and R. de Vries (eds), *The Sage Handbook of Qualitative Methods in Health Research* (Los Angeles: Sage), 88–105.

5
Gender-sensitive Indicators for Healthcare

Vivian Lin and Helen L'Orange

Introduction

The use of gender-sensitive indicators is a critical component in the effort for effective gender mainstreaming. Gender mainstreaming was endorsed to promote equity between women and men at the Fourth World Conference on Women in Beijing in 1995, and more recently, in 2006, in a resolution of the Economic and Social Council (ECOSOC, 2006). International organizations regularly collect data from member states and publish voluminous collections of national statistics. The importance of this for gender mainstreaming has recently been underscored by Sen and colleagues in their report to the WHO Commission on Social Determinants of Health, Knowledge Network on Women and Gender Equity, which proposed the following strategy:

> Ensure collection of data disaggregated by sex, socioeconomic status, and other social stratifiers by individual research projects as well as through larger data systems at regional and national levels, and the classification and analysis of such data towards meaningful results and expansion of knowledge for policy. (Sen et al., 2007: x)

Concern about the lack of sex-disaggregation of routinely collected statistics has led to attempts to develop indicators for gender equity and health at the global, national and sub-national level (Beck, 1999; UNIFEM, 2000). Comprehensive women's health surveillance reporting, such as report cards, have also been attempted in some countries, along with concerted global efforts to engender the Millennium Development Goals (MDGs) (UNIFEM, 2008).

This chapter will review these developments, including: how gender-sensitive indicators are defined; how indicators of gender equity and health might be chosen; how they might be linked to decision-making processes; and how an effective monitoring system might be constructed. The challenges in developing and using gender-sensitive indicators will also be canvassed. It should be noted that much of the work globally has focused on women and women's health – rather than on the health of men – and this is the orientation reflected in this chapter.

What are gender-sensitive health indicators?

Based on the work of Beck (1999) and the United Nations Development Fund for Women (UNIFEM, 2000), gender-sensitive indicators can be defined as:

> ... those that enable us to identify, examine and monitor gender-related changes in society over time [and] constructed so as to compare the position of women and men so to focus on gender gaps. (Lin et al., 2007b: S28)

As comparing information about women's status to that of men may give an incomplete picture of their experiences, goals and interests (Austen et al., 2000), a full analysis may also require the use of sex-specific indicators – such as those conditions experienced by one sex – to ascertain absolute levels of health as well as gender gaps (UNIFEM, 2000). Health indicators can be described as 'statistics or parameters that provide information on trends and changes in the condition and status of health' (Tudiver et al., 2004: 2). However, the frameworks and theoretical constructs used to understand health critically influence the indicators developed, as do assumptions about women and their roles. Although health is a composite of biological make-up and socio-economic circumstances, the traditional use of a biomedical approach combined with particular assumptions about women has resulted in a number of limitations to existing health indicators. Many indicators focus on illness/disease rather than on health and well-being and/or assume gender neutrality (Abdool and Vissandjée, 2001; Eckermann, 2000). Conversely, they tend not to be concerned with health-seeking behaviours and strategies for achieving positive health (AbouZahr and Vaughn, 2000; Tudiver et al., 2004).

Making health indicators gender-sensitive involves identifying an appropriate existing conceptual framework for understanding health which both links social determinants and health outcomes and includes gender as a central component. Criteria to guide the assessment or development of gender-sensitive indicators have been developed by Beck (1999) and supported by other authors (for example, Abdool and Vissandjée, 2001; Lin et al., 2007a). These include:

- Data should be easy to use and understand. Indicators should be phrased in readily understandable language, and should be developed at a level relevant to the institutional capabilities of the country.
- Data should be relatively reliable and reliability checks should be carried out. Indicators should be reliable enough to use as a time series, and the time span clearly specified.

- Indicators should be about something measurable and ideally something where intervention can lead to change. Concepts such as 'women's empowerment' or 'gender equity' may be difficult to define and measure. Instead, proxy indicators, for example relating to greater choice for women in accessing healthcare, may have to be used.
- Indicators should be collected using internationally accepted definitions as they enable international comparison.
- Indicators should involve comparison to a norm, for example, the situation of men in the same country or the situation of women in another country, to focus on questions of gender equity rather than only on the status of women.
- Data should be disaggregated by sex, and wherever possible, national-level indicators should also be disaggregated by age, socio-economic grouping and locality in order to inform a broader analysis of the social forces within a society which have brought about the particular status of women and men.
- Indicators should, where feasible, measure the outcome or impact of a situation rather than the input. For example, women's literacy is often a better measure of women's educational status than female enrolment rates. Female mortality rates are a better measure of women's health status than access to healthcare.

Why use gender-sensitive health indicators?

The key reason for using gender-sensitive health indicators is to provide a rigorous information base for decision-making and policy actions that can improve health outcomes and reduce inequities (Coleman, 2003). They can assist the monitoring of equity trends in health status and healthcare access and utilization and can support policy by answering the key questions: 'Is the gap in health status improving or worsening over time?' and 'How are policies and interventions working to narrow the gap?' (Evans et al., 2001: 5).

Indicators generally 'point to key questions rather than provide answers' (Beck, 1999: 9) and do not provide analysis of broader social patterns and context, such as how gender relations have been shaped in particular ways, and how these relations could be altered. A complementary gender-based analysis is needed as a component of the indicator interpretation process. Box 5.1 provides an example of the successful development of gender-sensitive indicators concerning eye diseases.

How adequate are current indicators used by international organizations?

To foster gender-based analysis in mainstream health systems, it is necessary to ensure mainstream health indicators are gender-sensitive. A health

Box 5.1 Promotion of the equitable use of eye services and reduction of eye disease and blindness in Tanzania

Background

Nearly two thirds of blind people worldwide are women and girls. In many places, men have twice the access to eye care as women. Of the 30 million blind people in China, India and Africa, 20 million are women. Women bear about 75 per cent of trachoma-related blindness. Compared to men, women are 1.8 times more likely to have trichiasis and account for about 70 per cent of all trichiasis cases.

Relevant gender-sensitive health indicators and their findings

Sex-disaggregated data enabled identification of gender as an issue by pointing to the association between gender and blindness, which in turn led to the identification of potential reasons for differences, particularly local factors associated with use of services. A key finding was the unequal utilization of eye-care services for cataract, trachoma and congenital/developmental cataract, including:

- women consistently have lower rates of utilization of cataract surgical services compared to men;
- the barriers that restrict the use of eye-care services by men and women are different due to differences in gender roles and behaviours;
- young girls who become blind due to congenital cataract are much less likely than boys to be brought to hospital for surgery.

Strategies adopted and impact

These findings have been used by the Kilimanjaro Regional Eye Care Strategy; this is a partnership between the Tanzanian Ministry of Health, Kilimanjaro Christian Medical Centre (KCMC) Hospital, and a number of donors to develop gender-sensitive strategies to improve utilization and to achieve equity of eye-care services and reduce blindness. Strategies include:

- creating a bridge between communities and the hospital to reduce problems associated with travel access, need for transport and so on;
- negotiating with hospital/s to reduce price of surgery to make it affordable for most families;
- improving awareness, access and acceptance of eye-care services in a gender-sensitive fashion in the community;

(Continued)

Box 5.1 (Continued)

- eye-care services implemented systematically at 20 different referral sites in reach of every village; these sites are visited every three to six months;
- reduction of hospital-based barriers to utilization of services;
- counselling of eye disease patients to improve decision-making and acceptance by family members – particularly for elderly females.

The Kilimanjaro data showed that by the third site visit, more females than males were attending the clinics for treatment. The programme has encouraged Tanzania to be the first African country to build a gender focus into its national five-year Vision 2020 Plan.

Source: Courtright, 2008.

information framework can be used to map indicators that relate to health and its determinants. Work by Lin and colleagues (2003) builds on, and adds a gendered dimension to, the mainstream health information framework – developed by Canada and adapted by Australia, the Organization for Economic Development and Cooperation (OECD) and the International Standards Organization (ISO). The four tiers of the Health Information Framework (Figure 5.1) can be populated with indicators used by various agencies to clarify what information is available and what needs to be monitored. This information framework and others like it do not replace conceptual frameworks for gender equity and health, as causal pathways cannot be tracked between 'tiers'. It is, however, a mechanism for examining the comprehensiveness of indicators sets as equity indicators can be explicitly included in each tier of the health information framework in order to assess the extent to which mainstream indicators incorporate gender sensitivity.

In an audit of 1095 health indicators commonly used by international organizations Lin and colleagues (2007a) found deficiencies in the indicators' technical quality, underlying conceptual bases, and coverage across the tiers of the above health information framework. In terms of technical construction, most routine indicators lacked sufficient specificity to contribute to gendered and equity analyses of health and healthcare systems. Gender-relevant indicators related to health system performance, gender equity and health were particularly limited, indicating a major gap in data collection at global and national levels. Specific findings from Lin and colleagues (2007a) on the 1095 indicators included the following:

- Most routine indicators, including basic health indicators such as infant mortality, were not disaggregated by sex or age, although sex-disaggregation

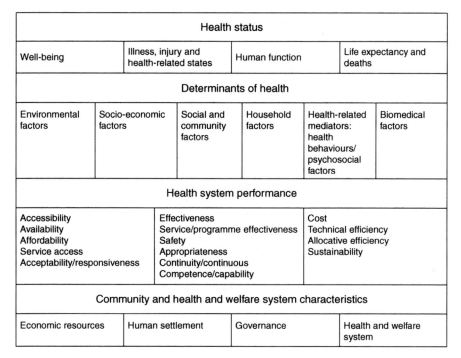

Health status			
Well-being	Illness, injury and health-related states	Human function	Life expectancy and deaths
Determinants of health			
Environmental factors	Socio-economic factors	Social and community factors	Household factors	Health-related mediators: health behaviours/ psychosocial factors	Biomedical factors
Health system performance			
Accessibility Availability Affordability Service access Acceptability/responsiveness	Effectiveness Service/programme effectiveness Safety Appropriateness Continuity/continuous Competence/capability	Cost Technical efficiency Allocative efficiency Sustainability
Community and health and welfare system characteristics			
Economic resources	Human settlement	Governance	Health and welfare system

Figure 5.1   The health information framework
Source: Lin et al. (2007a).

was reported in indicators on life expectancy, education, workforce and democracy;

- Most sex-specific indicators described women, and were age-limited to women of reproductive age, or described reproductive outcomes, for example, deliveries and births. Largely missing were indicators on the health problems of females out of reproductive age – older women, girls – or pertaining to non-reproductive states, for example, mental health;
- The depiction of men was just as limited: only four sex-specific topics describing males were found, including urethritis, violence, and un/ employment;
- There were no indicators disaggregated by ethnicity or socio-economic groups and comparisons of females to males – using the male as the norm – were found in only six topics, including literacy, education and employment;
- The dominance of reproductive health indicators, and the absence of indicators for health-related states and human function, reflects an embodied biomedical orientation to the concept of health.

The ready availability of indicators related to socio-economic determinants of health, in contrast to the limited information about household, social, community and psycho-social factors, suggests that women's status has received far more attention than other risk or protective factors for health. As women comprise the majority of health service consumers, carers, healthcare workers and citizens (in most countries), improving indicators for monitoring health system performance is receiving insufficient attention from a gender perspective.

What other indicator frameworks are currently in use for tracking gender equity in health?

The audit of health indicators used by international organizations (see Lin et al., 2003) represents one starting point for selection of indicators to use for monitoring gender equity in health. Other frameworks exist and some are outlined below. The large number of indicators in use and the wide array of frameworks for indicators raise questions about who uses them, and whether their application in advocacy and policy-making would be improved if there was a smaller list that could be tracked over time.

Reporting-driven and international convention-driven frameworks

One approach is to respond to the requirements of gender equity reporting by making reference to international conventions. The key amongst these are:

- *The Committee on the Elimination of Discrimination against Women* (CEDAW): Countries that have ratified or acceded to CEDAW are legally bound to put its provisions into practice. They are also committed to submit national reports, at least every four years, on measures they have taken to comply with their treaty obligations. There are 114 indicators to be reported against. For small nations CEDAW reporting can be very onerous.
- The eight *Millennium Development Goals* (MDGs) – which range from halving extreme poverty to halting the spread of HIV/AIDS and providing universal primary education, all by the target date of 2015 – represent priorities agreed to by all countries and the leading development institutions and have galvanized unprecedented efforts to meet the needs of the world's poorest. Although the MDGs were promulgated five years after the mainstreaming strategy was adopted at the 1995 Beijing Conference, they do not address gender adequately, nor major issues for people in many parts of the world.

Analysis of national reports on MDGs (UNDP, 2003) concluded that gender issues were 'ghettoized' to three goals – on gender equity, maternal mortality and HIV/AIDS, all of which were within women-specific sectors. The review of progress against each individual MDG also remains gender-blind given that most statistics are not sex-disaggregated, including, for example, data on net enrolment in primary education, child mortality, prevalence of HIV/AIDS and other diseases, and environment-related data and indicators (ESCWA, 2005). Furthermore, while such reviews can identify the gender gap as one of the key challenges, indicators alone cannot analyse the root causes and, consequently, cannot address how the gender gap should be addressed in each area.

Intervention-driven frameworks

A second approach is a core list of indicators tied to health intervention possibilities. In the USA, the Institute of Medicine (IoM) proposed *Leading Health Indicators* on the basis that they cover important public health issues, are readily available and can motivate action (see Chrvala and Bulger, 1999). It is interesting to note that most indicators reflect highly gendered patterns, such as physical activity, overweight and obesity, tobacco use, substance abuse, mental health, responsible sexual behaviour, injury and violence prevention, access to care, immunizations and environmental quality.

The US *National Report Card on Women's Health* (National Women's Law Centre and Oregon Health and Science University, 2007) evaluates 34 health status indicators and 63 health policy indicators, and assesses the progress, or lack thereof, of individual states and the nation as a whole in reaching key benchmarks related to the status of women's health (Box 5.2). The *Report Card* also provides an important overview of key disparities in the health of women based on race, ethnicity, sexual orientation, disability status and other factors. Although useful in a rich nation like the USA, this approach is beyond the resources of most nations.

While most countries have a plethora of indicators, the problem is how to choose an appropriate set and whether they can feasibly be used in resource-poor environments. A pilot conducted in China in 2004 found that data on most of the 32 proposed core indicators for gender equity and health (which span health status, health determinants and health systems performance) are available from the existing information system and can be collected at low cost (Liu et al., 2006).

Theory-driven frameworks

A third approach starts with a theoretical framework about gender equity. For example:

- The *Gender-related Development Index* (GDI) is an indication of the standard of living in a country, developed by the United Nations (UN). It is one of the five indicators used by the UN Development Programme in its annual Human Development Report. It aims to show the inequities between men and women in the following areas: long and healthy life, knowledge, and a decent standard of living (UNDP, 1995).

- The *Gender Empowerment Measure* (GEM) is a measure of inequities between men's and women's opportunities in a country. It combines inequities in three areas: political participation and decision-making, economic participation and decision-making, and power over economic resources (UNDP, 1995).

These types of measures can be useful for benchmarking, but they do not necessarily point to priorities for intervention, and are unlikely to engage decision-makers in the health sector.

How can gender-sensitive health indicators be linked to decision-making?

Despite increased attention to evidence-based health policy globally (Davies et al., 2000; Lin and Gibson, 2003), there exist general political and practical challenges beyond the issue of gender equity and health. It is well recognized that researchers – as generators of evidence – and policy-makers occupy two distinct worlds and their different imperatives and styles of decision-making make linkages difficult (Choi et al., 2005). Hanney and colleagues (2002) argue that a range of strategies is required for linking researchers to decision-makers – including, amongst others, long-term liaison, knowledge brokers, evidence champions, change agendas, diffusion networks, communication training. Deliberative processes that bring together different stakeholders to consider a wide range of evidence have also been proposed (CHSRF, 2006). Within such a participatory forum scientific and decision-maker communities can come together to examine different types of evidence to make values explicit and promote consensus where possible. The US *National Report Card on Women's Health* (Box 5.2) is an illustration of this.

Based on these general considerations, there are a number of key issues to consider when using indicators to inform research, policy, legislation and programme development, raise awareness and monitor systems performance:

- the focus should be on indicators that promote action;
- the types of decisions and decision-makers need to be clear;
- indicators should be recognized as only one input into decision-making;
- indicators need to lead to or link with gender-based analysis;
- indicators must engage the broader community.

In addition, the value of good quality and conceptually sound indicators is limited if there is not an appropriate monitoring system which incorporates a participatory process for examining and making sense of gender-sensitive indicators. This suggests that the following issues are important when linking gender-sensitive indicators to decisions.

Box 5.2 The US National Report Card on Women's Health

The report cards are designed to support the work of women's health advocates and are developed by collaboration between researchers and decision-makers. Health status indicators are selected on the basis of whether they have significant impact on women's quality of life, functioning and well-being and whether they affect a large number of women generally or a large number of women in a specific population and/or age group. The policy indicators are selected in conjunction with the health indicators based on whether they can have significant positive impact and whether they are measurable and comparable across states.

Along with reports released in 2001, 2004, and 2007:

- briefings have been held in both houses of US Congress;
- data have been used by over 100 organizations to support introduction of the Family Care Act of 2001 – to provide health insurance coverage for parents of eligible children;
- Delaware and Maryland have created Offices on Women's Health in response;
- Maine has introduced legislation to increase funding for women's health initiatives;
- Oregon and Alabama state health departments have used the reports to create education materials;
- Pennsylvania legislators held a hearing on women's health;
- health insurance in Georgia created an advisory group to determine how they can better address women's health issues.

Source: National Women's Law Centre and Oregon Health and Science University, 2007.

The focus should be on indicators that promote action

The US Institute of Medicine (IoM) proposes that indicators chosen for monitoring should be ones which:

- are worth measuring as they are an important and salient aspect of the public's health;
- can be measured for diverse populations as they are valid and reliable for the general population and diverse population groups;
- are understood by people who need to act, whether on their own behalf or that of others. They should be able to readily comprehend the indicators and know what action will improve their status;

- can galvanize action at the national, state, local and community levels by individuals, organized groups, and public and private agencies;
- create actions that lead to anticipated, proven and feasible improvement (such as changes in personal behaviours, implementation of new policies, and so on) that can alter the course of the indicators when widely applied; and
- reflect results of action when measured over time showing tangible improvements in various aspects of the nation's health. (Chrvala and Bulger, 1999: 6)

Both the types of decisions and decision-makers must be clear

The nature of decisions to be taken will influence the indicators chosen. Different levels of decision-making – and different decision-makers – attempt to solve different problems. In many countries the primary care clinic and the hospital are concerned with patient-level and organizational-level decision-making. Local governments and regional health authorities make allocative decisions across the community; national governments make trade-offs between regions, sectoral issues and population groups. Thus, the evidence required by, or given to, these levels must be appropriate to the problems concerned (Lin et al., 2005). Box 5.3 illustrates how different types of information are useful at different levels and for different purposes within a federal system.

Indicators should be recognized as only one input into decision-making

Indicators can be used for all aspects of a policy cycle – from identification of the problem, to setting policy objectives, to implementing policy and evaluating policy outcomes. But it is important to recognize that the policy, programme and legislative processes do not rely on indicators alone. Surveillance and monitoring activities are only one input into evidence-based decision-making. Contextual factors such as research orientation, professional judgment and community opinions are all legitimate inputs into forming the knowledge base for decision-making – and these inputs reflect more fundamental values, expectations and cultures of communities. Furthermore, decision-makers often find that evidence is difficult to interpret, not specifically relevant to the policy being considered, not timely enough, and contradictory in relation to other expert opinions (Tranmer et al., 1998).

These contextual factors will mesh with each other in complex ways and may be the most important determinant of whether indicators will be used to inform policy-making, while the evidence plays only one part (Lin, 2008). To improve the uptake of data into decision-making requires attention be given to a range of social and organizational factors (Oldenburg et al., 1997). Dissemination efforts will need to be well-targeted, and linkage systems between data producers and users are needed to ensure adoption.

Box 5.3 Preventing domestic violence in Australia

Qualitative data was used in the 1970s and early 1980s by women's advo-cacy groups to bring the issue of domestic violence to the attention of policy-makers and decision-makers. This led to the establishment of the first services and some policy changes.

As reforms and programmes were implemented, indicators and their measurement were built at the NSW Bureau of Crime Statistics and Research (BOSCAR) and the Women's Coordination Unit worked with the police to design forms to collect useful data as part of the 'apprehended violence order' process. In 1989, BOSCAR reported that 99 per cent of individuals seeking these protection orders against a spouse or de facto spouse were women.

The Commonwealth/State Supported Assistance Program (SAAP) now funds 150 women's refuges. In 1989, twice-yearly census data were collected; data were used to formulate policies such as the 1992 National Strategy on Violence against Women.

- In 1990, the Australian Bureau of Statistics initiated a survey of victims of crime. In 1996, the ABS conducted a major Violence against Women Survey. In 1997 the Council of Australian Governments initiated Partnerships against Domestic Violence, with 12 strategies and 13 indicators.
- In 2004, the Victorian Health Promotion Foundation released a research report, *The Health Costs of Violence: Measuring the Burden of Disease Caused by Intimate Partner Violence*. Finding that nine per cent of all medical problems that beset women under 45 were caused by domestic violence, the Victorian State Government accompanied the release of the Report with a set of strategies.
- In 2009 The Australian Government released *Time for Action*, the major report of the National Council to Reduce Violence against Women and their Children, stating that the Government's position on vio-lence against women is zero tolerance. Research commissioned by the National Council had found that violence against women would cost the Australian economy around $13.6 billion this year, rising to $15.6 billion in 2021/22 if appropriate action is not taken. The implementa-tion of the Plan will take a whole-of-government approach, involving nine portfolios.

Source: National Council to Reduce Violence against Women and their Children, 2009.

Indicators need to link with gender-based analysis

Data alone are insufficient. To achieve the intended purposes of using health indicators, there is a need for an iterative and participatory process of reviewing the data, to make sense of their meaning in context. When coupled with gender-based analysis, indicators can better inform policy and programme development to improve the tailoring and targeting of health programmes and services for individuals and communities based on answering policy relevant questions such as the following: Why did this trend or pattern occur? What are the short and long-term implications for the health of women and men and for particular sub-groups? What specific policies and interventions are likely to be most effective in achieving improved health outcomes and reducing health inequalities? (see Östlin et al., 2007; Tudiver et al., 2004).

For example, health statistics revealed that aboriginal men in Australia have high mortality from chronic disease and high rates of smoking and alcohol consumption. However, they do not adopt advice from healthy lifestyle health promotion campaigns, and self-management programmes do not work. Rather than intervening on specific diseases and risk factors, a gender analysis led to the development of non-pathologizing approaches to health promotion (known as the Mibbinbah Project), through facilitated men-only discussions in worksheds as a way to reach and work with these men on the psycho-social issues and social conditions which determine their health status and health behaviour (CRCAH, 2009).

Indicators must engage the broader community

The importance of communicating the data cannot be underestimated. Data and indicators need to provide appropriate information to the target audience (such as local, trend data), be up-to-date, timely for decision-making and presented in an appropriate format (such as via geographical information systems). Data should engage a wide range of stakeholders, and be readily analysed by interested parties. Data also becomes more accessible when accompanied by people's stories, providing real-life contexts for the statistics. An effective accessible surveillance system would ensure that interested communities and civil society groups become empowered.

What are the key challenges and possible strategies in developing and using gender-sensitive health indicators?

If gender mainstreaming is to be promoted as a social policy approach for all countries, it is incumbent upon international organizations to undertake international organizational assessment. Gender equality within development organizations can be assessed not only in relation to the gender-sensitivity of their policies and programmes but also in regard to internal organizational structure, procedures, culture and human resources (Moser, 2007). In 2008, the WHO conducted a baseline assessment of the WHO Gender Monitoring and Evaluation Framework in support of the strategy – the Gender Strategy 2008–2013 – for integrating gender analysis and actions into WHO's work (WHO, 2008). This is a first step towards identifying whether there were opportunities for promoting use of sex-disaggregated data and gender analysis. Strategies for developing and using gender-sensitive health indicators should focus on improving the conceptual basis and infrastructure for gender-sensitive health indicators; building linkage mechanisms between producers and users of data; and developing an effective monitoring system.

Improving the conceptual basis and infrastructure for gender-sensitive health indicators

There is a challenge for health information systems to adopt an expanded concept of health, as administrative data collections on which indicators are often built typically do not incorporate the full range of health interventions, nor the social influences that shape health outcomes. The development of alternative data collection strategies to include the gendered reality of the health experience is, however, both costly and unlikely to be used by decision-makers in most health systems. Hence, there is a challenge about how to integrate such strategies into the mainstream.

Improving the existing health information infrastructure would entail:

- adequate and sustainable human and financial resources for additional collection, analysis and reporting;
- capacity-building mechanisms and processes at multiple levels to train and support enhanced understanding of the meaning and the action potential of gender-sensitive health indicators; and
- an ongoing process for accountability that brings together key stakeholders at various levels to review and discuss action requirements.

Mechanisms to link data producers and users

Collection and analysis of gender-sensitive data is insufficient to support the ongoing links between production and use of indicators for decision-making. Enhancing the uptake of data will require consideration of how to build on existing capacities and link local knowledge with more global research evidence. It can also challenge mindsets and power differentials while finding ways for players who respond to different incentives to stay engaged in the longer term (Blagescu and Young, 2006). A number of mechanisms are commonly advocated for reducing the gap between research and policy and these can be usefully applied to improving uptake of data about gender equity and health (Buse et al., 2005; Lin, 2003):

Table 5.1   Practical steps for improving linkages between researchers and policy-makers

Steps to be taken by researchers	Steps to be taken by policy-makers
Communicate research findings simply through newsletters, summaries, etc.	Set up advisory mechanisms to help identify priorities for gender analysis
Hold briefings, seminars and workshops for policy-makers	Monitor and benchmark programmes and budgets, and publish findings
Discuss policy implications or include policy recommendations in research	Ensure funding of strategic, priority-driven research to monitoring outcomes
Target opinion leaders for dissemination	Develop a culture of a 'learning organization' within government departments, including regular seminar programmes and sabbaticals for policy analysts
Involve policy-makers in key stages of the monitoring process	Ensure in-house units have analytical capacity, including for gender
Conduct more policy-relevant research, including more action research, evaluation research and systems research	Establish policy research institutions that have ongoing involvement in gender analysis, policy monitoring and analysis
Offer training to policy-makers on surveillance and gender analysis	Provide training for researchers on, and involve them in, policy development processes

Source: adapted from Lin (2008).

Capacity-building efforts are needed across the network of players as knowledge transfer requires a more explicit recognition that a range of individuals are likely to play different roles in that process (Thompson et al., 2006), but there can be challenges in bringing community members into apparently highly technical processes of indicator development (Hochfeld and Bassadien, 2007). There needs to be a balance between expert-led processes and an inclusive process, and between technical criteria and value-based perspectives. Participation needs to continue from indicator development through to the monitoring process.

An effective monitoring system

For gender-sensitive health indicators to be influential, there is a need to build systems for monitoring and information uptake. The optimal structure and process of monitoring systems should have the following features (based on WHO Kobe Centre, 2003):

- *Relevance*: link with governance processes, including with other reporting and monitoring systems, for example CEDAW and MDGs at the international level; and link with and contribute to health system development and health sector reform processes through indicator development and analysis which addresses key policy concerns and potential for action.

- *Efficient data collection*: build on existing systems for data collection and indicators proposed through key international consensus and reporting frameworks, such as the *World Health Report*, the *Human Development Report* and *The State of the World's Children*; work on both improving specificity of national reporting and harmonizing of regional data systems (through common data definitions and standards); and use proxy indicators when collecting additional data is not feasible.
- *Effective reporting*: a regular reporting time-frame, for example not less than two years, with an accessible, appealing, user-friendly reporting style that engages stakeholders; offer specificity, including, where possible, sex, ethnicity, age, socio-economic status, and highlight action potential; provide quantitative and qualitative indicators and analyses which enable local contexts to be taken into account in the reporting system while using benchmarks for performance monitoring where possible; enable analysis and reporting of trend data on core sets of indicators, and by appropriate peer groupings for comparative performance assessment.

Conclusion

In this age of evidence-based policy formulation and performance measurement, the time has come for mainstream health systems to act in a concerted way to engender the indicators they use. Routine reporting by international organizations has offered little to enable monitoring of gender equity and health. Current information systems and infrastructure continue to perpetuate existing foci for data collection and reporting. Women's health advocates have, therefore, offered a plethora of alternative frameworks (see also Chapter 24 by Armstrong). Yet the strengths of currently used indicators, especially those using international standards, lie in their histories of use as comparative data to assess trends over time and across different countries. There is, thus, clearly a need to improve the adequacy of current indicators as well as to develop new types of indicators. The challenge is to retain comparability while developing standard indicators that provide more complex information including gender-sensitive and equity-sensitive perspectives.

If gender is ever to be at the heart of health policy and practice then a small set of gender-sensitive indicators needs to be agreed to, and used consistently, by international organizations and nations. This would provide the most cost-effective system by building on the existing infrastructure for data collection and analysis, as well as linking with mainstream policy and management decision-making. Indicators do not speak for themselves. They need to be interpreted, understood and acted upon. Gender integration needs to be strengthened in both the implementation and monitoring/evaluation phases of the planning and programme cycle. This includes the use of gender-sensitive indicators with sex-disaggregated data leading to or linked with gender analysis. A social process of monitoring is essential.

Summary

- Gender-sensitive indicators can alert governments and the public to policy and programme successes and failures, and are most effective when linked to gender analysis.
- There is a need to develop gender-sensitive health indicators which go beyond the reproductive health of women, and more attention needs to be paid to men's health.
- If gender-sensitive indicators are to be useful for decision-making, a small, manageable set of gender-sensitive indicators needs to be agreed upon that assesses health system performance and key social influences on health.

Key reading

Lin, V., S. Gruszin, C. Ellickson, J. Glover, K. Silburn, G. Wilson and C. Poljski (2007) 'Comparative Evaluation of Indicators for Gender Equity and Health', *International Journal of Public Health*, 52 (Supplement 1), S19–S26.

Mehra, R. and G. Gupta (2006) *Gender Mainstreaming: Making it Happen* (Washington, DC: International Center for Research on Women).

Williams, S., J. Seed and A. Mwau (1994) *The Oxfam Gender Training Manual* (Oxford: Oxfam Publishing).

References

Abdool, S. and B. Vissandjée (2001) *An Inventory of Conceptual Frameworks and Women's Health Indicators* (Montreal: Centre of Excellence for Women's Health).

AbouZahr, C. and J. Vaughn (2000) 'Assessing the Burden of Sexual and Reproductive Ill-Health: Questions Regarding the Use Of Disability-adjusted Life Years', *Bulletin of the World Health Organization*, 78, 655–66.

Austen, S., T. Jefferson and A. Preston (2000) *The Challenges of Defining and Measuring Women's Social and Economic Progress* (Perth: Women's Economic Policy Analysis Unit, Curtin University of Technology).

Beck, T. (1999) *Using Gender-sensitive Indicators: A Reference Manual for Governments and Other Stakeholders* (London: Commonwealth Secretariat).

Blagescu, M. and J. Young (2006) *Capacity Development for Policy Advocacy: Current Thinking and Approaches among Agencies Supporting Civil Society Organisations*, Working Paper 260 (London: Overseas Development Institute).

Buse, K., N. Mays and G. Walt (2005) *Making Health Policy* (Maidenhead: Open University Press).

Choi, B.C.K., T. Pang, V. Lin, P. Puska, G. Sherman, M. Goddard, M. J. Ackland, P. Sainsbury et al. (2005) 'Can Scientists and Policy-Makers Work Together?', *Journal of Epidemiology and Community Health*, 19 (8), 632–7.

Chrvala, C. and R. Bulger (1999) *Leading Health Indicators for Healthy People 2010*, Final Report (Washington, DC: Institute of Medicine).

CHSRF – Canadian Health Services Research Foundation (2006) *Weighing Up the Evidence: Making Evidence-informed Guidance Accurate, Achievable, and Acceptable* (Ottawa: Canadian Health Services Research Foundation).

Coleman, R. (2003) *A Profile of Women's Health Indicators in Canada*, prepared for the Women's Health Bureau (Ottawa: Health Canada).

Courtright, P. (2008) 'Gender and Blindness Introduction. Women Bear 2/3 of the World's Blindness. What Can We Do?', at: www.kcco.net/gendblindintro.html, accessed 17 August 2009.

CRCAH – Cooperative Research Centre for Aboriginal Health (2009), at: www.crcah.org.au/research_progam_areas/downloads/114185_mccoyFactSheet-0308.pdf, accessed 28 August 2009.

Davies, H., S. Nutley and P. Smith (2000) *What Works? Evidence-based Policy and Practice in Public Service* (Bristol: Policy Press).

Eckermann, L. (2000) 'Gendering Indicators of Health and Well-Being: Is Quality of Life Gender Neutral?', *Social Indicator Research*, 52 (1), 29–54.

ECOSOC – United Nations Economic and Social Council (2006) Council Resolution 2006/36.

ESCWA (2005) *Millennium Development Goals in the Arab region*, at: www.escwa.un.org/information/meetings/editor/Download.asp?table_name=eventDetails&field_name=id&FileID=1335, accessed 28 August 2009.

Evans, T., M. Whitehead, F. Diderichsen, A. Bhuiya and M. Wirth (2001) *Challenging Inequities in Health: From Ethics to Action* (New York: Oxford University Press).

Hanney, S., M. Gonzalez-Block, M. Buxton and M. Kogan (2002) *The Utilisation of Health Research in Policy-making: Concepts, Examples, and Methods of Assessment* (Geneva: WHO).

Hochfeld, T. and S. R. Bassadien (2007) 'Participation, Values and Implementation: Three Research Challenges in Developing Gender-sensitive Indicators', *Gender and Development*, 15 (2), 217–30.

Lin, V. (2003) 'Improving the Research and Policy Partnership: An Agenda for Research Transfer and Governance', in V. Lin and D. Gibson (eds), *Evidence-based Health Policy: Problems and Possibilities* (South Melbourne: Oxford University Press), 285–97.

Lin, V. (2008) 'Evidence-based Public Health Policy', in K. Heggenhougen and S. Quah (eds), *International Encyclopedia of Public Health* (San Diego: Academic Press), 527–36.

Lin, V. and B. Gibson (eds) (2003) *Evidence-based Health Policy: Problems and Possibilities* (South Melbourne: Oxford University Press).

Lin, V., H. L'Orange and K. Silburn (2005) *Developing Gender-sensitive Indicators: Relevance and Uses*, Bureau for Gender Analysis and Women's Health (Ottawa: Health Canada).

Lin, V., S. Gruszin, C. Ellickson, J. Glover, K. Silburn, G. Wilson and C. Poljski (2007a) 'Comparative Evaluation of Indicators for Gender Equity and Health', *International Journal of Public Health*, 52 (Supplement 1), S19–S26.

Lin, V., H. L'Orange and K. Silburn (2007b) 'Gender-sensitive Indicators: Uses and Relevance', *International Journal of Public Health*, 52 (Supplement 1), S27–S34.

Liu, Y., L. Zhang, Z. Zhang and R. Pang (2006) *Piloting Proposed Core Gender-sensitive Health Indicators – Experience in China* (Beijing: Foreign Loan Office, Ministry of Health).

Moser, A. (2007) *Gender and Indicators* (Sussex University: Institute for Development Studies).

National Council to Reduce Violence against Women and their Children (2009) *Time for Action: The National Council's Plan for Australia to Reduce Violence against Women and their Children, 2009–2021* (Canberra: Commonwealth of Australia).

National Women's Law Centre and Oregon Health and Science University (2007) *National Report Card on Women's Health,* at: http://hrc.nwlc.org, accessed 17 August 2009.

Oldenburg, B., M. O'Connor, M. French and E. Parker (1997) *The Dissemination Effort in Australia: Strengthening the Links between Health Promotion Research and Practice* (Canberra: Australian Government Publishing Service).

Östlin, P., E. Eckermann, U. S. Mishra, M. Nkowane and E. Wallstam (2007) 'Gender and Health Promotion: A Multisectoral Policy Approach', *Health Promotion International,* 21 (S1), 25–35.

Sen, G., P. Östlin and A. George (2007) *Unequal, Unfair, Ineffective and Inefficient. Gender Inequality in Health Care: Why It Exists and How We Can Change It,* Final Report to the WHO Commission on Social Determinants of Health, at: www.eurohealth.ie/pdf/WGEKN_FINAL_REPORT.pdf, accessed 15 May 2009.

Thompson, G., C. Estabrooks and L. Degner (2006) 'Clarifying the Concepts in Knowledge Transfer: A Literature Review', *Journal of Advanced Nursing,* 53 (6), 691–701.

Tranmer, J., S. Squires, K. Brazil, J. Gerlach, J. Johnson, D. Muisiner, B. Swan and R. Wilson (1998) 'Factors that Influence Evidence-based Decision-Making', in Canada Health Action (ed.), *Building on the Legacy,* Evidence and Information, Volume 5 (Ottawa: Editions MultiMondes), 19–91.

Tudiver, S., M. Kantiebo, J. Kammermayer and M. Mavrak (2004) 'Women's Health Surveillance: Implications for Policy', *BMC Women's Health,* 4 (Supplement 1), S31.

UNDP – United Nations Development Programme (1995) *Human Development Report* (New York: UNDP).

UNDP – United Nations Development Programme (2003) *MDGs: National Reports – A Look Through a Gender Lens* (New York: UNDP).

UNIFEM – United Nations Development Fund for Women (2000) *Progress of the World's Women* (New York: UNIFEM).

UNIFEM – United Nations Development Fund for Women (2008) *Making the MDGs Work for All* (New York: UNIFEM).

WHO (2008) *Gender Strategy 2008–2013: Integrating Gender Analysis and Actions into WHO's Work* (Geneva: WHO).

WHO Kobe Centre (2003) *Report of the Expert Working Group on Gender-sensitive Leading Health Indicators* (Kobe: WHO Centre for Health and Development), at: www.who.or.jp/library/cm_report.pdf, accessed 15 May 2009.

6
Gender Assessment: European Health Research Policies

Ineke Klinge

Introduction

In the late 1980s concerns were raised in the United States that by conducting research mainly on white young men biomedical and health research was not adequately meeting the needs of women and for that matter of the elderly, children and persons from ethnic minorities. At this time insights emerged that the one-size 'male norm' in health research did not fit all people. Researchers thus started to realize that sex differences and gender effects were crucial in health research. An overview produced for the Canadian Institutes of Health Research lists the initiatives that have been implemented subsequently to promote or support research to take account of gender and sex differences (Caron, 2003; see also Chapter 24 by Armstrong). This includes initiatives in the USA taken by the National Institutes of Health (NIH) and the Food and Drug Administration (FDA) as well as initiatives in Canada and European countries. In the USA, NIH guidelines required the inclusion of women and (ethnic) minorities in clinical research (NIH, 1994). In 1993 the FDA had recommended that clinical studies should include enough men and women to detect clinically significant sex differences in drug efficacy and safety, and that sex differences should be reported.

With a focus on biomedical research, this chapter will describe developments in Europe and in particular highlight the health research policy of the European Commission (EC) as implemented in consecutive Framework Programmes for Research and Development. The Framework Programmes are the most important policy platform and the biggest source of funding for EU research and increasingly also set the agenda in the member states. As 'think tanks' the Framework Programmes are highly relevant when it comes to gender policies in science (see, for example, European Commission, 2001; 2004). This chapter asks the important question: What has the EC done to guarantee that the health research it funds aims to address adequately the health needs of both men and women? After having introduced the EC gender equality policy for research and its accomplishments, the chapter will use illustrative case studies to provide an up-to-date insight into what new research data have been produced by sex- and gender-sensitive research designs; the examples used here are selected from research carried out by the author and other colleagues (see, for example, Klinge, 2007a; 2007b). The subsequent section deals with further developments in EC gender equality policy for research focusing on the most recent Framework Programme (FP7). Finally, challenges and opportunities of making sex and gender central to healthcare are discussed.

EU gender equality policy for research

An important innovation in European health policy was the translation of the EU gender equality policy, enshrined in consecutive treaties, to research. The Communication *Women and Science: Mobilising Women to Enrich European Research,* issued by the European Commission in 1999, had placed the 'gender and science' issue on the research agenda (European Commission, 1999). The Communication acknowledged the severe underrepresentation of women in science and, more importantly, defined the policy task of promoting gender equality in terms of three dimensions seen as characteristic of the relationship between gender and science: science *by, for* and *about* women. Thus a distinguishing feature of this gender equality policy for research was that it was aimed at addressing two issues: first, the participation of women in research at all levels and second, the contents of research.

Gender impact-assessment studies

The Framework Programmes for Research and Technological Development are multi-annual programmes describing the research priorities for European Research for the associated years. The Programme as a whole is made up from various research domains called thematic priorities or themes. The first steps towards the innovation of EU health research policy were the Gender Impact Assessment Studies of FP5 launched by the EC in 2000 (European Commission, 2001; see Klinge and Bosch, 2001; 2005). The 'by, for and about' motto was to guide the analysis and seven teams were charged with a gender assessment of the implementation of FP5. The analysis aimed to investigate the participation of women in FP5 research at all levels and to explore whether the research themes, methods and issues that are prioritized affect women and men differently. Using two newly developed methodological instruments – a Gender Impact Resource (based on international literature) and a Gender Impact Assessment Protocol – the results of our Gender Impact Assessment demonstrate that the attention paid to sex and gender in the work programmes and, as a consequence of this, in the funded research, turned out to be fairly limited (Klinge and Bosch, 2001). In particular, the composition of research populations was often not argued for, which might have led to underrepresentation of women and to taking males as the norm. Similarly, data collection methods were not proven to be suitable for women and men. Data were often not disaggregated according to sex. Projects appeared to possess little awareness of how the outcome of a research project could differentially affect men and women. In short, 'the evaporation of gender was evident' (European Commission, 2001: 25). Thus the recommendations developed in the Gender Impact Assessment Study of the Life Sciences Research Programme became the basis for the new guidelines for applicants to FP6 in the health field (Klinge and Bosch, 2005).

New guidelines for FP6

With FP6, the motto of 'by, for and about' women of the EU gender equality policy was changed into a new 'formula', summarized as GE = WP + GD (European Commission, 2003). The idea expressed in this formula is that the promotion of gender equality (GE) concerns two issues: first, the stimulation of women's participation in research at all levels (WP), and second, the consideration of the gender dimension of the research content (GD). For the domain of biomedicine and health, it was obvious that the gender dimension should be understood as considering the impact of biological sex differences as well as the possible effects of social gender in biomedical and health research. The possibility of gender/sex differences must therefore be considered in all areas of health research, unless it can be demonstrated that gender/sex is inappropriate, with respect to the health of the subjects or the objectives of the research. Gender/sex issues should now be considered in:

- the formulation of research hypotheses, the development of research protocols, choice of research methodologies and analysis of results;
- biological pre-clinical and epidemiological behavioural research/studies on both human and animal subjects;
- the use of cells, tissue and other specimens, where appropriate; and
- the choice for a particular study population should be thoroughly justified and the sex of the participants described in full (for details, see European Commission, 2003).

These aspects were taken into account in the process of evaluating applications to FP6. As a special condition for submitting proposals, large collaborative projects had to write a so-called Gender Action Plan (GAP) as part of the project, describing the measures the consortium (comprising all partners in a particular project) would take to pay attention to women's participation in the projects (WP) and how to consider sex and gender aspects in research (GD).

A need for practical tools

Attention to sex and gender had become firmly inscribed in important EC documents as the work programme and guide for FP6 research applicants. However, it was not difficult to imagine that the research community would face a number of challenges of various types – conceptual, methodological, practical and ethical – to integrate sex and gender into their research and that they might need practical tools and relevant examples. This was the aim of the GenderBasic project, which was funded by the EC in 2005 and ran until 2008 (for details, see Klinge, 2008).

The main steps of this project and methodological issues addressed were as follows. First, investigators of selected running FP6 projects were interviewed to explore problems or challenges they encountered in executing the compulsory Gender Action Plan. Second, knowledgeable researchers at high-level life sciences European Research Institutes were interviewed on (possibly) existing institutional policies regarding the integration of sex and gender aspects into research. This part of the project aimed at exploring how institutes outside the realm of EU research policy would practice the integration of sex and gender. A major activity of the project was the commissioning of review articles on the various methodological aspects of integrating sex and gender into various types of biomedical and health research (basic, translational, clinical and public health). Basic research is research 'at the bench' in which scientists study disease at a molecular or cellular level. Translational research transforms scientific discoveries arising from laboratory studies into clinical applications 'at the bedside'. Reviews were also commissioned on health conditions that were in urgent need of addressing in terms of sex and gender aspects, such as, for instance, asthma, metabolic syndrome, nutrigenomics, osteoporosis, anxiety disorders and work-related health. High-level scientists were invited to write state-of-the-art reviews and to offer solutions for methodological challenges. Comments on these reviews were solicited from peers and the results were discussed in a workshop which included the review authors, referees and selected stakeholders (they were subsequently published in a special issue of the journal *Gender Medicine*; see Klinge, 2007b).

During this workshop, the practical examples on the relevance and explanatory power of gender served as an eye-opener, especially for biomedical researchers. Especially, the conceptual distinction of gender from biological sex was welcomed, since the majority had become 'socialized' by biomedicine to use the terms sex and gender interchangeably, which leads to unwanted confusion, as is visible in much biomedical literature. Despite many efforts by important institutional actors, such as the US Institute of Medicine (IoM), WHO and Health Canada, to 'educate' basic and biomedical researchers on the distinction between sex and gender, this has still not become standard practice.

The achievements of the GenderBasic project were threefold: it stimulated research into: 1) sex differences; 2) the workings, mechanisms and effects of gender in particular for understanding masculinity and male gender roles and their effects on individual health; and 3) the interaction of sex and gender (Klinge, 2007b). The following section provides an illustration of the innovative potential of this approach.

'Male' and 'female' diseases: the problematic gender bias in healthcare

Two conditions in which sex and gender differences are highly relevant have become widely known and have triggered many detailed studies; namely; cardiovascular disease and osteoporosis, which are commonly known as 'male' and 'female' diseases respectively. Cardiovascular disease (also often defined as coronary heart disease, CHD) was for a long time known as a 'male disease' affecting middle-aged men in stressful jobs (for details, see Chapter 10 by Riska on CHD). However, sex differences exist in the kind of symptoms experienced. Whereas men most often experience a crushing pain in their chest, women more often experience nausea and back pain (for details, visit, for instance, www.genderandhealth.ca). Taken together with the labelling of CHD as a 'male disease' and gender effects in communication patterns between doctors and patients, women historically have been under-diagnosed and under-treated. This under-treatment has become known as the 'Yentl Syndrome', meaning that a woman has to masquerade as a man in order to get the same attention from medical professionals (Healy, 1991). Several authors have singled out the various sex differences and gender effects at diagnosis and treatment, and extensive campaigns have also been launched in primary care settings to redress the existing situation.

Osteoporosis represents the opposite of the case of cardiovascular disease. Here, it is men who have been neglected in research and under-diagnosed in primary care, a phenomenon often called 'candidacy' in the literature (White, 2008: 5). The principle behind the idea of candidacy is that public and health professionals alike come to see an illness or health problem as being particularly likely to occur within one population group and, therefore, a person outside of that segment of society would not be considered a likely candidate. In the case of osteoporosis the likely candidate is an older woman, but now we recognize that men are at much greater risk than was previously thought (White, 2008). In addition, Geusens and Dinant (2007) have reviewed relevant sex differences in osteoporosis related to sex hormones. Still today there exist more screening opportunities for women; older men, who live alone and lack social support, face more implications for recovery from fractures.

How sex and gender matter on different levels of health research

The following cases highlight the potential of the tools for sex- and gender-sensitive approaches on different levels of research, including animal, clinical and public health research – and also illustrate the different ways sex and gender matter. The examples are selected from the GenderBasic project (Klinge, 2007b).

Animal models

A first example concerns basic or pre-clinical research, a level where sex and gender aspects only recently have attracted research interest. Holdcroft (2007) points, first of all, to the relevance of very small differences between the sexes that may, however, produce clinical treatment effects as a consequence of additive or synergistic effects and therefore have to be investigated. Several current obstacles prohibit discovering small differences; for example, oestrogen effects are levelled out due to variability in the hormonal cycle among females and in consequence are lost. Holdcroft (2007) argues that sex hormones, level of oestrogens and the menstrual cycle are complex to consider, yet may be active in multiple ways and should be taken into account. Current research hardly considers the importance of progesterone or other neurosteroids that vary during the oestrus cycle, and levels of testosterone are not measured at all. Thus, animal models are needed that are adequate for studying human disease; the current models cannot consider co-morbidity, age-related changes or use of contraceptives.

Existing research suggests two things: first, the need to record the age and weight of male and female animals and, for females, to determine their reproductive status and ovarian cycle phase as accurately as possible; and second, to determine the sex of origin of biological research materials and to disclose it on publication (Holdcroft, 2007). Although most people would agree that socio-cultural gender effects are not at stake at the level of animal research, Franconi (2007) has drawn attention to several environmental effects that are relevant to consider. She argues that social interactions and environment are relevant for laboratory animals, and thus may have important consequences in pre-clinical research. She points to early-life social interactions such as diet, mother-pup interaction and neonatal handling that affect males and females differently. Furthermore, life experiences, such as pregnancy and lactation, should be studied in pharmacological research, and an animal model is needed that is similar to humans and includes oral contraceptive use (Franconi, 2007).

Asthma and food allergy

Asthma is a complex disease and the relative influence of genetic, hormonal, social and cultural factors remains to be studied. It is a chronic inflammatory airway disease that has a higher prevalence in boys than in girls before puberty and a higher prevalence in women than in men in adulthood. Postma (2007) highlights several sex differences and various gender effects. To begin with, sex differences in the development of the pulmonary system are visible in utero. It has been demonstrated that the lungs of the female foetus mature more rapidly than those of the male foetus and surfactant production in female foetuses also starts earlier compared to male foetuses. Taken together, the results imply that female newborns have increased airflow rates compared with male newborns and are less likely to develop respiratory distress syndrome. Hormonal changes and genetic susceptibility are likely to contribute to the change in prevalence around puberty.

The role of gender is also visible. In parental reporting about symptoms of their sons and daughters, it has been described that boys' symptoms are more often reported and that more boys receive treatment. The consequences of this bias affect recruitment to research studies and clinical data. Thus a possible under-diagnosis may exist in girls, especially in low-income groups. Bias in diagnosis by physicians is also described: adult women are diagnosed with asthma, men with chronic obstructive pulmonary disease (COPD). Postma (2007) hypothesizes that men and women may respond differently to treatments due to biological, environmental and social influences. Furthermore, gender identity and gender role socialization are also important in therapy compliance. Williams (2000) demonstrates how peer pressure causes boys to hide their asthma from peers, thus restricting their use of inhalants when in company; by contrast, girls incorporate their asthma in their social circle and thus show better therapy compliance. Postma (2007) concludes that the relative contribution of genetic disposition, hormonal influences and social environment (gender role behaviour) in asthma is under-researched. Future topics to be studied are possible differences in breastfeeding of boys versus girls and in smoking behaviour of the mother or father affecting the child, and the role of differences between boys and girls in outdoor play.

Similar sex and gender effects have been demonstrated in food allergy research. Food allergy is an adverse immunological reaction that may be due to IgE or non-IgE-mediated immune mechanisms accompanied by serious symptoms, the worst of it being an anaphylactic shock that may cause death. Gender effects have to be considered with respect to parental reporting on how a child's food allergy affects the quality of life. Here, mothers and fathers may differ in their perception of risk, and consequently the answers given in questionnaires may be different (DunnGalvin et al., 2006).

Anxiety disorders

Anxiety disorders fall in the area of mental health, a domain where gender issues have long been recognized (see Chapter 11 by Busfield). Anxiety disorders are more prevalent among women than among men overall, for subtypes, across lifetime and over various countries, and are independent of specific healthcare settings. Also, co-morbidity is higher in women and symptoms of anxiety more severe compared to men (Bekker and van Mens-Verhulst, 2007). Women are 'allowed' by society to show fear and anxiety, while masculinity is not compatible with showing emotions. As a consequence, men internalize fear which then may erupt in (domestic) violence and suicide. Bekker and van Mens-Verhulst (2007) identify various different aetiological models underlying anxiety disorders in the literature, namely genetic differences (neurotransmitters), physiological differences (hormones and cortisol secretions), classical and operant conditioning paradigms, social role expectations, and differences between men and women in environmental exposures to stimuli.

Bekker and van Mens-Verhulst (2007) also discuss three theories to explain prevalence data – learning theory, a sex/gender role perspective and attachment and schema theory – and examined the degree of attention paid to gender by each theory. The findings reveal that gender role socialization is of influence in three areas: 1) self-reporting and lower willingness to report in men; help-seeking behaviour was lower in men; 2) higher use of anxiety-reducing drugs in women and alcohol in men; and 3) more difficulties in avoiding behaviour for men with agoraphobia compared to women, as traditional gender roles have assigned the outside world as the work domain of men, but the home as a woman's world of work.

Bekker and van Mens-Verhulst (2007) conclude that widespread attention has been paid to differences between men and women in the prevalence of anxiety disorders and their possible origins, but that scant attention has been given to these differences in terms of treatment. Of special concern is the fact that mental health research is conducted using instruments that are susceptible to gender effects, such as self-report questionnaires and surveys. An example is the under-reporting of health complaints by men as influenced by gender role prescriptions to be strong (see also Chapter 14 by Hunt et al.). Another problem is conceptual complexity; differences in reporting health are embedded in a cultural context of gendered notions and gender 'mandates' for women and men. Here, a synoptic model is suggested that reviews determinants in five dimensions: body, gender, differential diagnostics, male–female differences in exposure, and person-related vulnerability factors. This model links to an interdisciplinary approach into sex and gender factors in anxiety disorders, including genetic, neurobiological and bioenvironmental factors (Bekker and van Mens-Verhulst, 2007).

A further example is depression, which has been studied extensively by gender researchers and has also inspired basic researchers. Here, too, sex and gender are relevant in different ways and on different levels; to name only a few results, under-diagnosis in men, due to the traditional masculine gender role to tough it out (Branney and White, 2008); diagnostic bias, as the dominant symptoms investigated seem to reflect feminine behaviour patterns, leading to under-recognition of symptoms mentioned by men (Noordenbos, 2007); and the possibility – based on research in rats – that there perhaps exist two types of depression, dependent on involvement of different neurological pathways in males and females (Kozicz, 2007).

Nutrigenomics

Nutrigenomics is a research field aimed at the health of the entire popula-tion and research into sex differences in genetic polymorphisms is a relatively new area. Ordovas (2007) highlights the interplay between sex, genes and disease susceptibility that is even more complicated by intersections with environmental and behavioural factors, such as dietary habits, smoking and alcohol consumption; together, these factors modulate the balance between health and disease. This complexity underlies the poor replication obtained for most candidate gene association studies examining common diseases and their predisposing factors. Recent research into cardiovascular disease and obesity sheds light on the role of sex and gender within these complex relationships (Ordovas, 2007). Some firmly established research data on polymorphisms of apolipoprotein E (APOE) – involved in lipid metabolism and risk for cardio-vascular disease – and perilipin (PLIN) – involved in obesity risk – support the role of sex-specific polymorphisms in the differential response to environmental factors. Regarding the relationship between PLIN haplotypes and obesity, risk differences were demonstrated *within* the group of women; by studying this relationship in Chinese, Malay and Asian Indian groups, the PLIN locus turned out to be an ethnic-dependent modulator of obesity risk in humans.

A better understanding of the mechanisms involved in energy metabolism, especially in fat metabolism, is vital to providing better therapeutic tools for the control of obesity at both the personal and population level. Put in simple words: establishing someone's genetic profile concerning the polymorphisms involved may be used as a tool to predict whether a particular dietary inter-vention will be effective; for example, a diet containing a high amount of unsaturated fatty acids or a low-energy diet. Ordovas (2007) argues that a better understanding and greater recognition of the significance of specific disease-associated genetic polymorphisms in the context of sex is of critical public health and clinical importance. Important gender effects in nutrigenomics concern the dietary questionnaire, a widely used instrument in population studies. It remains to be determined whether the validity of such questionnaires is similar for men and women. Should men or women provide less reliable information, this would be an important confounder for the outcome of these studies. Also, differences between women and men in dietary compliance and adherence to dietary recommendations remain to be studied; this is also true for differences in exercise, smoking and alcohol intake as effects of gender influencing gene–diet interactions.

Mainstreaming gender equality in EU health research

The adoption of the policy strategy of mainstreaming gender equality marks a fundamental step and prerequisite for innovating EU health research. However, implementing this in health research policy has been neither smooth nor easy. Notwithstanding serious efforts made, and results obtained by individual actors, mainstreaming gender equality in EU health research policy and practice as dealt with in consecutive Framework Programmes has met various barriers. The ambitious Gender Action Plans of FP6 have not fulfilled the high expectations. Monitoring studies demanded by the Commission for all thematic priorities report a number of problems encountered by individual research consortia (European Commission, 2008a; 2008b; Expert Group, 2009). The concept 'gender dimension' was poorly understood and interpreted in different ways. The monitoring studies show that measures taken and efforts made by individual consortia focused primarily on promoting women's participation by various means among which mentoring was especially popular. The Commission's Science and Society Report states, 'gender issues are weakly addressed across all priorities' (European Commission, 2007: 35), and highlights some reasons for this:

> ... as well as a poor understanding of the concept (the gender dimension) and practical ways of integrating gender aspects in research, there are some indications that there is a lack of willingness to address it. Some projects automatically dismiss the relevance of gender to the research topic or instrument used, without analysis of whether it might be relevant. (European Commission, 2007; 36)

Research further highlights that addressing sex and gender issues with respect to the *content* of research was especially problematic (Klinge, 2008). Amongst other things, execution of the Gender Action Plan was often allocated to a person not knowledgeable on gender issues as an 'add-on' task and without a specific budget. Only occasionally was the message about the relevance and possible influence of sex and gender taken on board; a positive example is the state-of-the-art review on sex and gender factors in food allergy research (DunnGalvin et al., 2006). We can learn from this experience about the importance of considering the integration of sex and gender aspects right from the inception of a research project and not as an extra 'requirement' and of the responsibility of the research coordinator in order to comply with the policy aims of the Commission. Also, appropriate integration of sex and gender in research implies an early incorporation into the design of a project, in the framing of hypotheses, choice of research population, methods and instruments to be used, ways of analysis and so on, by those who will actually carry out the research. It remains to be seen as to whether and how the most recent EU training programmes (Toolkit Gender in EU-funded research) for gender sensitivity impact in future research.

Different research paradigms

This chapter has focused to a large extent on biomedical research. Public health research has been much less addressed. Yet it is interesting to consider both research domains and the respective research focus – biomedical factors versus socio-cultural factors – as well as the priorities and differences between the two underlying discussions in the literature on whether attention to sex differences in biomedical research is 'a good thing to do'. Contributions to this debate have been made by various institutional actors and researchers. From the perspective of wanting to abolish the 'white male norm' in biomedical research, attention to sex differences is a 'good thing'. Indeed, a 'sexy' wave of interest in studying sex differences has emerged, although the term 'gender differences' is still used in publications. However, critical points have also been put forward.

Epstein (2007) questions the 'inclusion paradigm' of, among others, the US National Institutes of Health to include women and minorities in clinical research. He argues that a focus on sex *differences* may lead to dangerously inaccurate understandings of the causes of health disparities. Following these arguments the direct relationship between social class and health status can be obscured by a focus on bodily differences, that is: sex differences. Epstein points to the limits of biological explanations for health disparities between men and women, with longevity (higher in women) as an important example. Thus it is not biology but social factors that may fuel the differences between men and women.

Within the aim of public health policies to target health inequalities, Epstein identifies two styles or genres: first, talking about *disparities*, which implies talking about social injustice and a call for its elimination; and second, talking about *differences*, which implies a more neutral understanding whereby differences should be recognized, addressed and so on. He warns of the risk of interpreting disparities as differences and illustrates this by an example from molecular genetic research in toxicology. According to Epstein, causes for ill-health used to be looked for and found in the environment, in living conditions, such as, for example, living in neighbourhoods close to polluting industry. Nowadays causes are often looked for in genetic susceptibility. Here, the problem is that the individual gets blamed and genes are made responsible, and in turn, attention to environmental factors disappears while living in a polluted area is made your own responsibility. Therefore Epstein concludes that the question is not *whether* to study sex differences but *how* to study them. Consequently, a medical policy of inclusion, including studying sex, can only achieve its intended effects if it is connected to a complex approach towards health disparities.

The issue of how to address biological processes, including sex differences, has also raised debates within gender studies (see, for example, Clarke and Olesen, 1998). Feminist biologists, in particular, have expressed their concerns in this respect. They have questioned the lack of attention given to processes inside the body in many gender theories as well as in social science studies of the body. Of particular interest is the work of Lynda Birke and of Anne Fausto-Sterling. Birke (1999: 2; see also 153–6) states that 'feminist theory is only skin deep'. She firmly rejects biological determinism but argues the need for more contextual ways of describing and explaining biological processes and the development of interactive models of causality. Fausto-Sterling expresses a similar drive. She introduces a developmental systems theory highlighting that:

> ... instead of setting nature against nurture we reject the search for root causes and substitute a more complex analysis in which an individual's capacities emerge from a web of mutual interactions between the biological being and the social environment. (2003: 123)

In summary, more critical approaches to the inclusion of sex differences into biomedical research highlight that the most interesting area of research is not the study of differences per se but the study of how differences develop.

Conclusion

This chapter has explored the challenges and opportunities of making sex and gender central to health and healthcare, especially looking at European health research policies and biomedicine. I have introduced the concept of gender assessment and explored the related practical tools for implementation. Within this context I have also highlighted some problems with understanding sex and gender aspects in medicine and the critical connections between sex differences and gender effects. The case studies presented here clearly highlight the need for mainstreaming gender into biomedical and health research. Furthermore, and most importantly, the examples direct our attention towards the need for more complex approaches that take into account biological and social factors of health at all levels of research, from animal models and genetics to issues of public health.

Sex- and gender-sensitive biomedical and health research has ethical and social implications. Increasing the quality and quantity of evidence of the influence that sex and gender have on health outcomes and healthcare will add to better medical care at an individual level. By considering sex and gender, healthcare policies will become more effective in ensuring gender equity in the health of populations. However, the example of European health research policy has also highlighted that this is not an easy mission and gender policies face several different hurdles when applied to practice. In closing, I would like to highlight some specific current challenges and opportunities for medical and healthcare research into sex and gender factors.

Challenges

Shifting policy frames: The change from FP6 to FP7 entailed a major restructuring of the Programme for Research and Technological Development. A new part called IDEAS was added to the Programme. Proposals within this part of the Programme are evaluated based on 'excellence only' criteria, secured by the newly created European Research Council. Other criteria, in particular the 'horizontal requirements', including gender equality actions, are not compulsory in this part. Consequently, the requirement to take account of sex and gender issues that had been raised in FP6 evaporated in the IDEAS part of FP7. Such shifts over time in policy frames are also visible in a change in focus from sex and gender to ethnicity, and then to youth. Shifting the focus is perhaps part of a policy's life cycle, but if not evaluated properly before jumping to a new focus, this runs the risk of losing sight of valuable commitments, in this case to mainstreaming gender equality.

Individual level versus population level: Debating the one best approach to improve health is not fruitful. Instead, research strategies incorporating sex and gender in various fields – basic research, clinical care and public health – are the most innovative. Of course the central focus will vary; for example, in basic molecular research, sex differences in genetic polymorphisms will get more attention than in studies on help-seeking behaviour for depression. However, the core message should be that the eventual health outcome will always be dependent on the interaction between sex and gender – and for that matter between other dimensions of difference.

Opportunities

Pioneering research: Sex- and gender-sensitive research is attractive to newcomers, among them early researchers and women professionals, because of its pioneering character.

Higher ethical standards and accountability of professionals: Equity issues and the connected attention to sex and gender aspects in research may be linked to an overall trend towards improving ethical standards and accountability of professionals in healthcare.

Reform of curricula: An ongoing reform has started in Europe at various locations aiming at the incorporation of new sex- and gender-sensitive knowledge into biomedical curricula (see also Chapter 24 by Lagro-Janssen and Chapter 25 by Cheng et al.). For instance, a consortium of seven universities in Europe has successfully applied for the development of a module in gender medicine. The aim is to implement the module in various curricula – ranging from molecular medicine to health sciences – and also to offer it as post-initial training for professionals. This will bring together the diverse activities at a number of places in Europe and facilitate the implementation of sex- and gender-sensitive knowledge in care practices.

Moving towards an intersectional approach: Moving forward in the way of addressing not only sex and gender aspects in biomedical and health research but also other dimensions of difference in their dynamic interaction can effectively reduce any potential risk of biological or racial essentialism.

Summary

- European health research policies have overall furthered sex and gender research in the area of biomedicine; gender assessment brings opportunities and risks into perspective.
- Incorporating sex and gender in various fields – basic research, clinical care and public health – and at all levels of research is innovative and helps to improve the quality of healthcare.
- Critical debates, especially feminist approaches, on the inclusion of sex differences in biomedical research highlight that the most interesting area of research is not the study of differences per se but the study of *how* differences develop.
- Addressing not only sex and gender aspects in biomedical and health research but also other dimensions of difference in their dynamic interaction can effectively reduce any potential risk of biological or racial essentialism.

Key reading

Epstein, S. (2007) *Inclusion. The Politics of Difference in Medical Research* (Chicago: University of Chicago Press).

European Commission (2001) *Gender in Research. Gender Impact Assessment of the Specific Programmes of the Fifth Framework Programme – An Overview* (EUR 20022) (Brussels: Directorate-General for Research).

Healy, B. (1991) 'The Yentl Syndrome', *New England Journal of Medicine*, 325 (4), 274–6.

Klinge, I., for the GenderBasic Project (ed.) (2007) 'GenderBasic: Promoting Integration of Sex and Gender Aspects in Biomedical and Health-related Research', *Gender Medicine*, 4 (Supplement B), S59–S193.

References

Bekker, M. H. J. and J. van Mens-Verhulst (2007) 'Anxiety Disorders: Sex Differences in Prevalence, Degree, and Background, But Gender-neutral Treatment', *Gender Medicine*, 4 (Supplement B), S178–S193.

Birke, L. (1999) *Feminism and the Biological Body* (Edinburgh: Edinburgh University Press).

Branney, P. and A. White (2008) 'Big Boys Don't Cry: Depression and Men'. *Advances in Psychiatric Treatment*, 14 (4), 256–62.

Caron, J. (2003) *Report on Governmental Health Research Policies Promoting Gender or Sex Differences Sensitivity* (Ottawa: Canadian Institutes of Health Research).

Clarke, A. E. and V. L. Olesen (1998) *Revisioning Women, Health and Healing. Feminist, Cultural and Technoscience Perspectives* (New York: Routledge).

DunnGalvin, A., J. O. Hourihane, L. Frewer, R. C. Knibb, J. N. Oude Elberink and I. Klinge (2006) 'Incorporating a Gender Dimension in Food Allergy Research: A Review', *Allergy*, 61 (11), 1336–43.

Epstein, S. (2007) *Inclusion. The Politics of Difference in Medical Research* (Chicago: University of Chicago Press).

European Commission (1999) *Communication: Women and Science: Mobilising Women to Enrich European Research* (Brussels: European Commission).

European Commission (2001) *Gender in Research. Gender Impact Assessment of the Specific Programmes of the Fifth Framework Programme – An Overview* (EUR 20022) (Brussels: Directorate-General for Research).

European Commission (2003) *Vademecum: Gender Mainstreaming in the 6th Framework Programme – Reference Guide for Scientific Officers/Project Officers* (Brussels: European Commission).

European Commission (2004) *Gender Action Plan in Integrated Projects and Networks of Excellence. Compendium of Best Practices* (Brussels: Directorate-General for Research).

European Commission (2007) *Final Report of the Study on Integration of Science and Society Issues in the Sixth Framework Programme* (EUR 22976) (Brussels: European Commission).

European Commission (2008a) *Monitoring Progress towards Gender Equality in the Sixth Framework Programme. Nanotechnologies and Nanosciences, Knowledge-based Multifunctional Materials and New Production Processes and Devices* (EUR 23341) (Brussels: European Commission).

European Commission (2008b) *Monitoring Progress towards Gender Equality in the Sixth Framework Programme. Synthesis Report: Science and Society, Citizens and Governance in a Knowledge-based Society* (EUR 23342) (Brussels: European Commission).

Expert Group of the European Commission (2009) *Evaluation of the Sixth Framework Programmes for Research and Technological Development 2002–2006*, Report of the Expert Group to the European Commission, unpublished.

Fausto-Sterling, A. (2003) 'The Problem with Sex/Gender and Nature/Nurture', in S. J. Williams, L. Birke and C.-A. Bendelow (eds), *Debating Biology: Sociological Reflections on Medicine, Health and Society* (London: Routledge), 123–32.

Franconi, F. (2007) 'The Invisible Woman', paper presented at the *GenderBasic Expert Meeting*, Maastricht, 26–27 January 2007.

Geusens, P. and G. Dinant (2007) 'Integrating a Gender Dimension into Osteoporosis and Fracture Risk Research', *Gender Medicine*, 4 (Supplement B), S147–S161.

Healy, B. (1991) 'The Yentl Syndrome', *New England Journal of Medicine*, 325 (4), 274–6.

Holdcroft, A. (2007) 'Integrating the Dimensions of Sex and Gender into Basic Life Sciences Research: Methodologic and Ethical Issues', *Gender Medicine*, 4 (Supplement B), S64–S74.

Klinge, I. (2007a) 'Bringing Gender Expertise to Biomedical and Health-related Research', *Gender Medicine*, 4 (Supplement B), S59–S63.

Klinge, I., for the GenderBasic Project (ed.) (2007b) 'GenderBasic: Promoting Integration of Sex and Gender Aspects in Biomedical and Health-related Research', *Gender Medicine*, 4 (Supplement B), S59–S193.

Klinge, I. (2008) *Promoting Integration of the Gender Dimension in Biomedical and Health-related Research. Gendered and Translational Approaches in Basic, Clinical and Public Health Research, GenderBasic Final Report* (Maastricht: Centre for Gender and Diversity and Caphri School for Public Health and Primary Care), at: www.genderbasic.nl, accessed 12 August 2009.

Klinge, I. and M. Bosch (2001) *Gender in Research. Gender Impact Assessment of the Specific Programmes of the Fifth Framework Programme. Quality of Life and Management of Living Resources* (EUR 20017) (Brussels: European Commission).

Klinge, I. and M. Bosch (2005) 'Transforming Research Methodologies in EU Life Sciences and Biomedicine: Gender-Sensitive Ways of Doing Research', *European Journal of Women's Studies*, 12 (3), 377–95.

Kozicz, T. (2007) 'On the Role of Urocortin 1 in the Non-Preganglionic Edinger-Westphal Nucleus in Stress Adaptation', *General & Comparative Endocrinolgy*, 153, 235–40.

NIH – National Institutes of Health (1994) *Guidelines on the Inclusion of Women and Minorities as Subjects in Clinical Research, NIH Guide* (Washington, DC: National Institute of Health).

Noordenbos, G. (2007) 'Worden mannen over het hoofd gezien? Sekseverschillen in de diagnostiek en behandeling van depressie', *Tijdschrift voor Genderstudies*, 10, 16–28.

Ordovas, J. M. (2007) 'Gender, a Significant Factor in the Cross Talk between Genes, Environment, and Health', *Gender Medicine*, 4 (Supplement B), S111–S122.

Postma, D. S. (2007) 'Gender Differences in Asthma Development and Progression', *Gender Medicine*, 4 (Supplement B), S133–S146.

White, A. K. (2008) 'Osteoporosis and the Problem of Candidacy. Commentary', *GM2 Geriatric Medicine: Midlife and Beyond*, 38 (Supplement 3), 5.

Williams, C. (2000) 'Doing Health, Doing Gender: Teenagers, Diabetes and Asthma', *Social Science & Medicine*, 50 (3), 387–96.

7

Gender and the Medicalization of Healthcare

Susan E. Bell and Anne E. Figert

Introduction

Medicalization is a key concept of modernity, ubiquitously used in the social and medical sciences since the 1970s. We begin by adopting what sociologist Peter Conrad calls its essential meaning: *'defining a problem in medical terms, usually as an illness or disorder, or using a medical intervention to treat it'* (Conrad, 2005: 3, emphasis in the original). In this large and growing field, scholars generally agree that medicalization was a critical – if not fundamental – transformation of the 20th century. As we will show in this chapter, scholars disagree about its definitions, its connection with the dynamics and conceptual apparatuses of modernity and a global economy, and its cultural situatedness.

There are dangers of writing critically about medicalization. One of the dangers, resulting from its conceptual origins, is to assume the binaries of men/ women, femininity/masculinity and sex/gender. Another is to get stuck in a Eurocentric frame and to focus empirically on studies of its processes in North America, the UK and 'the west' more generally. This limits the development of medicalization theory. Just as medical anthropologists are increasingly examining US/western biomedicine as sites of ethnographic and cultural analysis, so should sociologists turn their gaze to more international and global concerns.

Although it is a gender-neutral term, the concept of medicalization historically has been linked to women. Most of the early work in sociology was about the medicalization of women's bodies; focused on the process by which conditions were defined and treated from a 'top down' perspective; and gave attention to Anglo-American settings. Recent feminist and gender scholarship has begun to re-imagine what medicalization is, to consider how medicalization affects men and women, and how gendered medicalization is more complicated than dichotomous views allow (Clarke et al., 2003). These reconsiderations reflect developments in sexuality scholarship and the turn in social science research to the study of global processes.

This chapter incorporates specific examples in gender and sexuality studies to reflect upon the political and theoretical significance of medicalization in people's lives and the implications for global healthcare policy. We ask how men's bodies are medicalized and how this process is similar to or different from women's experience. When sexuality enters into the debate, how do we think about transgendered people and their bodies? How has categorical thinking about gender and sex limited understandings of gendered medicalization?

Much of the early research was guided by theories of professional dominance and/or social construction. Current scholarship has refocused our analytic gaze from the power and authority of the medical profession to consider the active participation of individual patients/consumers/users individually and collectively (Figert, 2010). Informed by this refocus we ask how medicalization occurs within the increasingly complex healthcare system, erosion of physician control and professional dominance, and the expansion of expert patients. What happens when medicalization is actively sought instead of challenged? How have patterns of direct-to-consumer advertising and risk trafficking in some economies (notably the USA and New Zealand), and the global circulation of pharmaceuticals and biomedicine, influenced policy and practice? Pharmaceuticalization, biomedicalization and geneticization are concepts developed to describe and explain these complexities.

Tracing medicalization

The process of medicalization has a long and varied history. Historians and anthropologists document its beginnings in 17th-century western modernization and the application of scientific knowledge (Lock, 2004). The location of medicalization within large-scale social processes, such as modernization, the rise of a positivistic framework for understanding social problems, public health programmes of the modern state, and the emergence of science and the professions, is echoed throughout the historical and anthropological literature. To simplify, medicalization is a process associated with modernity.

The term medicalization itself has its roots in mid- to later 20th-century scholarship in the social sciences and humanities. The early sociological work of the 1970s focused upon the technically competent power and authority of physicians in modern society to define and treat individual patients. At the macro-level, it was pointed out that physicians and their organizational representatives have the authority and professional power in modern society to define and control what is formally recognized as a disorder, sickness or deviance; sociological analyses traced the medicalization process from the top down (Conrad and Schneider, 1980; Zola, 1972). The concept of control was prominent, used to explain consumers' demand (to control and improve upon their physical bodies) as well as medical imperialism (to control deviance through surveillance and the rational application of science to everyday life) and the turn to treatment as opposed to incarceration or punishment for deviance and mental illness (Lock, 2004).

While successful in documenting the process of medicalization in modern medicine, the focus on deviance (from badness to sickness) and on authority and professional control resulted in gender being relatively absent from this early sociological work (Plechner, 2000). Supported by a burgeoning body of feminist scholarship on women's bodies and the concurrent rise of the Women's Health Movements in the USA and western societies, historians, anthropologists and sociologists focused upon the connections between women's bodies and the greater control/medicalization of them by a predominantly male medical profession and a gendered scientific knowledge base. This research initially focused upon gender-specific processes such as childbirth and women's reproductive cycles (Leavitt, 1984; McCrea, 1983).

Most of the sociological scholarship in the 1980s and 1990s continued to take more of a social constructionist approach to medicalization in its examination of the construction of diagnostic categories, professional process and social control of behaviours. Articles by Riessman (1983) and Bell (1987) are noticeable exceptions to the early medical sociology work on medicalization and were important in challenging the idea that medicalization is entirely a top-down process and that women were passive recipients (as opposed to active proponents) of medicalization by a primarily male medical profession. However, feminist work in medical sociology in this period continued to emphasize the unique ways in which women's bodies were more susceptible to medicalization than men's bodies through processes such as childbirth, premenstrual syndrome (PMS) and menopause (Figert, 1996; Plechner, 2000). The literature since the late 1990s has taken a more expansive view of sex/gender to include men's bodies and intersex/ transbodies and of recent feminist thought – in particular intersectionality and attention to international, global and transnational processes. Thus Conrad writes:

> Men and masculinity have often been omitted from analyses of medicalization, in part because of the belief that men are not as vulnerable to medical surveillance and control (e.g., monitoring and intervention for medical conditions) as women. But ... such a belief is no longer tenable. (2007: 43–4)

In Conrad's work, the absence of a specific mention about men's bodies does not mean that men were absent from the analysis. Men and male bodies were the focus of a few early medicalization studies in sociology, notably of Conrad's own research about hyperactivity and alcoholism, but these studies did not use gender as a lens for understanding (Conrad and Schneider, 2000).

Masculinities and medicalization

As the above statement by Conrad (2007) points out, medicalization studies are now turning their analysis to the male body in order to remedy the equation of gender with women in sociological work. Thus scholars no longer ask *whether* men's bodies are medicalized but how, why and under what circumstances (Riska, 2003). Just as earlier studies of women expanded their focus beyond the reproductive realm, studies of men and medicalization have moved away from the initial focus upon the definition and control over sexuality to address how boys and men are medicalized through attention deficit hyperactivity disorder (ADHD) pharmaceuticals, sexual dysfunction and post-traumatic stress disorder (PTSD) treatments, and the development of the diagnostic category of 'andropause' to apply to ageing male bodies (Rosenfeld and Faircloth, 2006). Scholarly attention to the medicalization of men's sexuality continues, but the focus is less on the definitions and professional control of homosexuality than on the medicalization of heterosexual male sexuality, specifically, pharmaceutical interventions for male erections (Loe, 2004). Annandale and Riska argue that:

> [a]lthough the empowerment of consumers and the increased importance of the pharmaceutical industry – the so-called medical industrial complex – have been identified as independent actors in the construction of disease categories in general and medicalization in particular ... the gendered implications of this development have been insufficiently realized to date. (2009: 127)

So where to go with this burgeoning field? All of these works on both men and women still assume sex and gender as categories of modernity. That is, studies distinguish sex from gender; they take for granted the biological category of recognized (and fixed) sex differences and the socially constructed categories of those we call men and women or homosexual and heterosexual. As Epstein points out:

> In biomedicine as in our culture generally, sex is almost always treated as if it were a simple dichotomous variable. The presumptions are that one is either male or female and that the correct designation is not hard to determine – it can, in effect, be 'read off' the body. But nature knows no absolute distinctions. There is no unambiguous dividing line between the two sexes, and every criterion of differentiation that might be invoked, from genitalia to

hormones to chromosomes, fails to perform a strict demarcating function. (2007: 253)

Early studies in the field of sexuality unpacked the meanings of sex, sexuality and sexual identity and traced the social construction of the categories of homosexuality and heterosexuality. The contribution of these studies to understanding medicalization and masculinity is that they demonstrate the social construction of sexuality, sexual identity and homosexuality and begin to unpack the binaries of heterosexuality/homosexuality and man/woman.

Sexualities and medicalization

It is important to understand how and why men's bodies are also medicalized, but this area of scholarship does not necessarily problematize the sex of the human body. The work in the field of sexuality studies and the history of the medicalization of homosexuality which treats sex and the human body as problematic is foundational to our understanding of trans- and intersex today (Foucault, 1978).

Whereas homosexual behaviours are known to exist in the historical record and in all societies, and the category of homosexual was created and medicalized from the 19th century, transsexuals did not appear or were conflated with homosexuals before the 20th century. As Anne Fausto-Sterling (2000) argues, the 'modern' transsexual could not exist until the availability of hormones and surgery for changing bodies, and these technologies were developed and controlled by medicine. Before the availability of hormones and surgery for changing their bodies, women could pass as men (and vice versa) with clothing, appearance and performance. After the technologies were developed the possibility of 'transsexuals' emerged, but only by gaining access to these technologies. Access was secured when:

> ... transsexuals convinced their doctors that they had become the most stereo-typical members of their sex-to-be. Only then would physicians agree to create a medical category that transsexuals could apply in order to obtain surgical treatment. (Fausto-Sterling, 2000: 253)

Much like the early literature on women and medicalization, sexuality scholars are quick to point out that trans people were not 'medical dupes' (Rubin, 2006). Transsexuals were dependent on their medical care providers, but their use of the conceptual and material apparatus exemplifies how medicalization became a strategy for those wishing to become transsexuals (Rubin, 2006).

Harry Benjamin introduced the medical category of transsexual in the 1950s to advocate for and to treat people who wanted to permanently change their physical bodies into those of a different gender. Today 'gender identity disorder' is found in the latest version of the official diagnostic manual of the American Psychiatric Association (APA, 2000). A new generation of trans activists and mental health practitioners points out harmful effects of the medicalized (psychiatric) 'disorder'. Samons writes:

> In its current diagnostic form, only a small minority of transgender people benefit from the mental health diagnosis of gender identity disorder. Only a very few have [health] insurance that will pay for any kind of treatment [...] It is a dubious benefit that only a few receive but for which the entire population of transgender people pays the price: the social stigma that results from this labeling of transgender as a mental illness through the existence and use of this diagnosis. (Samons, 2009: xxvi)

To put it in terms of medicalization and gender, many transgender people are actively choosing not to pathologize or medicalize their bodies at the same time that they are actively challenging western and modern concepts of what it means to connect bodies with (sexual and gender) identities. 'Agnes' is one of the more famous cases of trans identity that was documented by the sociologist Harold Garfinkel in the 1960s. As told by Garfinkel (2006[1967]: 58), Agnes presented herself to the Gender Identity Clinic in Los Angeles as someone who was 'a girl' born in a male body that had 'spontaneously begun to feminize at puberty'. Agnes was diagnosed by the doctors at the clinic as having a rare intersexual condition, 'testicular feminization syndrome'. As a result of this diagnosis, Agnes was *allowed* to have a sex reassignment. It was later revealed that Agnes had deliberately lied to her doctors and had taken feminizing hormones before coming to the clinic in order to get past the diagnoses required for the operation (Garfinkel, 2006 [1967]).

While Agnes lied about her body, there are babies born every year with either ambiguous genitalia or where their genitalia are not consistent with their sex chromosomes. Estimates vary widely, but forms of intersexuality have always existed in the written human record (see Fausto-Sterling, 2000). Trans activists challenge the medical and scientific concept of sex and gender binarism, but as Preves points out, sexual surgery is not simply a practice resulting from medical imperialism: 'People who are sexually ambiguous and their families (may) also desire some semblance of normalcy in relation to social expectations of sex and gender' and seek sexual surgery to achieve 'gender binarism', and adopt medical language and categories to make sense of and talk about their experiences (Preves, 2003: 39). This acceptance of medicalized sexuality can make it difficult for intersex individuals 'to question medical opinion or authority, or to seek alternative care' (Preves, 2003: 45).

Expanding the medicalization frame: pharmaceuticalization, biomedicalization and geneticization

Today, scholars are questioning the usefulness of 'medicalization' as a sufficient framework 'in an age dominated by complex and often contradictory inter-actions between medicine, pharmaceutical companies, and culture at large' (Metzl and Herzig, 2007: 697). Physician power and authority (so important to early theories of medicalization) is changing in the west and indeed waning as a result of healthcare reforms and direct-to-consumer advertising of pharmaceuticals (in the USA and New Zealand) (Rose, 2007). Scholars are demonstrating the differential impact of biomedicalization and pharmaceuticalization across the globe such as found in demands for safe and cost-effective drug treatments for tuberculosis and HIV/AIDS (Petryna et al., 2006). To put it bluntly,

> some people are more medically made up than others – women more than men, the wealthy differently from the poor, children more than adults, and … differently in different countries and regions of the world. (Rose, 2007: 700)

Whereas some populations in some areas of the world are (over)medicalized, other populations in other parts of the world are undermedicalized, and medicalization scholarship suffers from insufficient attention to these differences and their consequences for global health and healthcare. During their travels through the disciplines and among different sociological cultures, scholars have expanded the definition of medicalization and introduced new terms to capture its dynamics in more subtle and nuanced ways (Clarke et al., 2010). Notable among these terms are pharmaceuticalization (Biehl, 2004), biomedicalization (Clarke et al., 2003) and geneticization (Lippman, 1991), which overlap with and provide an analytical focus to particular strands in medicalization.

Pharmaceuticalization

Williams and colleagues have defined pharmaceuticalization thus:

> [it] refers to the transformation of human conditions, capacities or capabilities into pharmaceutical matters of treatment or enhancement. As such it overlaps with but extends far beyond the realms of the medical or the medicalised, and serves further to blur the boundaries between treatment and enhancement. (Williams et al., 2008: 850)

Pharmaceuticalization maps on to global patterns of wealth and poverty, power and inequality and extends the concept of medicalization beyond the influence of the medical profession on a person's health or body to include dynamics among states, NGOs and pharmaceutical companies (Busfield, 2006;

Petryna et al., 2006). Attention to the global dynamics of pharmaceuticals is not new, although the dynamics have been transformed in the 50 years since feminist scholars and activists in Women's Health Movements looked critically at the development of the birth control pill and other reproductive technologies (Boston Women's Health Book Collective, 1973; Hartmann, 1987; Roberts, 1997). A recent study of the emergence and contested use of the human papillomavirus (HPV) vaccine for cervical cancer illustrates how the new pharmaceuticalization frame can be applied to understanding the permeation of sexual and reproductive technologies 'with meanings of sex/gender' and their role in the politics of gender and sexuality in social relations (Casper and Carpenter, 2008: 886). In richer countries, pharmaceuticalization combines

> the biological effect of a chemical on human tissue, the legitimacy of a condition as a disease, the willingness of consumers to adopt the technology as a 'solution' to a problem in their lives, and the corporate interests of drug companies. Together, these factors [transform] aspects of daily life into disease categories alongside the pharmaceutical agents that 'treat' them. (Fox and Ward, 2008: 865)

In these settings, pharmaceutical companies are either highlighting daily life choices, such as sleeping through the night, or publicizing new conditions and illnesses to gain more customers or consumers of their products (Fox and Ward, 2008). For example, the HPV vaccine is being widely marketed to girls and young women (but not boys or men) in the USA and UK, although most (80–85 per cent) of the annual deaths from cervical cancer are in developing countries (Casper and Carpenter, 2008). Direct-to-consumer advertising (DTCA) reflects global inequalities and contributes to medicalization in many ways. Conrad and Leiter state:

> Direct-to-consumer advertising for prescription medications has fuelled the medicalization that analysts noted as increasing in Western societies in the 1980s ... DTCA has become a major source of expanding medical markets and public engagement with medical solutions for life's conditions and problems. (2008: 829)

In addition, DTCA has 'changed the ways physicians and patients speak and listen to each other' (Metzl, 2007: 704). DTCA has also amplified, and in some cases changed, cultural expectations about illness and health, medication prescription and use and, in some ways, normalized the medicalization of the gendered body. Currently, television and radio broadcast advertising of prescription drugs or pharmaceuticals directly to consumers is permitted only in the USA and New Zealand. It is prohibited in the UK and most developed countries.

The globalization of pharmaceutical development has also produced new subjectivities through medicalization. The first is the creation of a need for pharmaceutically naïve subject populations to sustain clinical research and development and the expansions of markets (Petryna et al., 2006). This in turn opens the possibility for individuals and communities to gain access to resources and power and opportunities for citizenship. Other new subjectivities produced through pharmaceuticalization are 'pharmaceutical citizenship' or 'therapeutic citizenship', which can be tools for gaining access to resources and power (Biehl, 2004; Nguyen, 2005).

AIDS policy in Brazil illustrates how pharmaceutical citizenship through the medicalization of HIV/AIDS can be a new democratic tool for individuals, activist groups and states (Biehl, 2004). The Brazilian government joined with the World Bank in 1992 to create a National AIDS Program and by 1996 had begun to provide free antiretroviral drugs to all registered AIDS cases in the country. People with HIV/AIDS who were previously marginalized (noncitizens), claimed 'a new identity around their politicized biology, with the support of international and national, public and private funds' and through their social and biomedical inclusion became 'biomedical citizens' (Biehl, 2004: 122, 123). More importantly, AIDS activists successfully forced the Brazilian government to allow compulsory licensing of patented drugs during a declared public health crisis. In this respect, this therapeutic citizenship comes to represent a biomedicalized form of the state (Nguyen, 2005). Biological notions of citizenship – such as being HIV-positive – are used to ascribe an essentialized identity such as sex or race (Nguyen, 2005). An important effect of selective forms of biomedical citizenship such as the one in Brazil is that they systematically make some people visible and others invisible: 'bureaucratic procedures, informational difficulties, sheer medical neglect and moral contempt, and unresolved disputes over diagnostic criteria' all contribute to turning some people into 'absent things' (Biehl, 2004: 119).

Making visible these macro-processes and their gendered dimensions is key to disentangling how pharmaceuticalization and medicalization are connected, as well as to understanding how they can contribute to the creation of new democratic tools for individuals, activist groups and states and to new possibilities for entering into the grip of (medical) power. Because pharmaceuticalization has occurred so recently, we are just beginning to see how medicalization might work differently (or similarly) for global pharmaceuticalization processes and what the gender implications of this are.

Biomedicalization

Gender is inherently built into the framework of biomedicalization theory. The era of biomedicalization emerged in the mid-1980s along with changes in high-tech biomedical interventions designed not only for treatment but also for health maintenance, enhancement and optimization (Clarke et al., 2010). Biomedicalization regulates bodies not only by offering

> 'control over' one's body through medical intervention (such as contraception), but also by 'transformation of' ones' body, selves, health. Thereby new selves and identities (mother, father, walker, hearer, beautiful, sexually potent person) become possible. (Clarke et al., 2003: 182)

According to Clarke and colleagues, the addition of the prefix 'bio' to 'medicalization' produces a concept that encompasses

> the transformations of both the human and nonhuman made possible by such technoscientific innovations as molecular biology, biotechnologies, genomization, transplant medicine, and new medical technologies. (Clarke et al., 2003: 162)

A significant proportion of scholarship in this field takes a feminist approach to biomedicalization, in part because of the commitment to feminist health scholarship by those who developed the concept. As Mamo and Fosket put it, 'female corporeality and subjectivity are understood as constituted in and through (cultural) practices of (techno)science' (2009: 927). That is, bodies are simultaneously 'objects and effects of technoscientific and biomedical discourse' (Mamo and Fosket, 2009: 927). Biomedicalization has been employed to examine how gendered subjectivities and forms of embodiment are produced in lesbian practices of assisted reproduction, breast cancer prevention technologies, pharmaceutical interventions for male erections, and contraception/menstruation (see Fosket, 2004; Mamo, 2007).

Proponents of biomedicalization argue that, whereas gender is conceived of categorically in medicalization scholarship, gender is an effect of power, 'produced in relations'. This conception of gender is aligned with postmodern feminist scholarship in which gender is not a stable, given status but an outcome of performance. Gender is also not a privileged status, but one that is produced in intersections with race, 'class, sexuality, disability, and so on' as a result of 'selective and uneven biomedical efforts to transform, regulate, and optimize bodies and futures' (Clarke et al., 2010). Although the concept of biomedicalization does not necessarily privilege gender, it takes gendered bodies seriously. To date most scholarship in this field has given attention to the study of biomedicalization processes in the USA and is only beginning to look transnationally. Whereas pharmaceuticalization scholarship is de-emphasizing gender and emphasizing transnational processes, biomedicalization is inherently gendered but more western in its focus.

The challenge of biomedicalization for gender and medicalization studies is very persuasive. It came into being as process and concept along with postmodernity, and is capable of tracking multistranded workings of gendered power and knowledge. At the same time, because biomedicalization has begun to circulate so recently, maybe it is too soon to know how fully it captures what is going on in the postmodern world and to know whether it will take off and be taken up among scholars in the way medicalization has.

Geneticization

Geneticization is a concept proposed in the early 1990s by Abby Lippman to capture a new way of seeing and solving problems that reduces individual differences of race, gender and nationality to DNA codes:

> [It is] an ongoing process by which differences between individuals are reduced to their DNA codes, with most disorders, behaviors and physiological variations defined, at least, as genetic in origin. It refers as well to the process by which interventions employing genetic technologies are adopted to manage problems of health. (Lippman, 1991: 19)

Lippman observed that in popular discourse genetic variations were increasingly defined as problems for which there were medical solutions. At the time when she proposed the concept of geneticization, prenatal testing was the most widely used and familiar genetic activity; Lippman gave attention to women's stories about prenatal diagnosis to exemplify geneticization. This line of work has continued (Finkler, 2001) and its gender dimensions expanded to include men and men's stories about their responses to premarital carrier matching and other genetic tests (Raz and Atar, 2004).

Scholars disagree about the extent to which the processes of geneticization and medicalization overlap, but all of them agree that there are important differences between the two. Gusterson (2001: 252) argues that medicalization 'cannot convey the novelty and power' of the processes and a new way of seeing made possible by genetic research. Conrad distinguishes between medicalization, which does not 'require specific claims about cause, although the assumption is often biological' and geneticization, which 'is very specific about where at least part of the cause lies' (2000: 329). In a recent study of the relationship between medicalization and genetics in mental illness, homosexuality and susceptibility to chemical exposures, Shostak and colleagues (2008: S310) identify different patterns: 'genetic information does not always lead to geneticization, nor does geneticization inevitably lead to medicalization.' But where geneticization is a useful concept for us lies in its potential to link both gender and transnational processes of medicalization. For example, the development and circulation of Assisted Reproductive Technologies, so important in the development of geneticization as a concept within a US/western framework, has been recently studied in a range of different populations, from lesbians in the USA and UK, to Bedouin Muslim women in Israel, and throughout the world (Inhorn, 2006; Mamo, 2007; Raz and Atar, 2004).

Conclusion

We have argued in this chapter that medicalization is a capacious concept, but it does not fully capture the related but unique processes of biomedicalization, pharmaceuticalization and geneticization, especially when examining issues of sex, gender and sexuality in relation to health and healthcare. There is certainly a fair amount of overlap, but even such a powerful term as medicalization is not quite adequate to fully capture what is going on in the globalized world at the start of the 21st century precisely because its very definition is rooted in modernity and categorical thinking. At the same time, the concept of medicalization is worth holding on to. It is widely accepted and employed not only among scholars but also among the public. It wields cultural authority and can explain how control over medical phenomena is produced, accomplished, resisted and transformed. Its connection with modernity and modern processes of control, regulation, knowledge and power make its reach and impact partial. In a world where postmodern forms of knowledge and power circulate, medicalization as a process is too simple and as a concept too narrow for capturing the gendered circulation of pharmaceuticals, genetics and technoscience. We argue that we still need to use the concept of medicalization as our starting point or analytic wedge to explore the larger question of 'what has happened to gender?'.

Early critiques of medicalization repeatedly demonstrated its gendered dimensions by pointing out how and why women's bodies, life cycles and experiences are more likely to be medicalized than men's. As we have argued, connections between women's health and medicalization continue to be a rich resource for scholarly work, but more recent critiques have expanded the category of gender to include boys, men and transgendered people.

In the social sciences and the history of women's health, there is a long and established tradition of explaining the medicalization of women's bodies. Women have been both active participants in this medicalization and the object of sexist, racist and class-based policies and practices, especially surrounding reproductive issues. These gendered concerns have continued and elaborated with the conceptual tools offered by pharmaceuticalization, geneticization and especially biomedicalization. In addition, gender scholars have pushed the binaries of sex/gender/sexuality, and their work has informed that of medicalization scholars. The real danger, however, arises if this expansion allows scholars to turn away from the study of women and the various ways that the new processes of biomedicalization, pharmaceuticalization and geneticization continue to impact women as well as men, and trans and intersex bodies. With the disintegration of categorical frameworks and the expansion of subjectivities, how can gender be privileged and women included?

Although scholarship about medicalization is generally sharply critical, medicalization is not always a bad thing. For example, for those women globally who want to become mothers, participation in medicine (technology, services, knowledge) can be a strategy to accomplish what they perceive to be in their best interests. Childbearing is a key practice; evidence repeatedly shows how, why and with what consequences women seek medical assistance to achieve (biological) motherhood. In this case, medicalization is strategic (Inhorn, 2006). Additionally, new subjectivities are produced through the processes of medicalization and the conceptual frameworks for understanding them. These include 'transsexual', 'naive subjects', and 'pharmaceutical or therapeutic citizenship'. As Lock relates,

> paradoxically, [the process of] medicalization has actually promoted ... reflection by presenting people with choice, although globalization rather than medicalization per se has no doubt been the major driving force for change. The result is that older hegemonies have crumbled, only to give way to new ones, most often in the form of knowledge that comes under the rubric of science. (2004: 119)

Medicalization is sometimes, but not always, the right tool for the job of understanding complicated, global, multi-sited processes of gendered biomedical transformations today. Gender shows us how and why we need to fine-tune our thinking when we try to understand, intervene in, and improve healthcare. By continually expanding the concept of medicalization we risk losing its power to capture the processes and consequences of defining problems in medical terms and using medical interventions to treat them. At the same time, without the nuance provided by concepts such as biomedicalization, pharmaceuticalization and geneticization, we also risk losing the ability to capture these very real processes. Medicalization is a capacious concept that is a beginning but not the end of understanding gender and the medicalization of health and healthcare.

Summary

- Medicalization theory has shifted away from the initial focus on professional dominance to include active participation of patients/consumers.
- Medicalization theory has expanded. It has moved away from its initial focus on women to include men and it has moved away from a

dichotomous view, for example, of homosexuality/heterosexuality, to sexualities that include trans and intersex.
- Medicalization is now a global process.
- The processes of geneticization, pharmaceuticalization and biomedicalization overlap with and extend beyond the processes of medicalization.

Key reading

Busfield, J. (2006) 'Pills, Power, People: Sociological Understandings of the Pharmaceutical Industry', *Sociology*, 40 (2), 297–314.
Clarke, A., E. L. Mamo, J. R. Fishman, J. K. Shim and J. R. Fosket (2003) 'Biomedicalization: Technoscientific Transformations of Health, Illness, and U.S. Biomedicine', *American Sociological Review*, 68 (April), 161–94.
Conrad, P. (2007) *The Medicalization of Society: On the Transformation of Human Conditions into Treatable Disorders* (Baltimore: Johns Hopkins University Press).
Rosenfeld, D. and C. Faircloth (eds) (2006) *Medicalized Masculinities* (Philadelphia: Temple University Press).

Acknowledgements

We would like to acknowledge Allan Brandt, Ellen Annandale and Ellen Kuhlmann who gave us valuable comments on a draft of the chapter. Susan Bell is grateful for support from the Fletcher Research Fund, Bowdoin College.

References

APA – American Psychiatric Association (2000) *Diagnostic and Statistical Manual of Mental Disorders, Fourth Edition (DSM-IV)* (Washington, DC: American Psychiatric Association).
Annandale, E. and E. Riska (2009) 'New Connections: Towards a Gender-Inclusive Approach to Women's and Men's Health', *Current Sociology*, 57 (2), 123–33.
Bell, S. E. (1987) 'Changing Ideas: The Medicalization of Menopause', *Social Science & Medicine*, 24 (6), 535–42.
Biehl, J. (2004) 'The Activist State: Global Pharmaceuticals, AIDS, and Citizenship in Brazil', *Social Text*, 22 (3), 105–32.
Boston Women's Health Book Collective (1973) *Our Bodies, Ourselves* (New York: Simon and Schuster).
Busfield, J. (2006) 'Pills, Power, People: Sociological Understandings of the Pharmaceutical Industry', *Sociology*, 40 (2), 297–314.
Casper, M. J. and L. M. Carpenter, (2008) 'Sex, Drugs, and Politics: The HPV Vaccine for Cervical Cancer', *Sociology of Health and Illness*, 30 (6), 886–99.
Clarke, A., E. L. Mamo, J. R. Fishman, J. K. Shim and J. R. Fosket (2003) 'Biomedicalization: Technoscientific Transformations of Health, Illness, and U.S. Biomedicine', *American Sociological Review*, 68 (April), 161–94.
Clarke, A., J. Shim, L. Mamo, J. R. Fosket and J. R. Fishman (eds) (2010) *Biomedicalization: Technoscience and Transformations of Health, Illness and US Biomedicine* (Durham, NC: Duke University Press).

Conrad, P. (2000) 'Medicalization, Genetics, and Human Problems', in C. E. Bird, P. Conrad and A. M. Fremont (eds), *Handbook of Medical Sociology, Fifth Edition* (Upper Saddle River: Prentice Hall), 322–33.

Conrad, P. (2005) 'The Shifting Engines of Medicalization', *Journal of Health and Social Behavior*, 46 (1), 3–14.

Conrad, P. (2007) *The Medicalization of Society: On the Transformation of Human Conditions into Treatable Disorders* (Baltimore: Johns Hopkins University Press).

Conrad, P. and V. Leiter (2008) 'From Lydia Pinkham to Queen Levitra: Direct-to-Consumer Advertising and Medicalisation', *Sociology of Health and Illness*, 30 (6), 825–38.

Conrad, P. and J. Schneider (1980) *Deviance and Medicalization: From Badness to Sickness* (St Louis: Mosby).

Epstein, S. (2007) *Inclusion: The Politics of Difference in Medical Research* (Chicago: University of Chicago Press).

Fausto-Sterling, A. (2000) *Sexing the Body: Gender Politics and the Construction of Sexuality* (New York: Basic Books).

Figert, A. E. (1996) *Women and the Ownership of PMS* (Hawthorne: Aldine de Gruyter).

Figert, A. E. (2010) 'The Consumer Turn in Medicalization: Future Directions with Historical Foundations', in B. Pescosolido, J. Martin, J. McLeod and A. Rogers, (eds), *The Handbook of the Sociology of Health, Illness and Healing: Blueprint for the 21st Century* (New York: Springer).

Finkler, K. (2001) 'The Kin in the Gene: The Medicalization of Family and Kinship in American Society', *Current Anthropology*, 42 (2), 235–63.

Fosket, J. R. (2004) 'Constructing "High-Risk" Women: The Development and Standardization of a Breast Cancer Risk Assessment Tool', *Science, Technology and Human Values*, 29 (3), 291–313.

Foucault, M. (1978) *History of Sexuality, Vol. 1, An Introduction* (New York: Random House).

Fox, N. J. and K. J. Ward (2008) 'Pharma in the Bedroom ... and the Kitchen ... the Pharmaceuticalisation of Daily Life', *Sociology of Health and Illness*, 30 (6), 856–68.

Garfinkel, H. (2006 [1967]) 'Passing and the Managed Achievement of Sex Status in an "Intersexed" Person', in S. Stryker and S. Whittle (eds), *The Transgender Studies Reader* (New York: Routledge), 58–93.

Gusterson, H. (2001) 'Comment: The Kin in the Gene', *Current Anthropology*, 42 (2), 251–2.

Hartmann, B. (1987) *Reproductive Rights and Wrongs: The Global Politics of Population Control and Contraceptive Choice* (New York: Harper and Row).

Inhorn, M. C. (2006) 'Defining Women's Health: A Dozen Messages from More than 150 Ethnographies', *Medical Anthropology Quarterly*, 20 (3), 345–78.

Leavitt, J. W. (ed.) (1984) *Women and Health in America* (Madison: University of Wisconsin Press).

Lippman, A. (1991) 'Prenatal Genetic Testing and Screening: Constructing Needs and Reinforcing Inequities', *American Journal of Law & Medicine*, 17 (1&2), 15–50.

Lock, M. (2004) 'Medicalization and the Naturalization of Social Control', in C. W. Ember and M. Ember (eds), *Encyclopedia of Medical Anthropology: Health and Illness in the World's Cultures*, vol. 1 (New York: Lower Academic/Plenum Publishers), 116–24.

Loe, M. (2004) *The Rise of Viagra* (New York: New York University Press).

Mamo, L. (2007) *Queering Reproduction: Achieving Pregnancy in the Age of Technoscience* (Durham, NC: Duke University Press).

Mamo, L. and J. R. Fosket (2009) 'Scripting the Body: Pharmaceuticals and the (Re)Making of Menstruation', *Signs*, 34 (3), 926–49.

McCrea, F. (1983) 'The Politics of Menopause: The "Discovery" of a Deficiency Disease', *Social Problems,* 31 (1),111–23.

Metzl, J. M. (2007) 'If Direct-to-Consumer Advertisements Come to Europe: Lessons from the USA', *The Lancet,* 369, 704–6.

Metzl, J. M. and R. M. Herzig (2007) 'Medicalisation in the 21st Century: Introduction', *The Lancet,* 369, 697–8.

Nguyen, V. (2005) 'Antiretroviral Globalism, Biopolitics and Therapeutic Citizenship', in A. Ong and S. J. Collier (eds), *Global Assemblages: Technology, Politics, and Ethics as Anthropological Problems* (Malden: Blackwell), 124–44.

Petryna, A., A. Lakoff and A. Kleinman (eds), (2006) *Global Pharmaceuticals: Ethics, Markets, Practices* (Durham, NC: Duke University Press).

Plechner, D. (2000) 'Women, Medicine, and Sociology – Thoughts on the Need for a Critical Feminist Perspective', *Research in the Sociology of Health Care,* 18, 69–94.

Preves, S. E. (2003) *Intersex and Identity: The Contested Self* (New Brunswick: Rutgers University Press).

Raz, A. E. and M. Atar (2004) 'Upright Generations of the Future: Tradition and Medicalization in Community Genetics', *Journal of Contemporary Ethnography,* 33 (3), 296–322.

Riessman, C. K. (1983) 'Women and Medicalization: A New Perspective', *Social Policy,* 14 (Summer), 3–18.

Riska, E. (2003) 'Gendering the Medicalization Thesis', *Advances in Gender Research,* 7, 61–89.

Roberts, D. (1997) *Killing the Black Body: Race, Reproduction, and the Meaning of Liberty* (New York: Vintage Books).

Rose, N. (2007) 'Beyond Medicalisation', *The Lancet,* 369, 700–2.

Rosenfeld, D. and C. Faircloth (eds) (2006) *Medicalized Masculinities* (Philadelphia: Temple University Press).

Rubin, H. (2006) 'The Logic of Treatment', in S. Stryker and S. Whittle (eds), *The Transgender Studies Reader* (New York: Routledge), 482–98.

Samons, S. (2009) *When the Opposite Sex Isn't: Sexual Orientation in Male-to-Female Transgender People* (New York: Routledge).

Shostak, S., P. Conrad and A. V. Horwitz (2008) 'Sequencing and its Consequences: Path Dependence and the Relationships Between Genetics and Medicalization', *American Journal of Sociology,* 114, S287–S316.

Williams, S. J., C. Seal, S. Boden, P. Lowe and D. L. Steinberg (2008) 'Waking Up to Sleepiness: Modafinil, the Media and the Pharmaceuticalisation of Everyday/Night Life', *Sociology of Health and Illness,* 30 (6), 839–55.

Zola, I. (1972) 'Medicine as an Institution of Social Control', *Sociological Review,* 20 (4), 497–504.

Part II
The Social Patterning of Health by Gender

8
Changing Gendered Patterns of Morbidity and Mortality

Chloe E. Bird, Martha E. Lang and Patricia P. Rieker

Introduction

The dictum, 'women get sicker but men die quicker' is often treated as an established fact. However, historical demographic data demonstrate that women have not always outlived men. Moreover, current data from developing countries demonstrate that war, epidemic, disease and extreme poverty can diminish, or even reverse, women's advantage in life expectancy (see National Center for Healthcare Statistics, 2009; World Health Organization, 2008). Thus the apparently paradoxical gender differences in morbidity and mortality are neither universal nor invariant within and across societies (Annandale, 2009).

In this chapter, we briefly review gender differences in morbidity and mortality and how they have changed over time. We also discuss current debates about the biological and social explanations of these differences, and consider factors that widen or narrow the gender gap in physical health status and longevity. We argue that understanding the factors that affect health and shape health disparities is critical for both research and policy aimed at improving population health. Although many disciplines examine gender differences in health and mortality, substantial knowledge gaps remain when it comes to informing interventions and policy.

To address knowledge gaps, Bird and Rieker (2008) developed a framework of 'constrained choice' which provides a new direction for discourse, research and policy. Constrained choice describes how decisions made and actions taken at the levels of family, work, community and government shape men's and women's opportunities to pursue health. In this chapter, mainly with reference to the USA, we elaborate on the theoretical underpinnings of constrained choice as a process through which structural inequalities play out in disparities in individual and population health. We also consider how constrained choices relate to the social patterns of two important health problems: cardiovascular disease (CVD) and HIV/AIDS. In so doing, we begin with a broader discussion of how race, class and/or sexual orientation can and often do interact with gender to constrain choice in ways that limit individual agency by creating differential opportunities for a healthy life.

Gendered patterns in health and mortality

As Verbrugge and Wingard (1987) note, much of women's higher morbidity and lower mortality compared to men can be explained by gender differences in disease prevalence. In most industrialized nations, men develop more life-threatening conditions (for example, cancer and cardiovascular disease) at younger ages than do women. In contrast, women have higher rates of chronic debilitating disorders such as autoimmune diseases and rheumatoid disorders as well as irritating but less life-threatening diseases such as anaemia, arthritis, migraines and thyroid disease (Verbrugge and Wingard, 1987; NCHS, 2009). Even though women experience more physical illness, sick days and hospitalizations than men (even excluding reproductive related care), studies report mixed findings as to whether women experience worse self-rated health than men (Crimmins et al., 2002; Macintyre et al., 1996).

Women's mortality advantage is a fairly recent development. When life expectancy was lower, women did not typically outlive men and were at significant risk of dying in childbirth or subsequently from related infections. In fact, at the turn of the 20th century, the United States exhibited the public health characteristics similar to that of a developing country today: the three leading causes of death were infectious diseases: pneumonia, tuberculosis and infant diarrhoea (Omran, 1977). In 1901, the difference in life expectancy for males and females at birth was less than three years (48.3 vs 51.1 years for whites and 32.5 vs 35.0 for blacks) (Department of Commerce, 1921). Over the next 50 years, infectious death rates dropped markedly in the United States and other industrialized nations as a result of improved sanitation, vaccinations, nutrition and living conditions. With this epidemiologic transition, life expectancies increased for all major population subgroups, and degenerative diseases such as cardiovascular disease (CVD) and cancer became the leading causes of death. By 2004, life expectancy for industrialized nations had increased significantly with a marked jump in female mortality advantage. Japan led with life expectancy rates of 78.6 for males vs 85.6 for females, followed by Hong Kong (79.0 vs 84.7) and Switzerland (78.6 vs 83.7). In 2004, the United States ranked 26th among these nations at 75.2 vs 80.4. Since 1901, racial differences in US life expectancy have been reduced by half, but still remain statistically significant (75.7 vs 80.8 years for whites and 69.8 vs 76.3 for blacks) (NCHS, 2009: 201–3).

Data from Zimbabwe further demonstrate that gains in life expectancy are not necessarily permanent or universal. Whereas in 1990 women's life expectancy in Zimbabwe was about 64 years and men's about 60 years, by 2006, life expectancy was only 43 years for women and 44 for men. For example, as a result of the HIV epidemic the total fertility rate for the eastern region of Zimbabwe is eight per cent below the normally expected rate for that area. In addition to its obvious mortality effects, HIV infection also lowers women's fertility (Joint United Nations Programme on AIDS, 2008: 47). As UNAIDS and others have noted, these severe declines in life expectancy are due in large part to the spread of HIV/AIDS (Rieker et al., 2010; Velkoff and Kowal, 2007).

Moreover, in an examination of inequities in premature mortality rates in the United States between 1960 and 2002 Krieger and colleagues (2008) found that as population health improves the magnitude of health inequalities can either rise or fall and concluded that the reasons for these observed trends are unclear. Yet because such research is generally conducted at the population level without consideration of gender differences or gaps, it sheds little light on the impact on gender differences in health and mortality.

Biological and social explanations of gender differences in morbidity and mortality

Current social and biological science approaches to understanding gender differences in health each demonstrate some explanatory power in addressing the apparent mortality–morbidity paradox. Yet, the two approaches are most often presented as 'either/or' instead of integrated into a unified framework (Rieker et al., 2010). Researchers have only recently begun to articulate precisely how social and biological factors interact to create gender-based mortality and morbidity differentials (Fausto-Sterling, 2005). However, there is a general consensus on several key social and biological factors that shape physical health, stress and longevity.

Biological explanations

Biological explanations emphasize the contribution of differences in men's and women's physiology. For example, women appear to experience some biological advantages related to reproduction which reduce their risk of cardiovascular disease prior to menopause. In particular, women's more flexible circulatory system both allows for higher blood volume during pregnancy and reduces the risk of and impact of higher blood pressure. Biological explanations tend to focus on factors such as stress responses, genetic traits and hormonal differences (Bird and Rieker, 2008). Biological factors may also play a role in female mortality advantage at the beginning and end of life. In most human populations, approximately 105 boy babies are born to 100 girl babies each year, with a slightly narrower ratio in several European nations (Davis et al., 1998). This difference is due to infant males having higher rates of congenital abnormalities and X chromosome-related immune disorders (Abramowicz and Barnett, 1970). Furthermore, in their review of European mortality measures, Di Giulio and Pinnelli (2007) suggest that women in most developed nations live approximately five years longer than their male counterparts.

Stress research explores how the biological processes created by ongoing stressors shape health outcomes and how each gender adapts to stress. Traditional arguments attributed men's lower life expectancy to higher levels of strain from social role expectations of being a provider or breadwinner and to gender differences in coping, such as doing less emotional work in relationships (Wood, 2009). Much of early stress research suggested that women faced fewer stressors than men because most of their lives were spent in the private sphere of home and family (for example, Bradburn, 1969). However, current stress research from the United States focuses on coping mechanisms and demonstrates that men and women face both a variety of different stressors and have different resources to draw on in coping with these stressors (Dedovic et al., 2009).

Social explanations

Social explanations can be grouped into social stratification effects, social structure affects and gender-specific normative behaviours. The social structure of a given society is particularly important in shaping gender mortality and morbidity differentials. Social structure is arguably a manifestation of social norms, making it difficult to discern where social structure ends and gender roles begin. We therefore focus our discussion of social structure on the institutions of work and family.

In the United States and other industrialized nations, men have traditionally worked in manual labour jobs, served in the military and performed other high-risk endeavours. Women have been more likely than men to hold desk jobs or work in service occupations. This occupational structure gives men better access to many well-paid jobs but also places them at higher risk for many types of injury and accidents. While the women's rights movement reduced occupational gender segregation, these patterns continue to affect men's and women's incomes – particularly in the USA where the initial struggle addressed equal access to occupations rather than income equality across occupations (see England, 2005) – and exposure to many types of risks. Moreover, the gender divisions of labour at work and at home reinforce each other in ways that slow the trend toward similar work jobs and roles for men and women.

Both men and women also actively engage in the project of 'doing gender' by acting in accordance with normative expectations that reinforce traditional gender roles (Kimmel, 2008). These behaviours can contribute to gendered patterns of health and mortality. For example, in the United States, men have higher rates of both violent and accidental deaths, more reported alcoholism and more tobacco-related diseases than women in part because risk-taking, drinking and smoking are often encouraged as masculine behaviours (see also Chapter 1 by Payne and Doyal, and Chapter 16 by Schofield). Gender norms can even shape health-related information and recommendations. For example, Dworkin and Wachs (2009) demonstrate how fitness recommendations in health and fitness magazines are designed to encourage the development of idealized male and female bodies rather than health or even functionality. They document the extent to which advice and images aimed at men focus on building upper body strength, whereas advice to women emphasizes thinness and 'getting your body back' following a pregnancy.

Liberal and constructivist feminist approaches to health inequalities emphasize the ways in which unequal gendered social roles, health behaviours and healthcare treatment have contributed to differences in men's and women's health. Along with a focus on the impact of reproduction and the traditional institution of family, an extensive feminist literature considers the impacts of patriarchy on women's lives and health (Hall and Lamont, 2009). By limiting women's options, patriarchy has at times affected women's education, income and life chances in many ways that have contributed to poor health. However, when patriarchal norms restricted women's behaviour with the expectation that 'ladies don't smoke', they also protected generations of women from the direct hazards of tobacco use (Elliot, 2001). As these norms changed, women's smoking rates increased rapidly. Consequently, in the United States lung cancer became the leading cause of cancer mortality in women (Jemal et al., 2005). From its inception, the feminist movement has also questioned the gendered power dynamics of doctor–patient interactions (for example, Munch, 2004) and the lack of information made available to women to inform their reproductive and other health decisions. Feminist work also assesses the mental and physical health impact of women's care-giving roles which encourage prioritizing caring for others over self-care.

Marxist/socialist feminist approaches emphasize the relationships between class structure, the distribution of social and economic resources and health outcomes. Both poverty and income inequality are associated with decreased life expectancy and poorer health outcomes for those with low incomes (see, for example, Doyal, 1995). However, the relationship between income inequality and gender differences in health is complex because one cannot easily parse out the relative contribution of gender/sex and income. Moreover, gender differences still exist within income levels. Thus, we contend that the socio-economic gradient alone cannot explain the apparent mortality–morbidity paradox in men's and women's health (Bird and Rieker, 2008).

Multicultural and intersectional feminist approaches go farther, arguing that broader frameworks are needed to understand gender, socio-economic and racial/ethnic disparities in health and healthcare and to capture the ways in which these factors interact. Thus this line of work emphasizes the intersections of race, class and gender. Researchers in this area have built upon the work of theorists such as Nakano-Glenn (1999) and Hill Collins (2000) to demonstrate the complex and multiplicative nature of these intersections. These complexities result in straightforward, quantifiable health disparities such as decreased healthcare access, non-standard or substandard treatment and more complications and disability from treatable chronic conditions. These disparities appear consistently across a variety of public and privately administered healthcare settings (see Schulz and Mullings, 2006). Intersection theory has therefore proven invaluable in creating frameworks for addressing disparities in healthcare and health outcomes for sexual minorities (see Crenshaw, 1993; Fish, 2008).

Constrained choice

Despite their many strengths, liberal and constructivist feminist, marxist/ socialist feminist, and multicultural and intersectional feminist approaches do not provide a sufficient foundation for action aimed at improving population health and reducing health disparities. Specifically, each of these approaches is a critique of the structure of society and as such was not intended to identify points for health intervention. In fact, few theorists have offered approaches that explain the mechanisms through which social inequalities contribute to health disparities. Moreover, as we have noted above, few theorists have offered models that integrate the role of social and biological factors. Thus, while these theories are very useful in describing aspects of the social patterning of men's and women's lives, their application to integrated interdisciplinary research and policy remains to be developed.

To address the knowledge gaps, we developed our framework of 'constrained choice' which provides a new direction for discourse, research and policy (Bird and Rieker, 2008). The constrained choice model (shown in Figure 8.1) offers a platform for prevention and is based on four premises. First, decisions made and actions taken at every level of society including government, community, work and family can enhance or limit individual health behaviours and choices. In other words, these decisions can increase or reduce individual agency (see Chan, 2009). Second, these decisions have both intended and unintended consequences that lead to constrained choices thereby socially patterning individual lives in ways that contribute to gender, race/ethnicity and/or social class differences in health. These patterns shape the impact of exposure to stressors and health behaviours.

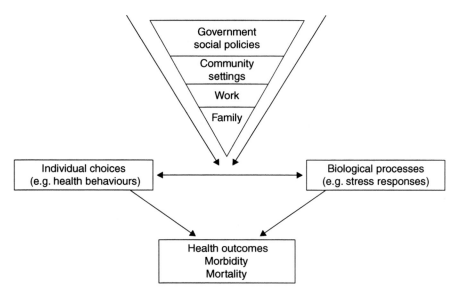

Figure 8.1   Constrained choice model
Source: adapted from Bird and Rieker (2008: 64)

For men and women additional physiological differences also contribute to these social patterns. Third, given the impact of decisions beyond the level of the individual, we contend that the production of health is a shared responsibility of decision-makers at each level. Fourth, the more marginalization an individual faces in society, the more limited his or her health choices will be. Thus combinations of disadvantages can make it more difficult or costly for individuals to pursue a healthy life and thus more likely that an individual will suffer poor health and a shorter life.

Applying constrained choice: two case examples of health conditions

To illustrate how constrained choices at each level of society contribute to health differences between and among men and women, we consider cardio-vascular disease (CVD) and HIV/AIDS. These conditions were selected because they are a primary cause of differential premature mortality among men and constitute a substantial health burden in terms of differential morbidity among women. In addition, they are useful for illustrating how race/ethnicity and gender interact to shape health risks and behaviours as elaborated below. We begin by describing the patterns of each disease in the USA and then apply the constrained choice model to understanding the incidence and trajectories by gender and race/ethnicity.

Cardiovascular disease

Cardiovascular disease (CVD) is the leading cause of morbidity and mortality for both men and women; it includes coronary heart disease (CHD) as well as vascular disorders such as arteriosclerosis and stroke. The prevalence of CVD and related mortality in the USA is higher in men than women due in part to earlier onset in men (National Center for Healthcare Statistics, 2009). However, more women than men ultimately die from and suffer the quality of life burdens of CVD because of their greater life expectancy.

As one would expect, CVD mortality rates increase substantially with age (CDC/NCHS, 2008). Within each age group, CVD mortality rates are higher for men than women, and for blacks than whites. Men demonstrate earlier onset of CVD morbidity and greater excess CVD mortality in middle age and early old age. However, the gender differences in CVD mortality narrow at older ages (over 74). The differences between black and white CVD mortality are pronounced and statistically significant. Black men aged 45 to 54 have a mortality rate twice as high as their white male counterparts and black women have a mortality rate three times higher than their white female counterparts. In later age cohorts excess black mortality drops off but does not disappear (CDC/NCHS, 2008).

HIV/AIDS

While men represent a larger percentage of people living with HIV/AIDS, consistently 26 per cent of all cases occur among women in the USA, though current indicators suggest that their numbers may be increasing. Since its first appearance in 1981, the social marginalization of HIV/AIDS sufferers has contributed to the disease's stigma and shaped related public policies. In the past 12 years, treatment innovations have shifted the medical understanding of HIV/AIDS from a terminal medical condition to a serious but treatable chronic disease. HIV/AIDS presents a unique set of challenges to existing health outcome paradigms (see also Chapter 12 by Gilbert and Selikow). Compared to men with HIV, HIV-positive women tend to receive less aggressive and effective treatment, progress to AIDS faster and have lower survival rates (African Services Committee et al., 2009; Shapiro et al., 1999). These patterns are even more markedly pronounced in black women with HIV/AIDS (James et al., 2008).

By 2006, an estimated 1.1 million people in the United States had HIV/AIDS, for a relatively low nationwide adult prevalence rate of 0.6 out of 100,000 persons (Centers for Disease Control, 2008b). Marginalized populations have not fared nearly as well. Although blacks and Latinos make up 13 per cent and 15 per cent of the United States population respectively, together they constitute 65 per cent of all people living with HIV/AIDS. Since the late 1980s, white men and women have made up a decreasing proportion of HIV/AIDS cases. From the beginning of the epidemic, black men have been disproportionately affected, making up approximately 25 per cent of all male cases in the first five years of the epidemic and currently constituting at least 45 per cent of all male cases. Since the beginning of the epidemic black women have constituted a majority of all female cases. Currently, they represent 65 per cent of all women living with HIV/AIDS. Below we discuss how the constrained choices approach can help us to understand these gendered patterns of CVD, HIV/AIDS and inform interventions to improve health and reduce disparities.

Levels of constrained choice

Every day, individuals make numerous choices that affect their health. These choices are not made in isolation but within the contexts of family, work and community settings, as well as broader public policy. Moreover, an individual's personal agency may at times be impeded or empowered by their gender, class, race/ethnicity or sexual orientation. This combination of social structures and individual agency can shape and constrain health behaviours and health choices (Rieker et al., 2010). Here we present examples from the US context.

Individual constraints

In trying to meet multiple obligations, individuals make routine everyday choices which do not promote health – such as working through lunch and eating at one's desk rather than going for a walk or eating convenience or fast food instead of preparing a healthier meal. Taken separately, these actions or choices are not necessarily gender-specific nor will they create major health consequences. Yet such choices are often made in the context of men's and women's gendered social roles and role expectations. The health impacts of daily actions are also mediated by innate and acquired differences in male and female biology. For example, as we noted above, women's more flexible circulatory system reduces both their risk of high blood pressure and its effects prior to menopause. Due to this biological difference, some of the negative health effects of a high sodium diet or a sedentary lifestyle may be more delayed in women compared to men. In addition, there is evidence that indicates that men and women metabolize both nicotine and alcohol differently which can lead to differential health outcomes (Bird and Rieker, 2008).

Whereas diet, exercise and exposure to stress are central to cardiovascular disease risk, the negotiation of safe sex practices is key to AIDS prevention. A broad body of work has established the gendered issues around requesting or requiring the use of condoms and other safe sex practices. Specifically, women are often disadvantaged in negotiating condom use due to unequal socio-economic status and power relative to their partner, or even a lack of knowledge that they are not in a monogamous relationship.

Many of the same behaviours that reduce health risks also improve resiliency and coping; for example, exercise, eating properly, limiting alcohol intake and maintaining social ties affect physical and mental health through multiple pathways. Consequently, individuals with few resources and stressful lives are at increasing risk of developing health conditions and, in turn, of experiencing poor health trajectories. Here differences in socio-economic status and in caregiver burdens, including lone parenting, expose women to higher levels of chronic stress. However, men may experience greater stress than women in attempting to fill the role of primary breadwinner. Gendered prevalence of specific types of negative coping, such as drinking and risk-taking in men or eating and self-blame in women, may exacerbate the differences in the impact of psychosocial stress on health.

Additional layers of complexity are added when one considers how the intersections of race/ethnicity and socio-economic status affect the range of options available to the individual and the extent of agency they have in making such choices. For example, in the USA black males typically face substantially higher unemployment rates than whites or black women. Such disadvantages further reduce life expectancy in black men, but also add to the socio-economic burdens on black women as lone parents and breadwinners. In the extreme case, multiple disadvantages or societal marginalization may eliminate choice altogether for both men and women.

Work/family

Much of men's and women's gendered experience is rooted in differences in work and family roles and role expectations. Work and its attendant social roles create expectations, form routines of daily living, and create norms of social interaction. All of these contribute to stress levels, health behaviours and coping mechanisms. Although differences in men's and women's roles in United States society have diminished in recent decades, women still more often perform roles of care-giving to children and to aging parents, while balancing many of the household duties.

Thus work and family can affect one's opportunities for positive health behaviours and the extent to which one is exposed to stressful situations or work over which one has limited autonomy or control, each of which can over time affect CVD risk through increased exposure to stress hormones including cortisol (Marmot, 2004). Less obvious perhaps is the extent to which norms and expectations shape one's options and even the meaning of requesting or requiring safe sex practices within marriage or other relationships which are presumed to be monogamous. Moreover, for many of those living on low or subsistence incomes or who are not in a monogamous relationship, traditional gender norms present a significant barrier to positive health behaviours, particularly safe sex.

Community impact

At the level of community, we focus on the impact of state and local policy and of the built environment. It is worth noting that many policies which are made at a national level in some European and other countries occur at the state and local levels in the United States. This includes many laws and regulations regarding smoking in public places and those regarding food, such as whether restaurants can use transfats, which are known to greatly increase CVD risk (Angell et al., 2009). Smoking rates in the United States were already declining more markedly in men than women, so recent smoking ban policies may ultimately yield greater benefits to women in reduced CVD and cancer risk. However, men typically eat fewer fruits and vegetables and thus may experience greater gains from the reduction of dietary transfats. Thus, community settings can have a substantial impact on individuals by shaping their day-to-day lives and activities by directly encouraging or facilitating positive health choices and behaviours, but the impact of specific policies will differ by gender due to differences in and among men's and women's lives. Similarly a city with good public transportation as well as streets and sidewalks built to accommodate pedestrians and bicyclists will improve public health directly by lowering its level of pollutants and encouraging individual exercise and/or active commuting. Such actions may also indirectly lower the level of stress in individuals' lives (Fitzpatrick and La Gory, 2000).

Alternatively, community settings and design can also impede health and health choices. For example, community planning that emphasises sprawling street designs that separate residential areas from goods and services discourage walking and offer limited alternatives to driving and long commutes. Some policies also have mixed health effects, such as legalized gambling which can bring money and jobs to an area, but may also increase gambling addiction and related problems.

While it is clear how local policies – such as bans on smoking in both indoor and outdoor public spaces, or requirements for the provision of bicycle lanes – affect health behaviours related to CVD, it may be less obvious that differences in local policies also are related to the incidence and outcomes of HIV/AIDS. However, some communities in the United States have embraced efforts to reduce the spread of HIV/AIDS and other diseases through needle exchange programmes which have been shown to effectively reduce HIV risk for drug users and addicts (Tempalski et al., 2007). Other communities have fought such programmes because they might in some way encourage or condone illegal drug use. Moreover, such programmes have a differential gender impact on HIV risk, particularly since very poor women often resort to trading sex for food, drugs or protection and thus are both exposed to risk as well as being in a difficult position to negotiate safe sex practices.

Government social policies

An essential tenet of constrained choice is that social and economic policy at the national level affect individual health and health choices, even if these policies may not be specifically health-related. Since the United States lacks national health insurance and exhibits significant gaps in public health policy, individuals and social groups with fewer social and economic resources (including but not limited to health insurance) experience higher morbidity and mortality rates. For example, currently 15 per cent of people who live in the United States lack health insurance. Men are more likely than women to have private insurance and to have obtained insurance through their employment, whereas women are more likely to have public insurance through Medicaid which primarily serves disadvantaged women and their children (Glied et al., 2008).

Not surprisingly, countries that have strong policy commitments to public health and welfare, such as Norway, Sweden and Canada, generally have higher life expectancy rates for both women and men than the United States and a relatively smaller gender gap (Bird and Rieker, 2008). Moreover, a comparative study of the health status of US and UK residents aged 55 to 64 (Banks et al., 2006), which used both disease biomarkers and self-reports, found that the US population, regardless of gender, was less healthy. The differences persisted after controlling for standard health behaviours. Although a health gradient existed in both countries and the largest disparities were reported for the bottom of the income and education hierarchy, for many of the diseases individuals at the top of the US socio-economic distribution were less healthy than their UK counterparts. The authors suggested that the greater link between health and economic resources in the United States may be due to the lack of health-protective welfare policies.

Perhaps the clearest example of the potential for national policy to shift gender differences in health behaviour in the United States is the Title IX programme, which was passed by Congress in 1972. Title IX prohibits any education programme or activity receiving federal financial assistance from discriminating on the basis of sex, and applies specifically to physical education, intramural sports (competitions within and among designated regional schools) and recreation, and athletics in elementary and secondary schools and colleges (Carpenter and Acosta, 2004). Although much debate continues about the full extent of its intended and unintended consequences and how far we are from gender equity in this regard, Title IX dramatically increased young women's physical education and opportunities.

The United States government has not made a commitment to conduct gender-based analyses of policies or to require it in federally funded health-related research. Many countries, such as Canada, for example, require gender-based analyses to assess whether and how a wide range of social policies affect both men and women, with the explicit intent of reducing inequity for women. However, few countries have made a systematic effort to assess possible disadvantages to men or have otherwise used such analysis to address men's earlier mortality. The Canadian Institutes for Health Research (CIHR) also has a commitment to gender-based analysis in the research they fund, irrespective of whether the investigators hypothesize that they will find such gender differences (CIHR, 2009; see Chapter 24 by Armstrong). This policy is intended to help overcome years of exclusion of women from biomedical studies and to more rapidly identify gender differences in treatment effects. Taken together, such policies form a systematic effort to identify sources of gender inequity.

National policies can also contribute to constraints on choice and individual agency that have a direct impact on both the spread of HIV and the disease trajectory of those who are HIV-positive. Moreover, the impact of these policies interacts with constraints at other levels. HIV/AIDS first appeared in the United States in the 1980s, an era of conservative federal politics with an emphasis on shrinking national government and national social programmes. The first groups diagnosed with what would eventually be called AIDS included men who have sex with men (MSM), IV drug users, sex workers, Haitians and people with haemophilia. While this mix at first appeared unlikely, each group was already stigmatized due to behaviour, race and/or disability status.

The marginalization of the groups first diagnosed with HIV/AIDS affected both the development and dissemination of policies and programmes aimed at treatment as well as prevention. Whereas the gay community organized and was able collectively to reduce some of the barriers to care, raise attention for their healthcare needs and assert rights in employment and other arenas, other marginalized groups (both men and women) with lower socio-economic status and less social agency did not benefit equally from these efforts, nor were they able to organize for their own needs (African Services Committee et al., 2009).

Conclusion

The constrained choice approach offers a systematic framework for addressing the apparent gender and health paradox by understanding how decisions made at multiple levels limit individual agency and collectively affect the opportunity to pursue a healthy life. This approach requires researchers and theorists to examine the relative contribution of women and men's biology, the social organization of their lives, the interaction among race/ethnicity and income, and the role of policy decisions and personal agency.

Although multiple theories have been offered to explain the various aspects of social inequalities and health, most fail to incorporate the combination of social and economic factors that directly and indirectly affect the gendered health patterns we describe in this chapter. Moreover, few provide insight into the interplay of social and biological processes that lead to changing gender patterns in morbidity and mortality. We argue that a broad framework and a multidisciplinary dialogue is essential for health researchers who aim not only to describe the social epidemiology of health and the factors that contribute to differences in men's and women's health (as well as health disparities among men and among women), but also to improve individual and population health by informing business practices and social and economic policies.

Perhaps the greatest challenge is to persuade policy-makers of the necessity and ultimate value of incorporating gender-based analysis and health effects into the decisions made and actions taken at various contexts – national policy, community or state policies, and employment settings. It is equally important for both families and individuals to develop a gendered health consciousness when making everyday life decisions. Recognizing that health is a shared responsibility will increase the opportunities to take both gender and health into account in schools, at work, in communities and in families.

Summary

- Gender differences in morbidity and mortality vary with changes in the leading causes of death and with changes in the social organization of men's and women's lives, which can impede or enhance their opportunities to pursue a healthy life.
- Many of the same constraints that put individuals at increased risk of disease incidence also place them at increased risk of poorer health trajectories. Consequently, social policies and actions at different levels of decision-making can contribute to population health and even shift gender differences in morbidity and mortality.
- Policy decisions can shape factors far beyond the control of individuals; these directly affect health, and include the safety and quality of the food supply, exposure to cigarette smoke in public spaces, and even the prevalence of HIV in high-risk populations in the local community.
- Gender-based analysis is central to assuring that social policies serve the population as a whole without exacerbating gender differences in health, including the practice that health research be applicable to both men and women.

Key reading

Annandale, E. (2009) *Women's Health and Social Change* (Abingdon: Routledge).

Bird, C. E. and P. P. Rieker (2008) *Gender and Health: The Effects of Constrained Choice and Social Policies* (New York: Cambridge University Press).

Schulz, A. J and L, Mullings (eds) (2006) *Gender, Race, Class and Health: Intersectional Approaches* (San Francisco: Jossey-Bass).

References

Abramowicz, M. and H. L. Barnett (1970) 'Sex Ratio of Infant Mortality', *American Journal of Diseases of Children*, 119 (4), 314–15.

African Services Committee, AIDS Alabama, Alliance of AIDS Services, Center for HIV Law and Policy et al. (2009) *Critical Issues for Women and HIV: Health Policy and the Development of a National AIDS Strategy*, Recommendations to the Office of National AIDS Policy (ONAP).

Angell, S. Y., L. D. Silver, G. P. Goldstein, C. M. Johnson, D. R. Deitcher, T. R. Frieden and M. T. Bassett (2009) 'Cholesterol Control beyond the Clinic: New York City's Trans Fat Restriction', *Annals of Internal Medicine*, 151 (2), 129–34.

Annandale, E. (2009) *Women's Health and Social Change* (Abingdon: Routledge).

Banks, J., M. Marmot, Z. Oldfield and J. P. Smith (2006) 'Disease and Disadvantage in the United States and England', *Journal of the American Medical Association*, 295 (17), 2037–44.

Bird, C. E., A. Fremont, A. Bierman, S. Wickstrom, M. Shah, S. Rector, T. Horstman and J. J. Escarce (2007) 'Does Quality of Care for Cardiovascular Disease and Diabetes Differ by Gender for Enrollees in Managed Care Plans?', *Women's Health Issues*, 17 (3), 131–8.

Bird, C. E. and P. P. Rieker (2008) *Gender and Health: The Effects of Constrained Choice and Social Policies* (New York: Cambridge University Press).

Bradburn, N. M. (1969) *The Structure of Psychological Well-being* (Chicago: Aldine).

Carpenter, L. J. and R. V. Acosta (2004) *Title IX* (Champaign: Human Kinetics Publishers).

CDC – Centers for Disease Control and Prevention (2008) 'HIV Prevalence Estimates – 2006', *Morbidity and Mortality Weekly Report*, 57, 1073–6.

CDC/NCHS – Centers for Disease Control and Prevention, National Center for Health Statistics (2008) *Compressed Mortality File 1999–2005*, CDC WONDER On-line Database, compiled from Compressed Mortality File 1999–2005 Series 20 No. 2K, at: http://wonder .cdc.gov/cmf-icd10.html, accessed 6 July 2009.

Chan, C. K. (2009) 'Choosing Health, Constrained Choices', *Global Health Promotion*, 16 (4), 54–7.

CIHR – Canadian Institutes for Health Research (2009) *Gender and Sex-based Analysis in Health Research: A Guide for CIHR Researchers and Reviewers*, at: www.cihr-irsc.gc.ca/ e/32019.html, accessed 29 May 2009.

Crenshaw, K. (1993) 'Mapping the Margins: Intersectionality, Identity Politics, and Violence against Women of Color', *Stanford Law Review*, 43 (6), 1241–79.

Crimmins, E. M., J. K. Kim and A. Hagedorn (2002) 'Life with and without Disease: Women Experience More of Both', *Journal of Women & Aging*, 14 (1–2), 47–59.

Davis, D.L., M. L. Gottlieb and J. R. Stampnitzky (1998) 'Reduced Ratio of Male to Female Births in Several Industrial Countries: A Sentinel Health Indicator?', *Journal of the American Medical Association*, 279 (13), 1018–23.

Dedovic, K. M., M. Wadiwalla, V. Engert and J. C. Pruessner (2009) 'The Role of Sex and Gender Socialization in Stress Reactivity', *Developmental Psychology*, 45 (1), 45–55.

Department of Commerce, Bureau of the Census (1921) *United States Life Tables: 1890, 1901, 1910, and 1901–1910*, Prepared by J. W. Glover (Washington, DC: Government Printing Office).

Di Giulio, P. and A. Pinnelli (2007) 'The Gender System in Developed Countries: Macro and Micro Evidence', in A. Pinnelli, F. Racioppi and E. Rettaroli (eds), *Genders in the Life Course: Demographic Issues* (Dordrecht: Springer), 25–50.

Doyal, L. (1995) *What Makes Women Sick: Gender and the Political Economy of Health* (New Brunswick: Rutgers University Press).

Dworkin, S. and F. Wachs (2009) *Body Panic: Gender, Health and the Selling of Fitness* (New York: New York University Press).

Elliot, R. (2008) *Women and Smoking since 1890* (Abingdon: Routledge).

England, P. (2005) 'Gender Inequality in Labor Markets: The Role of Motherhood and Segregation', *Social Politics*, 12 (2), 264–88.

Fausto-Sterling, A. (2005) 'The Bare Bones of Sex: Part 1 – Sex and Gender', *Signs*, 30 (2), 1491–1526.

Fish, J. (2008) 'Navigating Queer Street: Researching the Intersections of Lesbian, Gay, Bisexual and Trans (LGBT) Identities in Health Research', *Sociological Research Online*, 13 (1), at: www.socresonline.org.uk/13/1/12.htm, accessed 10 August 2009.

Fitzpatrick, K. M. and M. La Gory (2000) *Unhealthy Places: The Ecology of Risk in the Urban Landscape* (New York: Routledge).

Glied, S., K. Jack and J. Rachlin (2008) 'Women's Health Insurance Coverage 1980–2005', *Women's Health Issues*, 18 (1), 7–16.

Hall, P. A. and M. Lamont (eds) (2009) *Successful Societies: How Institutions and Culture Affect Health* (New York: Cambridge University Press).

Hill Collins, P. (2001) *Black Feminist Thought: Knowledge, Consciousness and the Politics of Empowerment* (New York: Routledge).

James, C. V., A. Salganicoff, M. Thomas, R. Ushan, M. Lillie-Blanton and R. Wynn (2008) *Putting Women's Health Care Disparities on the Map: Examining Racial and Ethnic Disparities at the State Level*, Kaiser Family Foundation, at: www.kff.org/minorityhealth/upload/7886.pdf, accessed 10 July 2009.

Jemal, A., E. Ward and M. J. Thun (2005) 'Contemporary Lung Cancer Trends among US Women', *Cancer Epidemiological, Biomarkers & Prevention*, 14, 582–5.

Joint United Nations Programme on AIDS (2008) *Report on the Global HIV/AIDS Epidemic 2008*, at: www.unaids.org/en/KnowledgeCentre/HIVData/GlobalReport/2008/2008_Global_report.asp, accessed 7 August 2009.

Kimmel, M. S. (2008) *The Gendered Society*, Third Edition (New York: Oxford University Press).

Krieger, N., D. H. Rehkopf, J. T. Chen, P. D. Waterman, E. Marcelli and M. Kennedy (2008) 'The Fall and Rise of US Inequalities in Premature Mortality: 1960–2002', *PLoS Medicine*, 5 (2), 0227–0241.

Macintyre, S., K. Hunt and H. Sweeting (1996) 'Gender Differences in Health: Are Things as Simple as They Seem?', *Social Science & Medicine*, 42 (4), 617–24.

Marmot, M. (2004) *The Status Syndrome* (New York: Henry Holt and Company).

Munch, S. (2004) 'Gender-biased Diagnosing of Women's Medical Complaints: Contributions of Feminist Thought, 1970–1995', *Women & Health*, 40 (1), 101–21.

Nakano-Glenn, E. (1999) 'The Social Construction and Institutionalization of Gender and Race: An Integrative Framework', in M. M. Feree, J. Lorber and B. B. Hess (eds), *Revisioning Gender* (Lanham: Altamira Press), 3–43.

NCHS – National Center for Health Statistics (2009) *Health, United States, 2008, with Chartbook* (Hyattsville: National Center for Health Statistics).

Omran, A. R. (1977) 'Epidemiologic Transition in the United States: The Health Factor in Population Change', *Population Bulletin*, 2 (2), 1–42.

Rieker, P. P., C. E. Bird and M. E. Lang (2010) 'Understanding Gender and Health: Old Patterns, New Trends and Future Directions', in C. E. Bird, P. C. Conrad, A. M. Fremont and S. Timmermans (eds), *The Handbook of Medical Sociology, Sixth Edition* (Nashville: Vanderbilt University Press).

Schulz, A. J and Mullings, L. (eds) (2006) *Gender, Race, Class and Health: Intersectional Approaches* (San Francisco: Jossey-Bass).

Shapiro, M. F., S. C. Morton, D. F. McCaffrey, J. W. Senterfitt, J. A. Fleishman, J. F. Perlman, M. A. Leslie, L. A. Athey et al. (1999) 'Variations in the Care of HIV-Infected Adults in the United States: Results from the HIV Cost and Services Utilization Study', *Journal of the American Medical Association*, 281 (24), 2305–15.

Tempalski, B., P. L. Flom, S. R. Friedman, D. C. Des Jarlais, J. J. Friedman, C. McKnight and R. Friedman (2007) 'Social and Political Factors Predicting the Presence of Syringe Exchange Programs in 96 US Metropolitan Areas', *American Journal of Public Health*, 97 (3), 437–47.

Velkoff, V. A. and P. R. Kowal (2007) *Current Population Reports, P95/07–1 Population Aging in Sub-Saharan Africa: Demographic Dimensions 2006*, United States Census Bureau (Washington, DC: Government Printing Office).

Verbrugge, L. M. and D. L. Wingard (1987) 'Sex Differentials in Health and Mortality', *Women & Health*, 12 (2), 103–45.

Wood, J. T. (2009) *Gendered Lives: Communication, Gender and Culture*, Eighth Edition, (Boston: Wadsworth).

Wood, S. F., A. Dor, R. E. Gee, A. Harms, D. R. Mauery, S. Rosenbaum and E. Tan (2009) *Women's Health and Health-care Reform: The Economic Burden of Disease In Women*, George Washington University, Jacobs Institute of Women's Health and Department of Health Policy, at: www.wellwoman09.org/materials/GWReport-CostBurdenofChron icIllnessFINAL.pdf, accessed 2 July 2009.

World Health Organization (2008) *World Health Statistics: Mortality and Burden of Disease*, at: www.who.int/whosis/whostat/EN_WHS08_Table1_Mort.pdf, accessed 4 July 2009.

9
Reproductive Regimes: Governing Gendered Bodies

Elizabeth Ettorre and Carol Kingdon

Introduction

This chapter examines the intersections between biological and social dimensions of gender and health with special reference to reproduction. We explore the notion of reproductive regimes through the consideration of four case studies that exemplify how contemporary women's reproductive bodies may engage with biomedicine. A major assumption running throughout the chapter is that, whilst the processes of reproduction may emerge as regulatory regimes for all bodies, women more than men have been viewed and managed as 'foetal containers'. Today there are social and cultural forces that afford pregnant women the opportunity to make 'choices' that challenge this notion of passivity. As the principle of patient choice becomes widespread in public and private healthcare systems across the developed countries of the western world and feminism increasingly operates in arenas of entitlement and individualism nevertheless the question remains: How is women's agency constrained by gendered disciplinary processes in the field of reproduction?

First, we discuss why an awareness of the sex/gender binary alongside the above biological and social intersections provides a 'backstory' to understand governing reproductive bodies. Next, we define reproductive regimes and analyse gendered disciplinary processes that evoke simultaneously the language of choice and control upon birthing bodies with reference to the rise of caesarean section (CS). We then consider genetic screening as a reproductive regime; we explore the stigmatization of deviant pregnant bodies with reference to substance misuse and outline future directions in biomedical surveillance within the context of public health and pregnancy.

The sex/gender binary and the challenges of fluid corporeality

A strong tradition of feminist work in the field of reproduction has a variety of constituents, including those that:

- draw attention to the ways in which women's reproductive bodies have long been regulated by the male-dominated medical profession;
- are concerned about the inadequacy of either an uncritical position that defers without question to the advances of science, or a pessimistic position that sees in contemporary reproductive technologies an unmitigated attack on women;
- focus on the global abuse of women's reproductive capacities, especially rape with its general health risks and risks of the spread of HIV/AIDS (Farmer, 2005);
- emphasize significant divisions between women in a now global market of reproductive body parts – such as ova and embryos – and services.

The authors' own contributions to the field of reproduction are overtly feminist and 'embodiment orientated'. Ettorre's (2002; 2007) work focuses on how female bodies are shaped and controlled through reproductive genetics as well as how pregnant bodies are designated as 'embodying deviance' through substance use. Works by Kingdon et al. (2006; 2009) explore women's embodied agency during pregnancy and birth, retaining a critical edge in relation to questions concerning *how* knowledge about reproductive bodies is produced, by whom, and with what consequences.

With regards to the above, feminist writing on the body is complex, varied and vast. One distinctive argument has replaced the assumption that inequalities between the sexes are derivative of 'nature' and fixed in biology – such as sex – with the notion that inequalities are derived from nurture and maintained by culture – such as gender (Price and Shildrick, 1999). More recently, feminist scholars of science have revealed how cultural ideas about maleness and femaleness are attributed to bodily parts that have no gender (Martin, 1991). Others recognize that irrespective of science's misrepresentations of the human female body as gendered, subordinate and defective, women are bodies in ways men are not – their unique capacity to gestate and birth young should be celebrated. This appreciation of real sexual difference is often criticized for essentialism but is nevertheless key (Annandale, 2009).

In recent years, the sex/gender binary conceptualization of body politics has broken down, while there exists a simultaneous trend to posit a corporeality that is fluid in its investments, meanings and performativities (Butler, 1993). In both feminist and masculinist scholarship on the body there is now widespread recognition of how culture can shape and alter the physical body (Bordo, 1993); thus the body is increasingly conceptualized as 'concurrently socially constructed and organically founded' (Turner, 1992: 17). Specifically in the field of reproduction, feminists influenced by the claims of post-structuralist scholars and others contend that gender has emerged as a powerful social institution that employs prescriptive moral claims and is fuelled by discursive practices charged with regulating bodies (Lorber, 1994; Rothman, 1994).

Defining reproductive regimes: the governance of pregnant bodies

Similar to gender (Lorber, 1994), reproduction as a component of culture is exhibiting signs of a social institution. As reproduction ascends as a social institution, it develops into a system of governance further surrounded by attendant regulatory regimes, focused on the replication of bodies which must exemplify completeness, health, well-being, individual potential and the future welfare of society (Ettorre, 2002). Reproduction is socially organized around a set of values, norms, activities and social relations that symbolize notions of able-bodiedness, human survival, progress and individual potential. At the same time, reproductive bodies, especially female reproductive bodies, become more valorized than ever before through reproductive regimes and the surveillance of their pregnant wombs in and through biomedicine.

There is a multiplicity of practices guiding pregnant bodies as they are gathered together in a systematic way under the flag of reproduction. The symbol of reproduction as an emergent social institution (and regulatory regime) is the pregnant body; the body of a woman producing a baby, as well as the chemicals, hormones, eggs, cells, genes, blood, foetal tissues – all gathered, drawn, scraped, tested, examined and, at times, discarded within reproductive medicine. Women are reproductive containers and science's (mis)representation of the female body shapes our whole understanding of how reproduction 'works', and has been and continues to be gendered throughout the life course from conception onwards. An assortment of disciplinary strategies – for example, biomedical knowledge, technologies, public health discourses and so on – attends to the pregnant body to construct and normalize it. This process is carried out under the supposedly benevolent gaze of the physician. Here, reproductive regimes exist as systems and processes structured around regulating reproductive bodies whether pregnant or not. They include the complex methods of governance, linking, submerging and sometimes fusing women's reproductive bodies with assortments of medical technologies and biomedical discourses, defining what are 'normal' and 'deviant' pregnant bodies as well as 'tried and tested' procedures.

For the purposes of this chapter, the term 'reproductive regimes' affirms the sociality of reproduction; directs attention to governmentality through which pregnant women play an active role in their own pregnancies; highlights power dynamics, the organized practices (mentalities, rationalities and techniques) through which pregnant women are governed; establishes material bodies; recognizes the 'conflictual' nature of reproduction; and makes links with both micro and macro levels.

Our conceptualization of reproduction as an institution or regulatory regime has feminist roots in scholarship on the body and reproduction and also draws from Turner's work (1987), which directs attention to the body as the focus of the medical profession with its overwhelming forms of surveillance and control. Turner (1987: 206) considers 'medicalization as an aspect of the rationalization of society through the dominance of scientific categories'. It is a process whereby medicine exerts social control by standardizing illness into phenomena that can be managed by bureaucratic organizations. Women have long been recognized as particularly vulnerable in this process; arguably nowhere is this more evident than in the medicalization of childbirth.

In the following discussions, we look at four contemporary case studies or existing reproductive regimes which illustrate the complexities involved when women's reproductive bodies confront a variety of biomedical practices and discourses. These cases highlight different dimensions of governance and general trends relevant to many women – for instance, those involved in caesarean section (CS) and the fit pregnancy genre – and some women – for instance, those engaging with reproductive genetics and drug use during pregnancy.

Regimes of medicalization and the rise of caesarean childbirth

The medicalization of childbirth can be traced to 17th-century western Europe, where metaphors of machine production were first used to describe a labouring woman's uterus and mechanical tools (most notably forceps) were first employed (Martin, 1987). A combination of the social forces associated with industrialization and with the Enlightenment began the process of redefining childbirth as a medical event rather than a social one. It facilitated male birth attendants' incursion into what was hitherto a woman's domain and first introduced the hospital as an alternative to birth at home. During the 1970s and early 1980s there was a proliferation of feminist interest in the medicalization of childbirth (Oakley, 1980). For many scholars then, as today, 'the issue is not that medicine has no place within maternity care, but that all pregnancies are medically managed, all of them are viewed as inherently pathological or risky, and normality is only ever defined in retrospect' (Henley-Einion, 2003: 177). This is particularly evident in the multiplicity of practices that now surround labour and vaginal childbirth that seek the safe delivery of the foetus preferably in hospital and usually within a medically defined timescale, for instance, using induction and augmentation. However, at the beginning of the 21st century it is unnecessary CS that has been described as the quintessential example of the medicalization of childbirth (Wagner, 2001). Figure 9.1 illustrates the dramatic global rise in CS rates.

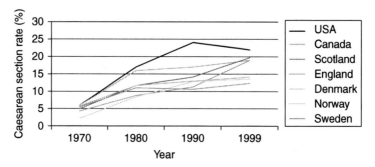

Figure 9.1   International caesarean section rates
Source: adapted from the National Sentinel Caesarean Section Audit Report (Thomas and Paranjothy, 2001: 2).

Globally, Latin America has the highest rates of CS. In Brazil, for example, the national CS rate is around 36 per cent, although it is not uncommon for private sector health clinics to report rates of 80 to 90 per cent (Hopkins, 2000). In stark contrast, it is estimated that in West Africa between 3.5 to 6.5 per cent of pregnant women need a CS for maternal or foetal problems (for example, protracted labour, placental abruption, malpresentation) but only 1.3 per cent delivers this way (Dumont et al., 2001). The World Health Organization advocates that there is no justification for any region to have a CS rate higher than 10 to 15 per cent (WHO, 1985). It has long been recognized that variations in CS rates may reflect obstetric attitudes and policies as much as any variation in need.

The new language of choice: caesarean section for maternal request

In addition to caesarean sections that are performed for ambiguous medical indications, a new kind of unnecessary CS has recently emerged. Caesarean delivery for maternal request (CDMR) has been defined as a subset of elective CS, performed not by medical necessity or indication, but on the request of the pregnant woman (National Institutes of Health, 2006). Arguably, what better way could there be to render the female reproductive body docile than to bypass the physiological process of labour and vaginal childbirth entirely and replace it with a planned medical procedure where an incision is made into a woman's abdomen and uterus, and the baby is delivered through her abdominal wall. However, one of the main criticisms of the medicalization thesis is that there are some real clinical and symbolic benefits of medicalization, with a number of feminist authors highlighting that some women may actively participate in the medicalization process to meet their own needs and exert control over their bodies during childbirth (Davis-Floyd, 1994). This raises the question: 'Who seeks control over the reproductive body during CDMR?' Is it women themselves, their clinicians, their partners, their foetus or another, such as, for instance, insurance companies?

Arguably, the most important disciplinary processes contributing to the rise of CDMR are associated with the medical appropriation of the language of 'choice'. Obstetric proponents of CDMR not only find support in contemporary healthcare policy discourses, but have reinvented neoliberal rhetoric of 'a woman's right to choose' from the reproductive rights movement of the 1970s (see comments by Professor Nick Fisk of Queen Charlotte's Hospital, London, in Revill, 2006). This powerful discourse not only implies that CDMR is 'what women want', but elevates its significance in public discourse. Despite successive international studies reporting that few women request CS (Kingdon et al., 2006), debate about CDMR continues, based on the premise that 'maternal request' is a valid concept with high or even moderate rates taken as given (Young, 2006). Convenience, avoidance of the pain associated with labour, alleviation of the risk of damage to the perineum (pelvic floor) and fear of vaginal birth are commonly reported reasons as to why women prefer CDMR. Thus, CDMR is constructed as a healthy alternative to vaginal birth with emphasis on preserving a woman's pelvic floor, reflecting 'new' medical knowledge of the problems following vaginal deliveries (some of which are iatrogenic) coupled with gendered discourses advocating maintenance of 'the vaginal tone of a teenager' as a new feminine ideal (Iovine, 1995, quoted in Wagner, 2000: 1677).

In the UK, research shows that, whilst many women support the principle of choice, in practice their autonomy is limited and all women feel that concerns about their baby's health should take precedence over any personal preference for vaginal or caesarean childbirth (Kingdon et al., 2009). In Nigeria, research found that, whilst previous infertility and advanced maternal age at first pregnancy were important reasons for CDMR, the perception that CS is the surest way toward a live birth was the critical factor underlying women's choice (Chigbu et al., 2006). This suggests an element of morality where, for women, making the 'right choice', or being seen to make the right choice, for their foetus is the most important thing, reflecting medicalized moral discourses that prioritize the foetus and gendered feminine ideals, including 'good mother(ing)' discourses.

Technologically mediated pregnancies

Sociological research has shown obstetricians to be the most active participants in the ongoing construction of a culture of CS in Brazil (Hopkins, 2000), Chile (Murray and Elston, 2005) and the UK (Simpson, 2004). However, professional opinion on the ethics of CDMR is divided (see ACOG, 2003; Schenker and Cain, 1999), suggesting more subtle medicalized regimes may be fuelling rising

CS rates generally and rates of CDMR specifically. In developed countries fertility is declining as more women delay childbirth and have fewer children. At the same time the medical gaze is ever-present, with the widespread use of real-time visual and aural technologies originating in the clinic circulating across society. Duden (1993) suggests that public images of the foetus have become part of the mental equipment of our time, serving to elevate the status of the foetus both prior to and during an individual pregnancy. Studies show that pregnant women now expect to 'meet their baby' on the ultrasound screen (Mitchell and George, 1998).

According to Haraway (1997: 177) in 'many contemporary technologically mediated pregnancies expectant mothers emotionally bond with their fetuses through learning to see the developing child on screen during a sonogram'. Selves and subjects are produced in such 'lived experiences', whilst the mother's testimony to the movement of the unseen child-to-be in her womb loses the authority it once had under modes of embodiment that are not technologically mediated. During pregnancy many women not only come to prioritize their foetus above their own health, but they may trust technologically mediated medical assessments of the welfare of their foetus more than their own instinct. This ill-equips them for labour and a vaginal birth without regular medical surveillance and intervention. In the UK, women's willingness to accept birth technology has increased significantly since the late 1980s, whilst women who have a negative antenatal attitude to birth interventions are less likely to have a CS (Green and Baston, 2007).

CDMR may remove the uncertainties of vaginal childbirth for clinicians and some women, but it also creates new ones, the implications of which are yet to be realized. Ultimately women can only birth safely by CS with medical regimes, whereas most women will birth vaginally with little or no medical assistance. A feminism that recognizes it is not wrong for some women to demand CDMR must not negate the needs of other women for whom CS remains a last resort. Also, feminism must recognize the threat CS currently poses to women's unique capacity to birth at a time when attention has shifted from the medicalization of childbirth to the politics of biomedicalization and newer reproductive technologies.

Reproductive genetics as forms of disciplinary biotechnologies

Biomedical discourses on the body and biotechnologies have become entrenched in contemporary cultures as our bodies have been, time and again, shaped by notions embedded in Cartesian dualism. Living bodies have been treated as no different from a piece of equipment, while this powerful and far-reaching discourse has consistently obscured considerations of sentient bodies. From this viewpoint reproduction emerges as a normative, standardizing system, which disciplines, controls and scrutinizes the actions of procreative bodies – both male and female. But female more than male bodies are constructed as reproductive and female procreative bodies tend to be subject to more medical surveillance, control and 'technologizing' than the procreative bodies of males. Given that the long process of conception and gestation is internal to the female body, the reproductive body stands for something essentially female (Shildrick, 1997).

With regards to the replication and production of bodies, biotechnology has had a major impact on present-day notions of reproduction. Wajcman (1991) argues that in no other area of social life is the relationship between gender and technology more vigorously disputed than in the sphere of human biological reproduction. Indeed, 'technological fixes' have been increasingly applied to pregnant, female bodies.

Some of the 'newer' reproductive technologies (RTs) can be designated as 'pre'-prenatal technologies – for example, in terms of the site for foetal development – and include a variety of techniques. For example, in-vitro fertilisation (IVF) in conjunction with superovulation, ultrasound, laparoscopic egg retrieval and embryo transfer as well as gamete intrafallopian transfer (GIFT) have allowed infertile women or women beyond childbearing age to experience pregnancy, if not give birth to a child. In the UK, where the first IVF baby was born in 1978, licensed clinics undertook 41,827 assisted conception cycles (33,051 patients) resulting in 9,655 births in 2006 (HFEA, 2008). The first IVF conception in the United States occurred in 1983. By 2000, 35,025 babies were born using assisted conception techniques, and 40,687 babies in 2001 (Thompson, 2005).

Figure 9.2 shows the increasing number of women undergoing assisted conception treatment cycles in the UK. There has been work written specifically by feminists which addresses the complex issues related to 'conception assisting' RTs for infertile women. While genetic technology is related to these RTs – for example, the genetic composition of eggs, sperm and embryos are monitored before implantation – prenatal screening and diagnosis tend to be focused on already pregnant women. All of these practices can be seen as assisting the birth of a 'normal', 'non-afflicted' baby/child. Feminists began to undertake research addressing how these technologies raised issues for women at a structural level, whilst simultaneously offering real solutions for infertile women at the level of individual agency.

The application of reproductive technologies and other biotechnologies mark a paradigmatic shift in our understanding of the body. Bodies become commodified and fragmented and potential bodies discarded. Furthermore, a hidden morality surrounds pregnant bodies as they may be drawn into an ethically suspect discourse when sex selection becomes normalized. The politics of sex selection in Asian countries is widely recognized (George, 2006; see

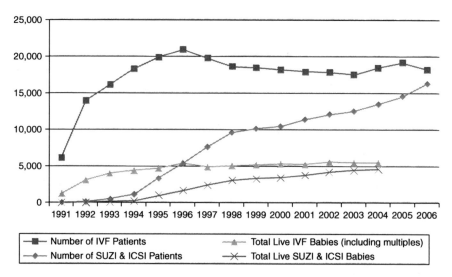

Figure 9.2   Human Fertilisation and Embryology Authority (UK) register data for IVF and ICSI

Source: a long-term analysis of the HFEA Register Data 1991–2006, at: www.hfea.gov.uk/docs/latest_long_term_data_analysis_report_91_06_pdf.

also Chapter 18 by Patel) and research in Arab countries also shows a trend of preference for boys over girls (Al-Akour et al., 2009).

The culture of medicine and specifically the professional practices of physicians with regard to reproduction have changed dramatically with these rapid biotechnological developments, generated by geneticists, embryologists and molecular biologists. The contribution of genetic factors to the entire range of diseases is being recognized, while the public hears that a greater proportion of childhood disease is genetic in origin. However, the medical profession's use of genealogical pedigrees to demonstrate that heredity was involved in the aetiology of a particular pathology can be traced to the mid-19th century (Resta, 1999). In many countries today medical experts contend that all pregnant women should undergo prenatal diagnosis and be screened for genetic disorders; see, for example, the screening choices for routine antenatal care in the National Health Service in the UK (www.screening.nhs.uk/an). At the same time, men and women in the general population believe that these sorts of techniques can be helpful in eliminating many serious diseases. These technologies erode the distinction between what is natural and what is not. Arguably, some women have gained through the implementation of these technologies, whilst other women have lost.

In this process we need to see pregnant bodies as not only foetal containers but also gendered sites where knowledge of genes, foetuses, reproductive processes and biomedicine converge. It is important to recognize that pregnant bodies are not gender-neutral systems. One difficulty with this work is to show *how* ideas about genetic codes in bodies, models about healthy and diseased genes, and data about appropriate kinds and levels of reproductive performances are culturally dependent 'embodied processes'.

To understand the importance of developing a feminist perspective is to recognize the powerful interplay between the field of genetics, modern medicine and the bodies of women. Is it fair that some women condemn themselves to shame because they do not measure up to society's image of what it means to be a good reproducing mother? The obvious answer is no. However, that these questions need to be asked demonstrates that reproductive genetics has profound ethical implications. If women's reproductive processes continue to be ranked according to genetic information, the field of genetics needs to become more gender-sensitive than it is at present and we need to see that gender, bodies and ethics go hand in hand.

Reproductive regimes of stigmatization: pregnant drug-using bodies within the somatic society

Reproduction regimes are important aspects of social and cultural corporeality in our somatic society in which bodies are the central organizing principle: they are simultaneously constrained by and resisting the principal fields of cultural and political activity (Turner, 1992). Women's bodies, and specifically their prenatal, reproductive spaces, became construed over time as the battlefield for the social body's survival (Stormer, 2000). These reproductive bodies become the substance of our ideological reflections on human life in a contemporary world of risk, danger, insecurity and disorder. In the 19th century women's reproductive organs began to coincide with colonial nation-states' perception that their material landscapes were apparently lacking sufficient white populations (Stormer, 2000). In western societies today the white majority's heterosexual, able-bodied, young, female wombs perform a functional role by normalizing prenatal space in a society obsessed with regulating reproductive bodies. In countries of the global south, basic human reproduction can often be surrounded by danger, disease and even death as pregnant women, distanced from organized medicine, battle for health against such threats as tuberculosis, famine and HIV/AIDS.

Within the regulatory regime of biomedicine, biopolitics revolve around controlling reproduction rather than increasing production. Biopolitics regulate the spaces between bodies – to monitor the interfaces between bodies, societies and cultures as well as to legislate the tensions between the habitus and the body. Turner (1992) contends that most if not all cultures want to close up bodies by promoting safe sex, using clean needles and so on. In this closing-up process the pregnant drug user becomes a visible feature or even a potent symbol of somatic society. She exposes how the personal and public problem of 'drug addiction' during pregnancy can reflect an unresolved tension between an embodied desire for an unfettered womb as an open ingesting body and the cultural need for bodily restriction, control and regulation. Of course, her race, class and age will govern both the formulation of her desires and the way culture controls these seemingly uncontrollable desires.

In the somatic society treating women as mere uterine environments that can be invaded or punished involves the kind of blaming-the-victim mentality that can only seem proper when one completely ignores the complex social conditions surrounding prenatal harm to future persons. Blaming pregnant drug users is all about wanting to close up these 'deviant' female bodies and regulate them physically and psychologically while at the same time denying that self-surveillance within the context of a desire for a positive foetal outcome may exist for many if not all of these women. In the UK, research shows that heroin is the main drug of pregnant drug users (Hall and van Teijlingen, 2006), while an estimated 7.5 babies per 1000 live births in the northeast of England were born to drug-using mothers (NEPHO, 2002).

From a feminist point of view a series of noteworthy uncertainties can be raised, given that the disciplinary power of western drug treatment systems often operates to adjust these pregnant drug-using women to dominant gender, race and class structures as well as depoliticizing and individualizing their situations. One can rightly ask: 'Who really benefits from these types of drug treatment systems?' Surely, it is not pregnant women. Indeed, previous research in this area has shown that pregnant women in drug treatment, similar to non-drug-using pregnant women, go through the developmental process of achieving a 'maternal identity' (Pursley-Crotteau and Stern, 1996). However, this research revealed that these women's psychological and biological needs conflicted often with the treatment philosophy that was on offer to them. Simply, the 'maternal' expectations of professionals and pregnant drug-users clashed.

If, as implied above, the ideal body in the somatic society is a conforming and not a deviant body, a drug-using body, particularly a female pregnant one, falls short of this conforming body ideal. On the one hand, the pregnant body is constructed both as a docile subject, submitting to invasive medical scrutiny and, as an active agent, responsible for optimizing foetal health. On the other hand, for the pregnant drug-using body, a woman's docility and active agency appear as questionable, if not vigorously denied, by society. This denial may be one reason why attempts are made in the drug treatment system to give pregnant drug-users treatment priority: these women are constructed as being wild, out-of-control bodies. This cultural denial of these women's agency and normality implies that their bodies as well as their foetuses are worthless and bad/deviant.

A whole series of discourses and practices shape the drug-using body as somatically different from the non-drug-using body. When a foetus is added to this equation, the moral character of the pregnant female body is called into question – she is a polluted foetal container (Murphy and Rosenbaum, 1999). She is viewed not only as behaviourally aberrant but also as socially disruptive by the very fact that she uses drugs while pregnant. She embodies disgust both by being pregnant and by consuming illegal drugs. The cultural fear is that by embodying disgust, she will reproduce something disgusting – a foetus – which will be ghastly, deformed or less than normal.

While cultural representations of pregnant women depict their bodies as vulnerable and in need of protection, pregnant drug-users are perceived as consciously forsaking that sort of protection and putting their bodies and foetuses in jeopardy. The pregnant drug user is the embodiment of risk. She appears in society as doubly disgusting – she carries a pregnancy in a polluted body because she consumes drugs which are 'dirty'. There is an assumed transparency of pregnant bodies, and for pregnant drug-users this means that 'seeing' into her womb or visualizing her embodiment reveals not only foetal but also cultural damage. And so, the stigmatizing goes on.

Reproductive regimes and the epidemiological gaze: future directions

The regimes that stigmatize pregnant drug-using bodies are being extended in public discourse to all pregnant women and even potential future child-bearers. Women of reproductive age are subject to increased surveillance with regulatory regimes that encompass women who smoke, drink alcohol, have poor diets, take little exercise or are labelled 'obese'. Within this regime, biopolitics extend to controlling the quality of reproduction, regulated by the modern apparatus of public health or what has been called the 'epidemiological gaze' (Klawiter, 2008: 23) and women are explicitly targeted as foetal containers. Public health discourse is saturated with health education campaigns that seek to deter women who are pregnant or planning pregnancy from using alcohol, drugs or tobacco and encourage vitamins (like folic acid), healthy eating and regular, moderate exercise.

In the UK for example, the *Health in Pregnancy Grant* – introduced by the Department of Health in April 2009 (http://campaigns.direct.gov.uk/money-4mum2be/) – requires pregnant women to access midwives and doctors who simultaneously prescribe biomedical regulation and individual responsibility for health. However, medically infused public discourses are known to disregard the diverse ways that individual women negotiate foetal health risks, and existing research has shown how regimes that seek to control pregnant women's smoking are gendered and foetal-centric (Oaks, 2001). Under these regimes non-compliance with medical advice is construed as deviant and the only socially, morally and legally acceptable parents-to-be – especially mothers-to-be – are those who act on behalf of their 'babies-to-be'.

Pregnancy is now a condition of hyper-visibility that was unimaginable less than 20 years ago. Annie Leibovitz's photograph of the actress Demi Moore on the cover of *Vanity Fair* (August 1991) provided the catalyst for the new visibility of pregnant embodiment across a range of different cultural media and has spawned new pregnancy markets. According to Tyler (2005) a 'fit pregnancy genre' is emerging with distinct pregnancy diets, keep-fit programmes, fertility control and fashion that couples 'good mother(ing)' discourses with new feminine ideals of pregnant beauty. The fit pregnancy genre endorses a normative pregnant form, constitutive of a relatively new reproductive regime in which bodies marked by difference (ethnic, racial, able-bodiedness and so on) do not 'fit'. These new ideals of pregnant beauty and the extension of the epidemiological gaze to all potential future child-bearers seek to exert control and physically shape future reproductive bodies.

Post-2000 there has been an identifiable change in tone and focus in feminist scholarship on reproduction that cautions against simplistic readings of physicians and scientists (Thompson, 2005). We extend this caution to simplistic readings of (pre)pregnant women, procreative bodies, technologies, procedures, services and popular discourses, all of which have an active role in shaping new and emerging reproduction regimes. Thus an important challenge arises from the possibility of exploring these reproductive regimes further and that is the need to appreciate their multi-layered complexities, which unquestionably require engaging with women and healthcare professionals and popular discourses, whilst at the same time endeavouring to retain a critical feminist lens that challenges gender inequalities. Meeting these challenges involves ensuring that important gains are maintained for procreative bodies embedded in reproductive regimes and real choices become a distinct possibility for improving reproductive health for all.

Conclusion

In this chapter we have defined and developed the concept of reproductive regimes, exposing some of the gendered processes that serve to control women during (pre)pregnancy and childbirth. We have explored the continued relevance of the notion of women as foetal containers in the context of caesarean section, reproductive genetics, pregnant drug-users and a new 'fit pregnancy genre'. This demonstrates how during pregnancy and birth women's reproductive bodies are principally constructed as foetal containers rendering vaginal childbirth as unhealthy and CDMR as preferable; symbolizing women's bodies as gendered sites of 'good' or 'bad' genes; stigmatizing pregnant drug-users' bodies as polluted; and designating all potential reproductive bodies as (un)healthy sites to be shaped and controlled.

Also, we have highlighted how foetal concerns may embody male/medical concerns and that consequently reproduction is a gendered regulatory process involving, at a deep level, corporeal morality. The discursive practices of modern medicine are now universal, yet shape individual women's reproductive bodies differently depending on their corporeality, geography, affluence and access to healthcare.

Summary

- Reproduction as a component of culture is exhibiting signs of a social institution and reproductive regimes exist through a variety of practices that inscribe pregnant bodies.
- Physicians' appropriation of choice discourses may serve to extend pregnant women's support for medicalization and contribute to the rise in caesarean section rates.
- Through reproductive genetics, pregnant women can be divided into those with 'good' and 'bad' genes.
- Drawn into powerful moral discourses on the body, pregnant drug-users are viewed as 'polluted' foetal containers.
- The regimes that control pregnant bodies are being extended in public discourses beyond pregnant women to all future child-bearers.

Key reading

Duden, B. (1993) *Disembodying Women: Perspectives on Pregnancy and the Unborn* (Cambridge, MA: Harvard University Press).

Ettorre, E. (2002) *Reproductive Genetics, Gender and the Body* (Abingdon: Routledge).

Ettorre, E. (2007) *Revisioning Women and Drug Use: Gender, Power and the Body* (Basingstoke: Palgrave).

Kingdon, C., J. Neilson, V. Singleton, G. Gyte, A. Hart, M. Gabbay and T. Lavender (2009) 'Choice and Birth Method: Mixed-method Study of Caesarean Delivery for Maternal Request', *British Journal of Obstetrics and Gynaecology*, 116 (7), 886–95.

References

ACOG – American College of Obstetricians and Gynecologists Committee Opinion (2003) 'Surgery and Patient Choice: The Ethics of Decision Making', *Obstetrics and Gynecology*, 102, 101–6.

Al-Akour, N., M. Khassawneh, Y. Khader and E. Dahl (2009) 'Sex Preference and Interest in Preconception Sex Selection: A Survey among Pregnant Women in the North of Jordan', *Human Reproduction*, 1 (1), 1–5.

Annandale, E. (2009) *Women's Health and Social Change* (Abingdon: Routledge).

Bordo, S. (1993) *Unbearable Weight: Feminism, Western Culture and the Body* (Berkeley: University of California Press).

Butler, J. (1993) *Bodies that Matter* (New York: Routledge).

Chigbu, C. O., I. V. Ezeome and G. C. Iloabachie (2006) 'Cesarean Section on Request in a Developing Country', *International Journal of Gynecology and Obstetrics*, 96 (11), 54–6.

Davis-Floyd, R. (1994) 'The Technocratic Body: American Childbirth as Cultural Expression', *Social Science & Medicine,* 38 (8), 1125–40.

Duden, B. (1993) *Disembodying Women: Perspectives on Pregnancy and the Unborn* (Cambridge, MA: Harvard University Press).

Dumont, A., L. Bernis, M. H. Bouvier-Colle and G. Bréart for the MOMA study group (2001) 'CS rate for Maternal Indication in Sub-Saharan Africa: A Systematic Review', *The Lancet,* 358, 1328–33.

Ettorre, E. (2002) *Reproductive Genetics, Gender and the Body* (Abingdon: Routledge).

Ettorre, E. (2007) *Revisioning Women and Drug Use: Gender, Power and the Body* (Basingstoke: Palgrave).

Farmer, P. (2005) *Pathologies of Power: Health, Human Rights, and the New War on the Poor* (Berkeley: University of California Press).

George, S. M. (2006) 'Millions of Missing Girls: From Fetal Sexing to High Technology Sex Selection in India', *Prenatal Diagnosis,* 26 (7), 604–9.

Green, J, M. and H. A. Baston (2007) 'Have Women Become More Willing to Accept Obstetric Interventions and Does This Relate to Mode of Birth. Data from a Prospective Study', *Birth,* 34 (1), 6–13.

Hall, J. L. and E. R. van Teijlingen (2006) 'A Qualitative Study of an Integrated Maternity, Drugs and Social Care Service for Drug-using Women', *BMC Pregnancy and Childbirth,* 6, 19.

Haraway, D. (1997) *Modest_Witness@Second_Millennium. FemaleMan©_Meets_Oncomouse™: Feminism and Technoscience* (London: Routledge).

Henley-Einion, A. (2003) 'The Medicalization of Childbirth', in C. Squires (ed.), *The Social Context of Birth* (Oxford, Radcliffe Medical Press), 173–86.

Hopkins, K. (2000) 'Are Brazilian Women Really Choosing to Deliver by Cesarean?', *Social Science & Medicine,* 51 (5), 725–40.

HFEA – Human Fertilisation and Embryology Authority (2008) *Facts and Figures 2006: Fertility Problems and Treatment* (London: HFEA).

Iovine, V. (1995) *The Girlfriends' Guide to Pregnancy: Or Everything Your Doctor Won't Tell You* (New York: Pocket Books).

Kingdon, C., L. Baker and T. Lavender (2006) 'Systematic Review of Nulliparous Women's Views of Planned Cesarean Birth: The Missing Component in the Debate about a Term Cephalic Trial', *Birth,* 33 (3), 229–37.

Kingdon, C., J. Neilson, V. Singleton, G. Gyte, A. Hart, M. Gabbay and T. Lavender (2009) 'Choice and Birth Method: Mixed-method Study of Caesarean Delivery for Maternal Request', *British Journal of Obstetrics and Gynaecology,* 116 (7), 886–95.

Klawiter, M. (2008) *The Biopolitics of Breast Cancer: Changing Cultures of Disease and Activism* (Minneapolis: University of Minnesota Press).

Lorber, J. (1994) *Paradoxes of Gender* (New Haven: Yale University Press).

Martin, E. (1987) *The Woman in the Body: A Cultural Analysis of Reproduction* (Boston: Beacon Press).

Martin, E. (1991) 'The Egg and the Sperm: How Science Constructed a Romance Based on Stereotypical Male-Female Roles', *Signs: Journal of Women in Culture and Society,* 16 (31), 485–501.

Martin, P. Y. (2004) 'Gender as a Social Institution', *Social Forces,* 82 (4), 1249–73.

Mitchell, L. and E. George (1998) 'Baby's First Picture: The Cyborg Fetus of Ultrasound Imaging', in R. Davis-Floyd and J. Dumit (eds), *Cyborg Babies: From Techno-sex to Techno Tots* (London: Routledge), 105–24.

Murphy, S. and M. Rosenbaum (1999) *Pregnant Women on Drugs: Combating Stereotypes and Stigma* (New Brunswick: Rutgers University Press).

Murray, S. F. and M. A. Elston (2005) 'The Promotion of Private Health Insurance and Its Implications for the Social Organisation of Healthcare: A Case Study of Private Sector Obstetric Practice in Chile', *Sociology of Health and Illness*, 27 (6), 701–21.

NIH – National Institutes of Health (2006) 'State-of-the-Science-Conference: Cesarean Delivery on Maternal Request: Final Statement', *Obstetrics and Gynecology*, 107, 1386–97.

NEPHO – North East Public Health Observatory (2002) *Drug Misuse in Pregnancy in the Northern and Yorkshire Region* (Leeds: NEPHO).

Oakley, A. (1980) *Women Confined: Towards a Sociology of Childbirth* (Oxford: Martin Robertson & Co).

Oaks, L. (2001) *Smoking and Pregnancy: The Politics of Fetal Protection* (New Brunswick: Rutgers University Press).

Price, J. and M. Shildrick (1999) 'Openings on the Body: A Critical Introduction', in J. Price and M. Shildrick (eds), *Feminist Theory and the Body* (Edinburgh: Edinburgh University Press), 1–14.

Pursley-Crotteau, S. and P. N. Stern (1996) 'Creating a New Life: Dimensions of Temperance in Perinatal Cocaine Crack Users', *Qualitative Health Research*, 6 (3), 350–67.

Resta, R. (1999) 'A Brief History of the Pedigree in Human Genetics', in R. A. Peel, (ed.), *Human Pedigree Studies* (London: Galton Institute), 62–84.

Revill, J. (2006) 'Why Mothers Should Be Offered Caesareans', *The Observer*, 5 March, 14.

Rothman, B. K. (1994) *The Tentative Pregnancy: Amniocentesis and the Sexual Politics of Motherhood* (London: Pandora).

Schenker, J. G. and J. M. Cain (1999) 'FIGO Committee Report: FIGO Committee for the Ethical Aspects of Human Reproduction and Women's Health, International Federation of Gynecology and Obstetrics', *International Journal of Gynecology and Obstetrics*, 64 (3), 317–22.

Shildrick, M. (1997) *Leaky Bodies and Boundaries: Feminism, Postmodernism and (Bio)ethics* (London and New York: Routledge).

Simpson, J. (2004) 'Negotiating Elective Caesarean Section: An Obstetric Team Perspective', in M. Kirkham (ed.), *Informed Choice in Maternity Care* (Basingstoke, Palgrave Macmillan), 211–34.

Stormer, N. (2000) 'Prenatal Space', *SIGNS: Journal of Women in Culture and Society*, 26 (1), 109–44.

Thomas, J. and S. Paranjothy (2001) *The National Sentinel Caesarean Section Audit Report* (London: RCOG Press).

Thompson, C. (2005) *Making Parents: The Ontological Choreography of Reproductive Technologies* (Cambridge, MA: MIT Press).

Turner, B. (1987) *Medical Power and Social Knowledge* (London: Sage).

Turner, B. (1992) *Regulating Bodies: Essays in Medical Sociology* (London: Routledge).

Tyler, I. (2005*) '*Pregnant Beauty: The Changing Visual and Cultural Practices of Pregnant Embodiment', paper presented at the Maternal Bodies Workshop, IAS Lancaster, 2 November 2005.

Wagner, M. (2000) 'Choosing Caesarean Section', *The Lancet,* 356, 1677–80.

Wagner, M. (2001) 'Fish Can't See Water: The Need to Humanise Birth', *International Journal of Gynecology and Obstetrics*, 75 (Suppl.), S25–S37.

Wajcman, J. (1991) *Feminism Confronts Technology* (University Park: Pennsylvania State University Press).

WHO – World Health Organization (1985) 'Appropriate Technology for Birth', *The Lancet,* 326, 436–7.

Young, D. (2006) 'Cesarean Delivery on Maternal Request: Was the NIH Conference Based on a Faulty Premise?', *Birth,* 33 (3), 171–4.

10
Coronary Heart Disease: Gendered Public Health Discourses

Elianne Riska

Introduction

Heart disease is a public health concern in most western societies. The high mortality from coronary heart disease (CHD) has resulted in public health initiatives to prevent this disease and to lower the morbidity and the mortality figures. CHD has been framed as a 'men's disease' in public health discourse because men continue to more often die from this disease at younger ages than women. This chapter examines how CHD has been constructed in male gendered terms in public health discourse and discusses what kind of implications this gendered notion of the disease has had for women. The argument is that the early public health discourse on CHD was framed in the context of the United States and based on the medicalization of a certain type of masculinity. Later feminist health advocacy in this area has also had its origin in the US context. The gendered and cultural contexts of the public health discourses on CHD are important to consider when promoting policies to reduce gender inequalities in cardiac health.

This chapter on gender and CHD is divided into three parts. The first part will look at the early knowledge production about CHD and its male-focused content and male-only studies. US research in the early 1960s on Type A behavioural pattern (TABP) is an example of the construction of medical knowledge as seemingly gender-neutral and generic but which came to have implications for the health of men and women other than those white, middle-class men considered at risk. The second part of the chapter looks at the efforts to correct medical knowledge on CHD and in the spirit of feminist empiricism to test and add new knowledge on women's risk factors for CHD in order to produce more gender-specific knowledge on the disease. The third and concluding part will summarize the issues examined in the chapter and suggest a way forward for research on gender-specific health risks and CHD.

Coronary heart disease: 'A men's disease'

Heart disease as a white, middle-class men's disease

In the mid-1950s, Americans became concerned with the rising morbidity and mortality from CHD among white, middle-aged men. Dietary concerns were raised but the early research on risk factors did not seem convincing to some CHD researchers. Two San Francisco-based cardiologists, Ray Rosenman and David Friedman, began to explore alternative explanations and one explanation right from their own practice was particularly appealing: at risk of CHD were certain white, middle-class men who could not relax at work or at home but worked full speed ahead as they strived to succeed in their jobs. Rosenman and Friedman sketched a set of behaviours that they had observed among their male patients and suggested that these constituted risk factors for CHD. As they argued, 'We call this a behavior pattern because it is an overt and observable pattern that reflects an individual's characteristic responses' (Rosenman, 1978: 60). They named this action-behaviour complex the Type A behavioural pattern. The shorthand for this behaviour was TABP and the behaviour was characteristic for a certain personality named Type A.

This was the early years of stress research wherein stress at work was considered a new and risky aspect for white-collar men's health. Friedman and Rosenman's (1960) Type A thesis predicted that a certain type of behaviour, embodied in a male executive who was extremely competitive, inclined to work for deadlines and never stopped working in pursuit of more material gain, was doomed for a heart attack (Riska, 2000). For these researchers, white, middle-class men were the group at risk and it did not occur to them to consider other groups, such as other social classes of men or women, as groups also at risk of CHD.

The operationalization of TABP was by means of a specially designed instrument, the so-called Structured Interview (SI) which was assumed to provide an easy diagnostic tool for general practitioners, who could check whether the designated set of behaviours applied to the (male) patient presenting with anxiety and stress symptoms. The 'extreme Type A person' – a pathological and preclinical case – could be identified by using 12 behaviours, each divided into four graded subcategories. These behaviours are: handshake, attitude, general appearance, motor pace, speech hurrying, voice quality, rhythmic movements, hands/feet, facial expressions, laughter, fist clenching and sighing (Rosenman, 1978: 67). The sum of the points suggested whether the person was a Type A and this category was medicalized.

Type A was considered a generic type of behaviour but at issue was the emotional repertoire of white, middle-class men in the US gender order in the 1950s. Today sociologists would use the term hegemonic masculinity (Connell and Messerschmidt, 2005) to capture the emotional and behavioural complex that described the construct and measures of TABP. The testing of the predictive power of the Type A construct was done with samples of white, middle-class men only. The first empirical testing was conducted in a population-based follow-up study beginning in 1960. This was the Western Collaborative Group Study that included over 3500 healthy, white, middle- and upper-class male executives from 10 Californian companies. After eight and a half years it was found that the previously seemingly healthy Type A men were twice as likely as other men in the sample to develop heart disease (Rosenman et al., 1975). This result was considered to provide empirical evidence of the predictive power of the SI as an instrument to identify men at risk of CHD.

However, the Type A construct was gradually perceived as problematic for medicine for two reasons. First, it did not fit the criteria of psychopathology and therefore failed to fall within the domain of psychiatry. Second, it was not a socially deviant behaviour and did not therefore fall within the domain of criminology and the institutional agents of social control, such as for instance police and the law (Roskies, 1991). Hence the Type A concept was criticized for its ambiguity but not for is gender bias. As new studies were conducted, groups other than white, middle-class men were included, beginning, for example, with the so-called Framingham study. This study included women and the results indicated that Type A and its measurement device – the SI and its successors, the Bortner scale and the Jenkins Activity Survey (JAS) – were murky at best, and some charged that the Type A scales were invalid. Rosenman (1991: 3) agreed that there were problems with self-report measures for TABP assessment, but he claimed that 'there is remarkable consistency with the TABP construct in the cluster of traits that are measured by such scales'. Others were less convinced and argued that TABP was a multidimensional concept and that some of the dimensions had no negative impact on health, while other dimensions tapped the 'toxic' elements of the Type A construct, such as hostility and anxiety (see for instance, Edwards et al., 1990; Miller et al., 1996; Mudrack, 1999).

As the scales were tested for consistency and validity, the results did not look promising. The classical SI scale was impractical to use in large surveys and the JAS was not very reliable as the intercorrelations between the scales were found to be rather low. Although various standardized scales claimed to measure TABP, there were built-in measurement errors, and the scales contained different dimensions of TABP. As one team of researchers concluded in rather harsh terms in the early 1990s: 'We suggest that the Bortner scale, the Framingham scale, and the JAS should no longer be used in their current form' (Edwards et al., 1990: 452).

Gradually the crucial component to be singled out was hostility but this dimension was considered to have an emotional and a behavioural component. The behavioural component – aggression, also called 'anger-out' – was felt to be best measured by the classical SI scale which also tapped men's repertoire of hostility. The other component of hostility was emotional and called 'anger-in', which was found to capture women's expressions of hostility (Miller et al., 1996). Later research has distinguished between two related concepts. One is Achievement Striving (AS), which is considered a positive aspect and related to high performance and productivity. This concept has been found to be related to high job control, high job satisfaction and few (low) role conflicts. By contrast, the other concept is Impatience Irritability (II), which has been found to be related to stress and low life satisfaction; these dimensions are negative and measure anger-in and depression, which are assumed to be related to the development of CHD (Day and Jreige, 2002; Mudrack, 1999).

These findings and explanations belong to the control theory of Type A behavioural pattern. According to the control theory, Type A persons strive to control their environment when they are threatened with loss of control (Sturman, 1999). Rosenman, the initiator of the Type A concept, has reformulated his definition of Type A to now fit the interpretation that is based on control theory. Using control theory he suggests that: 'Type A behaviours appear to be enhanced performance to assert and maintain control over the environment, whenever this is challenged or threatened' (Rosenman, 1991: 3).

In short, the preventive approach to coronary heart disease pointed to specific, quantifiable and manageable mechanisms. The formula was simple: if the risk factors could be controlled, heart disease could be prevented (Aronowitz, 1998; Clarke et al., 2003). The risk-factor approach to men's CHD connected the emotional strains of executive work with the rising mortality of middle-class, middle-aged (white) men caused by the fatal outcome of heart disease (Ehrenreich, 1983; Helman, 1987; Riska, 2000; 2004). The proneness to heart disease was assumed to reside in the negative emotions of Type A men: hostility, anger and aggression were defined as the gendered health risks of hard work required in entrepreneurial and executive positions in the US business world. This was the first time that men's competitive and aggressive behaviour was seen in pathological terms rather than as the normal cultural repertoire of masculine behaviour.

The Type A thesis was short-lived and it was declared invalid by academic medicine in the mid-1980s (Riska, 2004). Yet the thesis of the toxicity of hyper-masculinity has survived in public discourse as a set of health beliefs or lay epidemiology about 'coronary candidacy' and CHD continued to be framed as a men's disease (Davison et al., 1991).

Race/ethnicity, social class and men's cardiac health

Early research on Type A was conducted primarily by using a study population of white, middle-class men. In the early 1980s, a special instrument to measure the links between personal predisposition and risk factors for the development of CHD among African-American men was introduced. Health psychologists invented a term for a personality syndrome called 'John Henryism', a construct designed to acknowledge racially based stressors and the masculinity script of African-American men (James et al., 1983). In the scientific discourse John Henryism was originally defined as 'an individual's self-perception that he can meet the demands of his environment through hard work and determination' (James et al., 1983: 263). This construct derives from a legend, transmitted as a ballad, of a steel-driving man working on railroad construction in the United States in the 1870s who competes with a mechanical steam drill, beats his opponent – the machine – but dies of overexertion. The construct emphasizes personal characteristics, especially personal commitment to a strong work ethic and desire to succeed, as the explanatory factors for a person's health status.

A high level of John Henryism means that a person believes that any obstacles can be overcome through hard work and a strong will to succeed. The so-called John Henryism thesis predicts that a person who scores high in the attitude called John Henryism but who has limited ways of coping because of low income will be prone to a health risk, for example, high blood pressure. For the identification of the syndrome, a 12-item scale has been designed which uses a five-point Likert-type scale with high summary scores identifying high levels of the attitude defined as John Henryism (see, for instance, Whitfield et al., 2006).

From the beginning the concept was slightly hard to understand: it measured personal characteristics but explained the result by external, material factors. More recently scholars have introduced another dimension to the construct: namely 'John Henry active coping', which is a strong behavioural predisposition to cope in an active, determined and hard-working manner with racially based stressors, like barriers to upward mobility (Bonham et al., 2004: 737; Fernander et al., 2005: 492). According to this view, John Henryism refers to the interaction effect of a high level of John Henry active coping and low socio-economic status (SES) indicators, such as low education and low income, which will result in negative health outcomes, for example, high blood pressure. By contrast, a high level of John Henryism and a high SES among African-Americans has been found to be related to good health (Bonham et al., 2004). This means of explaining the interaction between a certain personality and health has been questioned. For example, critics have fumed that 'by concluding that John Henryism "causes" better health outcomes, we place the burden of health on the individual' (Griggs and Mallinger, 2004: 1658).

The behavioural risk factors that have been related to men's likelihood of getting coronary heart disease can be depicted in the form of a typology of masculinities and their assumed relationship to cardiac health (Figure 10.1).

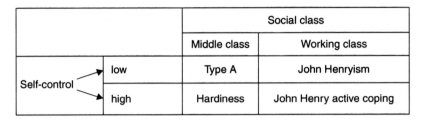

		Social class	
		Middle class	Working class
Self-control	low	Type A	John Henryism
	high	Hardiness	John Henry active coping

Figure 10.1 Typology of masculinities and CHD risks constructed in scientific discourse

The typology focuses on two dimensions of masculinity: a sense of control over the masculine self and men's location in the class structure (Riska, 2010). The first dimension medicalizes men's lack of control and assumes that lack of autonomy and a weak sense of a masculine self result in negative emotions, such as hostility, anger, anxiety and depression. The middle-class version of this man is Type A and the blue-collar and non-Caucasian version is John Henry man. The alphabet has continued to be used in recent research to explain negative emotions as risk factors for the likelihood for men to develop CHD, for example, Type D or the 'distressed' personality (Denollet and Pedersen, 2008).

The second dimension has introduced health-promoting factors linked to cardiovascular health and a refurbished version of the neglected Type B construct, which in the original Rosenman model was simply defined as the antithesis of Type A. A high sense of self-control, strong social ties and social support are assumed to have a buffering effect on cardiac health. In line with this reasoning, a personality type – called 'hardiness' – appeared in health psychology in the early 1980s. The 'hardy man' is a representation of a healthy white-collar (white) man who, regardless of a stressful situation, can cope with the anxieties and strains in executive work. Again in the empirical testing of this construct, only middle-class men were used as a study population (Riska, 2002). A blue-collar version of this 'healthy' masculine personality is displayed by a high level of John Henry active coping as described above.

The social categories of masculinities constructed in scientific discourse have medicalized certain masculine traits and declared other traits as 'healthy' masculinities. This traits approach is based on and tends to further confirm certain stereotypical notions of traditional masculinity.

CHD in public health discourse

A glance at the mortality statistics shows that the gender difference in CHD mortality varies widely between countries. The UK, Ireland, France, Italy, Germany, Sweden and Finland can be used as examples of differences between European (EU) countries. Mortality from coronary heart disease (also called

Table 10.1   Ischaemic heart disease mortality* by gender and country

Gender	UK	Ireland	France	Italy	Germany	Finland	Sweden
Women	65.1	71.2	22.4	45.2	71.8	90.4	68.3
Men	138.2	147.7	57.1	89.1	136.0	200.5	136.9
Men: women	2.1	2.1	2.5	1.9	1.9	2.2	2.0

Note: * Standardized death rates per 100,000 population, all ages in 2006.
Source: WHO Regional Office of Europe: European Health for All database (2009).

ischaemic heart disease) is twice as high among men as among women in all the countries listed in Table 10.1, but the gender gap is largest in France, the country that also has the lowest death rates for both men and women. Two other countries – Italy and Germany – have lower gender ratios, although Italy has a low mortality and Germany a relatively high mortality from this disease.

The UK, Ireland and Finland (see Table 10.1) have topped CHD mortality during the past 20 years among 15 EU countries. Although mortality from this disease declined for both men and women from 1985 to 2006 in the listed countries, the trends differed between them (O'Hara et al., 2008). The decline was fastest in Ireland, especially among women, while Finland showed the slowest decline in CHD mortality, both for men and women.

A decline in mortality from coronary heart disease CHD since the 1970s proved for many that the preventive measures taken had had a real impact and that the risk-factor approach to prevention would continue to lead to a downward trend (Waldron, 2000; O'Hara et al., 2008). The preventive measures for addressing the risk factors for CHD have more recently constituted a lowering of the diagnostic thresholds for the guidelines of high blood pressure and high cholesterol, two of the basic risk factors for CHD. The changing risk-factor definitions are assumed to further increase the prevalence of the risk factors for CHD and increase the drug costs and thereby national healthcare expenditures. Critics have argued that the benefits of the treatment for people not previously regarded to be at risk are not well known (Kaplan and Ong, 2007).

The public-health approach to CHD began in the 1950s, when the sudden high morbidity and mortality of heart disease, especially among white, middle-class, middle-aged men, made men the focus of prevention and research on how to halt what was perceived as a new health problem caused by the affluence of modern society – that is, rich, fatty food and a sedentary lifestyle. In the early 1990s, women's health advocates, such as Bernadine Healy, appointed the director of the US National Institutes of Health (NIH) in 1991, drew attention to the neglected high CHD morbidity and mortality among women and the lack of knowledge of the symptoms, diagnosis of and treatment for women with CHD (Bird and Rieker, 2008; Epstein, 2007). There were few clinical trials and preventive measures defined specifically for women in contemporary medical knowledge and public health policies.

CHD, women and the healthcare system

When the women's health movement and feminists brought attention to neglected aspects of women's health, at issue were women's reproductive health and biased notions about women's anatomy shaped by the tacit assumption that the male body was the standard and generic human body (Annandale, 2009; Kuhlmann and Babitsch, 2002). By aggregating male and female morbidity and mortality rates and the generation of medical knowledge based on all-male studies, empirical evidence concerning men was presented as generic and generalized to the entire population.

In the early 1980s, women's health advocates and equal-rights feminists began in the spirit of 'feminist empiricism' to demand new knowledge on women's health in the hope that such knowledge would correct the previously male-biased knowledge and create a more objective body of medical knowledge (Harding, 1991). In this reformist feminist endeavour, knowledge about heart disease was early on singled out as a chronic disease that was based on the knowledge of health risks and preventive and acute treatment guidelines related to men's health as the norm. For example, in the early 1990s a review on women and TABP noted that 'the understanding of the TA construct still remains primarily limited to male, middle-class men' and 'we do not at present have a very clear understanding, scientifically as well as clinically, of TA in women' (Thoresen and Low, 1991: 118).

That 'midlife men are seen as the archetypal coronary victim, while midlife women with equivalent symptoms receive less extensive diagnostic attention and fewer management actions' (Arber et al., 2006: 112) became a key concern for feminist researchers as well as women's health and public health advocates. Epstein (2007) has provided a sociological account of how the 'standard human' represented by white, middle-class, middle-aged men was challenged in American biomedical research practices in the early 1980s and replaced by a group-specific approach by the 1990s. Epstein calls the new approach the 'inclusion-difference' paradigm because it valorizes group-specificity, that is, specific knowledge on guidelines and policies related to gender, racial and ethnic differences in health. Epstein is concerned that this view on group-specific biology addresses health inequalities mainly with reference to biological differences. He and other critics have warned that this approach – with reference to gender called 'gender-specific medicine' – reinforces biological differences and diverts attention away from social practices and social structures that lead to ill-health in general and unequal health outcomes in particular (Epstein, 2007: 281; see also Annandale, 2009).

Recent examples of a group-specific approach to health have been the US Women's Health Study and the Women's Health Initiative, two disease-prevention research programmes launched in the USA in the early 1990s. These follow-up studies were very much a reaction against numerous past studies in the USA that had excluded women as all-male trials were used to examine risk factors related to CHD. Two US all-male studies had set the standards for the prevention of CHD. The first one was the Multiple Risk Factor Intervention Trial (acronym: MR FIT), which was initiated in 1972 to study special interventions to reduce health risks from smoking, high blood pressure and elevated cholesterol levels. It enrolled about 13,000 middle-aged males at risk of heart disease, half of whom were designated to a special interventions group and the other to a 'usual care' group. The study was not exactly a success because mortality was substantially lower than expected in both groups after seven years. The second study was the NIH-funded Physicians' Health Study which enrolled 22,000 male doctors from 1982 to 1988 (the study ended in 1995) for a follow-up study of the benefits and risks of low-dose aspirin and beta-carotene to prevent cardiovascular disease and cancer (Epstein, 2007). The results suggested that daily low-dose aspirin significantly reduced the risk of first myocardial infarction by 44 per cent but there was no significant effect on the risk of stroke and no effect on mortality from cardiovascular causes.

The two all-male studies – MR FIT and the Physicians' Health Study – have been viewed as the prototypes of the underrepresentation of women in clinical research, particularly in studies of CHD prevention and intervention trials. The two studies have also been set as examples of false universalism, a term that stands for the policy of using the experience of a dominant group's experience to represent the universal and the norm/standard rather than a particular experience (Epstein, 2007).

The task of generating knowledge on women's cardiovascular and cancer risks was met by the US Women's Health Study (WHS), conducted from 1993 to 2004. The WHS was a ten-year randomized, double-blind placebo-controlled study of the effects of a low dose of aspirin and vitamin E supplements on women. The WHS included nearly 40,000 healthy female health professionals 45 years and older whose health was monitored over 10 years. The findings showed that low-dose aspirin has no significant effect on either the risk of myocardial infarction or on the risk of death from cardiovascular causes but reduces the risk of stroke by 17 per cent. As an editorial in the *New England Journal of Medicine* reflected, 'what they find now is the inverse of what they found in men, and that is the puzzle' and the editorial pondered, 'the findings in men and women are opposite. How can this be?' (Levin, 2005: 1366).

Meanwhile another ambitious project was going on in the USA, the Women's Health Initiative (WHI), which began in 1992. The WHI was directed to post-menopausal women (about 68,000 women aged 50–79 were enrolled) to test four interventions: postmenopausal hormone therapy (oestrogen alone, oestrogen + progestin), dietary modification, calcium and vitamin D were used to treat the risk factors for the prevention of a wide range of diseases – CHD, breast cancer, colorectal cancer and osteoporotic fractures (Prentice and Andersson, 2007). Both hormone therapy interventions ended earlier than planned, one in 2002 and the other in 2004, when the health risks exceeded the benefits for the study population; for example, there was an increased risk of stroke from the oestrogen-alone intervention. It was concluded that hormone replacement therapy could not be used as an intervention in the prevention of coronary heart disease in women (Bird and Rieker, 2008). In a review of the trials, the WHI concluded that 'findings were not clear enough to support clinical decision making and public health recommendations' (Prentice and Anderson, 2007: 145).

What these US intervention studies on women and CHD proved was what past studies all the time had feared: when you include women in the clinical trials, especially in CHD intervention studies, things get complicated. But the studies on women also pointed out that the studies on men had been one-dimensional because they had not included various social classes of men. At issue was not only that the middle-class professional men in the Physicians' Health Study could not be used to generalize to women but in terms of education, income, and work conditions the study was not very representative of men either.

Conclusion

This chapter has looked at how CHD risks have been constructed in medical discourse as risks related to men's lives in modern society. The medical and public perception has been that CHD is a men's disease and leads to men's misfortune to die in middle-age. Men were therefore the target of the early prevention measures and follow-up studies. This genre of studies focused on high-risk individuals and one of the first prototypes of such a man was Type A of the early 1960s. Type A established the traits approach in identifying men at risk of developing CHD.

Type A man captured the traits of hegemonic masculinity (Connell and Messerschmidt, 2005) – aggression and self-centredness – and served as a representation of the health behaviour of hypermasculine men. This type of hypermasculinity was not hailed as a 'healthy' role model. In the 1950s and 1960s the rising prevalence of heart disease and increasing CHD mortality rates among men were perceived as threats to men's survival as breadwinners. The overconformity of the competitive and hyperactive Type A man was a medical concern and constructed as a pathological and hence medical category. The restoration of the hypermasculine Type A man to a 'hardy man' or Type B man would reaffirm the breadwinner function of traditional masculinity. As a review article on Type A in the early 1990s suggested, US society had entered an '"Age of Type B Behavior" requiring greater taming of extreme aggression and rugged individualism' (Van Egeren, 1991: 57).

The hardy man construct embodied the spirit – both the masculine and health aspects – of a 'healthy' traditional masculinity in the 1980s. Hardiness reaffirmed traditional masculinity by informing men that, if they could exert control over their masculine self at work, they could remain healthy. Hence, the construct of hardiness defines a new type of masculinity but confirms the core values of hard work, autonomy and self-control of traditional masculinity. Men are told that they can be committed to the work ethic without paying the health costs if they can remain in control (Riska, 2002).

The various constructs related to men's cardiac health – Type A, hardiness, John Henryism – were different types of masculinities evaluated within the risk-factor approach to proneness to heart disease. The risk factors were located in the conditions of work, its stresses and challenges for men. A more recent medical construct – the 'Viagra man' – is not framed within a social context nor to a specific social class or ethnic group, like Type A, hardiness and John Henryism (Riska, 2010). The focus of the pathology has been the Viagra man's failing sexual performance and his underachievement in the private and intimate sphere, while the health problem is identified as overachievement of Type A man in the context of work. In both constructs hypermasculinity serves as the medical norm: for Type A, hypermasculinity is man's doom at work, for Viagra man, it is his treasured goal in his leisure time.

The traits approach was used in the first phase of prevention studies that focused on high-risk individuals. These studies were mostly based on all-male, middle-class samples and the scales were designed to measure men's health-related behaviour, such as, for instance, Type A, the Bortner scale, the Jenkins Activity Survey and John Henryism. The traits approach has not been used to the same extent in evaluating women's risk factors for developing CHD. Instead research on women's cardiac health began in the second phase of prevention studies that represented a population-based approach.

The second phase of prevention studies that began in the 1970s was based on a population as a whole rather than on specific individuals whose personal traits increased their risk of CHD. As Epstein (2007) has shown, in the US context this phase resulted in the early 1990s in a group-specific approach and a demand to gather information about group-specific risk factors. The inclusion of women in clinical and cardiovascular prevention trials began in the 1990s and became part of the group-specific approach to generating new knowledge on cancer and cardiac health risks. For example, the aim of the US Women's Health Study and Women's Health Initiative was to get new knowledge on gender-specific risk factors for CHD for women. The US studies have been used here as examples not only because their public health and scientific histories have been well researched, but also because they have been important in setting national guidelines in other countries. From a gender and sociology-of-knowledge perspective, it would be important to examine and compare what kinds of gender approaches have characterized national CHD-prevention studies in Europe.

The US women-specific studies have generated new knowledge but also raised problems with evaluation studies that use a follow-up design. Economic, cultural and gender norms have changed since the early studies on men and the comparison and evaluation of the differences between the results are influenced by these changes. New treatment guidelines for CHD risk factors have identified new groups believed to be at risk, including younger age groups, but there is currently little evidence on the costs and benefits of the expanded definitions of disease when the guidelines for CHD risk factors have been changed (Kaplan and Ong, 2007). As the history of CHD prevention has shown, endeavours in this area of public health tend to have gendered implications.

Summary

- Coronary heart disease is a key area of public health; although relevant for men and women, it is fundamentally characterized by a 'masculinist' discourse.
- The needs of women are neglected; women face significant disadvantages in CHD care.
- A hegemonic male discourse also neglects the needs of other than white, male, middle-class men.
- The history of CHD prevention highlights that endeavours in this area of public health have gendered implications that need to be addressed in healthcare services.

Key reading

Kaplan, R. M. and M. Ong (2007) 'Rationale and Public Health Implications of Changing CHD Risk Factor Definitions', *Annual Review of Public Health*, 28, 321–44.

Prentice, R. L. and G. L. Anderson (2007) 'The Women's Health Initiative: Lessons Learned', *Annual Review of Public Health*, 29, 131–50.

Riska E. (2002) 'From Type A Man to the Hardy Man: Masculinity and Health', *Sociology of Health and Illness*, 24 (3), 347–58.

Riska, E. (2004) *Masculinity and Men's Health: Coronary Heart Disease in Medical and Public Discourse* (Lanham: Rowman & Littlefield).

References

Annandale, E. (2009) *Women's Health and Social Change* (Abingdon: Routledge).

Arber, S., J. B. McKinlay, A. Adams, L. Marceau, C. Link and A. O'Donnell (2006) 'Patient Characteristics and Inequalities in Doctors' Diagnostic and Management Strategies Relating to CHD: A Video-Simulation Experiment', *Social Science & Medicine*, 62 (1) 103–15.

Aronowitz, R. A. (1998) *Making Sense of Illness: Science, Society and Disease* (Cambridge: Cambridge University Press).

Bird, C. E. and P. P. Rieker (2008) *Gender and Health: The Effects of Constrained Choices and Social Policies* (New York: Cambridge University Press).

Bonham, V. L., S. S. Sellers and H. W. Neighbors (2004) 'John Henryism and Self-reported Physical Health among High Socioeconomic Status African American Men', *American Journal of Public Health*, 94 (5), 737–8.

Clarke, A. E., J. K. Shim, L. Mamo, J. R. Fosket and J. R. Fishman (2003) 'Biomedicalization. Technoscientific Transformations of Health, Illness, and U.S. Biomedicine', *American Sociological Review*, 68 (2), 161–94.

Connell, R. W. and J. W. Messerschmidt (2005) 'Hegemonic Masculinity: Rethinking the Concept', *Gender and Society*, 19 (6), 829–59.

Davison C., G. D. Smith and S. Frankel (1991) 'Lay Epidemiology and the Prevention Paradox: The Implications of Coronary Candidacy for Health Education', *Sociology of Health and Illness*, 13 (1), 1–19.

Day, A. L. and S. Jreige (2002) 'Examining Type A Behavior Pattern to Explain the Relationship between Job Stressors and Psychosocial Outcomes', *Journal of Occupational Health Psychology*, 7 (2), 109–20.

Denollet J. and S. S. Pedersen (2008) 'Prognostic Value of Type D Personality Compared with Depressive Symptoms', *Archives of Internal Medicine*, 168 (4), 431–2.

Edwards, J. R., A. J. Baglioni Jr. and C. L. Cooper (1990) 'Examining the Relationship among Self-report Measures of the Type A Behavior Pattern: The Effects of Dimensionality, Measurement Error, and Differences in Underlying Constructs', *Journal of Applied Psychology*, 75 (4), 440–54.

Ehrenreich, B. (1983) *The Hearts of Men: American Dreams and the Flight From Commitment* (Garden City: Anchor Press/Doubleday).

Epstein, S. (2007) *The Inclusion. The Politics of Difference in Medical Research* (Chicago: University of Chicago Press).

Fernander A. F., C. A. Patten, D. R. Schroeder, S. R. Stevens, K. M. Eberman and R. D. Hurt (2005) 'Exploring the Association of John Henry Active Coping and Education on Smoking Behavior and Nicotine Dependence among Blacks in the USA', *Social Science & Medicine*, 60 (3), 491–500.

Friedman, M. and R. H. Rosenman (1960) 'Overt Behavior Pattern in Coronary Disease', *Journal of the American Medical Association*, 173 (12), 1320–6.

Griggs, J. J. and J. B. Mallinger (2004) 'John Henryism – The Same Old Song', *American Journal of Public Health*, 94 (10), 1658–9.

Harding, S. (1991) *Whose Science, Whose Knowledge? Thinking from Women's Lives* (Ithaca: Cornell University Press).

Helman, C. G. (1987) 'Heart Disease and the Cultural Construction of Time: The Type A Behaviour Pattern as a Western Culture-Bound Syndrome', *Social Science & Medicine* 25 (9), 969–79.

James, S. A., S. A. Harnett and W. D. Kalsbeek (1983) 'John Henryism and Blood Pressure: Differences among Black Men,' *Journal of Behavioral Medicine*, 6 (3), 259–78.

Kaplan, R. M. and M. Ong (2007) 'Rationale and Public Health Implications of Changing CHD Risk Factor Definitions', *Annual Review of Public Health,* 28, 321–44.

Kuhlmann, E. and B. Babitsch (2002) 'Bodies, Health, Gender: Bridging Feminist Theories and Women's Health', *Women's Studies International Forum,* 25 (4), 433–42.

Levin, R. I. (2005) 'The Puzzle of Aspirin and Sex', *New England Journal of Medicine,* 352 (13), 1366–8.

Miller, T., T. W. Smith, C. W. Turner, M. L. Guijarro and A. J. Hallet (1996) 'A Meta-analytic Review of Research on Hostility and Physical Health', *Psychological Bulletin,* 119 (2), 322–48.

Mudrack, P. E. (1999) 'Time Structure and Purpose, Type A Behavior, and the Protestant Work Ethic', *Journal of Organizational Behavior,* 20 (2), 145–58.

O'Hara, T., K. Bennett, M. O'Flaherty and S. Jennings (2008) 'Pace of Change in Coronary Heart Disease Mortality in Finland, Ireland and the United Kingdom from 1985 to 2006, *European Journal of Public Health,* 18 (6), 581–5.

Prentice, R. L. and G. L. Anderson (2007) 'The Women's Health Initiative: Lessons Learned', *Annual Review of Public Health,* 29, 131–50.

Riska, E. (2000) 'The Rise and Fall of Type A Man', *Social Science & Medicine,* 51 (11), 1665–74.

Riska E. (2002) 'From Type A Man to the Hardy Man: Masculinity and Health', *Sociology of Health and Illness,* 24 (3), 347–58.

Riska, E. (2004) *Masculinity and Men's Health: Coronary Heart Disease in Medical and Public Discourse* (Lanham: Rowman & Littlefield).

Riska, E. (2010) 'Medicalization of Men's Health: Type A Man and Viagra Man', in M. Döring and R. Kollek (eds), *Emerging Diseases: Structure, Controversy and Change in the Scientific Making of Disease Patterns* (Bielefeld: Transcript Verlag).

Rosenman, R. H. (1978) 'The Interview Method of Assessment of Coronary-prone Behavior Pattern', in T. M. Dembroski, S. M. Weiss, J. L. Shields, S. L. Haynes and F. Manning (eds), *Coronary-prone Behavior* (New York: Springer), 55–69.

Rosenman, R. H. (1991) 'Type A Behavior Pattern: A Personal Overview', in M. J. Strube, (ed.), *Type A Behavior* (Newbury Park: Sage), 1–24.

Rosenman, R. H., R. J. Brand, C. D. Jenkins, M. Friedman, R. Straus and M. Wurm (1975) 'Coronary Heart Disease in the Western Collaborative Group Study: Follow-up Experience of 8½ Years', *Journal of the American Medical Association,* 233 (8), 872–7.

Roskies, E. (1991) 'Type A Intervention: Where to Go from Here?, in M. J. Strube, (ed.), *Type A Behavior* (Newbury Park: Sage), 389–408.

Sturman, T. S. (1999) 'Achievement Motivation and Type A Behaviour as Motivational Orientations', *Journal of Research in Personality,* 33 (2), 189–207.

Thoresen, C. E. and K. G. Low (1991) 'Women and the Type A Behavior Pattern: Review and Commentary', in M. J. Strube, (ed.), *Type A Behavior* (Newbury Park: Sage), 117–33.

Van Egeren, L. F. (1991) 'A Success Trap Theory of Type A Behavior: Historical Background', in M. J. Strube (ed.), *Type A Behavior* (Newbury Park: Sage), 45–58.

Waldron, I. (2000) 'Trends in Gender Differences in Mortality: Relationships to Changing Gender Differences in Behaviour and Other Causal Factors', in E. Annandale and K. Hunt (eds), *Gender Inequalities in Health* (Buckingham: Open University Press), 150–81.

Whitfield, K. E., D. T. Brandon, E. Robinson, G. Bennett, M. Merritt and C. Edwards (2006) 'Sources of Variability in John Henryism', *Journal of the National Medical Association,* 98 (4), 641–7.

WHO Regional Office of Europe (2009) *European Health for all Database,* at: http://data.euro.who.int/hfadb, accessed 23 February 2009.

11
Gender and Mental Health

Joan Busfield

Introduction

This chapter examines the way in which understandings of the linkages between gender and mental health have developed since second wave feminist research of the 1960s and 1970s. It examines the changing constructions and measures of mental disorder and the associated changes in the observed gender distribution of mental health and illness. From the female predominance noted in the 1960s and 1970s, subsequent studies have identified a more even gender balance in overall levels of mental health as they have incorporated a wider range of disorders. Yet there are still marked gender differences in the types of disorder identified, with women typically having far higher levels of depression and anxiety and men higher levels of alcohol and drug problems and the less common antisocial personality disorder. The chapter then examines some explanations for these observed differences, focusing in particular on gender differences in emotional expression and childhood sexual abuse.

1960s and 1970s feminist research

Interest in gender differences in mental health in western societies is particularly associated with the resurgence of feminist ideas in the 1960s and 1970s, although their existence but not their precise character is a global phenomenon (WHO, 2009). Betty Friedan in *The Feminine Mystique* described women's dissatisfaction with their lives as housewives as 'The problem that has no name' (1963: Chapter 1), pointing to the anxiety and depression that having to focus almost exclusively on their husbands and children could generate, as well as the high levels of divorce. Her critique of the gender division of labour, which then largely located women in the home and men in paid employment, was echoed by other feminists who sought to analyse women's situation and challenge gender inequality (see, for example, Gavron, 1968).

Such writings were not the first to suggest a link between gender and mental ill-health. Certain types of mental disorder had been seen as more or less female- or male-specific in western societies well before this. For instance, hysteria, initially viewed as a physical condition linked to the movement of the uterus, had by the end of the 19th century been transformed into a psychological illness, still considered far more common in women than men (Micale, 1995). Similarly the concept of involutional psychosis, introduced by Kraepelin at the end of the 19th century, was particularly applied to women who experienced anxiety, agitation and insomnia during the menopause (Zax and Cowen, 1976). Disorders considered largely male-specific have included masturbational insanity (Skultans, 1979) and shell-shock (Shepherd, 2000).

Phyllis Chesler, in *Women and Madness*, examined the links between gender and mental health more fully. Gender, she contended, was embedded in the very definition of what constitutes mental illness:

> What we consider 'madness', whether it appears in women or in men, is either the acting out of the devalued female role or the total or partial rejection of one's sex role stereotype. (1972: 56)

Hence there was a gender asymmetry in which women were much more likely to be identified as disturbed than men: 'Many men are severely "disturbed" – but the form their "disturbance" takes is either not seen as "neurotic" or is not treated by psychiatric incarceration' (Chesler, 1972: 38–9). This claim was supported by Broverman and colleagues' (1970) study which showed that clinicians' construction of mental health in a person whose gender was unspecified was far closer to that for men than that for women.

Analyses like Chesler's raise numerous questions: How are mental health and illness defined and identified? Are the definitions and processes of identification gender-neutral or are women more likely to be judged disturbed? Do men and women differ in the way they respond to difficulties? In order to consider such questions we need to start by analysing the key concepts before exploring the observed gender differences in the distribution and treatment of mental disorder and how they can be best understood.

Concepts

The distinction now usually made between sex and gender is attributed to Stoller (1984[1968]) who identified sex as the biological difference between men and women and linked gender to femininity and masculinity – to the characteristics considered appropriate to maleness and femaleness. This suggested a distribution of male and female characteristics across a linear dimension, which he viewed as independent of biology, though subsequent research suggests masculinity and femininity are two separate bi-polar dimensions not a single continuum (Shields, 2002: 52).

In Britain, Oakley's text *Sex, Gender and Society* (1972), did much to secure acceptance for the distinction between sex and gender in the social sciences, gender commonly replacing sex to refer to differences between men and women – the term indicating a rejection of biological determinism and an assertion of the importance of the social production of male–female differences and their variation across time and place. However, Oakley, like many subsequent authors, viewed gender, like sex, as primarily a binary category which, though not determined by biology, was still linked to biological sex. It is this sense of gender that permeated much academic and popular discourse. Of course, the salience of gender varies across time and place, but it is a fundamental dimension of social life. Moreover, like social class, and race or ethnicity, the concept usually also implies some form of stratification – unequal social relations and differences in power.

Concepts of mental health and illness have a longer history than the use of gender in the social sciences, and are more contested. In practice mental health is often defined negatively as the absence of mental illness, though more positive definitions have been formulated, such as the WHO's definition of mental health:

> ... a state of well-being in which the individual realises his or her own abilities, can cope with the normal stresses of life, can work productively and fruitfully, and is able to make a contribution to his or her community. (WHO, 2005: 2)

Note here the emphasis on social capacities – on being able to function in society. Such definitions suggest a dimensional view, where it is appropriate to identify an individual's location on a continuum stretching from excellent mental health to severe mental illness – a view incorporated into some measures of mental well-being.

In contrast, psychiatry (the medical specialty that deals with mental illness) uses a categorical model that differentiates types of mental illness in terms of distinctive symptom clusters and identifies the presence or absence of specific illnesses. However, notwithstanding the categorical model, psychiatry also distinguishes mental illnesses by their severity, with some considered more severe, with a more extensive impact on functioning and more limited chances of recovery (for example, schizophrenia or bi-polar disorder), and some as less severe, with a more limited impact on functioning and higher chances of recovery (for example, anxiety states and phobias). The most important of the current classifications that set the official boundaries of mental illness is the American Psychiatric Association's *Diagnostic and Statistical Manual of*

Mental Disorders (DSM), now in its fourth revised edition (American Psychiatric Association, 2000), which has had a global impact.

The contrast between mental health and mental illness, whether viewed as a continuum or categorical divide, incorporates a single binary opposition. Two further contrasts need to be borne in mind: that between physical and mental illness, and that between mental illness and social deviance or wrongdoing. The first is signalled by the addition of the term 'mental' to both health and illness – without the qualifier these terms are treated as referring to bodily rather than mental functioning. The second is a question of assumptions about agency. Whereas deviance contains a judgement about what someone *does,* for which there is assumed to be some individual responsibility, illness is a judgement about what *happens* to an individual to which agency is not attributed – in lay terms the contrast is between badness and madness. These contrasts help to illuminate the changing boundaries of mental illness – the transformation of hysteria from physical to mental illness is one example. The boundaries are portrayed in Figure 11.1 – the dashed lines indicating the shifting nature of the boundaries.

Historically in western societies and elsewhere some notion of madness was a feature of lay understandings, the term referring to conduct that appeared disturbed and inexplicable, lacking in reason and rationality; a form of 'unreason' as Foucault (1967) argued. If brought to medical attention, the diagnosis might have been one of mania or melancholia. Madness was, however, a narrow term, closer to what is now called psychosis; others with problems now viewed as psychological were, for instance, described in the 17th century as 'troubled in mind' or 'mopish' (MacDonald, 1981) or in the 19th century as suffering from 'shattered nerves' or 'nervous exhaustion' (Oppenheim, 1991: 5). Such problems were sometimes brought to medical attention, especially by the more affluent, but did not receive formal

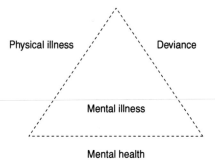

Figure 11.1 The changing boundaries of mental illness
Source: adapted from Busfield (1996: 55).

diagnostic labels. It was, however, the mad who, because of their sometimes violent and disruptive behaviour, were increasingly confined in institutions – a private madhouse, or a charitable or public asylum. Separate asylums for lunatics in turn became the places where a new medical expertise and specialism concerning madness – psychiatry – developed (Scull, 1993).

Yet it was largely developments in private medical practice outside the asylums that helped to broaden the boundaries of officially defined mental illness. On the one hand, disorders of emotion, most obviously forms of depression and anxiety, were added to the psychiatric lexicon – what, following Freud, were called the psychoneuroses and now more often the 'common mental disorders' because of their frequency. By this extension, being 'troubled in mind' or suffering from 'nerves' became a form of psychopathology, and the boundary of mental illness was expanded to incorporate a wide range of emotional problems. On the other hand, with the introduction of the concept of moral insanity in the mid-19th century, psychiatry started to incorporate a growing number of behaviour, conduct or personality disorders (Busfield, 2002), removing them from the category of wrongdoing. For instance, the 20th century witnessed a major shift in which the overuse of alcohol and drugs, commonly seen as reprehensible conduct, was increasingly defined as the mental disorders of alcohol and drug misuse and dependence (note the linguistic shift away from agency in the latter case).

Both boundary shifts have been highly contested – is sadness and misery a mental disorder? Is alcoholism best viewed as an illness? Horwitz and Wakefield (2007), for example, argue that much of the sadness now labelled depression is a proportionate response, in level and duration, to adverse circumstances and should not be viewed as mental illness unless disproportionate. Equally, many have argued that it is preferable to view alcoholism as a form of wrongdoing than as the pathology of alcohol dependence (see Conrad and Schneider, 1992). Given such debates, it is essential, when looking at empirical studies of the gendered distribution of mental health and illness, to examine the definitions used and their operationalization.

The gendered landscape of mental disorder

Epidemiological data from the 1960s and 1970s typically showed, as feminists had argued, that mental illness was more common in women then men. This was manifest both in patient statistics of treated cases and in community surveys using screening instruments to measure mental illness independently of whether or not an individual was in treatment. Gove and Tudor, using epidemiological tools, argued that this female predominance was a post-war phenomenon, resulting from the fact that married women's marital role had become 'more frustrating and less rewarding' (1972: 816) than men's – an analysis that supported the feminist claim that the gender division of labour disadvantaged women. They also noted that, whereas mental ill-health was considerably higher amongst the single and divorced than the married, the gender difference was much smaller, and if anything single and divorced men tended to have higher rates of mental illness than single and divorced women.

However, Bruce and Barbara Dohrenwend challenged this analysis, arguing that the gender differences were primarily the result of changes in 'the concepts and methods for defining what constitutes a psychiatric case' (1976: 1452), and that the increasing reliance on screening instruments that typically focused on neurotic symptoms, rather than the key informants and official records of the earlier studies, had generated the female preponderance. They also noted that rates of mental illness had increased markedly over time, contending that this was due to the increase in 'the breadth of our definitions of what constitutes a psychiatric case' (1976: 1450). In their view the significant gender difference was in the patterning of mental disorders with higher female rates of neurosis and manic-depressive psychosis and higher male rates of personality disorders, but no significant gender difference in rates of schizophrenia.

Subsequent studies have paid considerable attention to gender differences in the types of mental illness. The 1980–4 US Epidemiological Catchment Area survey used the Diagnostic Interview Schedule, designed to mimic clinical diagnosis across the spectrum of disorders, as a screening instrument. It found that taking the one-month, six-month and one-year prevalence measures, rates of mental illness were roughly equal in men and women (Regier et al., 1988). However, once the rates for specific illnesses were examined and the analysis more nuanced, gender differences were marked, as Table 11.1 shows.

The data also show very clearly how affective and anxiety disorders and alcohol and drug disorders, where gender differences are marked, are far more common than antisocial personality or schizophrenic disorders.

Subsequent US studies showed a similar picture. The 1990–2 US National Comorbidity Survey used the Structured Clinical Interview, developed to assist clinicians when using the *Diagnostic and Statistical Manual of Mental Disorders* (DSM) as its screening tool. Both this survey (Kessler et al., 1994)

Table 11.1 One-month prevalence of selected mental disorders, USA, 1980–4

Mental disorder	Women	Men
Affective and anxiety disorders	15.3%	8.2%
Alcohol and drug disorders	1.6%	6.8%
Antisocial personality disorder	0.2%	0.8%
Schizophrenic disorders	0.7%	0.7%

Source: Regier et al. (1988).

and its 2001–3 replication (Kessler et al., 2005) found little gender difference in the overall prevalence of mental disorders, but higher levels of anxiety disorder and depression in women (the latter said to be one of the most robust findings in psychiatric epidemiology) and higher levels of 'impulse control' and substance use disorders in men. These surveys also found that around one-third of those with one mental disorder had at least one other.

This gendered landscape has been observed in many other countries across the world (see, for example, Regier et al., 1988; WHO, 2009). A community survey of psychiatric morbidity in households in Britain in 1993 (Meltzer et al., 1995a) using a variety of screening tools, yielded a similar pattern to that of the US surveys. The results are given in Table 11.2.

The relatively high rates for neurotic symptomatology may reflect the fact that the time period covered was relatively short – a week – so 'symptoms' need not have lasted long and could well have been proportionate to some adverse event; typically, screening instruments do not examine the circumstances that may have given rise to particular feelings. A second British psychiatric morbidity survey in 2000 (Singleton et al., 2001) found a similar pattern, but this time a specific measure of personality disorder was included for a sub-sample and showed somewhat higher prevalence rates in men (4.4 per cent) than women (3.4 per cent).

A third survey, in England in 2007 (McManus et al., 2009), again showed higher prevalence rates of anxiety and depression in women (19.7 per cent) than men (7.5 per cent) in the previous week, and higher rates of alcohol dependence in men (9.3 per cent) than women (3.6 per cent). Two types of personality disorder were assessed in the survey – antisocial and borderline personality disorder – and one-year prevalence rates, though low, were higher in men (0.6 per cent) than women (0.1 per cent). The study also measured eating disorders using a special screening instrument and, as in other studies, found that women were more likely to have an eating disorder (9.2 per cent) in the previous year than men (3.5 per cent).

These surveys also collected some data on gender differences in contact with general practitioners (GPs) and the proportions in treatment. The 1993 British

Table 11.2   Prevalence rates of selected mental disorders, UK students 1993

Disorder	Women	Men
Neurosis – previous week	19.5%	12.3%
Alcohol dependence – previous year	2.1%	7.3%
Drug dependence – previous year	1.4%	2.9%
Psychosis – previous 12 months	0.4%	0.4%

Source: Meltzer et al. (1995a: Table 6.7).

psychiatric morbidity survey found that women were more likely than men to have consulted their GP for a mental complaint in the previous year (40 per cent against 27 per cent) (Meltzer et al., 1995b). The 2000 survey also found that of those with higher scores on the neurosis scale, women were more likely to have received treatment than men (29 per cent against 17 per cent) suggesting greater willingness by women to seek treatment for depression and anxiety (Singleton et al., 2001). The third survey showed that this also applied to the more 'male' substance use disorders (McManus et al., 2009). That women are more likely than men to have treatment for a given mental disorder has been observed worldwide (WHO, 2009). One consequence is that women are more likely to be using some form of psychotropic medication, with the attendant problems of side effects and dependency that this can generate, as well as issues concerning the doubtful efficacy of many psychotropic drugs (see, for example, Kirsch et al., 2008).

We can draw three main conclusions from such epidemiological data:

- First, there is considerable gender variation in psychiatric symptomatology, with women typically having higher levels of emotional problems and men typically having higher levels of behaviour and substance use disorders – a finding not restricted to western societies;
- Second, the extent of the overall gender difference in levels of mental health and illness clearly depends on how mental illness is defined and operationalized. Where the focus is on symptoms of depression and anxiety, as is frequently the case with simple screening instruments, then the observed rates of mental disorder are usually higher for women than for men. However, if substance use disorders are included the gender balance becomes more even;
- Third, women are more likely than men to be in treatment for a given mental disorder and so to be receiving some psychotropic medication.

One further point needs to be noted, however. Whilst community surveys do now often attempt to measure a broad spectrum of disorders, including substance use and antisocial personality disorders, thereby generating a more even gender balance, this does not always reflect actual mental health practice or indeed lay views. The 2007 psychiatric morbidity survey in England showed that those with higher depression and anxiety scores were more likely to be in treatment (24 per cent) than those with alcohol problems (14 per cent) (McManus et al., 2009). In part this difference may relate to service provision, with services often poor for those with substance use problems, but it may also reflect both lay views that individuals are more responsible for alcohol problems, and the greater stigmatization of the individuals involved (Link et al., 1997), suggesting that in practice substance misuse may often not be seen as a psychiatric disorder.

Explaining gender difference in mental illness

Symptom reports

The first consideration in any discussion of observed gender differences in mental health is whether the data are an artefact of the measures used. One aspect of this has already been explored through examination of the way the boundaries of mental illness are set, which clearly affects the observed gender differences. However, another crucial aspect needs to be examined: the extent to which men and women differ in their willingness to report psychological difficulties. This issue has been particularly raised in relation to symptoms measured via simple scales, such as the widely used General Health Questionnaire (GHQ), which concentrate on emotional problems. Do expectations of appropriate male and female emotional behaviour affect the responses to symptom surveys using self-reports or interviews?

A common cultural assumption in western societies is that women are more emotional than men. Indeed, greater emotionality is one aspect of cultural assumptions about femininity (Shields, 2002). Yet a recent analysis by Simon and Nath (2004), using data from the US General Social Survey (GSS), indicated that the frequency of everyday emotions men and women reported experiencing in the previous week was similar. The study found, however, two important gender differences. First, men reported experiencing more positive feelings than women, such as feeling contented, calm and happy, while women reported experiencing more negative feelings than men, such as feeling worried, sad or ashamed – a finding in line with women's higher levels of anxiety and depression in epidemiological studies. The authors contended that this is linked to differences in power and status which advantage men (see also WHO, 2009). Significantly, however, the study found no differences in the frequency of anger men and women reported experiencing.

Second, women were more likely than men to report expressing their feelings in some way – a finding the authors attributed to cultural socialization which they suggested has more impact on emotional *expression* than emotional *experience*. Emphasizing this distinction, they suggested that it may be women's greater tendency to express emotions that contributes to the cultural assumption that women are more emotional than men. Gender differences in emotional expression are clearly relevant to the issue of whether women are more willing to report psychiatric symptoms, and this is supported by other data. For instance, a recent survey of British social attitudes towards emotional support, based on self-reports, found that more women (39 per cent) than men (22 per cent) fell into the group of those more talkative about emotions (Anderson et al., 2009). Such data do suggest that women are more likely than men to admit to experiencing emotional problems. This tendency may be enhanced by the fact that screening instruments such as the GHQ have a more negative slant than the GSS questions on emotions – for instance, the GSS presented the listed emotions as normal and routine, whereas GHQ respondents are asked whether they have 'been losing confidence in yourself', or 'felt constantly under strain' or 'felt you couldn't overcome difficulties'. Because of this, social desirability factors may have had more impact on the latter than the former. Further, whereas the GSS covered emotions experienced in the previous week, the GHS talks loosely of health 'over the past few weeks' and of 'present and recent complaints', yet research suggests that self-reports are more likely to be influenced by gender stereotypes if questions are more general (Shields, 2002: 32).

A greater willingness to express and talk about emotions and emotional difficulties is also pertinent to differences in seeking treatment to which they contribute, as well as to the diagnoses received and treatments recommended. Moreover, whilst any diagnostic biases (see, for example, Broverman et al., 1970) of GPs and specialists are not pertinent to measures of mental disorder in community surveys, they are important to how disorders are actually identified and treated in clinical contexts.

Gender, stress and the channelling of emotions

A wide range of data provides evidence that stressful life events and chronic strains have an adverse impact on health and that the frequency of such events and strains increases as you move down the social scale (Mirowsky and Ross, 2003). A link between social class and mental ill-health is long established (Hollingshead and Redlich, 1956) and ideas about levels of stress have also been used to account for class differences. Similar ideas have also permeated discussions of gender differences in mental health and most early analyses concentrated on differences in the levels and types of stress faced by men and women. This was the type of argument put forward by Gove and Tudor when they claimed that marriage was 'more frustrating and less rewarding' (1972: 816) for women than men, suggesting thereby that men benefited more from marriage than women. This issue is of interest, notwithstanding the approximate gender balance identified in more recent community surveys, and is best explored using longitudinal data. Overall the beneficial effects of marriage on mental health are clear-cut. A longitudinal study of young adults by Horwitz and colleagues (1996) found, for example, that those who became and stayed married benefited in terms of their mental health compared with those who did not. They also found, contra Gove and Tudor (1972), that overall women benefited from marriage as much as men, with women reporting fewer alcohol problems and men less depression.

A further US longitudinal study by Simon (2002), using national panel data, also found that the emotional benefits of marriage applied equally to men and women, but that the negative consequences of marital loss differed in character – levels of depression increased in women, levels of alcohol abuse in men. Simon suggested that depression in women and alcohol problems in men are 'functional equivalents' – an idea put forward by previous authors. Such data indicate that we need to attend to gender differences in the *response* to difficulties – what has been termed 'emotional style' (Middleton, 1989).

Cloward and Piven, writing in 1979, used the sociological framework of deviance to argue that how people respond to stress is socially structured. They argued that whereas the focus of research had largely been on stressful conditions, which had been used to explain a wide range of deviant outcomes, too little attention had been paid to the responses to stress. These responses, they contended, are channelled by the normative rules of society – they are socially regulated. Hence we need to attend to the cognitive and moral framework through which stresses are interpreted. Resources and opportunities, as well as cultural expectations, have encouraged women either to passively endure stress or to engage in individualistic self-destructive forms of deviance, including mental and physical illness. In particular, Cloward and Piven argued that the rise of the healthcare system leads women 'to think of the tensions they experience as rooted in their health or mental health' and to 'search within their psyches and their bodies for the sources of their problems' (1979: 666, 668). In contrast, they suggested, male deviance tends to be more collective and to involve violence and aggression against others.

Although Cloward and Piven did not use this language, we can see here a contrast between turning feelings inwards and turning them outwards – an idea Freud developed, using the concept of internalization to refer to the taking in of the standards of others, especially parents, and externalization to refer to the turning outwards of feelings, especially aggression. Using a health rather than a deviance framework, psychiatrists and psychologists now often talk of two types of psychological disorder, the internalizing disorders typified by anxiety and depression, more common in women, and the externalizing disorders typified by aggressive and antisocial behaviour, but also including substance use disorders, more common in men – which in the case of alcohol may further encourage violence and aggression.

Simon and Nath's (2004) study of emotions is also relevant here. The authors analysed the responses to additional questions on anger and its expression, finding that women were just as likely as men (contra cultural expectations) to report experiencing anger. However, women reported more intense feelings of anger than men and of longer duration; they also reported coping with their anger in different ways. Women were more likely to talk about their angry feelings, including to the target of their anger, or to pray, whereas men were more likely to report dealing with their anger by having a drink or taking a pill (these responses were not differentiated).

One task, therefore, is to identify the factors that encourage the internalization or externalization of problems. Rosenfield and her colleagues have argued that what they call self-salience underpins these two types of responses – 'deviant directions' in the Dohrenwends' terms (1976: 1453): 'Self-salience is a set of relational schemas ranging from high levels that privilege the self over others to low levels that privilege others above the self' (Rosenfield et al, 2005: 323). Self-salience involves 'the primacy of the self relative to others in worth, boundaries and ranking ... [and] combines cognitive, emotional and moral components' (Rosenfield et al., 2005: 324). Its level is affected by gender socialization with men learning to privilege self over others and women others over self. And those with high self-salience (men) are, they suggested, likely to externalize their problems, those with low self-salience (women) to internalize them – a pattern supported by data from their study of adolescents which showed a relationship between low self-salience and internalizing problems and high self-salience and externalizing problems.

Whilst this approach has attractions, and the authors do link self-salience to factors like the level of power and socialization, nonetheless self-salience is constructed as largely a psychological dimension – an attribute of individuals – so that issues concerning power, resources, opportunities and cultural expectations are not placed centre stage.

Trauma and sexual abuse

Although recent work on gender differences has directed attention to responses to stress rather than to differences in the type or level of stress, certain adverse experiences have an especial impact on subsequent mental health. These might be better termed traumas than stresses to emphasize their severity. One is sexual abuse in childhood, which has been found in numerous studies to make depression in adulthood more likely. An extensive review of a large number of studies of the links between childhood sexual abuse, gender and depression found that childhood sexual abuse of girls was more common than sexual abuse of boys, and concluded that such abuse could 'predispose individuals to adult-onset depression' (Weiss et al., 1999: 816). The authors also noted that sexual abuse in childhood had more adverse effects than such abuse in adulthood – a reflection perhaps of the greater power imbalance in childhood.

A similar role is played by other traumatic events, though often the psychological consequences are more immediate. The concept of post-traumatic stress disorder (PTSD) incorporates the assumption that traumatic events can have psychopathological consequences, and is an exception to the rejection of aetiological assumptions in recent classifications of mental disorder. PTSD's history can be linked to the First World War concept of shell-shock, and its inclusion in the 1980 DSM-III followed campaigns from anti-Vietnam war veterans who wanted the psychological consequences of war to be properly recognized – an example of political influences shaping psychiatric classifications. The DSM symptoms of PTSD have some specificity and include persistently re-experiencing the traumatic event, persistent avoidance of stimuli associated with the trauma and increased arousal – all not present before the trauma but present for more than a month after (American Psychiatric Association, 2000). PTSD can follow 'exposure to an extreme traumatic stressor involving direct personal experience of an event that involves actual or threatened death or serious injury, or other threat to one's personal integrity' (American Psychiatric Association, 2000: 463), or witnessing such an event occurring to another person or learning about such an event that is unexpected and involves a family member or close associate.

This definition of traumatic stresses is potentially quite broad and, as the example of child sexual abuse indicates, such events may generate disorders other than PTSD, including those developing later in life.

The 2007 psychiatric morbidity survey in England found a third of the sample had experienced a traumatic event since the age of 16, with somewhat more men (35.2 per cent) than women (31.5 per cent) having experienced such a trauma – perhaps because male-on-male violence is common (McManus et al., 2009). As in the USA (Kessler et al., 1995), PTSD itself was marginally more common in women (3.3 per cent) than men (2.6 per cent), though the 2007 survey used a self-report measure of symptoms in the previous week – in contrast to the DSM's focus on symptoms lasting at least a month.

Implications for healthcare

Many of those people identified via screening instruments as having poor mental health are not in treatment and it is tempting to argue that more health services to treat common mental disorders and substance use disorders are needed, particularly for men, since the proportions of men in treatment are even lower than of women. However, the bulk of the mental health problems identified in community surveys are ones where we need to attend to the contextual factors in people's lives that are generating the misery, unhappiness, sleeplessness or irritability, or the resort to alcohol and drug misuse and dependence, that give individuals poor mental health scores rather than to their personal psychology and pathology. As Cloward and Piven (1979) argued, the healthcare system encourages people to search for the sources of their problems within themselves, yet the sources often lie in external social factors, such as being treated badly as a child, which can affect the individual's capacity to cope with difficulties, being made redundant, or being treated violently by one's spouse.

It is not possible in this chapter to explore adequately the social factors that generate mental ill-health, which vary from problem to problem; nonetheless it is clear that stresses and traumas play a major role in the genesis of anxiety, depression and substance use disorders. Given the doubtful efficacy and marked side effects of much psychotropic medication, which may well result from the failure to treat the social difficulties underpinning the psychological and behavioural difficulties, it is not at all clear that what is needed is more mental health treatment in the form of medication, sometimes excessive, provided by doctors, or indeed the cognitive behaviour therapy currently in vogue, which still focuses on the individual rather than their social circumstances. Directive counselling, practical advice and social support could well be more helpful than these treatments.

Conclusion

Since the feminist focus on gender differences in mental health in the 1960s and 1970s, there have been significant developments in three areas of scholarship, all of which have contributed to the understanding of gender differences in mental health. First, there have been major transformations in the classifications and attendant definitions of the boundaries of mental disorder and in its operationalization. These have been associated with the emergence of a more even gender balance in the overall level of mental disorders observed, alongside a greater interest in the varied gender landscape of mental disorders.

Second, there has been more work on men and masculinity that has contributed to increased attention to, and analysis of, mental disorders in men. And third, there has been new work on emotions, including the sociology of emotions, that is, enhancing understanding of the differences in emotional expression that contribute to the observed gender differences in types of mental disorder. However, the relationships between gender and mental disorder are not fixed or universal; rather, as gender relations change, including gendered differences in status, power, resources, opportunities and cultural expectations, so too does the gendered landscape.

Summary

- The way in which the concepts of mental health and illness are defined and measured affects the observed gender balance in overall levels of mental health.
- There is considerable gender variation in the psychological disorders commonly identified in men and women, with women typically having

> higher levels of emotional problems and men higher levels of behavioural and substance use disorders.
> - A range of factors contribute to the observed gender differences in types of mental illness. Culturally generated differences in emotional expression between women and men are of particular importance.
> - The healthcare system encourages people to search for the sources of their mental health problems within themselves; focusing on social circumstances and providing more practical social support may be more helpful.

Key reading

Busfield, J. (1996) *Men, Women and Madness: Understanding Gender and Mental Disorder* (London: Macmillan).

Cloward, R. A. and F. F. Piven (1979) 'Hidden Protest: The Channeling of Female Protest and Resistance', *Signs*, 4 (4), 651–69.

Horwitz, A. and J. C. Wakefield (2007) *The Loss of Sadness* (New York: Oxford University Press).

Simon, R. W. and L. E. Nath (2004) 'Gender and Emotion in the United States: Do Men and Women Differ in Self Reports of Feelings and Expressive Behaviour?', *American Journal of Sociology*, 109 (5), 1137–76.

References

American Psychiatric Association (2000) *Diagnostic and Statistical Manual of Mental Disorders*, Fourth Edition, Textual Revision (Washington, DC: APA).

Anderson S., J. Brownlie and L. Given (2009) 'Therapy Culture? Attitudes towards Emotional Support in Britain', in A. Park., J. Curtice, K. Thomson, M. Phillips and E. Clery (eds), *British Social Attitudes: The 25th Report* (London: Sage), 155–72.

Broverman, I. K., D. M. Broverman, F. E. Clarkson, P. S. Rosenkrantz and S. R. Vogel (1970) 'Sex Role Stereotypes and Clinical Judgments of Mental Health', *Journal of Consulting and Clinical Psychology*, 34 (1), 1–7.

Busfield, J. (1996) *Men, Women and Madness: Understanding Gender Madness* (London: Macmillan).

Busfield, J. (2002) 'The Archaeology of Psychiatric Disorder: Gender and Disorders of Thought, Emotion and Behaviour', in G. Bendelow, M. Carpenter, C. Vautier and S. Williams (eds), *Gender, Health and Healing* (London: Routledge), 144–62.

Chesler, P. (1972) *Women and Madness* (New York: Doubleday).

Cloward, R. A. and F. F. Piven (1979) 'Hidden Protest: The Channeling of Female Protest and Resistance', *Signs*, 4 (4), 651–69.

Conrad, P. and J. W. Schneider (1992) *Deviance and Medicalization* (Philadelphia: Temple University Press).

Dohrenwend, B. P. and B. S. Dohrenwend (1976) 'Sex Differences and Psychiatric Disorders', *American Journal of Sociology*, 81 (6), 1447–54.

Foucault, M. (1967) *Madness and Civilization* (London: Tavistock).

Friedan, B. (1963) *The Feminine Mystique* (New York: Dell).

Gavron, H. (1968) *The Captive Wife* (Harmondsworth: Penguin).

Gove, W. R. and J. F. Tudor (1972) 'Adult Sex Roles and Mental Illness', *American Journal of Sociology*, 78 (4), 812–35.

Hollingshead, A. B. and F. C. Redlich (1956) *Social Class and Mental Illness* (New York: Wiley).

Horwitz, A. and J. C. Wakefield (2007) *The Loss of Sadness: How Psychiatry Transformed Normal Sorrow into Depressive Disorder* (New York: Oxford University Press).

Horwitz, A., H. R. White and S. Howell-White (1996) 'Becoming Married and Mental Health: A Longitudinal Study of a Cohort of Young Adults', *Journal of Marriage and the Family*, 58 (November), 895–907.

Kessler, R.C., K. A. McGonagle, S. Zhao, C. B. Nelson, M. Hughes, S. Eshleman, H. Wittchen and K. S. Kendler (1994) 'Lifetime and 12 Month Prevalence of DSM-111-R Psychiatric Disorders in the United States', *Archives of General Psychiatry*, 51 (1), 8–19.

Kessler, R. C., A. Sonnega, E. Bromet, M. Hughes and C. B. Nelson (1995) 'Posttraumatic Stress Disorder in the National Comorbidity Survey', *Archives of General Psychiatry*, 52 (12), 1048–60.

Kessler, R. C., W. T. Chiu, O. Demler and E. E. Walters (2005) 'Prevalence, Severity and Comorbidity of 12-Month DSM-IV Disorders in the National Comorbidity Survey Replication', *Archives of General Psychiatry*, 62 (6), 617–27.

Kirsch, I., B. J. Deacon, T. B. Huedo-Medina, A. Soboria, T. J. Moore and B. Y. Johnson (2008) 'Initial Severity and Antidepressant Benefits: A Meta-Analysis of Data Submitted to the Food And Drug Administration', *PLoS Medicine*, 5 (2), 260–8.

Link, B. G., E. L. Struening, M. Rahav, J. C. Phelan and L. Nuttbrook (1997) 'On Stigma and Its Consequences: Evidence from a Longitudinal Study of Men with Dual Diagnoses of Mental Illness and Substance Abuse', *Journal of Health and Social Behavior*, 38 (2), 177–90.

MacDonald, M. (1981) *Mystical Bedlam* (Cambridge: Cambridge University Press).

McManus, S., H. Meltzer, T. Brugh, P. Bebbington and R. Jenkins (2009) *Adult Psychiatric Morbidity in England, 2007* (London: The Information Centre).

Meltzer, H., B. Gill, M. Petticrew and K. Hinds (1995a) *The Prevalence of Psychiatric Morbidity among Adults Living in Private Households* (London: HMSO).

Meltzer, H., B. Gill, M. Petticrew and K. Hinds (1995b) *Physical Complaints, Service Use and Treatment of Adults with Psychiatric Disorder* (London: HMSO).

Micale, M. S. (1995) *Approaching Hysteria* (Princeton: Princeton University Press).

Middleton, W. R. (1989) 'Emotional Style: The Cultural Ordering of Emotions', *Ethos*, 17 (2), 187–201.

Mirowsky, J. and C. E. Ross (2003) *Education, Social Status, and Health* (New York: Aldine).

Oakley, A. (1972) *Sex, Gender and Society* (London: Temple Smith).

Oppenheim, J. (1991) *Shattered Nerves: Doctors, Patients, and Depression in Victorian England* (New York: Oxford University Press).

Regier, D. A., J. M. Boyd, J. D. Burke, D. S. Rae, J. K. Myers, M. Kramer, M. Robins, L. K. George et al. (1988) 'One-Month Prevalence of Mental Disorders in the United States', *Archives of General Psychiatry*, 45 (11), 977–86.

Rosenfield, S., M. C. Lennon and H. R. White (2005) 'The Self and Mental Health: Self-salience and the Emergence of Internalizing and Externalizing Problems', *Journal of Health and Social Behavior*, 46 (December), 323–40.

Scull, A. (1993) *The Most Solitary of Afflictions: Madness and Society in Britain, 1700–1900* (New Haven: Yale University Press).

Shepherd, B. (2000) *A War of Nerves: Soldiers and Psychiatrists in the Twentieth Century* (London: Jonathan Cape).

Shields, S. A. (2002) *Speaking from the Heart: Gender and the Social Meaning of Emotion* (Cambridge: Cambridge University Press).

Simon, R. W. (2002) 'Revisiting the Relationships among Gender, Marital Status and Mental Health', *American Journal of Sociology,* 107 (4), 1065–96.

Simon, R. W. and L. E. Nath (2004) 'Gender and Emotion in the United States: Do Men and Women Differ in Self Reports of Feelings and Expressive Behaviour?', *American Journal of Sociology,* 109 (5),1137–76.

Singleton, N., R. Bumpstead, M. O'Brien, A. Lee and H. Meltzer (2001) *Psychiatric Morbidity among Adults Living in Private Households* (London: Office for National Statistics).

Skultans, V. (1979) *English Madness: Ideas on Insanity, 1580–1950* (London: Routledge and Kegan Paul).

Stoller, R. (1984[1968]) *Sex and Gender* (London: Karnac).

Weiss, E. L., G. James, M. D. Longhurst and C. M. Mazure (1999) 'Childhood Sexual Abuse as a Risk Factor for Depression in Women', *American Journal of Psychiatry,* 156 (6), 816–28.

WHO (2005) *Promoting Mental Health: Concepts, Emerging Evidence, Practice* (Geneva: WHO).

WHO (2009) *Gender Disparities in Mental Health,* at: www.who.int/mental_health/media/en/242.pdf, accessed 24 July 2009.

Zax, M. and E. L. Cohen (1976) *Abnormal Psychology,* Second Edition (New York: Holt, Rinehart & Winston).

12
HIV/AIDS and Gender

Leah Gilbert and Terry-Ann Selikow

Introduction

The global HIV/AIDS epidemic presents many challenges on practical as well as theoretical levels. The attempts to explain different epidemiological patterns of the epidemic have generated a great amount of literature ranging from biological to sociological theories (Hunt, 1996). Following the growing recognition of the significance of social and behavioural factors in the epidemic (Barnet and Whiteside, 2002; Treichler, 1999) this chapter adopts a sociological approach and argues that there is an overwhelming consensus that HIV/AIDS is a 'social epidemic' like no other in history. It is embedded in the social structures of societies and its development and impact reflect their cultural characteristics and material resources (Farmer et al., 1996).

Although the spread and impact of HIV/AIDS has been universal, the burden of this epidemic is not borne equally by the global community. The fault lines include gender, geographic location such as developed and less developed countries, social and cultural categories and material inequalities within countries. The above translate into differential access to general resources as well as to healthcare, resulting in varied vulnerabilities to infection and access to prevention, treatment and care (Gilbert and Walker, 2002). It has been claimed that the gendered aspects of HIV/AIDS have been neglected by clinicians, policy-makers and politicians. This, as argued by Squire (2007), was the case particularly in developed-world epidemics contracted among gay men and largely male drug users, while the 'feminization' of the epidemic in the developing world put women at the forefront of many local and national HIV/AIDS programmes. Since globally HIV/AIDS is not distributed evenly and not gendered in the same way, the questions it poses about gender are determined by the nature of the epidemic in specific regions.

This chapter gives an overview of the epidemic highlighting its social dimensions with a focus on gender. Using HIV/AIDS in South Africa as a case study in sub-Saharan Africa, it also aims to explain the differential vulnerabilities and analyse their implications in the context of healthcare. We conclude by calling for a particular focus on structural interventions on the material and cultural level in order to impact on the factors that facilitate the spread of the epidemic.

Global overview of the HIV/AIDS epidemic

The World Health Organization (WHO) and the Joint United Nations Programme on HIV/AIDS distinguish three stages of the HIV epidemic (Matjila et al., 2008):

1. A low-level HIV epidemic confined to individuals with high-risk behaviour such as sex workers, men who have sex with men (MSM) and injecting drug users, with HIV prevalence in these subpopulations of less than five per cent, and with no spread of HIV infection to the general population;
2. A concentrated HIV epidemic which is confined largely to the subpopulations with risk behaviour; there is a rapid spread of HIV transmission in these subpopulations with prevalence in at least one of these subpopulations exceeding five per cent. However, it is not yet spread widely to the general population;
3. The generalized HIV epidemic in which HIV infection is firmly established in the general population. The major method of HIV transmission is heterosexual networking; prevalence of HIV infection in pregnant women is more than one per cent.

According to the latest report on the global AIDS epidemic, an estimated 33 million people were living with HIV in 2007 (UNAIDS, 2008). Compared to the figures in 2006 there were 2.7 million new HIV infections and 2 million AIDS-related deaths. Although the rate of new HIV infections has fallen in several countries, these favourable trends are, at least partially, offset by increases in new infections in other countries. The global percentage of adults living with HIV has levelled off since 2000 (UNAIDS, 2008).

Gender distribution of HIV/AIDS outside sub-Saharan Africa

While the global gender distribution of people living with HIV/AIDS (PLWHA) indicates an equal number of men and women, it hides the inherent differences in the dominant patterns the epidemic follows. In the rest of the world – excluding sub-Saharan Africa – the estimate is that twice as many men as women are living with HIV/AIDS; 7,095,722 men as opposed to 3,464,734 of women (UNAIDS, 2008). This is most likely a reflection of the fact that gay men and MSM are the most vulnerable to HIV/AIDS in the rest of the world. This is confirmed by the volume of research devoted to the spread of, and impact of, the epidemic within this risk group as well as the clear emphasis on health programmes designed to reduce the risk among them since the onset of the epidemic.

Despite the initial successes in reducing the numbers of new infections, gay men are however still considered to be highly vulnerable. In the USA, the UK and a number of other European countries HIV and AIDS have affected young gay men more than any other group of people. There are also many other parts of the world where MSM, many of whom do not identify themselves as gay, are affected by HIV/AIDS (Avert, 2009). In the USA HIV infection and AIDS accounted for 71 per cent of all HIV infections among male adults and adolescents in 2005 (based on data from 33 states with long-term, confidential name-based HIV reporting), even though only about five to seven per cent of male adults and adolescents identify themselves as MSM. According to this report the recent overall increase in HIV diagnoses for MSM, coupled with racial disparities, strongly points to a continued need for appropriate prevention and education services tailored for specific subgroups of MSM, especially those who are members of minority races and ethnicities (CDC, 2007).

Globally, women account for half of all HIV infections; this percentage has remained stable for the past several years. However, according to an UNAIDS and UNFPA report (2004), since 1985 the percentage of women among adults living with HIV/AIDS has risen from 35 per cent to 48 per cent worldwide. It has been suggested that 98 per cent of HIV-positive women live in developing countries, and that sub-Saharan Africa is the most affected region. In sub-Saharan Africa almost 61 per cent of adults living with HIV in 2007 were women, while in the Caribbean that percentage was 43 per cent, compared with 37 per cent in 2001 (UNAIDS, 2008). The proportions of women living with HIV in Latin America, Asia and Eastern Europe are slowly growing as HIV is transmitted to the female partners of men who are likely to have been infected through injecting drug use or during unprotected paid sex or sex with other men. In Eastern Europe and Central Asia it is estimated that women accounted for 26 per cent of adults with HIV in 2007, compared with 23 per cent in 2001; in Asia that proportion reached 29 per cent in 2007, compared with 26 per cent in 2001 (UNAIDS, 2008).

Rising rates of HIV infection among women are therefore a major cause for concern, since, as indicated, there is evidence to suggest that HIV/AIDS is spreading from particular population groups – such as sex workers or injecting drug users – into the general population, with women and girls increasingly infected (UNAIDS and UNFPA, 2004).

Gender distribution of HIV/AIDS in sub-Saharan Africa: a different story

The figures in sub-Saharan Africa, a region that bears the brunt of more than 65 per cent of the global prevalence of HIV/AIDS, tell a distinct story. The latest estimates are that 12,022,986 women are living with HIV/AIDS compared to 8,243,177 men (UNAIDS, 2008). While in the rest of the world – although on the rise – the percentage of women infected with HIV/AIDS is lower than the percentage of men, in sub-Saharan Africa it exceeds 60 per cent (UNAIDS, 2008).

These data are in line with other studies indicating that in sub-Saharan Africa the epidemic is not confined to gay men, MSM, drug users and sex workers, but rather is a generalized heterosexual epidemic and that women are more vulnerable than men (Shisana and Davids, 2004; Susser and Stein, 2000). Specifically, the southern Africa region has a generalized high prevalence HIV epidemic and carries the highest burden of HIV infections in the world. In 2007 southern Africa accounted for 35 per cent of new HIV infections and 38 per cent of global AIDS-related deaths. In 2005 the national population-based HIV prevalence in eight countries in southern Africa – Botswana, Lesotho, Mozambique, Namibia, South Africa, Swaziland, Zambia and Zimbabwe – exceeded 15 per cent, a level that no other country in the world had reached.

The factors that have been identified as the main contributors to this pattern of the epidemic comprise biological, economic-structural and socio-cultural elements which have been dubbed a 'lethal cocktail' by a Southern African Development Community (SADC) expert think tank (Leclerc-Madlala, 2006: 29). Since similar forces seem to be fuelling and shaping the epidemic in the Republic of South Africa, which is used as a case study in this chapter, they will be discussed in further detail in the following sections.

The case of HIV/AIDS in South Africa

Like other sub-Saharan African countries South Africa is in the midst of a 'global epidemic' with 32 per cent of all people with HIV existing and 34 per cent of deaths due to AIDS occurring in South Africa (Hedden et al., 2008). Due to its relatively large population of over 40 million, South Africa as a country has the largest absolute number of persons – 4.9 to 5.7 million – living with HIV infection in the world. It is estimated that about a quarter of a million of these persons are children below the age of 15 years. An estimated 350,000 children and adults died in South Africa of AIDS in 2007 alone (Matjila et al., 2008).

The gender distribution of PLWHA in South Africa reflects the general pattern in sub-Saharan Africa of greater vulnerability among women (Shisana et al., 2005). The most disturbing fact, however, is that this difference is highest in the 15 to 24 age group where the prevalence of HIV/AIDS among women is 17 per cent as opposed to four per cent among men (UNAIDS, 2008). A recent population-based survey indicated that the risk of infection in women aged 20 to 29 years was 5.6 per cent; accordingly, women's risk is six times that of males of the same age group, which is 0.9 per cent. The survey also indicated that among persons of 15 to 24 years females accounted for 90 per cent of all recent HIV infections (see Rehle et al., 2007). This trend is of concern since the latest population study reveals that HIV prevalence remains disproportionally high for females overall in comparison to males. It peaks in the 25 to 29 age group, where 32.7 per cent were found to be HIV-positive in 2008 (Shisana et al., 2009).

These data are complicated by the differential distribution of PLWHA among 'racial' groups in South Africa. According to the figures published by the Human Sciences Research Council, based on their national study conducted in 2005, the prevalence among black people is 13.3 per cent as opposed to 1.6 per cent among the white population (Shisana et al., 2005), rendering a race/class dimension to the spread of the epidemic.

Explanations of differential vulnerability to HIV/AIDS

In order to avoid falling into the trap that Annandale and Riska (2009: 125) warn against of focusing on 'the social to the relative neglect of the role of biology', this section first draws attention to the universal biological explanations underlying the greater vulnerability of women to HIV infections and then proceeds with the distinctive social explanations applicable to the sub-Saharan African context, with a focus on South Africa.

Bio-medical explanations: There is a range of biological factors that predispose women to a higher susceptibility to sexually transmitted infections (STI) which in turn increases their risk to HIV during sex (Hedden et al., 2009; Sprague, 2008). The main reasons for women's higher susceptibility of STI are:

- a greater area of mucous membrane is exposed during sex that provides fertile ground for the virus to enter the woman's body; this is more so in the case of young women whose genital tracts are not fully developed;
- larger quantities of fluids are transferred from men to women during sexual intercourse;
- a higher viral content in male fluids compared to female fluids;
- women are exposed to infectious fluids for a longer time during the act;
- micro-tears can easily occur in women's vaginal tissue as a result of sex, particularly if it is forced or unwelcomed;
- individuals with an STI are six times more likely than other individuals to pass on or acquire HIV during sex;
- a genital sore caused by an STI increases the risk of becoming infected with HIV from a single exposure by ten to 300 times (WHO, 2008).

Socio-cultural explanations: Although it is biologically easier for women to contract HIV, a growing body of literature is providing convincing evidence to illustrate 'non-biological' factors that increase women's vulnerability to

HIV/AIDS. Therefore, while taking biology into account, social scientists focus on structural causes of HIV/AIDS. In particular, in sub-Saharan Africa, special attention has been given to the analysis of inequalities and women's socio-economic position that lead to economic dependency on men as well as the socio-cultural norms that encourage gender inequality and the power of men over women. The consequences of these material and cultural inequalities are manifested in a number of ways that increase women's vulnerability to HIV/AIDS (Gilbert and Walker, 2002). In South Africa, the key manifestations are:

- high levels of sexual violence against women;
- transactional sex;
- the construction of subservient femininities and 'dangerous' masculinities that endorse multiple partners and undermine women's ability to negotiate condom use.

These key drivers of the epidemic are the factors that constitute the 'lethal cocktail' since, combined with the unfavourable biological factors, they interact in complex ways to fuel and shape the epidemic in this region. The salience of these issues in the context of HIV/AIDS in South Africa is the focus of the section that follows.

The 'lethal cocktail' and the 'gender machinery'

Shefer and colleagues argue that 'in the post-apartheid era there is a large "gender machinery" present in South Africa, including a wide range of legal and constitutional mechanisms as well as material resources to actively promote gender equality and challenge women's oppression' (2008: 157). However, there is a dislocation between this and women's lived realities, as is manifested in the high HIV/AIDS prevalence amongst women. There is a large body of literature dealing with policy (Butler, 2005) and, although not the focus of this chapter, the importance of locating any gendered health analysis within a policy environment needs to be acknowledged, while understanding that 'lived realities' cannot be read from policy. Further, we cannot ignore the impact of the history of apartheid with its employment-related male migration, widespread social dislocation and long-term disruption of family and social organization when considering the current HIV/AIDS epidemic (Marks, 2008; Walker et al., 2004).

Drawing on an UNDP study, Hunter (2007) argues that globalization and the South African state's market-led economic policy have accentuated social inequalities. He pays attention to rising unemployment and social inequalities that leave some groups, especially poor women, extremely vulnerable. For example, overall illiteracy rates are higher among blacks but are the highest among rural black women (27 per cent). In 2001, 53 per cent of black women were (formally) unemployed compared to 42 per cent of males. These figures, however, are higher than in the white population, demonstrating the racial inequalities referred to earlier. Poor access to education combined with low rates of employment result in economic inequalities. These inequalities, in turn, lead to inadequate access to resources such as housing, health and social welfare services (Gilbert and Walker, 2002). Universally, patriarchal social structures have excluded women from those aspects of society that are responsible for leadership, policy formation, resource allocation and decision-making. The power inequalities associated with such exclusion are reflected in and maintained by the social conditioning of women and men where specific roles are considered gender-appropriate.

In post-apartheid South Africa there is much evidence that there is a normative hyper-masculinity that puts both women and men at risk of HIV infection. The 'real man' has been constructed as biologically programmed to have unconstrained needs for frequent sex with a variety of women. Moreover, many men's perceptions of manhood often lead them to refuse to use condoms as they feel condom use diminishes their sexuality and their view of themselves as men (Selikow, 2004). This construction of a real man is cemented by reference to culture and encourages and legitimates multiple partners and sexual violence (Ragnarsson et al., 2008). However, double standards exist in relationship to gendered sexualities and, amongst women, in particular young women, the hegemonic femininity elevates young men and mandates deferential behaviour to men obliging women to be obedient to their male partners and to focus on men's sexual pleasure, even if it increases their own risk of HIV infection.

The example of 'dry sex' is illustrative of a sexual practice that privileges men's pleasure and makes women biologically more vulnerable to HIV infection. It is a sexual practice of minimizing vaginal secretions by using herbal aphrodisiacs, household detergents or antiseptics, or by wiping out or placing leaves in the vagina. The goal of these activities is to make the woman's vagina dry and tight, supposedly to increase sexual pleasure for the man. However, these practices make sex very painful for the woman. 'Dry sex' is common in this region and is of concern as it increases the chances of transmitting STI, such as HIV, for both partners since it may lead to vaginal lacerations and suppresses the vagina's natural bacteria, both of which increase the likelihood of HIV infection and the tearing of condoms (Myer et al., 2004).

Further, the role of multiple and concurrent sexual partnerships (MCP) is increasingly recognized as important in heterosexual HIV transmission in southern Africa. The overall rate of both men and women in South Africa having concurrent partners is high; 45 per cent of males and 28 per cent of females aged 15 to 19 as well as 36 per cent of males and 21 per cent of females aged 20 to 24 reported being involved in MCP. Indeed, within the social construction of masculinity it has become normative to have MCP. Young girls often implicitly endorse the predominant male norm of MCP as they do not expect to be the only sexual partner, and are aware that boys have concurrent partners (Ragnarsson et al., 2008).

In addition, transactional sex has been identified as a one of the key drivers of the HIV/AIDS epidemic (Leclerc-Madlala, 2006). Put simplistically, transactional sex involves the exchange of sex for either a subsistence resource or for conspicuous consumption. Studies have found that in South Africa, transactional sex is common and widely accepted; recent studies have reported prevalence rates of transactional sex as being as high as 21 per cent in some communities in South Africa (Dunkle et al., 2004). In a contradictory context of both poverty and consumerism, where women have little access to resources, often their only resource is sex, hence the increase in transactional sex. Transactional sex is not only a central factor in driving MCP, it is also a sexual interaction where it is difficult for women to negotiate the use of a condom because when women do not perceive themselves to be sex workers they may perceive some level of intimacy or emotional involvement, hence making it less likely that a condom will be used (Preston-Whyte et al., 2000). Moreover, when 'rewards' are exchanged for sex, it is unlikely that women will succeed in negotiating a condom. Further, often transactional sex involves young women partnering with older men who have more resources; intergenerational sex – the 'sugar daddy phenomenon' – increases young women's HIV risk (Leclerc-Madlala, 2004).

There is a growing recognition that the patterns of HIV transmission in South Africa are structured by gender and social inequalities, within which violence against women and girls is embedded. South Africa's history has been characterized by violence against women by both strangers and within intimate relationships and this is still the case today, as attested to by many studies (Dunkle et al., 2004; Shefer et al., 2008). For example, South Africa has the highest incidence of reported rape of any country. In 2006 a study reported that close to one in four men surveyed had participated in sexual violence. Of the total, 16.3 per cent had raped a non-partner or had participated in gang rape, while 8.4 per cent had been sexually violent towards an intimate partner. Moreover, women with violent or controlling male partners are more vulnerable to HIV infection as abusive men are more likely to have HIV and to impose risky sexual practices on their partners (Urdang, 2006).

There is a strong correlation between gender-based violence and HIV/AIDS due to a number of factors; violence against women is both a consequence and a cause of HIV/AIDS (Eaton et al., 2003). However, despite the multiple vulnerabilities of women, it is imperative to not see women as merely 'passive victims'. Although it is beyond the reach of this chapter, there is a growing body of research into how women exercise power and resistance to male domination (Hunter, 2007; Selikow, 2004). Moreover, gender relations are not static and, as Shefer and colleagues maintain, 'shifts in power between men and women do not appear to be represented at the level of sexual negotiation in any consistent way, so it seems there are many hurdles undermining safe and equitable sexual negotiation' (2008: 173–4).

Impact of HIV/AIDS on women as caregivers

Thus far we have focused on the gender patterning of HIV/AIDS in South Africa, demonstrating why women are at greater risk of HIV/AIDS. There is, however, another dimension to this epidemic that is underreported and that is its *impact*, particularly on women. Universally, gender norms assign women the primary role in caring for HIV/AIDS orphans and people who are ill and dying from AIDS, frequently when they are ill themselves. By some estimates, up to 90 per cent of caring work related to the epidemic occurs at home (UNIFEM, 2009). Based on a study in South Africa and three other developing countries, a Voluntary Services Overseas (VSO) position paper concluded:

> In all four countries, women are shouldering a disproportionate burden of care. Women are more likely to give care and less likely to receive it. Women's traditional domestic roles are being expanded by having to care for sick relatives or members of the community. The increased poverty associated with HIV and AIDS means that many women are undertaking additional jobs as breadwinners. (2003: 20)

The 'gogos' or grannies in South Africa, and elsewhere in sub-Saharan Africa, are at the centre of caregiving for PLWHA. Since the elderly often live in multi-generational households, they become the primary caretakers of the sick, of the children of the sick and of the orphaned. In addition to providing the physical and emotional care to the sick they often carry the financial burden of the whole household as a consequence of the AIDS-related deaths of eco-nomically active members (Schatz and Ogunmefun, 2007).

In addition to women's role in the family, they also play a disproportion-ate role in the various stages of the disease trajectory within the structures of organized healthcare services. This is done in their professional capacity as nurses who play a major role in most prevention and treatment programmes as well as in a voluntary, unpaid or often poorly paid capacity as counsellors for Voluntary Counselling and Testing (VCT), peer educators or as Anti-Retroviral Therapy adherence counsellors (Gilbert, 2008). However, due to the severe nature of the disease, particularly at the later stages, the burden is most relentless when it comes to home-based care.

Currently community and home-based care, delivered with little support from the public health system, is the key response to the HIV/AIDS pandemic globally. A report in 2004 showed that 90 per cent of care for people living with AIDS takes place in the home and is usually unpaid, unsupported and unrecognized (UNAIDS, 2004). The vast majority of volunteers in home-based care programmes are women, who increasingly have to replace formal health-care as services buckle under the strain of HIV/AIDS. According to the evidence provided by VSO (2006), two thirds of primary caregivers in households surveyed in southern Africa are female and one quarter of these are over 60 years of age. Further, a South African national evaluation of home-based care found that 91 per cent of caregivers were women.

This situation is not always taken into account in policy design, which can lead to an increased burden on women. For example, in its framework for action on community home-based care in resource-limited settings, the WHO only briefly acknowledges that the majority of carers are women and young girls, and does not examine the implications of this (VSO, 2006). The key plan-ning questions put forward did not recognize that women and young girls may have particular needs related to their role, nor did it prompt policy-makers to consider how to support men who may wish to take on a more proactive role in this area. Note should be taken, however, that there is evidence to suggest an increase in male involvement in this area, with many community organi-zations focusing on training and supporting men to provide home-based care among other HIV/AIDS-related functions (VSO, 2006).

The heavy impact described so far is unsustainable due to lost opportunities and severe physical and psychological effects on women. A study in South Africa showed that 40 per cent of households had to take time off from work to care for the ill (VSO, 2006). Many of their income-generating activities were affected, resulting in households being pushed into poverty. In addition, many of the caregivers suffered from the stressful nature of the work with no support – which includes caring for dying people and orphans. Furthermore, they often experi-enced stigma related to their association with PLWHA, adding to their levels of stress (Gilbert and Walker, 2009).

The increased burden of care on women is a major problem in South Africa. Programmes focusing on palliative or home-based care risk adding to the burden on women unless these gender roles are acknowledged in programme design. In South Africa, where some support is available in the form of grants, there is often little knowledge of how to access them, or even that they exist (VSO, 2006).

A need for gender sensitive intervention strategies

The HIV/AIDS epidemic necessitates intervention strategies that address its gendered nature. In particular, it is important to focus on the way it plays out in specific social contexts. In South Africa, as in the rest of sub-Saharan Africa, women, by virtue of their subordinate position to men, are not in a position to control the practice of safe sex if they have to rely on the use of male condoms and be at the mercy of their partners who often fail to cooperate. For this reason much research has focused on devices such as female condoms that can help women protect themselves, but that still require some degree of male cooperation. There has also been an emphasis on microbicides – gels or creams that could prevent HIV infection which can be applied vaginally without the partner's knowledge. Although not as successful as was hoped, such inventions can potentially reverse the decision-making process in sexual relations and give women the power to decide on safe-sex practices. Needless to say, the development of these women-controlled prevention methods should take place in tandem with challenging women's material inequalities as well as the traditional cultural norms that put women in a disadvantageous position in the first place.

Circumcision can also be seen as a gendered public health intervention that targets men only. There is evidence to suggest that circumcision reduces the risk of HIV infection in men. However, the same risk reduction does not apply to partners of circumcised men (Matjila et al., 2008). Although it has been put forward by the WHO and UNAIDS as a recommended intervention strategy, it has generated significant controversy with regard to its implementation. The voices advocating caution argue that cultural issues surrounding male circumcision need to be considered and that traditional leaders should be involved as the custodians of culture before any large-scale public health rollout takes place. Others have wondered whether the male-centred intervention would have a disempowering effect on women and increase their HIV risk by giving men an excuse not to use condoms. An important concern raised in this context is that male engagement in HIV prevention should not be confined to surgical intervention and therefore all circumcision programmes must be accompanied by gender-transformative approaches to HIV/AIDS.

An urgent need for gender-sensitive approaches, although with different implications, is also obvious with respect to antiretroviral treatment (ART), which is a socially complex area. One aspect of this complexity is the fact that although, medically, men and women may respond differently to the medication and experience ART in a diverse manner, access to ART should be a dimension of HIV/AIDS that is gender-neutral. However, most programmes experience an underrepresentation of men, with fewer than expected men attending the clinics (Shisana et al., 2005). The factors put forward as potential barriers for men to access treatment include low uptake of testing for HIV/AIDS, emphasis on prevention of mother-to-child transmission, lack of programmes for specific groups such as MSM, stigma and discrimination and, in particular, the feminization of the epidemic. However, the fact that men are not accessing HIV prevention as well as treatment services has not been on the government's agenda for action in any of its public documentation – and this is cause for concern.

Conclusion

Although the spread and impact of HIV/AIDS has been universal, in this chapter it has been demonstrated that the burden of this epidemic is not borne equally by the global community. Epidemiological data clearly show that the highest prevalence rates are in sub-Saharan Africa. Less visible, however, is the complex combination of forces that fuel the epidemic. The epidemic in this region is increasingly 'feminized' as a growing proportion of infections occurs amongst and affects women. The gender distribution of HIV/AIDS in South Africa reflects a similar pattern. Using South Africa as a case study of one country in the sub-Saharan African region, the aim of this chapter has been to interrogate the contextual factors underlying the differential vulnerabilities between men and women. The analysis reveals that a 'lethal cocktail' of biomedical, political, economic and cultural forces shape the gendered dynamic of the epidemic in South Africa. The most common 'ingredients' of this cocktail are lack of access to material resources; cultural norms where women are subservient to men and where masculinity is defined in terms of multiple sexual partners; transactional sex; intergenerational sex; and patriarchy and power of men, combined with high levels of violence against women. In addition the chapter draws attention to the gendered impact of the epidemic where women bear the heavy load of caregiving for the sick and their families.

Since successful intervention strategies need to be tailored to specific contexts, we argue that it is important to make visible the ingredients of this 'lethal cocktail' and the gendered nature of caregiving to enable health professionals and policy-makers to address context-specific concerns. However, in the interest of sustainable transformation, we contend that, while not ignoring biology or individual behaviour, it is timely to focus on structural interventions at both the material and cultural level and alter the context in which HIV/AIDS is flourishing.

Summary

The following key recommendations should be highlighted:

- adopt a theoretical and practical 'gender inclusive' approach that focuses on all dimensions of the epidemic, including prevention, treatment and care;
- develop a broader conception of HIV/AIDS that is located within the socio-economic and cultural environment, rather than focusing on individualistic approaches;
- challenge gender-based power inequalities at both the macro-economic level as well as at the socio-cultural level;

- devise programmes that are based on an understanding that often both women and men adhere to traditional notions of gender roles, and of the construction of gender roles;
- recognize that women's economic dependence on men increases their vulnerability to violence and to HIV/AIDS and ensure that women have more access to general resources such as education, information and socio-economic opportunities;
- ensure that men are also responsible for the treatment and care of those affected by HIV/AIDS.

Key reading

Gilbert L. and L. Walker (2002) 'Treading the Path of Least Resistance: HIV/AIDS and Social Inequalities – A South African Case Study', *Social Science & Medicine*, 54 (7), 1093–1110.

Hunter, M. (2007) 'The Changing Political Economy of Sex in South Africa: The Significance of Unemployment and Inequalities to the Scale of the AIDS Pandemic', *Social Science & Medicine*, 64 (3), 689–700.

Shisana, O. and A. Davids (2004) 'Correcting Gender Inequalities Is Central to Controlling HIV/AIDS', *Bulletin of the World Health Organization*, 82 (11), 812.

World Health Organization (WHO) (2008) 'Women and HIV/AIDS', at: www.who.int/gender/hiv-aids/en/, accessed 16 March 2009.

References

Annandale, E. and E. Riska (2009) 'New Connections: Towards a Gender-inclusive Approach to Women's and Men's Health', *Current Sociology*, 57 (2), 123–33.

Avert (2009) *HIV/AIDS and Young Gay Men*, HIV/AIDS Information Sheets, at: www.avert.org/young-gay-men.htm, accessed 21 April 2009.

Barnet, T. and A. Whiteside (2002) *AIDS in the Twenty-first Century: Disease and Globalization* (New York: Palgrave Macmillan).

Butler, A. (2005) 'South Africa's HIV/AIDS Policy, 1994–2004: How Can It Be Explained?', *African Affairs*, 104 (107), 591–614.

CDC – Centers for Disease Control and Prevention (2007) *HIV/AIDS Fact Sheets: HIV/AIDS among Men Who Have Sex with Men* (Atlanta: Centers for Disease Control and Prevention), at: www.cdc.gov/hiv, accessed 22 April 2009.

Dunkle, K. L., R. Jewkes, H. Brown, G. E. Gray, J. A. McIntryre and S. D. Harlow (2004) 'Transactional Sex Among Women in Soweto, South Africa: Prevalence, Risk Factors and Association with HIV Infection', *Social Science & Medicine*, 59 (8), 1581–92.

Eaton, L., A. J. Flischer and L. E. Aaro (2003) 'Unsafe Sexual Behaviour in South African Youth', *Social Science & Medicine*, 56 (1), 149–65.

Farmer, P., M. Connors and J. Simmons (eds) (1996) *Women, Poverty, and AIDS: Sex, Drugs, and Structural Violence* (Monroe: Common Courage Press).

Gilbert, L. (2008) 'Public Health and Health Professionals in the Times of HIV/AIDS', *South African Sociological Review*, 39 (2), 301–16.

Gilbert L. and L. Walker (2002) 'Treading the Path of Least Resistance: HIV/AIDS and Social Inequalities – A South African Case Study', *Social Science & Medicine*, 54 (7), 1093–1110.

Gilbert, L. and L. Walker (2009) '"My Biggest Fear Was That People Would Reject Me Once They Knew My Status" – Stigma as Experienced by Patients in an HIV/AIDS Clinic In Johannesburg, South Africa', *Health and Social Care in the Community*, 18 (2), 139–46.

Hedden, S. L., D. Whitaker, L. Floyd and W. W. Latimer (2009) 'Gender Differences in the Prevalence and Behavioural Risk Factors of HIV in South African Drug Users', *AIDS Behavior*, 13 (2), 288–96.

Hunt, C. W. (1996) 'Social vs Biological: Theories on the Transmission of AIDS in Africa', *Social Science & Medicine*, 42 (9), 1238–96.

Hunter, M. (2007) 'The Changing Political Economy of Sex in South Africa: The Significance of Unemployment and Inequalities to the Scale of the AIDS Pandemic', *Social Science & Medicine*, 64 (3), 689–700.

Leclerc-Madlala, S. (2004) 'Transactional Sex and the Pursuit of Modernity', *Social Dynamics*, 29 (2), 1–21.

Leclerc-Madlala, S. (2006) 'What Really Drives HIV/AIDS in Southern Africa? Summary Report of SADC Expert Think-Tank Meeting in Maseru, 10–12 May 2006', *AIDS Legal Quarterly, Network Newsletter*, June 2006, 29–32.

Marks, S. (2008) 'The Burdens of the Past', in A. Ndinga-Muvumba and R. Pharoah (eds), *HIV/AIDS and Society in South Africa* (Durban: University of KwaZulu-Natal Press), 37–62.

Matjila, M. J., A. A. Hoosen, A. Stoltz and N. Cameron (2008) 'STIs, HIV and AIDS and TB: Progress and Challenges', in P. Barron and J. Roma-Readon (eds), *South African Health Review 2008* (Durban: Health Systems Trust), 89–102.

Myer, L., L. Denny, R. Telerant, M. de Souza, T. C. Wright and L. Kuhn (2005) 'Bacterial Vaginosis and Susceptibility to HIV Infection in South African Women: A Nested Case Control Study', *Sexually Transmitted Diseases*, 31 (3), 174–9.

Preston-Whyte, E., C. Varga, H. Oosthuizen, R. Roberts and F. Blose (2000) 'Survival Sex and HIV/AIDS in an African City', in R. M. Parker, M. Barbosa and P. Aggleton, (eds), *Framing the Sexual Subject: The Politics of Gender, Sexuality and Power* (Berkeley: University of California Press), 165–90.

Rehle, T., O. Shisana, V. Pillay, K. Zuma and W. Parker (2007) 'National Incidence Measure – New Insights into the South African Epidemic', *South African Medical Journal*, 97 (3), 194–9.

Ragnarsson, A., A. T. Onya, A. Thorson, A. M. Ekstrom and L. E. Aaro (2008) 'Young Males' Gendered Sexuality in the Era of HIV and AIDS in Limpopo Province, South Africa', *Qualitative Research*, 18 (6), 739–46.

Schatz, E. and C. Ogunmefun (2007) 'Caring and Contributing: The Role of Older Women in Rural South African Multi-generational Households in the HIV/AIDS Era', *World Development*, 35 (8), 1390–1403.

Shefer, T., M. Crawford, A. Strebel, L. Simbayi, N. Dwada-Henda, A. Cloete, M. R. Kaufman and S. C. Kalichman (2008) 'Gender, Power and Resistance to Change among Two Communities in the Western Cape, South Africa,' *Feminism and Psychology*, 18 (2), 157–82.

Selikow, T. (2004) '"We Have Our Own Special Language." Language, Sexuality and HIV/AIDS: A Case Study of Youth in an Urban Township in South Africa', *African Health Sciences*, 4 (2), 102–8.

Shisana, O. and A. Davids (2004) 'Correcting Gender Inequalities Is Central to Controlling HIV/AIDS', *Bulletin of the World Health Organization*, 82 (11), 812.

Shisana, O., T. Rehle, L. Simbayi, W. Parker, K. Zuma, A. Bhana, C. Connolly, S. Jooste et al. (2005) *South African National HIV Prevalence, HIV Incidence, Behaviour and Communication Survey 2005* (Cape Town: HSRC Press).

Shisana, O., T. Rehle, L. C. Simbayi, K. Zuma, S. Jooste, V. Pillay-van-Wyk, N. Mbelle, J. van Zyl et al. (2009) *South African National HIV Prevalence, Incidence, Behaviour and Communication Survey 2008: A Turning Tide among Teenagers?* (Cape Town: HSRC Press).

Sprague, C. (2008) 'Women's Health, HIV/AIDS and the Workplace in South Africa', *African Journal of AIDS Research*, 7 (3), 341–52.

Squire, C. (2007) *HIV in South Africa* (London: Routledge).

Susser, I. and Z. Stein (2000) 'Culture, Sexuality, and Women's Agency in the Prevention of HIV/AIDS in Southern Africa', *American Journal of Public Health*, 90 (7), 1042–8.

Treichler, P. A. (1999) *How to Have Theory in an Epidemic: Cultural Chronicles of AIDS* (Durham, NC: Duke University Press).

UN Economic and Social Council (2009), at: http://un.org/News/Press/docs/2009/wom1728.doc.htm, accessed 27 April 2009.

UNAIDS (2004) *Report on the Global AIDS Epidemic (4th Global AIDS Report)* (Geneva: United Nations).

UNAIDS (2008) *Report on the Global AIDS Epidemic* (Geneva: United Nations).

UNAIDS and UNFPA (2004) *Women and HIV/AIDS: Confronting the Crisis* (Geneva: United Nations).

UNIFEM (2009) *Care-giving in the Context of HIV/AIDS*, Briefing Sheet prepared for the 53rd Session of the Commission on the Status of Women, 2–13 March 2009.

Urdang, S (2006) 'The Care Economy: Gender and the Silent AIDS Crisis in Southern Africa', *Journal of Southern African Studies*, 30 (1), 165–77.

VSO – Voluntary Services Overseas (2003) *Gendering AIDS: Women, Men, Empowerment, Mobilisation*, AIDS Agenda: VSO Position Paper, at: www.impactaids.org.uk/newsletter/gendering_aids_exec.pdf, accessed 21 April 2009.

VSO – Voluntary Services Overseas (2006) *Reducing the Burden of HIV and AIDS Care on Women and Girls*, VSO Policy Brief, at: www.icw.org/files/AIDSAgenda/BurdenofCare/PolicyBriefAugust2006.pdf, accessed 10 March 2009.

Walker, L., G. Reid and M. Cornell (2004) *Waiting to Happen. HIV/AIDS in South Africa* (Boulder: Lynne Reinner Publishers/Cape Town: Double Storey Books/Juta).

WHO – World Health Organization (2008) *Women and HIV/AIDS*, at: www.who.int/gender/hiv-aids/en/, accessed 16 March 2009.

13
Gender and End-of-life Care

Alex Broom

Introduction

Despite many a scholar and philosopher presenting death and dying as, as Mark Twain famously said, 'the great leveller', the fact is that death and dying reflect, produce and articulate different social hierarchies, moral frameworks and cultural ideologies (Howarth, 2007a; Seale, 1998; Timmerman, 2010). How you die and the circumstances of your death are heavily shaped by aspects of your biography, including gender. Moreover, contemporary dying is a morally and politically laden social process that is deeply embedded in culturally specific gender relations (Broom and Cavenagh, 2010; Lawton, 2000). This chapter examines the wider patterning of death and dying internationally as well as some specific ways in which gender interplays with experiences of end-of-life care. Through an exploration of key issues related to morality, dignity, the right to die and 'the good death', the chapter seeks to unpack, at the organizational level *and* at the level of individual experience, some key issues at the intersection of gender and dying in western developed nations.

Gender is but one factor shaping end-of-life care. Other aspects of one's biography including such things as class, ethnicity, geography, sexuality and so on play equally important roles (Howarth, 2007a, 2007b). Yet, the interplay of gender and end-of-life care has received particularly little attention in the academic literature for a range of reasons (Broom and Cavenagh, 2010). The perception of death and dying as a leveller is perhaps one reason for the paucity of research on gender at end of life. Moreover, there has been a rather deterministic focus on *sex* differences within the palliative care literature (Dattela and Neimeyera, 1990; Donovan et al., 2008) rather than an exploration of the complex cultural scripts and gendered experiences that shape our dying processes (Howarth, 2007a).

More broadly, the emphasis of palliative care research has been firmly placed on psychological management and biomedical supportive care (Field et al., 1997). This has meant limited exploration of the challenges to gender identities in end-of-life care settings, including the relationality of dying and the moral codes operating within the end-of-life care settings (Froggatt, 1997; Kellehear, 2008). Yet, much like other healthcare contexts, gender has been shown to play a key role across and within end-of-life care settings, shaping patient transitions from primary care to palliative care and from community palliative care to in-patient hospice care (Broom and Cavenagh, 2011). In combination with other facets of individual biography, gender scripts and identities mediate individual preferences, interactions with clinical staff and intervention requests at the end of life (Broom and Cavenagh, 2010; Clark and Seymour, 1999; Field et al., 1997).

This chapter begins with an outline of gender and/or sex differences in life-expectancy, cause, and place of death in selected countries as well as a discussion of some of the factors that explain these patterns. In what follows the focus moves to an in-depth exploration of the gendered experiences of end-of-life care and how some men and some women may experience and engage in dying differently. It should be noted that the focus here is largely on the developed world as issues facing developing countries around death and dying are vastly different (Broom and Doron, 2011; Parry, 1994). Several of the case studies presented here are drawn from Australia, and represent the first studies of their kind in this particular area. The aim of this chapter is not to present a monolithic perspective of sex-related roles *determining* human experiences of dying. Rather, it is to provide a constructivist-driven review of the field that examines how gender constructs, scripts and identities interplay with contemporary death and dying.

Population trends on death and dying

One of the clearest indicators that gender shapes the character of contemporary death and dying is cross-cultural epidemiological data on how, where and why people die. Although substantial differences do exist across cultures, men and women die differently. That is, on a population level, they die in different locations, of different things and at different stages in their lives.

Gender differences in life expectancy

While life expectancy at birth for men and women has improved over the past century, it is still shaped according to whether you are born male or female (see also Chapter 8 by Bird et al.). As shown in Table 13.1, life expectancy at birth for men is significantly lower than for women across OECD nations. In the United States the overall difference in life expectancy between men and women has declined since 1979 (Kochanek et al., 2011: 29) yet a significant gap persists. Similar patterns can be seen in the United Kingdom (Office for

Table 13.1   Life expectancy at birth in selected countries, 2009

Life expectancy	Men	Women
Australia	79.7	84.2
France	77.8	84.8
Germany	77.7	82.7
Japan	79.6	86.5
United Kingdom	78	82.2
USA	76	80.9

Source: World Health Organization (2011)

National Statistics, 2010). It is important also to consider that while women can expect to live longer than men, they are also more likely to spend more years in poor health or with a disability (Kochanek et al., 2011: 29).

In Australia over the past 20 years life expectancy at birth has improved by 6.0 years for men and 4.3 years for women (Australian Bureau of Statistics, 2011a). The situation for indigenous/marginalized populations in many developed countries is even more concerning with the gap between life expectancy even greater. For example, in Australia, life expectancy at birth for Aboriginal men from 2005–7 was estimated to be 67.2 years compared with 72.9 years for women, a difference of nearly 5.7 years.

The reasons for these differences in life expectancy of men and women at birth are multiple and complex and there are a variety of perspectives on the legitimacy of particular explanations. Ultimately, most differences in life expectancy at birth relate to the socio-behavioural and environmental differences men and women are likely to have over the life course. Such differences in behaviour and exposure result in premature death amongst men, higher levels of disability and chronic illness amongst women in older age, and broader patterns in the eventual causes of death.

Gender differences in cause of death

One of the clearest indicators that gender impacts on health outcomes is the international data on cause of death. While there are consistencies between men and women in terms of causes of death – ischaemic heart disease (or also referred to as coronary heart disease; CHD) and cancer/neoplasms both dominate mortality statistics in developed countries – national data sets also consistently illustrate differences. Table 13.2 shows some of the key differences in the three leading causes of death in selected countries by sex.

To provide some context to Table 13.2, differences between men and women in major causes of death tend to relate to such things as levels of smoking (trachea/lung cancer), diet (ischaemic heart disease/CHD), alcohol intake (cirrhosis), drug use (unintentional injury) and depression (injury/suicide).

Table 13.2   The three leading causes of death in selected countries by sex

Causes of death	Men			Women		
	#1	#2	#3	#1	#2	#3
Australia*	CHD	Trachea/lung cancer	Stroke/ cerebrovasc. diseases	CHD	Stroke/ cerebrovasc. disease	Dementia/ Alzhiemer's
England and Wales**	CHD	Malignant neoplasm trachea/lung/ bronchus	Stroke/ cerebrovasc. diseases	CHD	Stroke/ cerebrovasc. disease	Dementia/ Alzhiemer's
USA†	CHD	Malignant neoplasms	Unintentional injury	CHD	Malignant neoplasms	Stroke/ cerebrovasc. diseases
Sweden††	CHD	Stroke/ cerebrovasc. disease	Prostate cancer	CHD	Stroke/ cerebrovasc. disease	Dementia

Sources: * Australia for 2009; Australian Bureau of Statistics (2011a)
    ** England and Wales for 2009; Office for National Statistics (2010)
    † USA for 2007; National Center for Injury Prevention and Control (2010a)
    †† Sweden for 2009; Official Statistics of Sweden (2011)

For example, in the United Kingdom (UK) the Office for National Statistics (2011b) found that the death rate from alcohol-related causes doubled for men from 9.1 per 100,000 in 1991 to 18.3 per 100,000 in 2006 whereas for women it increased from 5.0 to 8.8 per 100,000. Similarly, in 2006/07 use of Class A drugs was five per cent for men and two per cent for women (Office for National Statistics, 2011b). Such patterns of morbidity and mortality are deeply embedded in cultural understandings about, and the enactment of, gender (Courtenay, 2009).

Examining other forms of death, such as suicide, we see further examples of a particularly gendered cultural dynamic. As shown in Table 13.3, suicide rates are dramatically different according to sex. For example, in Australia men are over three times more likely to commit suicide than women, although Australian women are much more likely to have attempted suicide. While the processes underpinning these outcomes are complex and differ for each individual (Shiner et al., 2009), there is little doubt that cultural pressures and norms around both masculinities and femininities shape the acceptability of asking for help, in the context of mental illness, and thus the risk of suicide.

Place of death by gender

The relationship between gender and place of death has received relatively little attention in the academic literature and such dynamics are culturally

Table 13.3   Suicide rates (per 100,000) in selected countries by sex

Suicide rates	Men	Women
Australia (2009)*	14.9	4.5
UK (2009)**	17.5	5.2
USA (2007)†	18.4	4.7
France (2008)††	23.2	7.5
Germany (2009)††	15.1	4.4
Japan (2008)†††	35.1	13.5
Sweden (2009)††	17.7	7.1

Sources: * Australian Bureau of Statistics (2011b)
    ** Office for National Statistics (2011a)
    † National Center for Injury Prevention and Control (2010b)
    †† Eurostat (2011)
    ††† World Health Organization (n.d.)

variable. Yamasaki and colleagues (2008) surveyed 386 Japanese men and women and found that 50 per cent of all respondents preferred to die at home versus 38.8 per cent in a hospital or nursing facility. Of those surveyed, 60 per cent of men preferred to die at home and 70 per cent wanted to be cared for by their spouses. By comparison, only 40 per cent of women wanted to die at home and the majority wanted to be cared for by daughters, other family members or their spouses (Yamasaki et al., 2008).

Cohen and colleagues (2010) have researched death at home in the context of cancer in selected Western European countries. Their results reveal that men with cancer die at home more often than women in the majority of countries selected; the difference is statistically significant for the Netherlands and Norway, and interestingly, also within the UK between England and Wales. Gomes and Higginson (2008), drawing on England and Wales, have looked at the place of death for all causes of death, Their research highlights that, although in decline, higher rates of death at home for men have persisted over time.

These statistics reflect a gendered dynamic in and around death and dying. That is, gender dynamics and practices may shape an individual's preparedness to be cared for or 'burden' their partner or family in the dying process. Specifically, men may be more prepared to be cared for at home by their partner – situated within the traditional feminine carer role – whereas women may not be as willing to accept this shift in interpersonal dynamic (Yamasaki et al., 2008). Alternatively, men may experience a disintegration of self in institutional palliative care contexts and thus prefer a home setting (Broom and Cavenagh, 2010). Ultimately, statistical patterns indicate that, although personal preferences and degree of physical dependence will shape their desire for death at home or in a hospital, gender plays a significant role.

The gendered mediation of end-of-life care: three case studies

While epidemiological data around gender and sex differences in death and dying provide significant insight into how our social and cultural status – as men or women – may drive our particular ending, it is useful to engage in an in-depth and conceptually driven analysis of the gendering of dying. While there is a plethora of literature on so-called male and female preferences at end of life, specifically around the desire to end life, questions of pain relief and for supportive care (Dattela and Neimeyera, 1990; Donovan et al., 2008; Murray et al., 2003), such analyses have tended to depend on role-based models of behaviour. It can be more useful to examine the meanings of gender and expression of gender identities within the dying process and how differently positioned men and women experience bodily, identity and relational challenges in formalized care settings. That is, to engage in analyses of the emotional planes of experience and micro-practices of care that actually feed into these wider statistical patterns.

The following section provides a series of reflections on how experiences of end-of-life care and decisions about, and preferences for, dying are deeply embedded in gender constructs and forms of identity work. The first case study is the gendered character of obligation and reciprocity at end of life.

Reciprocity, obligation and the moral economies of dying

Academic debate has tended to centre on ethics and rights at end of life with relatively little work done on the relational expression and performance of moral codes (Chattoo and Ahmad, 2008; Lawton, 2000; see also Booth, 1994, on moral economy). Yet, research shows that in the context of gender and gender identities, dying represents a key site of moral practice (Broom and Cavenagh, 2010; Sayer, 2005). Within end-of-life care settings, notions of duty and rights in the form of social contracts between stakeholders heavily shape individual experiences (Meyer, 1995, 1989; Raja, 2009). Tensions between individual interest, like, for example, the desire for a quick death, and the common interest such as ideas about 'timely deaths', shape the possibilities and peculiarities of end-of-life care experiences and these relations are gendered in character. For example, in their study of an Australian hospice, Broom and Cavenagh (2010) found that ideas about 'good deaths' (for example, fought, natural, stoic, peaceful) have become an integral part of end-of-life care, and potentially serve to morally bind patient choice and desire so as to produce 'good patients' as well as 'good deaths'. They argue that doing 'the good death' has become centred on normative ideas about 'not giving up', 'fighting for your life' and 'ris[ing] to the occasion' (Broom and Cavenagh, 2010: 871–2). As one of their participants stated:

Participant: I know [wife's name] wants me to hang around as long as I can. Um, no, I've got no intentions of giving up, I've got every intention of fighting it for as long as I can. Um, you're fighting a losing battle, but what the hell, you've got to be in it! . . . My own preference, as I said, would've been to have a sudden death. But, you don't get your preference, you don't get a choice. You get whatever cards were dealt [male, terminal cancer]. (Broom and Cavenagh, 2010: 871)

This particular study and others in the context of end-of-life care (Chattoo and Ahmad, 2008), illustrate the potent moral framing of dying in formalized care settings – a pressure to 'to fight on' and 'not give up'. Such dynamics produce personal conundrums and inter-personal tensions, whereby the needs and desires of the dying person may conflict with those of the carer/s, family and clinical staff. Such tensions have, in turn, been shown to be mediated by gendered experiences of 'being a burden' (Broom and Cavenagh, 2010: 872; see also McPherson et al., 2007). That is, women at the end of life may find it problematic to accept being cared for given their historical or existing carer role in the family or relationship. Furthermore, men's role expectations around physicality, potency and control may be perceived to be eroded within the dying process or institutionalized palliative care setting. This experience was illustrated in the account of one male in in-patient hospice care:

Participant: Put it this way, nobody would ever say that they've, it's been their aim in life to get sick at the end of it and die in a certain particular way. I don't know, I can only put it from a male point of view, possibly, 'cause I know we men, and probably women too, to a great degree as well, we each of us all, we're all very proud of our own independence, our own abilities to, see ourselves through life, with ah, the provision of a roof over our head, and ah, bringing our children up, well fed and protected and sheltered, sort of thing. Owning your own home, it's sort of being a solid brick in the community sort of thing. So it's very, very hard when it comes to, when we start to get frail [male, terminal cancer]. (Broom and Cavenagh, 2010: 872)

Such findings illustrate the gendered character of dying, bodily disintegration, and receiving care, including the specific challenges end-of-life care presents within a wider cultural context of 'male' and 'female' roles (Broom and Cavenagh, 2010). Shown in the above excerpt, 'being a solid brick in the community', rather than a person in need of help, encapsulates the underlying grief of the loss of status. Such gendered practices and identities also shape perspectives on assisted dying and idealized deaths. That is, a swift and even self-determined death may be more appealing to many men within the context of cultural ideas about bodily potency, mastery, self-sufficiency and control (Broom and Tovey, 2009). While 'fighting on' may be considered virtuous, 'ending it now' reflects a masculine form of potency and self-determination; a 'fitting end' for a male not wishing to experience further erosion of the masculine self.

Ultimately, such research illustrates the intersectionality of moral practice and gender identities in end-of-life care settings (Field et al., 1997; Hart et al., 1998; Kellehear, 2008; Lawton, 2000). Moreover, such dialectics – struggle/virtue versus self-determination/autonomy – present those at end of life with a series of difficult, if not impossible questions. Should I 'die well', as culturally ascribed, or retain a sense of my authentic masculine/feminine self? What does 'struggling on' mean in terms of my role and sense of place within my family and my sense of self within relationships? Such gendered forms of relationality also shape the desire to hasten death and perspectives on euthanasia and assisted dying.

The gendered mediation of dignity and euthanasia or assisted dying

As suggested, end-of-life care settings often contain, imbue and reify a range of cultural scripts around obligation, reciprocity and 'the good death'. Such moral framings are often problematic in the context of gender identities, but are complicated further in combination with the politics of human dignity, that is, how an individual should be treated in the context of suffering, bodily disintegration and identity trouble. Dynamics and cultural codes around rights and responsibilities have their beginnings in the social contractual rights and obligations of modern constitutional democracies (Meyer, 1995). That is, a universally ascribed promise of life that the modern state is obliged to provide. Similarly, end-of-life care is largely embedded in a 'responsibilities' and 'rights' model. This includes institutionalized structures and beliefs that shape the perceptions on 'human dignity' and even extend to the production of 'timely deaths' (Parry, 1982, 1994). Research in this area suggests that such rights and obligations may be experienced differentially in and around gender. That is, the expression of rights and the conceptualization of dignity may be, in some ways and for some people, enmeshed in gendered expectations and discontents. For example, in Broom and Cavenagh's (2010) study, the male participants critiqued the governance of their deaths and idealized the quick death in the context of the 'male role':

Participant: Yeah, I mean, right now, if I had my choices, if you could pick the way to go, I would choose to go the way my grandfather did, which was coming out of the paddock to have breakfast, grabbed his little grandson, put him on his knee, said to grandma that he was ready for his porridge, and he put his brown sugar on his porridge, and his home-made butter, and was stirring it all in there, and dropped dead of a heart attack. Now that's the way to go if you've got a choice [male, terminal cancer]. (Broom and Cavenagh, 2010: 872)

Participant: [excerpt truncated from original] . . . well they're not allowed to [do euthanasia] by law to start with, is one of the things. Um, ah, why they didn't do it? Religion would be one, would be the main one, I should imagine. And just morally that it's wrong to take a life and so forth. But it's my decision, and I should have been left alone. I do believe this, and I have lots of friends, who my children said that to: 'You should have just left him alone. You go, you wanted to go. You've had your life.' I'm eighty-three in nine months [male, heart failure]. (Broom, 2012: 231)

Cultural ideas about men and masculinity combine with ideas about 'good deaths', perspectives on assisted dying, and conceptions of dignity (Seale, 1998). Moreover, they are in turn infected by the dual problematic of a moral accountability to do the 'good death' (contractual obligations) and a potential intolerability of undignified endings for gender identities. Within the palliative care model of dying, requests for euthanasia or assisted dying would, in fact, be disruptive of the 'natural order', and a threat to the body politic, if such requests or desires became widespread or accepted (Meyer, 1995). Being 'kept alive', in many respects, becomes a bureaucratic imposition of a treasured democratic right – the right to a timely death, protected by the state – but, paradoxically, a potential denial of human dignity. In saying this, ultimately, dignity, in the context of dying, can be viewed in multiple ways; each of which are embedded in the politics of morality, honour and obligation and gendered forms of relationality. That is, dignity at end of life can mean 'going out with poise' (stoicism) or it can mean being allowed to 'end it now' (self-determination). While culturally these different pathways may promote certain ideas about value and worth – and problematize relations of gift and honour – both contain and fulfil aspects of dignity. Such experiences and articulations of dignity may often be embedded in gender relations and identities.

This research illustrates the importance of considering the institutional delivery of end-of-life care (James and Field, 1992) and its complicity in the moral framing of contemporary dying (Chattoo and Ahmad, 2008). In many respects end-of-life care service providers produce and govern ideas about 'good' and 'timely' deaths, and in turn, frame gendered experiences in end-of-life care settings. Sociologically, there are dual processes evident. The first is a moral economy of dying (Booth, 1994) that, through cultural scripts around 'good deaths' and ideas about gift/obligation, provides a relational framework for 'dying well' (Broom and Cavenagh, 2011). Such moralities of dying ('closure', 'acceptance' and 'a natural end') produce interpersonal dilemmas about the responsibility: to live as long as one can; to reconcile existential questions before death; and, to accept one's end. Such dilemmas are gendered in character with men and women often making choices very differently in end-of-life care settings, or indeed not being provided with particular choices (euthanasia or assisted dying) that may be perceived to be more consistent with their gender identity.

Gender, self-responsibility and healing in advanced cancer care

In the context of cancer care, and particularly with advanced terminal cancer, the use of complementary and alternative medicine (CAM) has become extremely popular in many western nations; between 30 and 80 per cent of cancer patients use CAM depending on the given patient population (Broom and Tovey, 2008). Moreover, 'alternative medicine' as a social movement has been closely tied to women's social movements (Bix, 2004; see also Chapter 29 by Cant and Watts). Indeed, we see much higher levels of support for, and use of, CAM in female populations internationally (Luff and Thomas, 2000); a pattern some would argue is linked to the affinity of CAM with feminine ideas about the body, subjectivity and closeness to 'nature' (Sointu, 2006; Sointu and Woodhead, 2008). For example, Sointu (2006) argues that CAM practices more broadly enable women to perform and embody ideals such as self-responsibility and self-actualization. Similarly, much CAM discourse in the context of advanced cancer care endorses ideas about self-responsibility, self-help and the ability to 'heal' oneself (Broom, 2009a, 2009b; McClean, 2005).

Such discourses around 'work on the self' depart significantly from biomedical approaches to cancer care and can be empowering and useful to many men and women. The approaches taken by many naturopaths, herbalists, spiritual healers and so on arguably create a normative potential that can far exceed the potential held by the biomedical community (Scott, 1998). Thus, on the one hand, CAM practice and ideology have emerged from a wider feminist critique of biomedical control over women's bodies and emotions to refocus on 'care', narrativity and subjectivities (Broom, 2009c; Sointu, 2006). On the other hand, some forms of CAM present an emerging normative control over advanced cancer and end-of-life care experiences. Women participating in a study by Broom illustrated the contradictory effects of new discourses and practices around self-responsibility, self-determination and agency at the end of life:

> The bottom line is I think you have to have some control in all of this . . . The only thing you have control about, are things that you can put into your body that are easily accessible [Female, breast cancer, metastatic disease]. (Broom, 2009a: 78)

> I tend not to get desperate about things. I've gotta think positive and . . . [pauses and thinks for a while] I think that people who *have* to think positive, that deep down they're not. The fact that they've *gotta* force themselves to be positive, means that consciously they're being positive

but subconsciously . . . it just drips away [Female, breast cancer, advanced disease]. (Broom, 2009a: 81)

This study reflects an emerging awareness that ideas about terminality and dealing with a terminal prognosis may be embedded in wider gendered sensibilities. Moreover, ideas about 'being peaceful' and 'getting control', while useful for some men and women, may represent another moral framing and disciplinary device at the end of life; this time from CAM providers and imbued in CAM models of healing (Bishop and Yardley, 2004; McClean, 2005), that is, the 'think positive' and 'being vigilant' ideology that women in particular may be exposed to.

Vigilance in the context of women with advanced cancer, as opposed to men, may also be embedded in forms of maternal referencing and relational forms of obligation. In this same study by Broom (2009), the women often talked about their responsibility to their children or husband and the importance of survival therein. Such findings indicate that there is a willingness to pursue CAM self-healing practices amongst women, and secondly to embrace the ideas of self-responsibility and vigilance therein (see also Sered and Agigian, 2008).

These findings are particularly important in the context of women's historical and ongoing efforts to critique and move away from professional surveillance and control of the body and self (see also Chapter 7 by Bell and Figert, and Chapter 24 by Armstrong). CAM-derived ideas about well-being, self-help and self-responsibility (in the context of end-of-life care) may represent new sites of governance of the self and of health and illness (Rose, 1999). Given that women are much more prolific users of CAM for care more broadly and for cancer specifically, how CAM practices and ideologies are shaping women's experiences of advanced cancer and end-of-life care are critical issues for future investigation (see also Chapter 29 by Cant and Watts).

Conclusion

This chapter has examined some of the potential intersections of gender and end-of-life care as well as unpacking some of the moral, ideological and political underpinnings of 'modern dying'. At an epidemiological level, there are clear and persistent differences in morbidity and mortality between men and women internationally (see also Chapter 8 by Bird et al.). While the gap between men and women in terms of mortality is slowly getting smaller in the West, there are clear problems evident in the context of gender relations that impact on contemporary death and dying.

Formalized, institutionalized end-of-life care settings are presenting men and women with both opportunities and problems. These settings offer enhanced control over bodily disintegration and decay. Yet they raise questions about desirable deaths and the role of gendered sensibilities therein. How should I die? Where should I die? And how does this impact on my sense of self, identity and family structure? Moreover, forms and models of care have diversified and end-of-life care is becoming more pluralistic, incorporating models beyond that offered by biomedical palliative care. Across each of these themes are persistent inequalities and peculiarities significantly impacting on men and women's experiences of dying and of end-of-life care. Gendered cultural scripts are contributing not only to premature death and illness – or the prevalence of particular kinds of illness – but shape individual and interpersonal struggles in end-of-life care settings. The acknowledgement that death and dying are ultimately gendered in nature will be a welcome move toward better understanding and thus the improvement of end-of-life care for both men and women.

Summary

- End-of-life care is a morally and politically bound healthcare setting within which gender constructs play an important role.
- The forms of care that people pursue in the context of terminal diagnoses can be heavily influenced by gendered ideas about agency, self-responsibility and self-help.
- Dying takes place within the context of moral codes of reciprocity and obligation, and the power of the state, through various institutions, influences the definition of 'good' and 'timely' deaths.

Key reading

Broom, A. and J. Cavenagh (2010) 'Moralities, Masculinities and Caring for the Dying', *Social Science & Medicine*, 71 (5), 869–76.
Chattoo, S. and W. Ahmad (2008) 'The Moral Economy of Selfhood and Caring', *Sociology of Health and Illness*, 30 (4), 550–64.
Timmerman, S. (2010) 'There is More to Dying than Death: Qualitative Research and the End-of-Life', in I. Bourgeault, R. Dingwall and R. De Vries (eds), *The Sage Handbook of Qualitative Methods in Health Research* (Los Angeles: Sage), 19–33.

References

Australian Bureau of Statistics (2011a) *Leading Causes of Death by Gender*, at: www.abs.gov.au, accessed 17 May 2011.
Australian Bureau of Statistics (2011b) *Suicides – Key Characteristics, 3303.0 – Causes of Death, Australia 2009*, at: www.abs.gov.au, accessed 17 May 2011.
Bishop, F. and L. Yardley (2004) 'Constructing Agency in Treatment Decisions', *Health*, 8 (4), 465–82.

Bix, A. (2004) 'Engendering Alternatives. Women's Health Care Choices and Feminist Medical Rebellions', in R. D. Johnston (ed.), *The Politics of Healing: Histories of Alternative Medicine in Twentieth-century North America* (New York: Routledge), 153–80.

Booth, J. (1994) 'On the Idea of the Moral Economy', *American Political Science Review,* 88 (3), 653–67.

Broom, A. (2009a) '"I'd Forgotten about Me in All of This": Discourses of Self-healing, Positivity and Vulnerability in Cancer Patients' Experiences of Complementary and Alternative Medicine', *Journal of Sociology,* 45 (1), 71–87.

Broom, A. (2009b) 'Intuition, Subjectivity and le Bricoleur: Cancer Patients' Accounts of Negotiating a Plurality of Therapeutic Options', *Qualitative Health Research,* 19 (8), 1050–9.

Broom, A. (2009c) 'The Sociology of Complementary and Alternative Medicine', in J. Germov (ed.), *Second Opinion: An Introduction to Health Sociology* (Melbourne: Oxford University Press), 433–51.

Broom, A. (2012) 'On Euthanasia, Resistance and Redemption: The Moralities and Politics of a Hospice', *Qualitative Health Research,* 22 (2), 226–37, DOI: 10.1177/1049732311421181, accessed 14 September 2011.

Broom, A. & J. Cavenagh (2010) 'Moralities, Masculinities and Caring for the Dying', *Social Science and Medicine,* 71 (5), 869–76.

Broom, A. and J. Cavenagh (2011) 'On the Meanings and Experiences of Living and Dying in a Hospice', *Health: An Interdisciplinary Journal for the Social Study of Health, Illness and Medicine,* 15 (1), 96–111.

Broom, A. and A. Doron (2011) 'The Rise of Cancer in Urban India: Cultural Understandings, Structural Inequalities, and the Emergence of the Clinic', *Health,* DOI: 10.1177/1363459311403949, accessed 14 September 2011.

Broom, A. and P. Tovey (2008) *Therapeutic Pluralism: Exploring the Experiences of Cancer Patients and Professionals* (London: Routledge).

Broom, A. and P. Tovey (eds) (2009) *Men's Health: Body, Identity and Social Context* (Oxford: Wiley-Blackwell).

Chattoo, S. and W. Ahmad (2008) 'The Moral Economy of Selfhood and Caring', *Sociology of Health and Illness,* 30 (4), 550–64.

Cohen, J., D. Houttekier, B. Onwuteaka-Philipsen, G. Miccinesi, J. Addington-Hall, S. Kaasa, J. Bilsen and L. Deliens (2010) 'Which Patients with Cancer Die at Home? A Study of Six European Countries Using Death Certificate Data', *Journal of Clinical Oncology,* 28 (13), 2267–73.

Courtenay, W. (2009) 'Theorising Masculinity and Men's Health', in A. Broom and P. Tovey (eds), *Men's Health: Body, Identity and Social Context* (Oxford: Wiley-Blackwell), 9–32.

Dattela, A. and R. Neimeyera (1990) 'Sex Differences in Death Anxiety: Testing the Emotional Expressiveness Hypothesis', *Death Studies,* 14 (1), 1–11.

Donovan, K., A. Taliaferro, C. Brock and S. Bazargan (2008) 'Sex Differences in the Adequacy of Pain Management among Patients Referred to a Multidisciplinary Cancer Pain Clinic', *Journal of Pain and Symptom Management,* 36 (2), 167–72.

Eurostat (2011) *Death Due to Suicide, by Gender,* at: http://epp.eurostat.ec.europa.eu, accessed 17 May 2011.

Field, D., J. Hockey and N. Small (eds) (1997) *Death, Gender, and Ethnicity* (London: Routledge).

Froggatt, K. (1997) 'Rites of Passage and the Hospice Culture', *Mortality,* 2 (2), 123–36.

Giddens, A. (1991) *Modernity and Self-Identity* (Stanford: Stanford University Press).

Gomes, B. and I. Higginson (2008) 'Where People Die (1974–2030): Past Trends, Future Projections and Implications for Care', *Palliative Medicine,* 22 (1), 33–41.

Hart, B., P. Sainsbury and S. Short (1998) 'Whose Dying? A Sociological Critique of the "Good Death"', *Mortality,* 3 (1), 65–77.

Howarth, G. (2007a) *Death and Dying* (Cambridge: Polity Press).

Howarth, G. (2007b) 'Whatever Happened to Social Class? An Examination of the Neglect of Working Class Cultures in the Sociology of Death', *Health Sociology Review,* 16 (5), 425–35.

Illouz, E. (2008) *Saving the Modern Soul* (Berkeley: University of California Press).

James, N. and D. Field (1992) 'The Routinization of Hospice: Charisma and Bureaucratization', *Social Science & Medicine,* 34 (12), 1363–75.

Kellehear, A. (2008) 'Dying as a Social Relationship', *Social Science & Medicine,* 66 (7), 1533–44.

Kochanek, K., J. Xu, S. Murphy, A. Miniño and H. Kung (2011) 'Deaths: Preliminary Data for 2009', *National Vital Statistics Reports,* 59 (4), 1–51.

Lawton, J. (2000) *The Dying Process* (Routledge: London).

Luff, D. and K. Thomas (2000) 'Getting Somewhere, Feeling Cared For: Patient Perspectives on CAM', *Complementary Therapies in Medicine,* 8 (4), 253–9.

McClean, S. (2005) '"The Illness is Part of the Person": Discourses of Blame, Individual Responsibility and Individuation at a Centre for Spiritual Healing in the North of England', *Sociology of Health and Illness,* 27 (5), 628–48.

McPherson, C., K. Wilson and M. Murray (2007) 'Feeling Like a Burden: Exploring the Perspectives of Patients at the End of Life', *Social Science & Medicine,* 64 (2), 417–27.

Meyer, M. (1989) 'Dignity, Rights, and Self-Control', *Ethics,* 99 (3), 520–34.

Meyer, M. (1995) 'Dignity, Death and Modern Virtue', *American Philosophical Quarterly,* 32 (1), 45–55.

Murray, M., A. O'Connor, V. Fiset and R. Viola (2003) 'Women's Decision Making Needs Regarding Place of Care at End of Life', *Journal of Palliative Care,* 19 (3), 176–84.

National Center for Health Statistics (2011) *Health, US, 2010: With Special Feature on Death and Dying* (Hyattsville: National Center for Health Statistics).

National Center for Injury Prevention and Control (2010a) *WISQARS Leading Causes of Death Reports, 1999–2007,* at: http://webappa.cdc.gov/sasweb/ncipc/leadcaus10.html#AdvancedOptions, accessed 17 May 2011.

National Center for Injury Prevention and Control (2010b) *WISQARS Injury Mortality Reports, 1999–2007,* at: http://webappa.cdc.gov, accessed 17 May 2011.

Office for National Statistics (2010) 'Death Registrations by Cause in England and Wales, 2009', *Statistical Bulletin, 26 October 2010,* at: www.statistics.gov.uk/pdfdir/dth1010.pdf, accessed 18 May 2011.

Office for National Statistics (2011a) 'Suicide Rates in the United Kingdom, 2000–2009', *Statistical Bulletin, 27 January 2011,* at: www.statistics.gov.uk/pdfdir/sui0111.pdf, accessed 17 May 2011.

Office for National Statistics (2011b) 'Focus on Gender', *Statistical Bulletin,* at: www.statistics.gov.uk/focuson/gender/default.asp, accessed 17 May 2011.

Official Statistics of Sweden (2011) *Causes of Death 2009,* at: www.socialstyrelsen.se, accessed 4 May 2011.

Parry, J. (1982) 'Sacrificial Death and the Necrophagous Ascetic', in M. Bloch and J. Parry (eds), *Death and the Regeneration of Life* (Cambridge: University of Cambridge Press), 74–110.

Parry, J. (1994) *Death in Banaras* (Cambridge: University of Cambridge Press).

Raja, I. (2009) 'Rethinking Relationality in the Context of Adult Mother-Daughter Caregiving in Indian Fiction', *Journal of Aging, Humanities, and the Arts*, 3 (1), 25–37.

Rose, N. (1999) *Governing the Soul* (London: Free Association Books).

Sayer, A. (2005) 'Class, Moral Worth and Recognition', *Sociology*, 39 (5), 947–63.

Scott, A. (1998) 'Homeopathy as a Feminist Form of Medicine', *Sociology of Health and Illness*, 20 (2), 191–214.

Seale, C. (1998) *Constructing Death* (Cambridge: Cambridge University Press).

Sered, S. and A. Agigian (2008) 'Holistic Sickening: Breast Cancer and the Discursive Worlds of Complementary and Alternative Practitioners', *Sociology of Health & Illness*, 30 (4), 616–31.

Shiner, M., J. Scourfield, B. Fincham and S. Langer (2009) 'When Things Fall Apart: Gender and Suicide Across the Life-course', *Social Science & Medicine*, 69 (5), 738–46.

Sointu, E. (2006) 'Healing Bodies, Feeling Bodies', *Social Theory and Health*, 4, 203–20.

Sointu, E. and L. Woodhead (2008) 'Spirituality, Gender and Expressive Selfhood', *Journal for the Scientific Study of Religion*, 47 (2), 259–76.

Timmerman, S. (2010) 'There is More to Dying than Death: Qualitative Research and the End-of-Life', in I. Bourgeault, R. Dingwall and R. De Vries (eds), *The Sage Handbook of Qualitative Methods in Health Research* (Los Angeles: Sage), 19–33.

World Health Organization (n.d.) *Suicide Rates (per 100,000), by Gender, Japan, 1950–2008*, at: www.who.int, accessed 17 May 2011.

World Health Organization (2011) 'Life Tables', *Global Health Observatory Data Repository*, at: http://apps.who.int, accessed 17 May 2011.

Yamasaki, M., S. Ebihara, S. Freeman, T. Ebihara, M. Asada and S. Yamanda (2008) 'Sex Differences in the Preference for Place of Death in Community-dwelling Elderly People in Japan', *Journal of the American Geriatrics Society*, 56 (2), 376.

Part III
Equity and Access to Healthcare

14
Gender and Help-seeking: Towards Gender-comparative Studies

Kate Hunt, Joy Adamson and Paul Galdas

Introduction

The question of whether there are differences in the use that men and women make of healthcare services has occupied researchers for many decades (see, for example, Cleary et al., 1982; Mechanic, 1976; Nathanson, 1977). It is often taken as a given that men make lesser use of healthcare services than women (see, for example, White and Witty, 2009). Statements such as that 'men are less likely than women to actively seek medical care when they are ill, choosing instead to "tough it out"' (Tudiver and Talbot, 1999: 47) are common. Men's supposed 'underuse' or delayed use of healthcare is often taken to be a key part of the explanation for men's shorter life expectancy in comparison with women (White and Witty, 2009). Their underuse of the healthcare system is constructed as a social problem (O'Brien et al., 2005: 503) and has moved up the policy agenda in countries such as the UK, the USA, Australia and Canada in recent years (see also Chapter 16 by Schofield).

Such definitive statements have contributed to a 'strong public narrative' which emphasizes 'expectations that rather than seek help, men will be strong, stoical and often silent in matters relating to health and well-being' (Robertson, 2003: 112). However, this creates problems for how women's help-seeking behaviour is interpreted. An unfortunate implication of this public narrative is that, in presumed contrast to men, women will go to the doctor more readily and will consult with less serious complaints. Such assumptions can lead to women's problems being trivialized when presented to doctors.

In this chapter we outline the origins of these widely held beliefs about gender and help-seeking, and how these have been translated into a binary assumption that, given the same health problems, men will delay seeking help for longer than women. We highlight studies which have shown that the way that men talk about their help-seeking behaviour is linked to their presentations of masculinity, or how they 'do' gender (Saltonstall, 1993; West and

241

Zimmerman, 1986). We then consider exceptions to this dominant portrayal of the relationship between hegemonic masculinity and men's help-seeking behaviour (Connell and Messerschmidt, 2005) and present examples of gender-comparative research on help-seeking. Throughout the chapter we focus on research from Anglo-American countries. We conclude by agreeing, with others, that the 'research base in relation to the link between gender and use of health services is surprisingly poor' (Wilkins et al., 2009: 4) and outlining the reasons why it is important to conduct more gender-comparative studies if we are to better understand the links between gender and help-seeking.

Evidence for men's reluctance to seek help and some important exceptions

In the UK and other western countries, most data show that, *on average*, women consult their general practitioner (GP) more than men (McCormick et al., 1995). Gender differences in GP consultation rates overall are particularly marked in the reproductive years. For example, in Scotland in the 15 to 24 and 25 to 44 age groups women are twice as likely to visit a GP compared to men (ISD, 2000). This partly reflects the medicalization of childbirth, which means that most pregnant women see their GP several times for ante-natal and post-natal care, and many women rely on methods of contraception which are provided within primary care.

In the past two decades or so, following a period when interest in the links between gender and health was largely confined to issues with women's health, there has been increased interest in the links between men's health and their enactment of gender. The ways in which men adopt various expressions, or practices, of masculinity and how this is related to their health and health behaviours has been the focus of many fascinating studies. These have drawn on theoretical insights which have suggested that, although there are numerous expressions of masculinity and masculine identity, there is often a dominant form or hegemonic practice of masculinity in any given context which is recognized as being the most culturally valued (see, for example, Connell and Messerschmidt, 2005; Chapter 16 by Schofield).

Courtenay is one of the many scholars who has drawn a direct link between denial of weakness and the rejection of help as key practices of hegemonic masculinity. He has argued:

> The most powerful men among men are those for whom health and safety are irrelevant ... By dismissing their health care needs, men are constructing gender. When a man brags, 'I haven't been to a doctor in years', he is simultaneously describing a health practice and situating himself in a masculine arena. (Courtenay, 2000: 1389)

The observations of women's greater average use of primary care services *overall* – for all health problems and services combined – in interaction with studies of men which have examined the way that masculinities and health are linked, have led to a very widespread belief that men will delay seeking care longer than women whatever their underlying health problem. Galdas (2009) has recently reviewed a number of studies which demonstrate how notions of masculinity and help-seeking behaviours are intricately linked. Most of these are studies of men with male-specific illnesses (prostate or testicular cancer) or with coronary heart disease (CHD) which has often, erroneously, been character-ized in the popular and medical imagination as a disease that is more common amongst men (Emslie et al., 2001; see also Chapter 10 by Riska on coronary heart disease).

It is not unusual for studies which have investigated the views of men with a particular condition, such as prostate cancer, to generalize their findings to how men will deal with all conditions. As one example, George and Fleming (2004) studied the factors affecting men's help-seeking in relation to the early detection of prostate cancer. From interviews with 12 men who had attended a charity-based service for the early detection of prostate cancer in Northern Ireland they came to the common conclusion that 'men experi-ence social, psychological and structural barriers to help-seeking including a threat to masculinity, embarrassment, fear and guilt at using an under-resourced health service' (George and Fleming, 2004: 345). They go on to make the more sweeping assertion that 'men delay help-seeking when they are ill and under-use primary health care services' (2004: 346). Others have been a little more tentative in their conclusions. For example, Addis and Mahalik have argued that:

Men may experience barriers to seeking help from health professionals when they perceive other men in their social networks as disparaging the process. This is especially so if a) other men are perceived as unanimous in their attitudes, b) a large number of men express similar attitudes, c) men see themselves as quite similar to the members of the reference groups, and d) the members of the men's reference groups are important to them. (2003: 11)

Undoubtedly, many well-conducted qualitative studies of men in a range of countries (including the UK, the USA, Canada and Australia) have found that men often express a reluctance to seek care and have taken this to be an important, if not emblematic, expression of their masculinity. We turn next, however, to consider a few studies which have argued not that masculinity and help-seeking are unrelated, but that the ways in which masculinities and help-seeking are linked are more multi-faceted and complex.

Examples of studies challenging the universality of men's reluctance to seek help

O'Brien and colleagues (2005) studied the links between masculinity and health, and specifically examined how men spoke about help-seeking behaviours. A total of 59 men participated in 15 focus groups. The sample was diverse by age (range 15 to 72 years), occupational status, socio-economic background and health status. Some groups of men were expected to have had unremarkable experiences of masculinity and health; these were largely occupationally based groups, such as gas workers, fire-fighters and students. Other groups were recruited because they were known to have had health problems which might have prompted greater reflection on masculinity and health, for example, groups with men who had prostate cancer, coronary heart disease or mental health problems. The majority of the men lived in central Scotland, and just one focus group was conducted with men of Asian origin, reflecting the limited ethnic diversity in this part of Britain.

These focus group discussions suggested a 'widespread endorsement of a "hegemonic" view that men "should" be reluctant to seek help, particularly amongst younger men' (O'Brien et al., 2005: 503). For example, one member of a focus group, made up of students, said:

> ... the only time I have (gone) to hospital or seen a doctor ... was when I had been punched in the face (and) ... I needed stitches ... or a relative tells you that you've got to go .... even then I've been reluctant to go. (O'Brien et al., 2005: 507)

This man related his reluctance to consult to 'the whole idea about what constitutes a man. A real man puts up with pain and doesn't complain' (O'Brien et al., 2003: 507–8). However, whilst similar sentiments were very commonly expressed in the groups, some men clearly distanced themselves from this dominant portrayal. A fire-fighter, for example, challenged the hegemonic view of men who trivialized symptoms and dismissed the need for help as 'naïve, I wouldn't say that's masculine' (O'Brien et al., 2005: 513), and his colleague described a reluctance to consult amongst men as 'completely moronic, I mean, it's caveman stuff, but that is to a certain extent how guys still operate'. Indeed, the men in the fire-fighters' group agreed that seeking help at the first sign of symptoms and asking for preventative health checks were important to their continuing ability to work effectively.

O'Brien and colleagues argued such exceptions rarely get considered, although they noted that Robertson (2003: 112) has commented that men struggle with balancing 'a dilemma between "don't care" and "should care"'. However, O'Brien and colleagues noted that these exceptions were not unrelated to men's constructions of their masculinity. They argued that, for the fire-fighters, help-seeking was a way of *preserving* the strongly valued sense of masculinity that they gained through their occupational status. In their working environment at least, the fire-fighters felt able to critique the constraints of an 'old school mentality', and to reject it without consequence for their sense of masculinity.

Other exceptions to men's reluctance to consult could also be understood by reference to a 'hierarchy of threats' to masculinity. O'Brien and colleagues (2005) interpreted some men's discussion of their apparent readiness to consult with putative problems with their sexual performance as indicating that they would rather 'risk' their masculine status by consulting for a sexual health problem than put it in greater jeopardy by not being able to have sex. For some men (such as those with myalgic encephalomyelitis), they argued that consultation – and through it, a diagnosis which to some extent legitimated being unable to fulfil certain roles, like working, 'providing' for the family, which the men felt they were expected to meet as men – presented a potential means to *restore* a masculine identity that had been undermined by the nature of their illness. Finally, men who had survived episodes of illness which they perceived to be life-threatening (cardiac problems, prostate cancer) were more reflective and sometimes critical about men's general reluctance to seek help and appeared to have accepted that preserving their future health assumed a higher priority than preserving their masculinity.

O'Brien and colleagues acknowledged that these men's accounts of their attitudes to help-seeking may not reflect their actual past actions, but

> they poignantly describe a culture, a 'practice of masculinity', which most men felt they were expected to conform to and reproduce, or to justify their rejection of such practices. (O'Brien et al., 2005: 515)

Another qualitative study which also explicitly challenged the universality of men's reluctance to consult contrasted accounts of the decision to seek medical help for cardiac chest pain by 36 men of 'white' ethnicity and UK ancestry and 20 South Asian men (English-speaking men of Indian or Pakistani ancestry) living in the northeast of England (Galdas et al., 2007). The men were recruited from two coronary care units and six cardiology wards in two teaching hospitals. All participants had been admitted after experiencing chest pain which was subsequently confirmed as a first acute myocardial infarction or newly diagnosed angina pectoris. Participants were interviewed at their hospital bedside, and were asked to give their own account of the 'events and actions relating to their experience from the outset of pain to hospital admission', before being asked further questions on their 'views, common behaviours and premises about seeking medical help "as a man" that aimed to elicit information on how constructions of masculinity were associated with a participant's experience of seeking help'; this approach was taken to limit the effect of 'masculine "impression management"' (Galdas et al., 2007: 224).

In this study, the majority of 'white' men were noted to perceive a need to demonstrate that they had endured a high level of pain before seeking help for chest pain symptoms (as in earlier studies, for example, White and Johnson, 2000). However, the accounts provided by most of the South Asian participants were quite different. These men described how they had consulted quickly when they experienced persistent or recurrent chest pain. They considered pain to be a legitimate reason to seek medical help and none appeared to think that seeking help for their chest pain was either 'unmanly' or a sign of weakness. What is more, they placed great emphasis on their responsibilities for their families, which they felt they could not fulfil if they were seriously ill (or if they died). The majority of Indian and Pakistani men had discussed their symptoms with their family, in contrast to the majority of white men who suggested that they only disclosed their chest pain to others as a last resort, when they could no longer tolerate the pain or when they felt confident it was a sign that they had a 'legitimate' illness that they should be worried about.

Many of the white men talked with pride about the lengthy periods since their last visit to the GP and only one had consulted a GP before being admitted to hospital with his chest pain symptoms. In stark contrast, all but one of the 20 Indian and Pakistani men had visited their GP before being admitted to hospital. Thus, it was apparent in this study that seeking medical help was portrayed as a 'last resort' by the white men and avoiding 'being perceived as a hypochondriac or weak by others played a part in many white men's decisions to delay seeking help from a healthcare professional until they became certain their pain could not be coped with alone', whereas the willingness to seek medical help observed amongst most Indian and Pakistani men can be seen to 'signify men's retention of a culturally distinct, (non-dominant) form of masculinity' (Galdas et al., 2007: 227–8).

These interesting exceptions to the prevailing orthodoxy that men are always reluctant to present themselves as being willing to seek help for health problems are likely to be reflected in other studies. As Galdas has concluded:

> the simplistic notion of 'men' being consistently averse to seeking medical help in a timely manner is not wholly supported by the empirical evidence ... In developing an empirical basis from which to inform interventions to effectively engage men with health services, it is important to ... avoid universalising assumptions about hegemonic masculinity that propagate an essentialist discourse about the damaging affect of 'masculinity' on men's help-seeking behaviour. (2009, 77–8)

We would argue that two steps are essential to developing this empirical basis. The first is for researchers to critically investigate the particular circumstances in which men articulate or reject a link between reluctance and prevailing notions of appropriate demonstrations of their masculinity. Second, and perhaps most crucially, there is a need for many more studies to adopt a gender-comparative approach. These need to be of at least two kinds: 1) quantitative studies which compare patterns of help-seeking behaviours amongst men and women with similar underlying morbidity; and 2) qualitative research which critically explores the similarities and differences in the ways that women and men talk about their decisions to consult (or not) when faced with novel or ongoing symptoms. Such research is rare: most empirical investigations of gender and help-seeking have used single-sex samples and addressed problems that are either specific to men or specific to women (Annandale et al., 2007). In the next section we consider a few exceptions to this generalization.

Comparing patterns of healthcare use in men and women with similar conditions

Given the widespread and entrenched nature of the assumption that women consult more frequently, and more readily, than men, it is surprising how few studies have sought to systematically compare patterns of consultation amongst men and women with similar morbidity. We consider here a few exceptions. The first is a systematic review of two common symptoms, namely back pain and headache. Although these are often not indicative of serious underlying disease, they nonetheless can be troubling and disruptive and both symptoms contribute substantially to absence from work and to the burden of ill-health presented to primary care. The second is an empirical study which considers whether women are more likely to consult than men for particular groups of chronic conditions. The third considers gender and consultation prior to the diagnosis of one of the most common forms of malignancy, colorectal cancer, which is a major cause of death in most countries.

Gender and consultation for headache and back pain

Hunt and colleagues (2010) have recently undertaken a systematic review of consultation for headache or back pain in order to question the strength and consistency of evidence that women consult more frequently. To be eligible for inclusion, studies had to include both users and non-users of healthcare, have gender as an explanatory variable, and be based on epidemiological methods. The review was restricted to studies which were conducted in more developed countries and published in English. An extensive and systematic search identified just 14 publications (mostly reporting studies conducted in northern European countries, although four were from the USA, and one each from

Australia and Greece) which reported data on consultation amongst men and women with symptoms of back pain. Overall, evidence for greater consultation by women with back pain in comparison with men was weak and inconsistent. Amongst those who reported symptoms of back pain, the odds ratios for women seeking help, in comparison with men ranged from 0.6 (95 per cent confidence intervals 0.3, 1.2, adjusted only for age) to 2.17 (95 per cent confidence intervals 1.35, 3.57, unadjusted for other factors), although none of the studies with an odds ratio of less than 1.00 (which would indicate that men were more likely to consult than women) were statistically significant. Three of the four studies which reported a statistically elevated odds ratio (which would suggest that women were consulting more than men) examined recent consultation (within the last six months).

The evidence for women being more likely to consult for headache than men was a little stronger. Five of the 11 studies reporting on gender and consultation for headache showed a statistically elevated odds ratio (indicating that women were more likely to have consulted than men), and none suggested that men were more likely to consult than women for headache.

However, this review highlights the paucity of evidence on gender and consultation *for specific conditions and symptoms*. First, few studies had the question of whether consultation patterns differ for men and women as the main focus of their analysis. Mostly gender was included as one of a number of socio-demographic variables, and often the numbers of men and women in the study, or the sex-specific prevalence of symptoms or of consulting, were difficult to extract from the papers. Second, the studies varied greatly in their definitions of the symptom (including its severity and duration) and of help-seeking. Some included consultation over a relatively short period – for example, the last month – whereas others used 'ever consulted' as their outcome. Some confined themselves to consultation with a general practitioner whilst others included other healthcare professionals or alternative practitioners. Third, the studies were conducted in countries with very different healthcare systems (including those which rely heavily on private healthcare insurance, such as the USA, and countries with free access to healthcare, such as the UK, with its National Health Service). Fourth, all of the studies employed a cross-sectional design, and so are subject to potential methodological problems (such as differential recall or reporting of symptoms or of healthcare use); none prospectively followed a group of people with a given symptom to investigate how they dealt with their symptom over time.

This variability between studies limits the extent to which firm conclusions can be drawn about whether women and men differ in their healthcare utilization for the symptoms of headache and back pain and illustrates the need for well-designed studies which can accurately establish whether there are gender differences in consultation for specific symptoms and conditions. Despite these limitations, and given the strength of the assumptions that women consult more readily for common symptoms, what was striking was that the evidence for greater consultation amongst women was surprisingly weak and inconsistent, especially with respect to back pain.

Gender and consultation for chronic illness

In an analysis of general population data, Hunt and colleagues (1999) explicitly set out to examine gender differences in consultation when comparing 'like with like', as far as possible, by attempting to 'standardize' for presence and perceived severity of illness. This analysis used data from detailed face-to-face interviews with two cohorts (people born in the early 1930s and in the early 1950s, aged in their late thirties and late fifties when the data were collected for this analysis) of the West of Scotland Twenty-07 Study which included a much extended version of the British General Household Survey question on longstanding illness (LSI). Instead of asking simply whether a person had a longstanding illness and whether this caused limitation to their activities, further questions asked for the name of the conditions (so that LSI could be grouped to five condition groups [musculoskeletal, respiratory, digestive, cardiovascular and mental health] using the British Royal College of General Practitioners coding scheme [RCGP, 1986]), the frequency and severity of pain, and whether it had caused restriction to activities in the previous four weeks. As expected, overall women had consulted their GP more times on average than men in the previous twelve months – 3.48 vs 2.34 ($p < 0.01$) in the 1950s cohort; 4.38 vs 4.21 (NS) in the 1930s cohort; this included all consultations for any symptom, condition or advice.

However, a series of logistic regression analyses showed that amongst those who reported that they had a particular type of condition, women were no more likely to have consulted a GP for that condition in the past year for any condition group and *men* were *more* likely than women to consult if they reported a digestive condition (odds ratio 1.65, 95 per cent confidence limits (cls) 1.29–2.68). This pattern persisted when taking account of the severity of the condition. These results reinforced findings from an earlier analysis of participants in the Twenty-07 Study which examined consultation for 33 common symptoms (Wyke et al., 1998) and found that, when account was taken of who had experienced symptoms in the last month, there were no gender differences in GP consultation for any of the 33 symptoms in the 1930s cohort and gender differences for just three symptoms in the 1950s cohort (a female excess in consulting for headaches and skin problems, and a male excess for stomach problems or cramps). Hunt and colleagues concluded that:

> ... these data argue against the most widely accepted explanations for gender differences in consulting, namely that, once illness is recognised, women

are more likely to consult than men … It is important that the stereotype of women being more likely to respond to symptoms and chronic conditions by consulting general practitioners does not persist unchallenged. The limited evidence from … studies which have controlled for underlying pathology or symptomatology … lends little support to the view that women are more likely to over-rate and over-react to symptoms once recognised. (1999: 98–9)

Gender and consultation prior to the diagnosis of colorectal cancer

One limitation of the study by Hunt and colleagues (1999) was that, although it was able to take account of self-perceived severity and restriction of daily activities (which are known to be important predictors of help-seeking), it was only able to control for type of morbidity within broad groupings of conditions, such as respiratory, cardiovascular and so on. An exemplar study comparing consultation in men and women with colorectal cancer, and specifically the time from their first recognition of symptoms to their diagnosis, was conducted over 20 years ago (Marshall and Funch, 1987). Few similar studies have been conducted since. This study (conducted in and around Seattle, USA) used population-based survey methods to identify people who had been diagnosed with colorectal cancer. Adult men and women with a definitive diagnosis (confirmed by a tissue biopsy) of non-recurrent colorectal cancer participated in an interview which investigated when they had first noticed their symptoms, any actions they took before they sought medical treatment, their reasons for seeking or waiting to seek treatment, and any problems they had in obtaining treatment. In all 154 men and 153 women were interviewed.

Marshall and Funch reported that the most common symptoms for both men and women were rectal bleeding, general weakness and abdominal pain. Neither the number of symptoms nor the prevalence of any prediagnostic symptom differed by gender. Similarly, the reported severity of symptoms was comparable between men and women. They concluded that 'overall, these findings suggest that, for colorectal cancer patients, males and females report the same symptoms, and describe them in a similar manner' (Marshall and Funch, 1987: 74). Men's and women's actions before consulting were also similar: they reported similar levels of use of over-the-counter drugs, and of talking to other people (including their spouse and friends) about their symptoms.

They then examined 'patient delay' (the number of days between first noticing symptoms and contacting a doctor about the symptoms) and 'diagnostic delay' (the time between the patient's first visit or call to the doctor and a definitive diagnosis) overall, and in people with cancer of the colon and cancer of the rectum separately. When both cancers were considered together, there was no difference between patient delay (mean number of days: 180.0 for men, 198.7 for women, t-value 0.72, NS). For colon cancer there was a suggestion that men delayed slightly longer (mean number of days: 198.4 for men, 179.5 for women), although this difference was not significant (t-value – 0.29). However, for cancer of the rectum *female* patients delayed on average more than 100 days longer than men (mean number of days: 149.3 for men, 254.9 for women, t-value 2.37, p = 0.02).

There was also a substantial difference in diagnostic delay for colorectal cancer (mean number of days: for men 67.0, for women 106.1, t-value = 2.35, p = 0.02), which was due entirely to the greater diagnostic delay experienced by women with colon cancer (mean number of days: for men 71.7, for women 125.7, t-value = 2.49, p = 0.01). Further investigation showed that women who had longer diagnostic delays had visited their doctor more times before their diagnosis was made. Marshall and Funch concluded that their study

> [lends] little support to the common claim that women are more likely than men to respond to symptoms of illness by seeking medical care. Female colorectal cancer patients did not ... report with disease at earlier stages than those at which male colorectal cancer patients reported. Female colorectal cancer patients did not delay less than male patients in seeking medical care [...] They also experienced more delay than men securing definitive diagnosis subsequent to having consulted a clinician. (1987: 80)

Although this study was conducted more than two decades ago, it is clear that the conclusions have done little to dent the popular medical view that women are less likely to delay before presenting their symptoms to the medical profession. Furthermore, a recent systematic review of the influences on pre-hospital delay in the diagnosis of colorectal cancer concluded that there was no relationship between patient gender and the time between a patient first noticing a cancer symptom and presenting to primary care or between first presentation and referral to secondary care (Mitchell et al., 2008).

Conclusion

In this chapter we have attempted to demonstrate that the link between gender and help-seeking is much more complex than commonly portrayed. Whilst we recognize that many well-conducted studies of men recount numerous examples of men's reluctance to seek medical help when they experience symptoms or are worried that something may be wrong, we are concerned that there is a danger that an over-simplistic view of gender and healthcare use may lead to policies or interventions which may not best serve the health of either men or women. Failing to recognize contexts in which men engage in *timely* help-seeking consistent with their masculine identities may lead us to overlook ways that health practitioners and policy-makers could encourage more men to take more active care of their health.

However, we believe that there are more fundamental gaps in the evidence. Because most recent insights from research on men, masculinities and health have arisen from empirical studies of all-male samples, there is no opportunity to ask whether there are similar expressions of reluctance to seek healthcare amongst women. This is a surprising omission as some qualitative research (for recent examples, see Townsend et al., 2006; 2008) has shown that it is commonplace for both men and women (even those with high levels of morbidity) to represent their use of healthcare as a 'last resort' and to go to great lengths to present their management of their illness and their use of healthcare within a moral framework. Because of an often unconscious tendency to valorize distinctions rather than similarities between men and women, it is often presumed that *because* men are reluctant to consult, women are not, and because women are willing to use healthcare for some aspects of their lives (such as contraception and the monitoring of pregnancy and childbirth), they will be more willing to consult more quickly for all aspects of their health.

In the few examples that we have cited which have used gender-comparative methods to examine patterns of healthcare use in men and women with similar underlying morbidity, there is, at best, insufficient evidence that men consult less frequently or delay longer before consulting. The study by Marshall and Funch (1987), though over 20 years old, is not alone (Mitchell et al, 2008) in finding that men do *not* delay longer before consulting with symptoms of colorectal cancer, but is often overlooked. Their findings suggest that doctors may pay different attention to symptoms depending on the gender of the patient. Whilst this may often make good clinical sense (abdominal pain or bloating in a man could not be a symptom of cancer of the ovary in men, and frequent night-time urination could not be a symptom of prostate cancer in women, to take extreme examples), Arber and colleagues (2006) have found that a patient's gender may affect the initial assessment of the severity of symptoms and the need for further investigation. In an elegant experimental study, doctors assessing exactly the same presentation of potential symptoms of coronary heart disease by males and females asked fewer questions and recommended fewer examinations and further diagnostic tests when assessing female patients. They were less likely to think that their symptoms were due to CHD, and they had a lower threshold of certainty about their diagnosis. Arber and her colleagues (Arber et al., 2006; Adams et al., 2008) recognized that their findings may reflect stereotypical conceptualizations of CHD as a male disease. However, their results and those of Marshall and Funch (1987) could indicate that there is a danger that, because of the deep-rootedness of the assumption that women will consult more quickly and at lower levels of morbidity (despite a lack of robust scientific evidence), women's symptoms may be regarded as more trivial and less indicative of serious underlying disease than men's.

Appropriate use of healthcare is vital in maximizing individual health and longevity and in making the best use of resources that are increasingly over-stretched with increasing burdens of chronic ill-health. The goal is to increase rapid consultation with early symptoms of serious underlying disease that could respond to early medical intervention, whilst discouraging consultations for more commonplace symptoms which are not amenable to medical treatment. More empirical research is needed that includes and compares both men and women, and which examines the diversity of experience and attitudes *amongst* men and *amongst* women if we are to avoid misleading essentialist assumptions that because 'men' behave in one way, 'women' will behave in another.

Summary

- Although, on average, women consult in primary care more than men, particularly during the peak reproductive years, there is little robust evidence comparing rates of consultation in men and women experiencing the same illnesses.
- Although gender-comparative studies are rare, according to current evidence men do *not* delay longer in seeking help for colorectal cancer, a major contributor to premature mortality.
- Studies with all-male samples have noted a reluctance to consult amongst men which has been widely attributed to a desire to conform to dominant representation of masculinity. However, qualitative research also shows that *women* also commonly present healthcare use as a 'last resort'.
- More critical gender-comparative research is needed to understand the ways in which men and women's help-seeking is similar or different to avoid medical bias in consultations (based on false premises about readiness to consult) and to develop gender-sensitive policy and practice on the most appropriate use of healthcare resources.

Key reading

Adams, A., C. D. Buckingham, A. Lindenmeyer, J. B. McKinlay, C. Link, L. Marceau and S. Arber (2008) 'The Influence of Patient and Doctor Gender on Diagnosing Coronary Heart Disease', *Sociology of Health and Illness*, 30 (1), 1–18.

Annandale, E., J. Harvey, D. Cavers and M. Dixon-Woods (2007) 'Gender and Access to Healthcare in the UK: A Critical Interpretive Synthesis of the Literature', *Evidence and Policy*, 3 (4), 463–86.

Galdas, P. (2009) 'Men, Masculinity and Help-seeking', in A. Broom and P. Tovey (eds), *Men's Health: Body, Identity and Social Context* (London: Wiley), 63–82.

O'Brien, R., K. Hunt and G. Hart (2005) 'Men's Accounts of Masculinity and Help-seeking: "It's Caveman Stuff, But That Is to a Certain Extent How Guys Still Operate"', *Social Science & Medicine*, 61 (3), 503–16.

References

Adams, A., C. D. Buckingham, A. Lindenmeyer, J. B. McKinlay, C. Link, L. Marceau and S. Arber (2008) 'The Influence of Patient and Doctor Gender on Diagnosing Coronary Heart Disease', *Sociology of Health and Illness*, 30 (1), 1–18.

Addis, M. E. and J. R. Mahalik (2003) 'Men, Masculinity, and the Contexts of Help Seeking', *American Psychologist*, 58 (1), 5–14.

Annandale, E., J. Harvey, D. Cavers and M. Dixon-Woods (2007) 'Gender and Access to Healthcare in the UK: A Critical Interpretive Synthesis of the Literature', *Evidence and Policy*, 3 (4), 463–86.

Arber, S., J. McKinlay, A. Adams, L. Marceau, C. Link and A. O'Donnell (2006) 'Patient Characteristics and Inequalities in Doctors' Diagnostic and Management Strategies Relating to CHD: A Video-Simulation Experiment', *Social Science & Medicine*, 62 (1), 103–15.

Cleary, P. D., D. Mechanic and J. R. Greenley (1982) 'Sex Differences in Medical Care Utilization: An Empirical Investigation', *Journal of Health and Social Behavior*, 23 (2), 106–19.

Connell, R. and J. W. Messerschmidt (2005) 'Hegemonic Masculinity. Rethinking the Concept', *Gender and Society*, 19 (6), 829–59.

Courtenay, W. (2000) 'Constructions of Masculinity and their Influence on Men's Well-Being: A Theory of Gender and Health', *Social Science & Medicine*, 50 (10), 1385–1401.

Emslie, C., K. Hunt and G. Watt (2001) 'Invisible Women? The Importance of Gender in Lay Beliefs about Heart Problems', *Sociology of Health and Illness*, 23 (2), 203–33.

Galdas, P. (2009) 'Men, Masculinity and Help-seeking', in A. Broom and P. Tovey (eds), *Men's Health: Body, Identity and Social Context* (London: Wiley), 63–82.

Galdas, P., F. Cheater and P. Marshall (2007) 'What Is the Role of Masculinity in White and South Asian Men's Decisions to Seek Medical Help for Cardiac Chest Pain?', *Journal of Health Service Research and Policy*, 12 (4), 223–9.

George, A. and P. Fleming (2004) 'Factors Affecting Men's Help-seeking in the Early Detection of Prostate Cancer: Implications for Health Promotion', *Journal of Men's Health and Gender*, 1 (4), 345–52.

Hunt, K., J. Adamson, C. Hewitt and N. Nazareth (2010) 'Do Women Consult More than Men? A Systematic Review of Gender and Consultation for Back Pain and Headache', unpublished manuscript.

Hunt K., G. Ford, L. Harkins and S. Wyke (1999) 'Are Women More Ready to Consult than Men? Gender Differences in General Practitioner Consultation for Common Chronic Conditions', *Journal of Health Services Research & Policy*, 4 (2), 96–100.

ISD – Information Services Division, NHS Scotland (2000) Consultation rates per 1,000 population. Scottish Health Statistics, Section L1 (Edinburgh: ISD).

McCormick, A., D. Fleming and J. Charlton (1995) *Morbidity Statistics from General Practice. Fourth National Study 1991–1992*, OPCS Series MB5 no. 3 (London: HMSO).

Marshall, J. R. and D. P. Funch (1987) 'Gender and Illness Behavior among Colorectal Cancer Patients', *Women & Health*, 11, 67–82.

Mechanic, D. (1976) 'Sex, Illness Behavior, and the Use of Health Services', *Journal of Human Stress*, 2, 29–40.

Mitchell, E., S. Macdonald, N. Campbell, D. Weller and U. Macleod (2008) 'Influences on Pre-hospital Delay in the Diagnosis of Colorectal Cancer: A Systematic Review', *British Journal of Cancer*, 98 (1), 60–70.

Nathanson, C. A. (1977) 'Sex, Illness and Medical Care: A Review of Data, Theory and Method', *Social Science & Medicine,* 11 (1), 13–25.

O'Brien, R., K. Hunt and G. Hart (2005) 'Men's Accounts of Masculinity and Help-seeking: "It's Caveman Stuff, But That Is to a Certain Extent How Guys Still Operate"', *Social Science & Medicine,* 61 (3), 503–16.

Robertson, S. (2003) 'Men Managing Health', *Men's Health Journal,* 2 (4), 111–13.

RCGP – Royal College of General Practitioners (1986) *The Classification and Analysis of General Practice Data* (London: Royal College of General Practitioners).

Saltonstall, R. (1993) 'Healthy Bodies, Social Bodies: Men's and Women's Concepts and Practices of Health in Everyday Life', *Social Science & Medicine,* 36 (1), 7–14.

Townsend, A., S. Wyke and K. Hunt (2006) 'Self-managing and Managing Self: Practical and Moral Dilemmas in Accounts of Living with Chronic Illness', *Chronic Illness,* 2 (3), 185–94.

Townsend, A., S. Wyke and K. Hunt (2008) 'Frequent Consulting and Multiple Morbidity: A Qualitative Comparison of "High" Aand "Low" Consulters of GPS', *Family Practice,* 25 (3), 168–75.

Tudiver, F. and Y. Talbot (1999) 'Why Don't Men Seek Help? Family Physicians' Perspectives on Help-seeking Behaviour in Men', *Journal of Family Practice,* 48 (1), 47–52.

West, C. and D. Zimmerman, D. (1987) 'Doing Gender', *Gender and Society,* 1 (2), 125–51.

White, A. and M. Johnson (2000) 'Men Making Sense of Their Chest Pain – Niggles, Doubts and Denials', *Journal of Clinical Nursing,* 9 (4), 534–41.

White, A. and K. Witty (2009) 'Men's Under Use of Health Services – Finding Alternative Approaches', *Journal of Men's Health,* 6 (2), 95–7.

Wilkins, D., S. Payne, G. Granville and P. Branney (2009) *The Gender and Access to Health Services Study* (London: Department of Health).

Wyke, S., K. Hunt and G. Ford (1998) 'Gender Differences in Consulting a General Practitioner for Common Symptoms of Minor Illness', *Social Science & Medicine,* 46 (7), 901–6.

15
Gender Differences in Healthcare Utilization in Later Life*

Kakoli Roy and Anoshua Chaudhuri

Introduction

The discourse on gender and health frequently asserts that older women are universally more vulnerable to social, economic and health disadvantages than men. Most societies generally observe a nearly universal pattern of longer life expectancy among women, but in itself longer life conveys relatively little about the quality of life and burden of non-fatal disease during the extended years. Empirical studies from developed countries tend to observe that women report higher rates of morbidity and higher healthcare utilization than men. However, morbidity disadvantage among women diminishes with age; gender differences in self-rated health often vanish or are reversed in old age (Arber and Ginn, 1993). Although there is no similar debate regarding higher mortality rates among males, recent studies indicate that the pattern of gender differences in morbidity and healthcare utilization may be more complex, and they vary by measures of health, by symptoms, and across the life course (Macintyre et al., 1996; see also Chapter 14 by Hunt et al.).

The objective of this chapter is to examine the available evidence on gender differences in healthcare utilization among older adults in both developed and developing countries. Since health status is a critical factor impacting healthcare utilization, it is reviewed whenever relevant. Specifically, the chapter probes into the evidence and explanations for root causes of gender differences in health and inequities in healthcare utilization in different parts of the world, and its consequences on older populations. This includes examining evidence on whether improvements in socio-economic status and economic empowerment of women, by possibly enhancing their ability to undertake timely primary and secondary prevention during the life course, helps reduce observed gender gaps in old age.

Understanding the factors underlying gender differences in healthcare utilization among older adults might be critical for several reasons. First, continued population ageing in both developed and developing countries will have enormous impacts on their societies – the demands and pressures on old age security and healthcare systems being the most paramount (see also Chapter 21 by Burau et al.). Second, not only are health needs and health service utilization greatest among older adults, but with advancing age women generally outnumber men in most societies. Consequently, the lack of studies on healthcare utilization among older adults has been viewed by some feminist theorists as symptomatic of neglect of women's health issues. Third, a systematic re-examination would help assess whether gender differences described in one decade and in one context might offer lessons and perspectives that are generalizable across societies at different stages of development and with different cultural attitudes towards appropriate gender roles.

By tying together different strands of literature the chapter provides a comprehensive overview of healthcare utilization in later life. We begin by discussing empirical research and theoretical explanations in developed countries and then move onto consider developing countries. Finally, the chapter summarizes the challenges, as well as the opportunities, that meaningful policy interventions might provide in terms of improving the lives of vulnerable older populations all over the world.

The developed country perspective

Evidence on gender differences in health and healthcare utilization

The well-known empirical evidence that women live longer than men but, paradoxically, report being sicker in that they report higher rates of morbidity and disability has been widely confirmed in numerous representative health surveys in North America and Europe (Case and Paxson, 2005; Huisman et al., 2003). However, the greater morbidity among women is not a constant finding but varies considerably during the life course and across health measures (Strauss et al., 1993). In the reproductive age, the need for gynaecological care produces greater healthcare utilization among adult women, but gender differences in utilization tend to diminish at advanced ages. Specific studies on older adults indicate that older women generally report better or comparable self-assessed health but higher disability than same-aged men (Arber and Cooper, 1999; Marks, 1996).

It has been observed that the higher morbidity among women is accompanied by greater use of healthcare services. Greater utilization, however, often varies by symptom, or condition. For example, faced with a minor symptom – like discovery of a lump in the armpit two weeks after a cold – women are reported to seek medical attention more frequently than do men, yet there are no differences in the proportion of women and men that immediately seek medical advice when a major symptom, for example chest pain, appears (Adamson et al., 2003).

Gender differences in healthcare utilization, specifically among older adults, might also vary by type of service. For example, older women may be more likely than men to contact a general practitioner (Krasnik et al., 1997), but when it comes to hospital admissions there is either no gender difference or older men are likely to be hospitalized more frequently and have longer hospital stays than women (Bertakis et al., 2000). These findings could be explained by gender differentials in medical conditions where women are reported to have a higher incidence of less severe and acute chronic conditions than men, while men show excess morbidity for life-threatening conditions (Case and Paxson, 2005; Mathers and Loncar, 2006).

The Anderson Model of healthcare utilization

A conceptual model often applied to healthcare utilization among older adults is the health behaviour model developed by Anderson (1973). This model proposed that the decision to obtain healthcare can be influenced in varying degrees by three groups of factors: their need for such care (or illness level); their predisposition to use services; and non-health factors that either enable or impede the individual to obtain such services. Predisposing factors relate to an individual's propensity to seek formal healthcare and to his or her attitude towards receiving that care, while enabling measures relate to the availability and affordability of care, which depends on how the health system provides and finances healthcare. It is also hypothesized that the model of each type of health contact will be defined by a different set of variables. We describe two case studies that apply the Anderson framework to assess factors that might influence healthcare utilization among older adults in Spain.

A study by Fernández-Mayoralas and colleagues (2000) shows that there are gender inequalities in self-assessed health and in use and accessibility to healthcare services among a representative sample of older adults in Spain. A more recent study by Redondo-Sendino and colleagues (2006) on non-institutionalized older adults in Spain indicates that older Spanish women visited medical practitioners, received home medical visits and used a high number of medications more frequently than men, but there were no gender differences in hospital admission. The variables associated with greater need for healthcare services (specifically, number of chronic diseases and health-related quality of life) best explain the greater utilization by older women; and after adjusting for 'equal need', a certain inequality was observed in hospital admission in that it proved to be less frequent among women. The study results indicate that worse self-perceived health among older women compared to same-aged men would partly justify their greater use of a number of healthcare services. Data from other European countries show a similar pattern (Portrait et al., 2000).

Impact of gender differences in social roles and reporting behaviour

Various explanations have been postulated for the greater utilization of healthcare services by women. A hypothesis that has received considerable attention focuses on gender differences in social role obligations, health-reporting behaviour and health orientation which may influence illness behaviour through several channels. First, women may report more ill-health than men because the sick role is socially more acceptable for them and as a consequence they may be more likely to admit illness, discuss symptoms and seek help (Gijsbers van Wijk and Kolk, 1997). Second, women may also be more sensitive to bodily discomfort (Benyamini et al., 2000). Third, women possibly experience greater illness resulting, at least in part, from the stresses of their assigned social and nurturing roles, and the strains arising from their lower social positions (Verbrugge, 1986).

Overall, the evidence indicates that men and women take account of different constellations of factors when assessing their health and also when making decisions to obtain formal health services. What remains less clear is whether the higher symptom reporting among women leads to an increased use of healthcare services and whether gender differences in healthcare utilization is driven by gender differences in symptom perception. A study by Ladwig and colleagues (2000) on a representative sample of the German adult population in the age group of 25 to 69 years confirmed higher symptom reporting and higher health service utilization among women in all age groups. However, gender differences in utilization were found to be independent of symptom perception or symptom reporting across all age groups. Most importantly, the study confirmed that there are factors other than gender, particularly self-assessed health, poor social class status and chronic illness, which have a significant impact on symptom reporting. Several studies also indicate an association between occupational class and symptom reporting (Verbrugge, 1986).

Impact of gender differences in socio-economic status

In the three decades since Nathanson's (1975) seminal article leading to the widely accepted 'paradox' – namely, that women live longer but are sicker and use more healthcare than men – there have been far-reaching societal changes with enormous impacts on men's and women's lives, roles, employment, health and well-being. Recent studies seem to indicate that the observed higher utilization by older women compared to same-aged men might be much more modest than previously assumed (see also Chapter 14 by Hunt et al.). Since one possible explanation for this is inequality in material circumstances, a possible interpretation of declining gender gaps might be improvements in women's occupational and socio-economic status during the past few decades.

A study by Arber and Cooper (1999) using data on more than 14,000 older men and women from three years of the British General Household Survey reveals minimal gender differences in self-assessed health and long-standing illness coexisting alongside substantially higher levels of functional impairment among women. These findings persist even after controlling for differential social class, marital status and income. As hypothesized, class based on occupation during working life is strongly related to self-assessed health and disability among both men and women, but for a given level of physical disability, older women report better self-assessed health than same-aged men. Overall, despite minimal differences in morbidity, older women are still more likely to be socially and economically disadvantaged than men because of higher disability, lower occupational class and living arrangements where a greater proportion of women are widowed or living alone compared to men.

A recent longitudinal study prospectively examined the association between functional status and utilization of a wide variety of healthcare services among a representative, nationwide cohort of older adults in Spain (León-Muñoz et al., 2007). The findings indicate that limitation in instrumental activities of daily living (IADL) is prospectively associated with greater utilization of most healthcare services by older adults of both sexes, and with a lower use of visits to primary care physicians by women. The study highlights gender differences in the relationship between functional limitation and utilization. Compared with men without limitation in IADL, those with a limitation in one of five IADL made greater use of non-home services, specifically visits to primary care practitioners, hospitalization and emergency services. In contrast, among women, one limitation in IADL was positively associated with visits to hospital specialists. Where more than one IADL was limited, however, women showed a lower frequency of visits to the primary care practitioner. The results also suggest that visits by physicians or nurses to the patients' homes replace patient visits to the general practitioner when a number of limitations are present. Hence, reorienting the healthcare service model to include provision for long-term care might be a policy imperative for ageing societies.

Ageing societies and long-term care utilization

Long-term care becomes necessary when individuals experience aggravated disabilities or chronic disease, and are generally reserved for the elderly and provided until the end of life. The expected growth of the elderly population is expected to increase the demand for long-term care, possibly constraining or exceeding available resources. Informal care of the elderly by adult children, particularly daughters, is the most common and cost-effective long-term care and could reduce medical expenditures if it substitutes for formal care. However, the availability of informal caregivers may continue to shrink with increasingly fractured families, delayed childbearing, falling family size, and as more daughters enter the workforce. This might increase the demand for formal care arrangements which are far more costly than informal care. Thus, an important policy question surrounding long-term care is whether it would be fiscally prudent to create tax incentives for families to provide more informal care (see, for an overview, Chapter 21 by Burau et al.). Recent state and national policies in the United States have attempted to incentivize informal care, with current bills proposing substantial tax credits to encourage informal care. We summarize a few case studies to assess the effectiveness of informal care in terms of its impact on utilization and expenditures on formal care, identify underlying determinants and, most importantly, evaluate potential policies/ interventions that could boost informal care by family as an alternative to formal care, thereby limiting expenditures.

To evaluate the effectiveness of informal care policies, a study (Van Houtven and Norton, 2004) using the 1998 US Health and Retirement Survey assessed how informal care by adult children impacts use of formal care. The findings indicate that informal care reduces formal healthcare utilization among both elderly men and women by reducing paid home healthcare and delaying nursing home entry. Research studies from Europe also show informal care to be a net substitute for formal home care (Charles and Sevak, 2005). In a follow-up paper (Van Houtven and Norton, 2008), the authors probe further into utilization issues by examining whether informal care can reduce formal care expenditures. They also examine whether the effect of informal care varies across important subpopulations of both providers and recipients of care. First, they assess whether the effect is equally strong across married and unmarried elderly persons. They postulate that because spouses provide informal care to each other, informal care by children would have less effect on utilization of formal care among the married elderly. Second, they examine whether care provided by sons and daughters have similar effects on expenditures. Third, they examine whether other sources of informal care provided by friends or other relatives are as effective as care provided by adult children in terms of substituting for formal care. The results indicate that informal care by adult children significantly reduces long-term and inpatient care expenditures among the single elderly, but are less effective among the married elderly. In addition, for the single elderly, informal care effectiveness does not vary by the gender of the child, and child caregivers are more effective than other types of caregivers – like friends and relatives – in reducing the likelihood of home health expenditures and skilled nursing home expenditures.

Another interesting study (Hanaoka and Norton, 2008) examines the effect of child caregivers on utilization of formal care by the elderly in Japan. To meet the healthcare needs of the rapidly growing share of older adults, Japan introduced public long-term care insurance in 2000 (see Chapter 21 by Burau et al.). Nonetheless, children, particularly daughters, are the most common source of care for elderly persons. For married sons, the daughter-in-law has the primary responsibility for providing care for her parent-in-law. These traditional Japanese social norms make the context particularly interesting. The results indicate that the supply of child caregivers is not uniform in its relationship to elderly parents' long-term care utilization, but varies by gender of the child. The child's marital status and the opportunity cost of their time also play an important role. Interestingly, the hypothesis that under the traditional norm the daughter-in-law has to take on primary caregiving responsibilities is not supported even when the birth order of the son is taken into account. Furthermore, the traditional role of daughters as primary caregivers for their parents is changing.

It is important to highlight that the majority of the studies that we have discussed are based on nationally representative surveys that exclude older adults living in institutions. Since women are more likely to be widowed and to live alone than men, they may be more likely to enter an institution. Gender differences in health and healthcare utilization would have possibly been higher without gender-related selective institutionalization. A study (Portrait et al., 2000) on the Dutch elderly of determinants of long-term care that includes institutional care finds that emergence or aggravation of physical disabilities among the elderly reduces the probability of receiving informal care, and increases the need for formal or institutionalized care. This finding is confirmed by a recent study (Bossing, 2009) that analyses the impact of informal care by adult children on the use of long-term care by the elderly in Europe and the effect of the level of parent's disability on this relationship. The focus is on two types of formal home care that are the most likely to interact with informal care: paid domestic help and nursing care. The results indicate that informal care substitutes for formal home care, but the effect tends to disappear as the level of disability of the elderly person increases. However, informal care is a weak complement to nursing care, independent of the level of disability.

The developing country perspective

Gender difference in healthcare utilization: evidence and explanation

With recent improvements in life expectancy in the developing world, survival into older ages is becoming the norm for most countries with the exception of some in Africa. With growing populations of the elderly, evidence on the needs of the elderly is also slowly emerging. In general, studies from developing countries show that elderly women are more likely to report poorer health status than elderly men (Case and Deaton, 2006; Strauss et al., 1993; Zimmer and Kwong, 2004). However, although there are numerous studies that discuss inequities in healthcare utilization in developing countries, these are not specific to the elderly population, partly because of a lack of large-scale surveys of the elderly. A few studies that examine both gender differentials in health status and health utilization and the underlying reasons for these differentials are discussed next.

A study of rural Bangladesh (Young et al., 2006) used data from Matlab Health and Socio-economic Survey and Anderson's health behaviour model (discussed previously) to examine patterns of healthcare utilization by adults, utilization differences by age and gender, and the factors related to these utilization patterns. The authors found that women were twice as likely as men to be mobility-impaired and more likely than men to report poorer health status. Women also tended to seek more care in their reproductive years than men. However, beyond the reproductive years, the frequency of seeking care drastically dropped off for women compared to men. When non-fertility-related visits were examined it was found that approximately the same proportion of men and women were visiting a healthcare provider in their reproductive years, but substantially fewer women than men were getting healthcare visits in older ages. For men, particularly those in poor health, visits increased as they grew older. But for women with poor health, healthcare visits declined sharply as they grew older. The study explains that this gender difference in health utilization exists because men and women are valued differently according to their relative economic contribution to the household. Education and social norms may also affect women's healthcare utilization. Further, modesty norms in a predominantly Islamic society, such as in this study, may deter women from seeking care outside the household.

A study on health access and utilization in Pakistan (Shaikh and Hatcher, 2004), not restricted only to the elderly, discusses the role of women's autonomy in healthcare-seeking behaviours and provides similar conclusions as the Young and colleagues (2006) study. Segregation of the sexes, confinement of women to their homes and dependence on male family members to make decisions regarding whether and where to seek care deprive women of essential health information and care that they need. Distance to health providers becomes a disincentive for women to seek care especially because of their restricted mobility and the need to be accompanied by a male family member.

The gender disparity in resources available for women, women's health status and receipt of healthcare confers a relatively negative health impact on women; this may be a reason why Hosain and Begum's (2003) study from rural Bangladesh found a higher gender ratio of 148 men to 100 women in the age group 60 years and above. More men surviving in old age than women is a finding typical of countries such as Bangladesh and India (Rajan, 1989) but is in stark contrast to developed countries where women outlive and thus outnumber men in older ages.

A study on patterns of healthcare utilization in older ages in Brazil (Barretto et al., 2009) found that women overall are more likely to report temporary and permanent disabilities than men, but are more likely to access and utilize outpatient care. Men on the other hand are more likely to access and utilize inpatient care. The authors suggest that *machismo* may be a factor in men delaying healthcare utilization until hospitalization becomes necessary or that women tend to be more compliant with medications, counselling and seeking preventive treatment. An article examining health-seeking behaviour among Costa Rican elderly similarly found that it is common for older men to be unaware of chronic diseases such as diabetes, cancer and particularly hypertension (Méndez-Chacón et al., 2008). Elderly women are more likely to be diagnosed with chronic diseases than men and once diagnosed are more likely to seek care than men. Greater levels of chronic disabilities exist among poor older men compared to poor older women and the study suggests that this may be a result of differential exposure to risk factors such as unhealthy lifestyles (unhealthy diet, drinking and smoking) and poor working conditions in adult life.

Impact of gender differences in socio-economic status and empowerment

Greater survival rates among the elderly in higher income groups suggests that higher socio-economic status is positively associated with health and health-care utilization in developing countries. A study examining socio-economic inequalities in health and healthcare utilization among all age and gender groups in Thailand (Yiengprugsawan et al., 2007) found that the greatest socio-economic inequality in reporting recent chronic illness, poor self-reported morbidity and perceived health is among women aged 60 years or older. Further, even though older women are more likely to report illness compared to men, they are less likely to experience hospital admissions relative to older men.

The above findings are confirmed by a study by Roy and Chaudhuri (2008) which further explores the association between direct measures of socio-economic status and empowerment with gender disparities in health status and healthcare utilization among older adults in India. The findings indicate significant gender differences in health status and health utilization among older adults. Older women report worse self-rated health, higher prevalence of disabilities, and marginally lower chronic conditions than same-aged older men. This health disadvantage among women cannot be explained by demographics or the differential distribution of medical conditions. Controlling for education and income narrows the gender gap in both subjective and objective indicators of health status; however, statistically significant differentials still persist. Upon controlling for property ownership, the gender differential in functional health is reversed, and widens further with a successive control for economic independence. The female disadvantage in subjective health however persists but is narrower after controlling for property ownership, and disappears upon adding a successive control for economic independence. This implies that financially empowered older women in India might have equal or better health than otherwise similar men.

Despite the markedly poorer health status among women in India (Roy and Chaudhuri, 2008), the rates of healthcare utilization are also lower among women than men. This differential can largely be explained by gender differentials in socio-economic status and financial empowerment. Controlling for economic independence along with other socio-economic factors reduces the gender gap, because financially empowered and better-off older adults possibly have better health and need less inpatient care. These findings might imply that by enhancing their ability to undertake primary and secondary prevention during the life course, financial empowerment of women in developing countries like India can confer in older ages the female health advantage reflected in developed societies.

Parker and Wong (2001) use national data from Mexico to examine whether older women experience greater financial, social and health vulnerabilities compared to older men through worse living conditions and lower institutional support. The study finds that more elderly women than men live in extended households and those who are widows are likely to live in their children's households. This results in more women reporting better dwelling conditions than men and this gender gap increases in old age. Women are also slightly more likely to have better access to healthcare because of better health insurance coverage than men due to benefits received through insured spouses or through adult children. In Mexico and in many developing countries, adult children in the workforce can cover their dependent parents through their formal employment-based health benefits. Although the above-mentioned study does not look at health utilization explicitly, one could conjecture that women in families that are educated and employed in the formal workforce would not be disadvantaged in terms of healthcare access even if they never participated in the formal workforce themselves or lived as widows. This study provides important implications for old age policy. In countries that do not have state support for their elderly, one way to encourage informal support for the elderly through extended families would be through formal workforce policies or tax incentives.

Challenges and opportunities

Challenges for developed countries

The evidence generated from specific studies on older adults in developed countries indicates that while older women might have better or comparable self-assessed health than men, they generally report a higher prevalence of chronic conditions and functional impairments, which could possibly explain their higher healthcare utilization (Arber and Cooper, 1999; Macintyre et al., 1996). However, utilization varies by type of service, with older women being more likely than men to contact a general practitioner, but when it comes to hospital admissions there is either no gender difference or older men are more likely to be hospitalized and have longer hospital stays than women. This pattern could be explained by gender differentials in medical conditions where women are reported to have a higher incidence of less severe conditions, while men show excess morbidity for life-threatening conditions.

The studies also indicate that factors other than gender, particularly low social class/status, health-related quality of life and chronic illnesses and impairments, have a significant impact on healthcare utilization. Improvements in the socio-economic class/status experienced by current younger cohorts (compared to older cohorts) of older women might explain the narrowing gender gap in healthcare utilization in recent decades (Case and Paxson, 2005; Huisman et al., 2003). Upon controlling for gender differences in material circumstances, the majority of studies show that the predominant factor affecting higher utilization among older women is greater need (or, illness level). Utilization is also associated with access and availability of healthcare services. However, in most developed countries, with either universal healthcare – for example, the UK, Spain, the Netherlands – or some form of public insurance for the elderly – such as Medicare in the USA – greater utilization by older women could largely be due to their poorer health status (or need), particularly for curative care (like visits to the medical practitioner, hospitalization and use of emergency services) rather than preventive (for example, screening) or discretionary care (such as dental treatment). Nonetheless, it is critical to emphasize that, despite narrowing gender differences in morbidity and healthcare utilization among older adults in developed societies, older women are still more likely to be socially and economically disadvantaged than men because of higher disability, lower occupational class and living arrangements where a greater proportion of women are widowed or living alone compared to men.

Challenges for developing countries

Comparable evidence from developing countries indicates that inequalities in health and health utilization are intrinsically related to socio-economic inequalities. Poorer men and women not only have worse health but they also report worse healthcare access and utilization compared to more affluent men and women. These inequalities persist into later life because socio-economic disparities might increase among older adults in most developing countries. While both men and women are vulnerable in old age, female elderly in the developing world may be more disadvantaged for a variety of reasons. Because women are less likely than men to participate in the formal workforce, women are less likely to receive employment-related old age benefits. Moreover, women outlive men biologically, live longer as widows and thus resources available to women must last longer than for men. As a result, elderly women are more likely to live in poverty (Rajan, 1989). Women are also more likely to depend on informal sources of support from extended family compared to men.

A consensus appears to exist in the literature that although elderly women report worse health than elderly men they are less likely to seek care compared to elderly men in South Asian countries. This result is not true for other parts of the world such as in Brazil, where elderly women are more likely to report disabilities but are also more likely than elderly men to seek outpatient care (Baretto et al., 2009). Evidence indicates that older women tend to suffer from a disproportionate incidence of chronic conditions that are not life-threatening but are associated with functional impairments; these tend to be undervalued by health providers, resulting in lower hospital admissions compared to men (Rosenberg and Wilson, 2000). The overall findings from developing countries indicate that those who are better educated, have higher socio-economic status and are economically independent are better able to maintain good health and seek care when necessary throughout the life course, including in older ages (Roy and Chaudhuri, 2008). In contrast, the less privileged, be they defined by income, wealth, existence of children or social norms, lead a more vulnerable existence in their old age in these countries.

Finally, although the common understanding in developed countries is that better health utilization will improve health outcomes, this may not be true in the developing countries where providing basic living conditions such as clean water and sanitation may improve health status even more than increasing visits to a doctor. Further, a pluralistic system of western and traditional medicine exists in many developing countries, which makes it challenging to measure and improve health utilization by western standards.

Lessons learned and policy implications

Our review provides insights that have significant implications for old age policy around the world. The impact of lifelong patterns of socio-economic inequality on health outcomes and utilization affects men and women differentially in later life. Social security, pension assistance, financial empowerment, mandated support from extended family, and improvement of self-worth and status for women may be ways to reduce gender differentials in health status and utilization. For example, in the Langeburg study from South Africa (Case and Wilson, 2000) in which women started getting a pension at the age of 60 and men at the age of 65 years, there were significant improvements in self-reported health status for women and men at respective pension-eligible ages. In the developed world where there is some form of social security and public health insurance for the elderly, this lifelong inequality in resources gets levelled to a certain extent in old age. The lifelong inequality gets further exacerbated in old age with retirement and the loss of a regular income. Elderly women, especially those who never worked in the formal workforce, face even more hardships with longer lifespans, and through dependence on family members. Multisectoral development activities such as microcredit, education, teaching life-skills and non-formal education programmes are policies that have been shown to improve health status and health-seeking behaviours among women (Ahmed et al., 2003).

Evidence from both developed and developing societies also indicates that chronic impairments are a critical determinant of long-term care needs. Formal care and institutionalized care are expensive and are positively associated with income and education. With increased needs of an ageing population and socio-economic disparities within the ageing population, many state and family resources will be significantly strained. This will create a greater inequity in access to long-term care needs of the elderly unless a sustainable model can be implemented.

Informal care at home provided by family members is an important source of long-term care for the elderly and can be a substitute for more costly formal care. Informal care might also be successful in helping the elderly stay connected with their communities, and feel valued as productive and contributing members of society. In most developing countries, which lack affordable and sustainable formal care for the elderly, informal care by relatives is indispensable. However, with decreasing family size and increase in nuclear families, intergenerational support for the elderly is becoming a challenge in both developed and developing societies. For ageing societies struggling to find effective and sustainable long-term care policies for their growing elderly population, long-term care policy should factor in incentives for family members to take care of the aged, prolonging their participation in the community and preventing expensive institutionalization until it becomes absolutely necessary.

Conclusion

By providing a comprehensive review of evidence on gender differences in healthcare utilization among older adults in both developed and developing societies this chapter has highlighted that, despite universal commonalities, the specific factors that influence utilization are complicated, varying through time and across countries. Recent findings indicate that older women from developed countries generally report better or comparable self-assessed health but higher utilization due to greater chronic impairments. Comparable evidence from developing countries indicates that older women not only report (or experience) worse health, but they also report lower healthcare utilization than men. Nonetheless, what emerges as critical is that the reported higher utilization among older women for a given level of ill-health is not universal but there are subtle and complex variations across studies. From a policy perspective, it is important to recognize that there are considerable differences in health systems, as well as cultural mores, which impact gender-related variations in health awareness and care-seeking behaviours both within and across developed and developing countries, thereby making it difficult to generalize findings from any one country to other country settings.

The lack of a synthesized body of evidence on inequalities in healthcare utilization in later life has resulted in portraying an ageist image of the elderly as a homogenous group, who due to their declining health and higher healthcare utilization impose a financial burden on the rest of society. It is important to emphasize that maintaining good health is of central importance to the lives of elderly people, and a key determinant of their ability to remain independent and autonomous, and in predicting their overall life satisfaction. The nature and structure of gender differences in healthcare utilization in later life also depend on factors derived from an elderly person's current and prior productive role in society. Recent evidence indicates that financial empowerment enhances health and well-being among both older men and women; this has policy implications that extend beyond gender disparities.

For societies around the world, with shrinking social funds to care for their growing older population, economic empowerment of older adults could possibly be an effective mechanism for improving their health outcomes throughout the life course, lowering healthcare utilization and controlling long-term healthcare costs. Furthermore, paying attention to new, complementary and alternative modes of healthcare access and delivery may help generate valuable evidence in this area of study.

Summary

- Studies from developed countries indicate that older women generally report better or comparable self-assessed health but greater utilization due to higher prevalence of chronic conditions and functional impairments.
- Comparable evidence from developing countries indicates that older women not only report (or experience) worse health, but they also report lower healthcare utilization than men. While improvements in socio-economic status and financial empowerment might neutralize this gender difference, older women remain vulnerable because of longer life-spans, widowhood and financial and physical dependence on extended families.
- Despite certain universal commonalities, the specific factors that influence health and healthcare utilization among older adults are complicated, varying through time and across settings with considerable differences in health systems as well as cultural mores, thereby making it difficult to generalize findings from one country to other country settings.

Key reading

Arber, S. and H. Cooper (1999) 'Gender Differences in Health in Later Life: The New Paradox?', *Social Science & Medicine*, 48 (1), 61–76.

Roy, K. and A. Chaudhuri (2008) 'The Influence of Socioeconomic Status and Empowerment on Gender Differences in Health and Healthcare Utilization in Later Life: Evidence from India', *Social Science & Medicine*, 66 (9), 1951–62.

Van Houtven, C. H. and E. C. Norton (2004) 'Informal Care and Health Care Use of Older Adults', *Journal of Health Economics*, 23 (6), 1159–80.

Young, J. T., J. Menken, J. Williams, N. Khan and R. S. Kuhn (2006) 'Who Receives Health Care? Age and Sex Differentials in Adult Use of Healthcare Services in Rural Bangladesh, *World Health & Population*, 8 (2), 83–100.

Note

*The findings and conclusions in this report are those of the authors and do not necessarily represent the official position of the Centers for Disease Control and Prevention.

References

Adamson, J., Y. Ben Shlomo, N. Chaturvedi and J. Donovan (2003) 'Ethnicity, Socio-Economic Position and Gender – Do They Affect Reported Health-Care Seeking Behaviour?', *Social Science & Medicine*, 57 (5), 895–904.

Ahmed S. M., A. M. Adams, M. Chowdhury and A. Bhuiya (2003) 'Changing Health Seeking Behavior in Matlab: Do Development Interventions Matter?', *Health Policy and Planning*, 18 (3), 306–15.

Anderson, J. G. (1973) 'Demographic Factors Affecting Health Services Utilization: A Causal Model', *Medical Care*, XI (2), 104–20.

Arber, S. and J. Ginn (1993) 'Gender and Inequalities in Health in Later Life', *Social Science & Medicine*, 36 (1), 33–46.

Arber, S. and H. Cooper (1999) 'Gender Differences in Health in Later Life: The New Paradox?, *Social Science & Medicine*, 48 (1), 61–76.

Barreto, S. M., A. Kalache and L. Giatti (2009) *Gender Patterns of Health Care Use in Older Age*, Working Paper of Research Group on Ageing and Public Health, Medical School of the Federal University of Minas Gerais and Research Centre, Rene Rachou of the Oswaldo Cruz Foundation, Brazil.

Benyamini, Y., E. A. Leventhal and H. Leventhal (2000) 'Gender Differences in Processing Information for Making Self-assessments of Health', *Psychosomatic Medicine*, 62 (3), 354–64.

Bertakis, K. D., R. Azari, L. J. Helms, E. J. Callahan and J. A. Robbins (2000) 'Gender Differences in the Utilization of Health Care Services', *The Journal of Family Practice*, 49 (2), 147–52.

Bossing, E. (2009) 'Does Informal Care from Children to Their Elderly Parents Substitute for Formal Care in Europe?', *Journal of Health Economics*, 28 (1), 143–54.

Case, A. and C. Paxson (2005) 'Sex Differences in Morbidity and Mortality', *Demography*, 42 (2), 189–214.

Case, A. and F. Wilson (2000) *Health and Wellbeing in South Africa: Evidence from the Langeberg Survey* (Princeton: Princeton University Working Papers).

Case, A., and A. Deaton (2006) 'Health and Wellbeing in Udaipur and South Africa', in D. Wise (ed.), *Developments in the Economics of Aging* (Chicago: University of Chicago Press), 317–58.

Charles, K. K. and P. Sevak (2005) 'Can Family Caregiving Substitute for Nursing Home Care?', *Journal of Health Economics*, 24 (6), 1174–90.

Fernández-Mayoralas, G., V. Rodríguez and F. Rojo (2000) 'Health Services Accessibility among Spanish Elderly', *Social Science & Medicine*, 50 (1), 17–26.

Gijsbers van Wijk, C. M. T. and A. M. Kolk (1997) 'Sex Differences in Physical Symptoms: The Contribution of Symptom Perception Theory', *Social Science & Medicine*, 45 (2), 231–46.

Hanaoka, C. and E. C. Norton (2008) 'Informal and Formal Care for Elderly Persons: How Adult Children's Characteristics Affect the Use of Formal Care in Japan', *Social Science & Medicine*, 67 (6), 1002–8.

Hosain, G. M. and A. Begum (2003) 'Health Needs and Health Status of the Elderly in Rural Bangladesh', *Asia Pacific Journal of Public Health*, 15 (1), 3–9.

Huisman, M., A. E. Kunst and J. P. Mackenbach (2003) 'Socioeconomic Inequalities in Morbidity among the Elderly: A European View', *Social Science & Medicine*, 57 (5), 861–73.

Krasnik, A., E. Hansen, N. Keiding and A. Sawitz (1997) 'Determinants of General Practice Utilization in Denmark', *Danish Medical Bulletin*, 44 (5), 542–6.

Ladwig, K. H., B. Marten-Mittag, B. Formanek and G. Dammann (2000) 'Gender Differences of Symptom Reporting and Medical Health Care Utilization in the German Population', *European Journal of Epidemiology*, 16 (6), 511–18.

León-Muñoz, L. M., E. López-García, A. Graciani, P. Guallar-Castillón, J. R. Banegas, and F. Rodríguez-Artalejo (2007) 'Functional Status and Use of Health Care Services: Longitudinal Study on the Older Adult Population in Spain', *Maturitas*, 58 (4), 377–86.

Macintyre, S., K. Hunt and H. Sweeting (1996) 'Gender Differences in Health: Are Things Really as Simple as They Seem?', *Social Science & Medicine*, 42 (4), 617–24.

Marks, N. F. (1996) 'Socioeconomic Status, Gender and Health at Midlife: Evidence from the Wisconsin Longitudinal Study', in *Research in the Sociology of Health Care*, vol. 13 (New York: JAI Press), 133–50.

Mathers, C. D. and D. Loncar (2006) 'Projections of Global Mortality and Burden of Disease from 2002 to 2030', *PLoS Medicine*, 3 (11), e442.

Méndez-Chacón, E., C. Santamaría-Ulloa and L. Rosero-Bixby (2008) 'Factors Associated with Hypertension Prevalence, Unawareness and Treatment among Costa Rican Elderly', *BMC Public Health*, 8, 275.

Nathanson, C. A. (1975) 'Illness and the Feminine Role: A Theoretical Review', *Social Science & Medicine*, 9 (2), 57–62.

Parker, S. and R. Wong (2001) 'Welfare of Male and Female Elderly in Mexico: A Comparison', in E. G. Katz and M. C. Correia (eds), *The Economics of Gender in Mexico: Work, Family, State and Market* (Washington, DC: World Bank), 249–90.

Portrait, F., M. Lindeboom and D. Deeg (2000) 'The Use of Long-term Care Services by the Dutch Elderly', *Health Economics*, 9 (6), 513–31.

Rajan, S. I. (1989) 'Aging in Kerala: One More Population Problem', *Asia Pacific Population Journal*, 4 (2), 19–48.

Redondo-Sendino, A., P. Guallar-Castillón, J. R. Banegas and F. Rodríguez-Artalejo (2006) 'Gender Differences in the Utilization of Health-care Services among the Older Adult Population of Spain', *BMC Public Health*, 16 (6) (June), 155.

Rosenberg M. W. and K. Wilson (2000) 'Gender, Poverty and Location: How Much Difference Do They Make in the Geography of Health Inequalities?', *Social Science & Medicine*, 51 (2), 275–87.

Roy, K. and A. Chaudhuri (2008) 'The Influence of Socioeconomic Status and Empowerment on Gender Differences in Health and Healthcare Utilization in Later Life: Evidence from India', *Social Science & Medicine*, 66 (9), 1951–62.

Shaikh, B. T. and J. Hatcher (2004) 'Health Seeking Behaviour and Health Service Utilization in Pakistan: Challenging the Policymakers', *Journal of Public Health*, 27 (1), 49–54.

Strauss, J., P. J. Gertler, O. Rahman and K. Fox (1993) 'Gender and Life-cycle Differentials in the Patterns and Determinants of Adult Health', *The Journal of Human Resources*, 28 (4), 791–837.

Van Houtven, C. H. and E. C. Norton (2004) 'Informal Care and Health Care Use of Older Adults', *Journal of Health Economics*, 23 (6), 1159–80.

Van Houtven, C. H. and E. C. Norton (2008) 'Informal Care and Medicare Expenditures: Testing for Heterogeneous Treatment Effects', *Journal of Health Economics*, 27 (1), 134–56.

Verbrugge, L. M. (1986) 'Role Burdens and Physical Health of Women and Men', *Women and Health*, 11 (1), 47–77.

Yiengprugsawan, V., L. L. Y. Lim, G. A. Carmichael, A. Sidorenko and A. C. Sleigh (2007) 'Measuring and Decomposing Inequity in Self-reported Morbidity and Self-assessed Health in Thailand', *International Journal for Equity in Health*, 6 (1), 23.

Young, J. T., J. Menken, J. Williams, N. Khan and R. S. Kuhn (2006) 'Who Receives Health Care? Age and Sex Differentials in Adult Use of Healthcare Services in Rural Bangladesh', *World Health & Population*, 8 (2), 83–100.

Zimmer, Z. and J. Kwong (2004) 'Socioeconomic Status and Health among Older Adults in Rural and Urban China', *Journal of Aging and Health*, 16 (1), 44–70.

16
Men's Health and Well-being
Toni Schofield

Introduction

Men's health and well-being is a recent arrival on the international public policy and health scene, following in the wake of the women's health movement and the emergence of policy-making related to gender equity. To date, policy and research into men's health have proceeded on the basis that the object of their discussions and inquiries is self-evident: populations comprise males and females. Corresponding with this division are two differentiated arenas of health and health service experience that are specific to each sex: women's health and men's health. This chapter proposes, however, that this common-sense understanding is limited as a foundation for understanding the health and well-being of men. It oversimplifies and misrepresents the issues involved.

In embracing both health and well-being, the chapter not only addresses social processes and relations associated with patterns and experiences of diagnosable medical conditions (including injury, disability, disease and death) and healthcare provision but also those that are foundational for 'well-being'. Such a concept is obviously related to health but it suggests more than the absence of diagnosable medical conditions and healthcare provision. The diminishment of physical, mental and emotional suffering, a sense of human purpose, self-efficacy and of connectedness with others are some of the key dimensions that have been associated with it. Well-being, then, involves access to experiences that have been powerfully embodied and commonly associated, since the Enlightenment, with what it means to be a human being and a person.

While *both* health and well-being are intrinsically embodied, they are also quintessentially social insofar as people's access to and experience of them derives from the social dynamics and relations in which they are located. This means that how we experience ourselves in our physical, mental and emotional embodiment is a kind of individual inscription of our social embeddedness – of how we live and work, and the conditions under which we do so. Yet because of the disparities characterizing social organization and the barriers these create for many in accessing the material and symbolic resources to achieve health and well-being, the latter is an irretrievably political project. The political character of health and well-being is arguably nowhere more visible than in health policy-making and the claims by constituencies for financial support and validation by public authorities to secure their health and well-being (Schofield, 2004).

It is the claims of one of these constituencies – the men's health movement – and the discourse through which its claims are pressed that this chapter discusses. Based on empirical evidence, the chapter provides a critique of the prevailing representations of men's health, advancing an alternative conceptualization to describe, examine and discuss the 'real' trouble that some groups of men face in relation to their health and well-being. This approach focuses on gender as a dynamic social process that is played out symbiotically with other significant dynamics – namely class, ethnicity and indigeneity – in generating barriers for health and well-being among some groups of men. The chapter concludes with a discussion of men's use of and access to healthcare – an issue frequently addressed by prevailing men's health discourse as illustrative of gender inequity in health services policy and provision. Inequity among men, the chapter argues, certainly does operate in healthcare but it does not involve gender inequity as suggested by prevailing men's health discourse. The alternative framing of the problem of men's health proposed by the chapter aims to provide a more robust conceptual and empirical foundation for developing research and policy that will advance men's health and well-being.

The prevailing discourse of men's health

The term 'men's health' emerged in the 1990s and is basically the creation of public policy, research and popular media discourse. The proliferation of men's health policy development and research since then, especially in Australia, England, Ireland, Scotland and the USA (see Smith and Robertson, 2008), has meant that it is possible to refer to the collective commentary, analysis and discussion associated with it as 'men's health discourse'. Such discourse is by no means monolithic in its representation of 'the problem' of men's health, but there is nonetheless a prevailing or dominant approach which has as its conceptual bedrock the idea that sex difference, or the bodily 'reproductive distinction' between men and women (Connell, 2002: 10), creates two gender-based public health constituencies. Men's health is constructed by a contrast with women's health (Schofield et al., 2000: 248). What emerges as central to its representation is a robust binarism that relies mainly on statistical fabrication.

Biological and social binarism

From this perspective, women's health is basically constituted as a sex-based aggregate of measures related to women's reproductive illnesses and diseases, to their use of health services, and to their mortality, morbidity, disability and lifestyle practices (such as alcohol and tobacco use, and diet and exercise regimes). Corresponding with this representation is a collection of the same sorts of indicators but applied to men as a sex-based category – men's health. It is the margins of difference in the measurements between the two categories that are foundational for men's health discourse. If the magnitudes between the two are unequal then so too are the health statuses of men and women. Differential magnitudes signal the presence of a 'gender-specific' health issue. The absence of such difference, on the other hand, suggests gender neutrality and, in turn, no cause for gender-specific public interventions such as gender-specific policies, programmes and services.

This characterization of men's *and* women's health has been central to the development of men's health discourse and to the social movement that has advanced it. Indeed, the two have been inextricably related. The interdependence established between them has depended heavily on the representation of men and their health in terms of men as a sex that, in aggregate, has less favourable rates than women on a wide range of health indicators. Such a formulation has served as a basis for the public claim that men as a sex face specific health challenges that demand a sex-specific response.

Lending support to and legitimation of this framing of the problem of men's health is the emergent discipline of gender-specific medicine. It has developed in the context of a substantial critique of biomedical research and practice as having been gender-*in*sensitive. Researchers and practitioners in the field have appropriated the critique to establish themselves as a new and distinctive branch of medicine. They suggest that biomedical research has generally proceeded on the basis that women are 'small men' and, as a result, not needed to be included (Legato, 2004). It is evident that, like their counterparts engaged in men's health policy and research, the principal objective of gender-specific medicine is to advance knowledge of *sex differences* in systems medicine, and treatments for addressing them (Miller, 2005).

Men's health discourse, however, does not confine itself to biological sex differences. Men's health policy in particular has freely incorporated social understandings of men, forging a hybrid of biology and culture to create a sex-based public health constituency. Men, then, are constituted by the combination of male reproductive characteristics and engagement in the 'male role' or masculine practices that are socially determined. The latter are distinguished by their contrast with the 'female role' and feminine practices. Just as this approach imagines human embodiment as dimorphic, so too does it represent the social practices of human beings as taking 'the shape of a dichotomy between all-women and all-men' (Connell, 2002: 36). It proposes a match or homology between embodiment and culture. This binary is what men's health discourse understands as gender. Its incorporation of 'the social' is selective and partial, representing men and women as wholly distinct and mutually exclusive categories of people, and gender as the relationship that connects them as such – a conceptualization that has attracted sustained critique from within sociology and gender studies (see, for example, Annandale and Clark, 1996; Connell, 2002).

Like their counterparts in women's health, proponents of men's health insist that men have a collective interest and identity. However, in contrast to feminist approaches that have problematized the issue of a shared interest and identity among women in the face of significant differences among them (see, for example, Schofield, 2004; Young, 1997), men's health discourse simply adopts differentiation from the 'other' or 'opposite sex' as its conceptual foundation. The mere assertion of a bio-social sex dichotomy, then, is the theoretical basis for men's health claims of a collective problem. At the same time, however, within men's health discourse, the idea of a collective interest and identity among men in relation to their health goes hand-in-hand with the idea of a *plurality* of interests and identities among them. Although *all* men are represented as the subject, the discourse simultaneously emphasizes ways in which men's health disadvantage is not generalized among men (Courtenay, 2002). Certain groups of men are typically identified as bearing a particular burden: indigenous men, men from non-English-speaking ethnic backgrounds, African-American men (in the USA), men with disabilities, gay men, men of low socio-economic status and men in rural locations.

These differences are real and significant but positing them as central to men's health disadvantage creates conceptual tension within men's health discourse. On the one hand, to the extent that there is a shared interest and identity, all men as a whole have comparable or worse health than women as a whole. Yet on the other hand, while there are differences among men, only certain groups of men have comparable or worse health than women as a whole. Such a representation is intrinsically contradictory because both are not simultaneously tenable in the absence of a rational account of how this is possible. If it is the social disadvantage of *some* men that produces the rates of health differences between men and women, how can 'men's health' refer to men as a whole? (Schofield et al., 2000: 248).

The advancement of sex differences

A further distinctive feature of men's health discourse has been its mobilization of particular kinds of empirical evidence to support the conceptualization of men's health as a sex-differentiated category. Much of this evidence has been drawn from the vast international literature on sex differences in health, including mortality, average life expectancy, chronic illness, injury and disability from accidents, suicide and substance abuse. Some of the more unusual studies include rates of sex differences in snake bites, dog attacks and infections from eating with chopsticks (Connell et al., 1999). However, as an Australian government-commissioned study into men's health and sex differences commented:

> A finding of sex difference need not imply a difference between *all* men and *all* women. In fact, it usually does not. Quite small differences among a minority of the population may produce statistically significant differences in overall rates or averages. (Connell et al., 1999: 26)

The routine use of the sex differences literature in men's health discourse, however, serves as a mechanism for establishing men as a collective with a shared health interest and identity that policy-makers, researchers and practitioners need to address. Recognizing and referring to the many documented similarities between men and women in terms of their health, such as the major disease conditions they share in relation to mortality, does not produce a sex-differentiated constituency with gender-specific needs. Men's health discourse, then, has relied heavily on the empirical evidence of sex differences to advance the case for more public recognition and resources for men's health despite the fact that there is no evidence that the differences exceed the similarities in health (Connell et al., 1999).

The link between the advancement of sex differences in health and the pursuit of public recognition and funding for men's health is paradoxically evident in the discourse's recent turn towards evidence showing *similarities* between men and women in relation to domestic and 'intimate partner' violence. This development needs to be understood in the context of the international women's health movement and its success in introducing public sanctions against men's violence towards women in intimate relationships and households, and the allocation of public funding to support women in the face of such abuse. Underpinning these public interventions has been evidence of a longstanding relationship of the perpetration of domestic and intimate partner violence by men towards women (see also Chapter 2 by Abdool et al.). Men's health proponents are now challenging this evidence, arguing that public policy and services need to address the injuries that men incur through women's violence in intimate and domestic relationships. The evidence used in supporting this claim is drawn mostly from large quantitative studies or surveys internationally. Recent and illustrative examples are North American reviews of the literature on women who perpetrate intimate partner violence (Carney et al., 2007) and on partner violence by male and female university students in 32 nations (Straus, 2008). They indicate that while men typically express their physical violence towards their intimate partners by strangling them or beating them up, women also do so but mainly by slapping, punching, kicking, scratching and throwing things.

There are, however, some significant limitations associated with these studies, as reputable research-based critics have recently and comprehensively noted (Dobash and Dobash, 2004). For example, the alleged symmetry in men's and women's intimate violence is based on particular conceptualizations that view violence as discrete 'acts' regardless of who performs them, the circumstances in which they occur, and what they mean to the participants. As critics have commented:

> [The] 'act-based' approach must invariably equate the physical impact/consequences of a 'slap' delivered by a slight 5 ft 4 inch woman with the 'slap' of a heavily built man of 6 ft 2 inches. (Dobash and Dobash, 2004: 329)

Similarly, a woman's attempt to hit her partner while he is trying to hold her at arm's length having delivered a punch to her face is accorded equivalence to the punch. The evidence for the alleged convergence between men and women in relation to intimate partner violence, then, is thus surrounded by doubts regarding its *rigour* (Liamputtong and Ezzy, 2005: 34; Dobash and Dobash, 2004). As a recent discussion of measurement issues for violence against women commented, while surveys are a useful method for contributing to our understanding of intimate partner violence, the evidence they produce is often marred by inadequate reliability and validity (Desai and Saltzman, 2001). Moreover, the authors add, intimate partner violence is so complex and multifactorial that reliance on quantitative research results alone, no matter how widely or frequently the surveys are conducted and the results replicated, is likely to misrepresent the problem.

The use of empirical evidence in men's health discourse to assert sex differences in health outcomes and sex similarities in adverse health outcomes arising from violence between men and women is characterized by significant limitations. Further, the conceptualization of men's health advanced in men's health discourse (as discussed above) is seriously flawed. It is evident, then, that the prevailing model of men's health provides no grounds for advancing the idea that men, as a whole, share a set of health needs and that these disadvantage them *vis-à-vis* women as a whole. There are certainly groups of men with pressing health needs, but these are generally related to factors associated with men's class or socio-economic status, their indigeneity, ethnicity, sexuality and so on. Indeed, major health differences among men that are related to these factors, especially socio-economic differences, are usually much greater than those identified between men and women (Saurel-Cubizolles et al., 2009). The chapter now discusses the most significant of these differences in the context of an alternative dynamic social relations approach to understanding men's health.

A dynamic gender relations model of men's health

It has been argued that the limitations of prevailing men's health discourse stem from thinking of gender as two mutually exclusive categories of human beings. It proffers a static view, and one in which gender is basically a *noun* that refers to sex-differentiated characteristics, both biological and behavioural. Yet recent developments in the fields of gender studies and sociology suggest a new understanding of gender as a combination of dynamic social practices and relations that demands the dissolution of the match between sex-based, dimorphic human embodiment and culture. This does not mean that bodies do not count, especially in the reproductive distinction between them. This is, in fact, vital. But from a dynamic, social practice-based perspective, it is *how* this distinction is brought into play in determining who gets to participate where, how, under what conditions and with what kinds of material and symbolic consequences, including health outcomes, that is crucial (Schofield, 2004). In other words, a dynamic approach not only views gender as something that people do (West and Zimmerman, 1987), but as a principle of social organization that has significant implications for the social distribution and exercise of power (Alsop et al., 2002). This can be illustrated in relation to serious workplace injuries and deaths, and socio-economic status (SES), ethnicity and health.

Workplace health

In most capitalist countries throughout the world, workplace injuries occur overwhelmingly among men. The problem is usually represented as a simple correlation between the magnitudes of workplace injury and death, and the category 'men by occupation'. It is often accompanied by a further correlation between women's rates of workplace injuries and death and their occupational location in the workforce. Such correlations provide no explanation. They are purely descriptive of how men sustain worse workplace health than women by occupation. A dynamic gendered approach to this statistical relationship would explain it in the following way.

First, in addition to the disparity between men and women, it would also recognize that there are marked health differences *among* men that are related to their occupational location, just as there are among women. Men in traditional 'blue collar' jobs bear the lion's share of workplace injuries and deaths by comparison with their 'white collar' counterparts in managerial, administrative and professional jobs. This disparity among men arises largely as a result of the class-based organization of employment that men still dominate (Collinson and Hearn, 2005) despite women's increasing participation in the workforce since the 1960s. Working-class men incur a disproportionate rate of poor workplace health because they dominate participation in the most injurious areas of employment, such as mining, building and construction, transport and storage, and heavy manufacturing. Their dominance, however, is also gendered insofar as they rarely work alongside women who could be their girlfriends, partners, wives, sisters, mothers or daughters – in other words, working-class women. This is because working-class employment has developed through a gendered social process – that is, the incorporation of the reproductive distinction between bodies has been critical in the organization of work.

Being reproductively female or male has played a determining role in differential access to the labour market, occupational location, workplace conditions and rates of pay. As a result, working-class men historically have tended to occupy more of the available jobs, especially full-time, and have participated across a wider range of occupations than their female counterparts. Their greater and more diverse employment has gone hand-in-hand with more exposure to injurious and fatal work. The factor that has most influenced this outcome has been the adoption by both management and unions of aggressively exclusionary approaches to women's employment in hazardous jobs since the 19th century (Schofield, 2009a). This gendering of employment has seen a thoroughgoing masculinization of such work and men's experience of bodily damage in doing it.

The restructuring of developed capitalist economies since the mid-1970s, from manufacturing to 'services'-based industries, however, has meant that the overall number of serious occupational injuries and fatalities has declined and with it there has been an improvement in workplace health in these economies. Much of the toll of workplace injury and death has been redistributed to low and middle-income countries, such as China, India, Indonesia, Mexico and South Africa, where most of the world's manufacturing and a large proportion of its construction and mining now take place (Mylett and Markey, 2007).

At the same time, just as working-class women in developed capitalist societies have been afforded some greater protection from workplace health damage because of their more restricted access to hazardous employment arising from the operation of gender (Annandale, 2003), so too have women in middle and low-income countries. However, women's more restricted access to economic resources in these countries also has its downside as it has for their more privileged counterparts in high-income countries. In India, for example, where women have lower rates of employment and of education and earn markedly lower incomes and accrue a much smaller share of total property over their lifetimes, they are not only rendered more economically dependent in older age but also more vulnerable to chronic ill-health and more reliant on health services than their male counterparts (Roy and Chaudhuri, 2008; see also Chapter 15 by Roy and Chaudhuri). It is the gendered division in economic opportunity and education over the life course that advantages men and their health in older age in India.

Gendering in employment and economic life, however, is not simply confined to the organizational division of labour. It also involves how the social processes through which this organization is enacted render workers distinctively masculine or feminine (Connell, 2002). Men's relationships and activities at work are a social mechanism by which they bring themselves into being as men. A notable feature of this process historically is the relentlessness with which men have sought to segregate themselves from women in employment, frequently expressing their collective separateness in hostile and sometimes violent treatment of women. A graphic illustration is found in the aggressive harassment, abuse and exclusion by mining workers of women who have attempted to work side-by-side with men in mines in Australia, Canada and the USA, for example (Moore, 1996; Pini and Mayes, 2008).

Some have proposed that it is the masculinity of working-class men, especially those employed in injurious and lethal employment, that contributes significantly to their overall poorer health (for a critical review of this approach, see Paap, 2006). Such masculinity in the workplace allegedly takes the form of a range of high-risk activities such as participating in high-rise building construction without a safety harness, driving forklift and delivery trucks at high speed, and removing guards from dangerous machinery. These are strongly associated with serious injuries and deaths in industries with the worst occupational health outcomes. As recent developments in occupational health and safety (OH&S) legislation in Australia, the UK and the EU suggest, however, such practices are understood as being more indicative of failure by employers to ensure their employees adhere to OH&S regulation designed to ensure workplace health and safety (see, for example, Johnstone, 2004). Nevertheless, it is evident that some expressions of working-class masculinity are extremely health damaging to working-class men. As Emslie and Hunt relate:

> ... one way in which men can demonstrate culturally valued ... forms of 'masculinity' is by denying vulnerability, taking risks which may injure their health and rejecting health beliefs and behaviours which they associate with women. (2008: 808)

Working-class men's higher levels of substance abuse, especially alcohol and tobacco, constitute a well-known example (Lang et al., 2008). It is of course true that the gap between men's and women's consumption of tobacco and alcohol is closing (Annandale, 2003) but, again, class exerts a major force in this convergence:

> The remaining smokers in the developed countries are often socially marginalised, of low socioeconomic status and often have other co-occurrent issues such as mental illness and homelessness. (Greaves, 2007: 116)

It is among women of low socio-economic status in high-income countries (Graham et al., 2006) and women in low and middle-income countries (Greaves, 2007) that the increased use of tobacco among women, for instance, is mainly occurring. Meanwhile, the decline in smoking is being lead by men of high socio-economic status in high-income countries.

Socio-economic status, ethnicity and indigeneity

Socio-economic status is also powerfully implicated in men's higher rates of death and injury associated with motor vehicle accidents, crime and violence among men. Yet there are also pronounced sex differences in the incidence of such practices with men far outnumbering women in terms of the statistical score sheet (White, 2008). Such a relationship, however, as previously mentioned, simply indicates margins of difference that themselves require explanation. It is this imperative that necessitates a theoretical approach that is able to 'get behind', as it were, the statistical relationships used in men's health discourse to propose that men are in deep health trouble. Certainly men's higher rates of car ownership, their greater leisure time unencumbered by responsibilities for others, their more intensive development and use of skills in exercising aggression and physical force, and their more limited verbal development in communicating complex thoughts and feelings, are some of the gender dynamics at work in men's differentiation of themselves from women and as reflected in their higher rates of motor vehicle accidents, crime and violence. Yet it is the combination of these dynamics with those of class, indigeneity and ethnicity that provides a more complete and critical conceptual foundation for understanding the health carnage that men experience through their involvement with motor vehicles, crime and violence.

Criminologists have shown now for a very long time that socio-economic status or class is strongly implicated in men's involvement in injurious motor vehicle accidents, crime and violence towards other men (White, 2008). Precisely how and why is a complex issue but certainly the combination of aspects that characterize the lives of many working-class people such as limited education, low income, precarious employment or unemployment, substance abuse and the mental and emotional damage wrought by family violence, child abuse and neglect are profoundly formative. As the statistics on the higher rates of incarceration of African-American men in the USA (US Federal Bureau of Prisons, 2009) and indigenous men in Australia (Australian Bureau of Statistics, Australian Institute of Health and Welfare, 2008) also indicate, it is evident that men from some ethnic minorities, such as African-Americans in the USA, and from indigenous communities, such as Australian Aborigines, share many of the factors operating in the lives of working-class men that see them overrepresented in injurious motor vehicle accidents, crime and violence towards other men. It would appear, then, that some marginalized ethnicities and indigeneity involve further additions to the mix of dynamics that produces the adverse health outcomes men from working-class backgrounds experience through their high-risk activities. Dispossession and racist discrimination are the most likely culprits but there is still much to learn about precisely how these are operationalized in men's health-damaging practices.

Men's access to and experience of healthcare: a case of gender inequity?

Some groups of men, then, are in real health trouble, which stems basically from dynamics of class, indigeneity and ethnicity, combined with the practices in which these men engage in enacting and establishing their masculinities – a project largely generated by the mobilization of gender differentiation. Of paramount importance for understanding men's ill-health are the ways in which social practice becomes destructively embodied in men in the course of their lives. It is evident, for example, that if boys do not have the same opportunities as many girls to establish communicative attachments and develop capacities that allow them to verbalize and communicate complex thoughts and feelings, they are less likely to be able to negotiate and solve challenging problems interactively (Jalmert, 2003, cited in Lang et al., 2008). An embodied consequence of such deprivation is emotional frustration and anxiety, and an increased likelihood of physical abuse and violence.

Effective public policy responses and interventions based on a sound research base are needed to address the specificity and gravity of the health difficulties these men face. But as previously explained, men's health discourse, particularly in recent men's health policy, tends not to represent the problem of men's health in this way. In Australia and several other countries where men's health policies are presently being formulated and/or implemented, a dominant focus of the problem is healthcare (see, for example, Australian Department of Health and Ageing, 2008; Irish Department of Health and Children, 2008). The organization and delivery of mainstream health services are identified as being particularly inappropriate in responding to men's needs: they are not available outside men's working hours, they are not located near men's workplaces and waiting times are too long for men. According to this approach, healthcare is not 'men friendly'. As a result, men don't seek help or use the health services they need in order to deal with their poor health, and gender inequity characterizes the system. Accordingly, following the trail blazed by the women's health movement (US Office of Men's Health, 2009), recommendations are proposed for ensuring that health services are more 'men friendly' by being exclusively 'for men'. Providing government-funded, community-based screening services that are organized to administer health checks in such places as pubs and clubs, and using language that compares the body to a motor vehicle is common (see, for example, Irish Department of Health and Children, 2008: 68–9).

Again, however, what is worrying about men's health discourse is the absence of sound evidence to support the case that men are *not* using health services when they need to (Galdas et al., 2005; see Chapter 14 by Hunt et al.). This paucity of evidence is also reflected in the claim by men's health groups that mainstream health services are often inappropriate for men because they are largely 'feminized' spaces in which men feel uncomfortable. Doctors' surgeries, for example, are allegedly decorated in such a way that men feel they are not entering 'men friendly' territory (Banks, 2004: 157). Further, with the growth in numbers of women doctors, men are reported to be less able to communicate their health problems as well as they do with male doctors (Duncan and Hays, 2005).

It is certainly true that healthcare is an arena of major gender inequity in terms of the underrepresentation of men in the health workforce, and it is possible that this creates limitations for adequate service provision for some men. Accordingly, research into the low rate of men's participation in mainstream health services and its implications for the adequacy and appropriateness of such services for men could be undertaken to address men's health claims about the inappropriateness of health services for men. At the same time, proactive recruitment of men to healthcare professions and the implementation of measures to retain them could be piloted and evaluated. Such a proposal is entirely consistent with international gender equity policy and the role of gender mainstreaming in advancing its objectives (United Nations, 2000). It would also contribute to solving the global problem of attracting staff to the increasingly depleted ranks of the health workforce, especially over the forthcoming decades in the face of a predicted health workforce 'crisis' (Schofield, 2009b). Yet such an approach is notably absent in men's health policy recommendations for addressing the alleged problem of gender inequity in mainstream healthcare. The notable exception here is England and Wales, as a recent comparative analysis of men's health policy in Australia and the UK found:

> In the UK, incremental advances in men's health policy have been achieved by focusing on gender mainstreaming – an acknowledgement that gender equality is best achieved by integrating women's and men's health concerns into the formulation, monitoring and analysis of policies and programmes aimed at improving the health status of both men and women. Indeed, it has been argued that national public health strategies in the UK should address men's health needs by promoting gender-sen-

sitive policies, in contrast to a specific men's health policy. (Smith and Robertson, 2008: 286)

It would appear, however, that approaches to healthcare in which men are clearly differentiated from women in service provision have been a more powerful driver in the 'solutions' represented in men's health policy discourse as it has developed in other wealthy democracies such as Australia, Ireland and the USA. Prevailing men's health discourse frames gender inequity in ways that basically ignore the dynamism of gender and the centrality of power, as advanced by recent developments in sociology and gender studies. From a dynamic gender relations approach, gender may be understood as a social process in which the reproductive distinction is mobilized and incorporated in creating various kinds of relations, not only between men and women, but among them as well. Gender inequity is one of the most pervasive of the configurations arising from the process and involves the production of hierarchical relations between men and women such that men, in aggregate, share more of the available material and symbolic resources than do women (see also Chapter 1 by Payne and Doyal). The processes that generate gender equity are certainly implicated in the health and well-being of men but not in ways proposed by prevailing men's health discourse.

Gender inequity is not about patterns of sex-based measurements related to men's health outcomes and their access to and experience of healthcare. Health inequities do exist among men, deriving mainly from their class, indigeneity and ethnicity combined with the practices in which men engage in enacting their masculinities – a project largely generated by the mobilization of gender differentiation and the assertion of the sex distinction based on reproduction. Yet the trouble that some groups of men face in relation to their health and well-being as a consequence of this combination has little to do with inequitably gendered arrangements in healthcare. Claims of gender-inappropriate healthcare provision for men are rarely accompanied by sound evidence of what this means in relation to the organization and delivery of mainstream healthcare.

It is certainly the case that the health workforce and healthcare institutions are heavily dominated by women numerically, and it is possible, depending on adequate research and policy interventions, that this could be a problem and that it could be rectified through greater health workforce participation by men. But men's health discourse represents neither the problem of gender inequity in healthcare, nor its solution, in this way. Moreover, the inequities among men that derive from class, indigeneity and marginalized ethnicity and that impose barriers to mainstream healthcare for the men who have the worst health among men are subsumed by a discourse that names the problem as one of gender inequity.

Summary

- Men's health is constructed by a contrast with women's health. What emerges as central to its construction is a robust binarism that relies mainly on statistical fabrication. If the magnitudes between the two are unequal then so too are the health statuses of men and women.
- However, prevailing men's health discourse provides no conceptual or empirical grounds for advancing the idea that men, as a whole, share a set of health needs that disadvantages them *vis-à-vis* women as a whole.
- Some groups of men, however, are in real health trouble that stems basically from dynamics of class, indigeneity and ethnicity, combined with the practices in which these men engage in enacting and establishing their masculinities – a project largely generated by the mobilization of gender differentiation.
- While inequities related to class, indigeneity and marginalized ethnicity pose the most significant documented barriers to accessible and appropriate healthcare for men, it is possible that the underrepresentation of men in the health workforce creates major problems for adequate and appropriate healthcare for men.

Key reading

Courtenay, W. (2002) 'A Global Perspective on the Field of Men's Health: An Editorial', *International Journal of Men's Health*, 1 (1), 1–13.

Roy, K. and A. Chaudhari (2008) 'Influence of Socioeconomic Status, Wealth and Financial Empowerment on Gender Differences in Health and Healthcare Utilization in Later Life: Evidence from India', *Social Science & Medicine*, 66 (9), 1951–62.

Saurel-Cubizolles, M. J., J. F. Chastang, G. Menvielle, A. Leclerc and D. Luce for the EDISC Group (2009) 'Social Inequalities in Mortality by Cause among Men and Women in France', *Journal of Epidemiology and Community Health*, 63 (3), 197–202.

Schofield, T., R. Connell, L. Walker and J. F. Wood (2000) 'Understanding Men's Health and Illness: A Gender-relations Approach to Policy, Research, and Practice', *Journal of American College Health*, 48 (6), 247–56.

References

Alsop, R., A. Fitzsimons and K. Lennon (2002) *Theorising Gender* (Cambridge: Polity Press).

Annandale, E. (2003) 'Gender and Health Status: Does Biology Matter?', in S. Williams, L. Birke and G. Bendelow (eds), *Debating Biology: Social Reflections on Health* (London: Routledge), 84–95.

Annandale E. and J. Clark (1996) 'What is Gender? Feminist Theory and the Sociology of Human Reproduction', *Sociology of Health and Illness*, 18 (1), 17–44.

Australian Department of Health and Ageing (2008) *Development of a National Men's Health Policy: Information Paper*, at: www.health.gov.au/internet/main/publishing.nsf/Content/mhip-09, accessed 15 May 2009.

Australian Bureau of Statistics, Australian Institute of Health and Welfare (2008) *The Health and Welfare of Australia's Aboriginal and Torres Strait Islander Peoples 2008* (Canberra: Australian Institute of Health and Welfare and the Australian Bureau of Statistics).

Australian Institute of Health and Welfare (2009) *Health and Community Services Labour Force*, Catalogue No. HWL 43, Canberra.

Banks, I. (2004) 'New Models of Providing Men with Health Care', *Journal of Men's Health and Gender*, 1 (2–3), 155–8.

Carney, M., F. Buttell and D. Dutton (2007) 'Women who Perpetrate Intimate Partner Violence: A Review of the Literature with Recommendations for Treatment', *Aggression and Violent Behavior*, 12, 108–15.

Collinson, D. L. and J. Hearn (2005) 'Men and Masculinities in Work, Organizations and Management', in M. Kimmel, J. Hearn and R. Connell (eds), *Handbook of Studies on Men and Masculinities* (Thousand Oaks: Sage), 289–310.

Connell, R. (2002) *Gender* (Cambridge: Polity Press).

Connell, R., T. Schofield, L. Walker and R. Wood (1999) *Men's Health: A Research Agenda and Background Report* (Canberra: Commonwealth Department of Health and Aged Care).

Courtenay, W. (2002) 'A Global Perspective on the Field of Men's Health: An Editorial', *International Journal of Men's Health*, 1 (1), 1–13.

Desai, S. and L. E. Saltzman (2001) 'Measurement Issues for Violence against Women', in C. M. Renzetti, J. L. Edleson and R. K. Bergen (eds), *Sourcebook on Violence Against Women* (Thousand Oaks: Sage), 35–52.

Dobash, R. E. and R. P. Dobash (2004) 'Women's Violence to Men in Intimate Relationships: Working on a Puzzle', *British Journal of Criminology*, 44 (3), 324–49.

Duncan, A. K. and J. T. Hays (2005) 'The Development of a Men's Health Center at an Integrated Academic Health Center', *Journal of Men's Health and Gender*, 2 (1), 17–20.

Emslie, C. and K. Hunt (2008) 'The Weaker Sex? Exploring Lay Understandings of Gender Differences in Life Expectancy: A Qualitative Study', *Social Science & Medicine*, 67 (5), 808–16.

Galdas, P. M., F. Cheater and P. Marshall (2005) 'Men and Help-seeking Behaviour: Literature Review', *Journal of Advanced Nursing*, 49 (6), 616–23.

Greaves, L. (2007) 'Gender, Equity and Tobacco Control', *Health Sociology Review*, 16 (2), 115–29.

Hämäläinen, P., J. Takala and K. J. Sareela (2007) 'Global Estimates of Fatal Work-related Diseases', *American Journal of Industrial Medicine*, 50 (1), 28–41.

Irish Department of Health and Children (2008) *National Men's Health Policy 2008–2013: Working with Men in Ireland to Achieve Optimum Health and Wellbeing* (Dublin: Irish Department of Health and Children).

Jalmert, L. (2003) 'The Role of Men and Boys in Achieving Gender Equality: Some Swedish and Scandinavian Experiences', paper presented at the expert group meeting, 'The Role of Men and Boys in Achieving Gender', organized by the UN Division for the Advancement of Women, Department of Economic Affairs, Brasilia, Brazil, 21–24 October 2003, at: www.un.org/womenwatch/daw/egm/men-boys2003/documents.html, accessed 3 October 2009.

Johnstone, R. (2004) 'Rethinking OHS Enforcement', in L. Bluff, N. Gunningham and R. Johnstone (eds), *OHS Regulation for a Changing World of Work* (Sydney: Federation Press), 146–78.

Lang, J., A. Greig and R. Connell (2008) *Women 2000 and Beyond: The Role of Men and Boys in Achieving Gender Equality* (New York: UN Division for the Advancement of Women, Department of Economic and Social Affairs).

Legato, M. J. (ed.) (2004) *Principles of Gender-Specific Medicine, Vol. 1 and 2* (New York: Elsevier Academic Press).

Liamputtong, P. and D. Ezzy (2005) *Qualitative Research Methods*, Second Edition (Melbourne: Oxford University Press).

Miller, V. M. (2005) 'Book Review: Principles of Gender-specific Medicine, Vol. 1 and Vol. 2', *The Physiologist*, 48 (2), 67.

Moore, M. (1996) *Women in the Mines: Stories of Life and Work* (New York: Twayne Publishers).

Mylett, T. and R. Markey (2007) 'Worker Participation in OHS in New South Wales (Australia) and New Zealand: Methods and Implications', *Employment Relations Record*, 7 (2), 15–30.

Paap, K. (2006) *Working Construction: Why White Working-class Men Put Themselves and the Labor Movement in Harm's Way* (New York: Cornell University Press).

Pini, B. and R. Mayes (2008) 'Women and Mining in Contemporary Australia: An Exploratory Study', Annual Conference of the Australian Sociological Association 2008, 2 December 2008 (Melbourne: TASA), at: www.tasa.org.au/conferences/ conferencepapers08/rural.html, accessed 30 September 2009.

Roy, K. and A. Chaudhuri (2008) 'Influence of Socioeconomic Status, Wealth and Financial Empowerment on Gender Differences in Health and Healthcare Utilization in Later Life: Evidence from India', *Social Science & Medicine*, 66 (9), 1951–62.

Saurel-Cubizolles, M. J., J. F. Chastang, G. Menvielle, A. Leclerc and D. Luce for the EDISC group (2009) 'Social Inequalities in Mortality by Cause among Men and Women in France', *Journal of Epidemiology and Community Health*, 63 (3), 197–202.

Schofield, T. (2004) *Boutique Health?: Gender and Equity in Health Policy*, Australian Health Policy Institute, Commissioned Paper Series 2004/08 (Sydney: University of Sydney).

Schofield, T. (2009a) 'Workplace Health', in J. Germov (ed.), *Second Opinion: An Introduction to Health Sociology*, Fourth Edition (Melbourne: Oxford University Press), 111–29.

Schofield, T. (2009b) 'Gendered Organisational Dynamics: The Elephant in the Room for Australian Allied Health Workforce Policy and Planning?', *Journal of Sociology*, 45 (4), 1–18.

Schofield, T., R. Connell, L. Walker and J. F. Wood (2000) 'Understanding Men's Health and Illness: A Gender-relations Approach to Policy, Research, and Practice', *Journal of American College Health*, 48 (6), 247–56.

Smith, J. A. and S. Robertson (2008) 'Men's Health Promotion: A New Frontier in Australia and the UK?', *Health Promotion International*, 23 (3), 283–9.

Straus, M. A. (2008) 'Dominance and Symmetry in Partner Violence by Male and Female University Students in 32 Nations', *Children and Youth Services Review*, 30, 252–75.

United Nations (2000) *Beijing Declaration and Platform for Action with the Beijing+5, Political Declaration and Outcome Document* (DPI/1766/Rev.1) (New York: UN Department of Public Information).

US Federal Bureau of Prisons (2009) *Quick Facts about the Bureau of Prisons*, at: www.bop.gov/news/quick.jsp, accessed 15 May 2009.

US Office of Men's Health (2009) *Fact Sheet*, at: www.menshealthpolicy.com/OMH/fact Sheet.html, accessed 15 May 2009.

West, C. and D. H. Zimmerman (1987) 'Doing Gender', *Gender and Society*, 1 (2), 125–51.

White, R. (2008) 'Class Analysis and the Crime Problem', in T. Anthony and C. Cuneen (eds), *The Critical Criminology Companion* (Sydney: Hawkins Press), 30–42.

Young, I. M. (1997) *Intersecting Voices: Dilemmas of Gender, Political Philosophy and Policy* (Princeton: Princeton University Press).

17
The Healthcare Needs of Gay and Lesbian Patients

Jane Edwards

Introduction

A wealth of evidence documents non-heterosexuals' disadvantaged health status and healthcare access (Jillson, 2002; Sandfort et al., 2006; Tjepkema, 2008). While gender has become accepted as a 'routine' indicator of health inequality among the heterosexual population, non-heterosexuals' experience remains largely invisible (Leonard, 2002; NHS Scotland, 2003; Rogers et al., 2005; Wang et al., 2007). This is often (justly) attributed to the heterosexism and homophobia that characterize even societies considered otherwise liberal (such as Australia, the UK, Canada and western European nations). Yet the ways in which gender, sexuality and embodiment have been theorized are important, if less obvious, influences veiling the healthcare needs of non-heterosexuals.

This chapter outlines the way the conceptualization of gender and sexuality by biomedicine within women's health and in the men's health movement (in both its 'straight' and gay manifestations) has contributed to non-heterosexuals' relative invisibility. Data on the health status of non-heterosexuals are then reviewed; it must be noted that they are derived primarily from western settings, so caution must be exercised in extrapolation to other settings. The complexities of collecting and interpreting data on non-heterosexuals' health are outlined. Next, the chapter discusses the way gender and sexuality interacts to mediate health status. The chapter then describes the ways in which gender and sexuality combine to produce health needs that are different from those of heterosexuals. It also discusses the way in which different sub-groups in the non-heterosexual population have unique healthcare needs that often remain unrecognized. The range of factors that are barriers to healthcare access for non-heterosexuals are then outlined and their implications for the health status of this population are considered. Issues associated with non-heterosexuals receiving appropriate and acceptable care are also canvassed. The chapter also considers the complex strategies non-heterosexuals employ in negotiating healthcare and concludes with some strategies to improve healthcare provision.

Why has non-heterosexual health been invisible?

Biomedical epistemology formulated a received truth: gender is a biological state pivoting on the difference between men and women (Lacquer, 1990). While this view has been challenged in recent decades and exercises less hegemony than previously, it retains an insidious influence on thinking about gender and health (Kuhlmann, 2009; Schofield, 2008). The tethering of gender to embodiment shrouded the existence of gendered identities other than heterosexual men and women and cemented medicine's fixation with biology. Because medical epistemology and practice concentrate on the body and its pathologies, neglecting the life lived in and through that body (much less its socio-cultural context), all women are assumed to share a common biology and, therefore, to share the same health issues and needs (McDonald et al., 2003; McNair, 2003). An Australian general practitioner articulated this sensibility; 'lesbian women are just the same as any other women' (cited in McNair, 2008: 377).

The women's health movement (WHM), beginning in the late 1960s, deracinated the medical formulation of 'gender as embodiment'. It demonstrated that gender entails identities and behavioural scripts, social roles and cultural expectations, a system of power relations and access to resources that constitute and constrain what it means to be a woman (or, by implication, a man). Further, the women's health movement revealed how profoundly all these dimensions of gender have shaped women's experience of health and healthcare. Access to the labour market and education, socio-economic status, the domestic division of labour and other caring responsibilities profoundly influence women's health (Annandale and Hunt, 2000). This perspective on gender is therefore isomorphic with a paradigm that holds that morbidity and mortality have their roots in social relationships. Despite expanding the understanding of gender's influence on health status, the WHM nevertheless focused on gender as difference. This binary view inadvertently entrenched heterosexism, contributing to the ongoing obscurity of non-heterosexual women's needs (Annandale and Riska, 2009). Gender, not sexuality, was the trump card of the movement. Even a document that was a high-water mark for the women's health movement in Australia confidently asserted: 'Lesbian women in Australia have similar health needs to other women' (Commonwealth of Australia, 1989: 19).

Somewhat different factors contributed to the relative invisibility of non-heterosexual men's gendered health needs. An embryonic gay men's health movement existed prior to the onset of the HIV/AIDS pandemic in the 1980s.

Table 17.1   Areas of focus and areas of neglect in the health of non-heterosexual women and men

Group	Domain of focus	Domain neglected
Non-heterosexual women	Gender	Sexuality
Non-heterosexual men	Sexuality/biology	Gender

It was spawned by gay liberation, but drew much of its inspiration, assumptions and emphases from feminism; it generated a nascent analysis of the link between the social position of gay men (that is, their gendered existence) and their health, but it was stunted by the emergence of HIV/AIDS (Beehler, 2001; Scarce, 2000). This is because HIV/AIDS has been taken as the sum of non-heterosexual men's health issues; a single disease, understood through a thoroughly sexualized prism, defines their health (Beehler 2001; Sandfort et al., 2006; Scarce, 2000; NHS Scotland, 2003).

It has only recently been discovered that men, too, have a gender (Annandale and Riska, 2009). The 'mainstream' men's health movement (MHM), however, has done little to advance understanding of its impact on men's health. Reinstating a view of gender as mere sexual difference, it has concentrated on biomedical response to men's ailments and the structures shaping men's health are largely neglected (Hayes, 2003; Schofield, 2008; see also Chapter 16 by Schofield). This myopia is compounded by a focus on a narrow range of issues, notably sexual health (Annandale and Riska, 2009). To the extent that non-physical dimensions of men's health figure on the MHM's agenda, it conceptualizes them as psychological pathology (Annandale and Riska, 2009; Hayes 2003). While the acknowledgment of non-physical issues is laudable, rendering them psychological ailments both individualizes them and masks the influence of gender as a system of social relations. The gay men's health movement has pivoted on HIV/AIDS, spotlighting sexuality and obscuring gender. The mainstream men's health movement has focused on individual pathology, also sidelining gender. The influences shaping the invisibility of the health needs of non-heterosexual men and women are encapsulated in Table 17.1.

The health of non-heterosexual men and women

A gendered (and heterosexist) social order influences the status people are accorded, the power they can exercise and the life-chances open to them (Lorber and Moore, 2002). Lorber (1994) demonstrates that institutions, such as the family, medicine and even the economy and the polity are gendered. They are less obviously, but no less profoundly, heterosexed (Callahan et al., 2007). Moreover, gender is not a *thing*, in the way that binary understandings might imply; it is a *system* of social relations that hierarchically separate people into different gendered statuses. Contemporary western societies recognize four gendered subjectivities: heterosexual man; heterosexual woman; gay man and lesbian woman (Lorber, 1994). Other gendered subjectivities are possible, as Lorber (1994) points out. However, their existence is less visible and they are regarded with even less legitimacy than lesbians and gay men. The health of bisexuals, transgender and intersex individuals points to the need to expand the category of gender. This chapter will, for the most part, use the term 'non-heterosexual' as an inclusive term for same-sex-attracted people. When discussing people who claim an identity as gay or lesbian, however, these terms are employed. 'Non-heterosexual', however, may not accurately reflect the experience of transgender and intersex people; accordingly the term 'non-normative gender' is used. The acronym LGBTI (lesbian, gay, bisexual, transgender and intersex) is used to draw attention to diverse health and healthcare needs, not to suggest that it is a homogenous population.

Evidence indicates that non-heterosexuals and people of non-normative gender face particular challenges to their health and to accessing appropriate healthcare. The discrimination they experience gives rise to some common issues. In addition, sexual orientation and gender interact with social and biological processes to produce particular patterns of health and specific healthcare needs among lesbians, gay men, bisexuals, transgender and intersex (LGBTI) individuals (Leonard, 2002). Sandfort and colleagues (2006) propose three pathways that might mediate minority sexuality and/or non-normative gender, on the one hand, and poor health status on the other. One is via socially inflicted trauma due to heterosexism or flagrant discrimination. Another is inadequate use of health services and the final is a possible link between 'gay cultures' and adverse health outcomes, such as drug use among some non-heterosexual men (Sandfort et al., 2006) or alcohol use among non-heterosexual women (Hunt and Fish, 2008).

Non-heterosexual women

Population-based data on the physical health of non-heterosexual women are relatively scarce; they also exhibit some variance, which may reflect method-ological, conceptual and contextual differences. For instance, much of the research on non-heterosexual populations uses convenience samples, making generalization problematic (Sandfort et al., 2006). Studies frequently fail to differentiate between gay men and lesbians, on the one hand, and bisexual, transgender and intersex people on the other; despite emerging recognition that bisexual, transgender and intersex people have distinctive health issues (Bakker et al., 2006; Gay and Lesbian Medical Association and LGBT Experts, 2001; Pitts et al., 2006). Furthermore, some studies define sexual orientation by identity (whether an individual labels themselves as lesbian or heterosexual, for instance), while others focus on behaviour (for example, people who define themselves as heterosexual but engage in same-sex activity). Different findings may also reflect the social context in which study participants live. Sandfort and colleagues (2006) conjecture that, in some settings, the discrimination directed towards minority gender and sexual identities may influence some health-related behaviours. For instance, illiberal social environments might be conducive to higher levels of alcohol and tobacco consumption as a means of coping with stigma. This association is far from demonstrated but warrants further investigation.

Notwithstanding these minor incongruities, data from a range of settings suggest non-heterosexual women face greater risks to their health than their heterosexual counterparts. Lower consumption of fruit and vegetables has been noted (Jillson, 2002). Higher rates of obesity are widely documented (Cochran et al., 2001; Diamant and Wold, 2003; Gay and Lesbian Medical Association and LGBT Experts, 2001; Pitts et al., 2006). Behaviours conducive to poor health outcomes appear to be more frequent among non-heterosexual women. They are more likely to consume tobacco than other women (Cochran et al., 2001; Hunt and Fish, 2008; Pitts et al., 2006). However, evidence from a Dutch survey does not support this association (Sandfort et al., 2006). Higher rates of alcohol consumption have also been ubiquitously reported (Cochran et al., 2001: 593; Hunt and Fish, 2008; Pitts et al., 2006; Sandfort et al., 2006). These data suggest elevated risk levels for heart disease and some data do document a higher prevalence (Diamant and Wold, 2003; Gay and Lesbian Medical Association and LGBT Experts, 2001). It is not possible to know whether similar associations exist for non-heterosexual women in non-western settings because of lack of data.

Cancer registers in most countries do not include sexual and gender orientation, making it difficult to accurately assess differences in rates between women. However, non-heterosexual women face some distinctive risk factors for certain cancers. Lower rates of childbearing and oral contraceptive use, together with use of fertility drugs, heightens their risk of ovarian cancer (Cochran et al., 2001; Gay and Lesbian Medical Association and LGBT Experts, 2001). While the evidence about whether non-heterosexual women have higher rates of breast cancer is equivocal, they do face elevated risks, primarily due to lower rates of childbearing and higher alcohol intake (Cochran et al., 2001; Gay and Lesbian Medical Association and LGBT Experts, 2001).

Generally, non-heterosexual women have lower levels of self-reported good health than their heterosexual peers (Diamant and Wold, 2003; Pitts et al., 2006; Sandfort et al., 2006). Cochran and Mays (2007) posit that this may be associated with higher levels of psycho-emotional distress among non-heterosexual women. However, in their Dutch study, Sandfort and colleagues (2006) controlled for mental health status and a higher proportion of non-heterosexual women still reported elevated levels of chronic ailments. Poorer mental health among non-heterosexual women has been ubiquitously documented, particularly in relation to mood and anxiety disorders, in North America (Cochrane and Mays, 2007), England (Hunt and Fish, 2008), the Netherlands (Sandfort et al., 2006), Australia (Pitts et al., 2006), Scotland (NHS Scotland, 2003) and Canada (Tjepkema, 2008). Non-heterosexuals are more likely than other women to be taking medication for depression (Diamant and Wold, 2003). Eating disorders and self-harming practices are more common among non-heterosexual women (Hunt and Fish, 2008). Attempted suicide is also much more frequent (Jillson, 2002).

Non-heterosexual men

Not surprisingly, HIV/AIDS has dominated thought and practice about the health of gay men (Beehler, 2001; Sandfort et al., 2006; Scarce, 2000). Despite a period of declining prevalence, many countries are now reporting increased incidence of HIV (Guy et al, 2007). Non-heterosexual men also face higher risks of hepatitis B and C, are at elevated risk of anal cancer, and have higher rates of lymphoma (Gay and Lesbian Medical Association and LGBT Experts, 2001). They are also more likely to have elevated cholesterol and glucose levels and to be hypertensive than men in general (Wang et al., 2007). Rates of unsafe alcohol consumption are higher for non-heterosexual men and they are more likely to consume tobacco (Gay and Lesbian Medical Association and LGBT Experts, 2001; Wang et al., 2007). Sandfort and colleagues (2006), however, did not find associations between non-heterosexuality and tobacco and alcohol consumption in their Dutch study. Evidence does suggest that gay men are more likely to consume a range of illicit substances than the general male population (Gay and Lesbian Medical Association and LGBT Experts, 2001; Scotland NHS, 2003; Wang et al., 2007). Young gay men on both sides of the Atlantic are also more likely to have a negative body image and to develop eating disorders, which may persist into adulthood (Gay and Lesbian Medical Association and LGBT Experts, 2001; NHS Scotland, 2003).

As is the case for non-heterosexual women, non-heterosexual men's self-reported health status is worse than their straight counterparts; a finding replicated in diverse settings (see Pitts et al., 2006; Sandfort et al., 2006; Tjepkema, 2008; Wang et al., 2007). Non-heterosexual men report a greater prevalence of chronic complaints than their heterosexual counterparts even when controlling for mental health status (Sandfort et al., 2006). They also have higher levels of mental health problems, notably depression and anxiety. This finding is also replicated in numerous locations: Switzerland (Wang, 2007); North America (Jillson, 2002); the Netherlands (Bakker et al., 2006); Scotland (NHS, 2003); Canada (Tjepkema, 2008); and Australia (Pitts et al., 2006). US data indicate that non-heterosexual men are six times as likely to attempt suicide as their heterosexual peers (Jillson, 2002).

Transgender individuals appear to be at greater risk of a number of serious health conditions, including HIV/AIDS, being victims of violence, substance abuse and suicide (Jillson, 2002). They also experience disproportionately high rates of mental health problems (Jillson, 2002; Pitts et al., 2006; Scotland NHS, 2003). The American Public Health Association recommends recognizing transgender persons as a distinct group (Gay and Lesbian Medical Association and LGBT Experts, 2001). Some studies report that bisexuals' self-reported health status is worse than that of other groups and that they have more unmet health needs. Tjepkema (2008) found that bisexual women were least likely to have had screening for breast or cervical cancer in Canada. Another study (Diamant et al., 2000) suggests that, in the USA, bisexual women are the most likely group to not have a regular source of healthcare. Bisexual women and men also report high levels of psychological distress (Cochran and Mays, 2007; Tjepkema, 2008).

The healthcare needs of non-heterosexuals

These data reveal that gender and sexuality mediate health status. They also suggest many of the ailments afflicting non-heterosexuals, bisexuals and transgender people have their genesis in a heterosexist social order. This underscores the need to keep in play a 'social determinants of health' approach that includes gender and sexuality. These data emphasize the need to expand the repertoire of gender beyond bimodal renderings and to consider the ways these interact with various sexualities. Non-heterosexual women's needs have received most scholarly attention. Yet, too often, sexuality is regarded as an 'add-on' to gender and non-heterosexual women's health has frequently been reduced to a formula: gender + minority sexuality = compounded disadvantage. While acknowledging the disadvantage non-heterosexual women encounter, this glosses over the distinctive ways in which sexuality influences access to care, the quality of the care received and the complex engagement with health professionals. Non-heterosexual women have distinctive healthcare needs and experiences by virtue of being both women and non-heterosexual. Gay men, bisexuals, transgender and intersex people are also likely to have distinctive health and healthcare needs that result from the way gender and sexuality configure for each of them.

A perspective that regards non-heterosexual women (or, by implication, other sexual and gender minority groups) as just 'more disadvantaged' also overlooks the way legal constraints shape access to certain services (assisted reproduction or gender reassignment, for example) and the fact that certain benefits that go to heterosexual partnerships and families may be denied to the partners and families of non-heterosexuals and people of non-normative gender (Jillson, 2002). These factors place many non-heterosexuals and transgender and intersex people in a much more ambivalent relationship to medicine. Women may need assisted reproduction to become pregnant even if they are not infertile and transgender and intersex individuals may depend on medical intervention to have their preferred gender legally recognized. Furthermore, non-heterosexuals and people of non-normative gender are likely to have distinctive psycho-social needs from the mainstream population, such as the inclusion of partners in healthcare, recognition of a variety of family forms, specific needs following relationship break-down or the death of a partner, and having a gender legally documented (Hunt and Fish, 2008; Jillson, 2002; Pitts et al., 2006). Grief and bereavement are likely to be particular issues for non-heterosexual men in light of HIV/AIDS (Scotland NHS, 2003).

Healthcare access and utilization

Institutional barriers to service

Non-heterosexual women are less likely than heterosexual women to have health insurance, a significant barrier to healthcare access in the USA (Cochran et al., 2001; Diamant, 2000; Jillson, 2002). Little is known about levels of health insurance among non-heterosexual men. Transgender people in North America are especially prone to being uninsured or being underinsured, something which is concerning in view of the high cost of gender reassignment (Jillson, 2002). However, even where universal insurance exists, heterosexism and homophobia are formidable barriers to service utilization (Beehler, 2001; Mathieson et al., 2002). Heterosexism and homophobia are systemic factors, not just individual practices. For example, in North America, the UK and Australia it is legal, or has been until recently, to deny access to care to the partners of same-sex patients and to exclude them from decision-making (Hunt and Fish, 2008; Jillson, 2002; Pitts et al., 2006). Until recently, a majority of privately funded fertility clinics in the UK were unwilling to provide services to non-heterosexual women; the fact that discriminatory attitudes and behaviours may be illegal does not mean they are not exercised (Hunt and Fish, 2008; Scotland NHS, 2003).

Service utilization

Lower levels of health service use by non-heterosexual women are widely documented (Diamant and Wold, 2003; Hunt and Fish, 2008; Jillson, 2002; McNair, 2003). Women may forgo a service or delay using it until the problem can no longer be avoided, frequently intensifying its severity (Mathieson et al., 2002). The capacity to utilize services in a timely fashion is itself a criterion of equitable access (Jillson, 2002). Further, non-heterosexual women are less likely to have a regular healthcare provider, which predicts lower levels of service use and is also likely to thwart continuity of care (Jillson, 2002). Tjepkema (2008) found that lesbians and bisexuals in Canada were more likely than heterosexual women to have had an unmet healthcare need in the previous year.

Non-heterosexual women make less use of screening services for common forms of malignancy – notably cervical and breast cancers – despite having equivalent or elevated risks (Cochran et al., 2001; Hunt and Fish, 2008; Tjepkema, 2008). Notwithstanding their risk of heart disease, they are less likely than their heterosexual peers to have lipid and cholesterol screening (Jillson, 2002; McNair, 2003). While non-heterosexual women make less use of services to treat or prevent physical ailments, they are ubiquitously documented to make greater use of mental health services (Bakker et al., 2006; Pitts et al., 2006; Tjepkema, 2008).

Less attention is given to the experiences and needs of non-heterosexual men than women for issues other than HIV/AIDS. Further, many reports do not disaggregate the data on men and women and report results for LGBTI populations (see, for example, Gay and Lesbian Medical Association and LGBT Experts, 2001; Jillson, 2002; Leonard, 2002). This fails to distinguish the specific experiences and needs of non-heterosexual men. For instance, disparate healthcare settings document higher levels of service use by non-heterosexual men than either heterosexual men or non-heterosexual women. Thus non-heterosexual men in both the USA and the Netherlands were more likely to have seen a family physician or a specialist in the past 12 months for physical complaints (Bakker et al., 2006; Tjepkema, 2008). In Canada, non-heterosexual men were also more likely to have seen a psychologist, a nurse or an alternative care provider and to have participated in self-help groups (Tjepkema, 2008). Non-heterosexual men were just as likely as their heterosexual counterparts to have a regular service provider, unlike non-heterosexual women. This difference does not reflect socio-demographic variables or health status; it may reflect the salience of HIV for non-heterosexual men, making them more likely to seek preventive services and to be open about their sexuality (Tjepkema, 2008).

Bakker and colleagues (2006) found that greater use of health services by non-heterosexual men in the Netherlands was not related to HIV (the number of HIV-positive men in their sample was small, however, and caution should be exercised in interpreting this result). The role of HIV in this apparently greater use of health services is an issue for conjecture. Nevertheless, it points to the fact that little is known about whether non-heterosexual men's help-seeking is related to differences in health status, their attitudes to service utilization or socio-cultural factors that influence help-seeking. Greater use of mental health services by non-heterosexual men has been observed in a number of settings, but this too may be influenced by a range of factors, including HIV status (Bakker et al., 2006; Pitts et al., 2006; Tjepkema, 2008). Bakker and colleagues (2006) found no difference between the degree of confidence that non-heterosexual and heterosexual Dutch men had in the care they received. This contrasts with a lack of confidence in, and dissatisfaction with, care reported by non-heterosexual men in the USA (Bakker et al., 2006; Tjepkema, 2008).

This may reflect contextual and cultural factors and reveals the need to be sensitive to local context, despite the effects of globalization.

Interaction with healthcare providers

Tjepkema (2008) notes that attitudes to same-sex attraction are more important to non-heterosexual women than non-heterosexual men in choosing a doctor. This may be explained by Beehler's finding that non-heterosexual men do not regard 'coming-out' to healthcare providers with the same degree of risk as women (Beehler, 2001). Nevertheless, both groups attach importance to the relationship they have with practitioners and engage in active attempts to find practitioners who are 'friendly' to non-heterosexuals. Research shows that men and women use a referral network, usually among their non-heterosexual peers, to identify acceptable service providers (Beehler, 2001; Edwards and van Roekel, 2009). Transgender people also use such networks to locate knowledgeable and non-discriminatory service providers (Jillson, 2002). However, these strategies assume the availability of friendly providers. This may be unwarranted in some contexts, for example, rural settings or those where same-sex activity is illegal. Further, such techniques depend on access to a network of knowledgeable people and it is unlikely that all non-heterosexual and non-normative gendered people will be linked to such relationships, particularly in situations of marked discrimination.

The challenges to accessing care do not stop at a clinician's doorway. Non-heterosexual people exercise a vigilant, yet creative, agency in their interaction with service providers. Many non-heterosexuals would like their doctors to know about their sexuality, yet do not disclose it fearing it would compromise the quality of the care they receive (Beehler, 2001; Pitts et al., 2006). Information management is a central component of interaction with health professionals and men and women employ complex strategies to control information about themselves. Pitts and colleagues (2006) found that about two thirds of their (male and female) Australian respondents believed that their regular GP knew about their gender/sexual identity and one fifth believed that their GP did not know. Fifty per cent of non-heterosexual women in a UK study had not told their GP of their sexuality (Hunt and Fish, 2008). Levels of disclosure are very low among transgender and intersex individuals (Pitts et al., 2008). Few patients, it would appear, directly disclose their sexuality or gender orientation in healthcare settings. This may result in sub-optimal care because important information is withheld. Further, being 'out' to healthcare providers predicts more regular use of health services, so non-disclosure might also mitigate continuity of care (Tjepkema, 2008). The following two vignettes provide a window on some situations that might easily go unnoticed by health professionals.

Vignette 1

Emma is a 70-year-old woman. She has lived with her partner, Fiona, for the past 30 years. The nature of their relationship was not disclosed to friends or family; they merely said that they had decided to share a house after the end of the heterosexual marriages in which each of them had been involved. Recently, Fiona suddenly died and Emma is devastated. She feels she cannot share her grief with anyone. In addition, she is not sure if she has any legal claim to Fiona's estate; the house was in Fiona's name and her family now want it sold. Emma would like advice but this means publicly acknowledging the nature of her relationship with Fiona. Emma is sleeping poorly, has little appetite and is losing weight.

- What actual or potential health issues are posed by this scenario?
- What kinds of questions should a health professional ask of Emma to adequately understand her situation?
- What advice should health professionals give Emma?

Vignette 2

Michael is a first-generation immigrant. He is 39 years old, married to Hannah and has three teenage children. Michael loves his wife and children and feels enmeshed in his ethnic community. However, he experiences enormous guilt over the fact that he periodically has sex with other men, often without using a condom. His same-sex activity is frequently associated with illegal drug use. Michael lives in dread that his family, friends and community will discover his sexual activity with other men and he fears he may have acquired a sexually transmissible infection, but doesn't know to whom he should turn. He feels trapped.

- What are the actual or potential health issues posed by this scenario?
- What kinds of questions should a health professional ask of Michael to respond adequately to his situation?
- What advice should health professionals give Michael?

Acceptable, not just accessible, care

Competent and respectful care is a prominent concern for non-heterosexuals and people of non-normative gender. Discriminatory attitudes on the part of healthcare professionals are reported by non-heterosexual women and men in many contexts (Beehler, 2001; Jillson, 2002; Hunt and Fish, 2008; Mathieson et al., 2002; Scotland NHS, 2003). Fish and Hunt (2008) report that only 30 per cent of the women who disclosed their sexuality in their UK study felt that the practitioner refrained from making inappropriate comments and only 10 per cent felt that their partner was really included in the consultation process. Transgender individuals report high levels of insensitive and disrespectful attitudes and behaviour on the part of health professionals (Jillson, 2002; Scotland NHS, 2003) and there are instances of gay men and transgender people being denied services (Jillson, 2002).

Non-heterosexual women report being asked inappropriate questions by practitioners acting on heterosexist assumptions. When women acknowledge being sexually active, they are frequently railed with questions about contraceptive use and pregnancy (Hunt and Fish, 2008). Non-heterosexual men also report being inappropriately treated because of heterosexist presumptions (Beehler, 2001). The presumption of heterosexuality probably underpins widespread lack of knowledge about the healthcare needs of non-heterosexuals, especially those of women. For instance, there is an unfounded presumption that non-heterosexual women are not at risk of cervical cancer (McNair, 2003). Hunt and Fish (2008) found that 20 per cent of their UK respondents were told they were not at risk of cervical cancer and, more alarmingly, two per cent had been refused a test. The generally lower rate of cervical cancer screening noted among non-heterosexual women may be in part prompted by this belief. Likewise, it is often falsely assumed that non-heterosexual women are not at risk of sexually transmissible diseases and they are under-tested (Hunt and Fish, 2008; Mathieson et al., 2002; McNair, 2003). It may in fact be the case that they are at elevated risk for certain infections (Scotland NHS, 2003). Non-heterosexual men also complain that many practitioners are ignorant about their specific health needs, particularly HIV transmission, testing and management (Beehler, 2001). While health professionals are not well-informed about the healthcare needs of non-heterosexual women and men, they display a monumental ignorance about transgender and intersex populations (Jillson, 2002; Scotland NHS, 2003).

Conclusion

This chapter has sought to explain the health status of non-heterosexuals and to discuss the issues associated with their ability to access care that is appropriate and acceptable. I have argued for a gendered perspective that encapsulates an emphasis on the social production of ill-health to adequately understand and respond to non-heterosexuals' needs. In the conclusion I direct attention towards the way forward. A number of suggestions are frequently made to improve healthcare delivery to non-heterosexuals and people of gender diversity. These are outlined in Table 17.2.

Table 17.2   Steps to improve healthcare for LGBTI populations

Focus of attention	Strategies
Changed healthcare provider behaviour	Healthcare providers educated about the needs of LGBTI individuals
	Healthcare providers educated about the difference between: 1) identity and behaviour; 2) gender and sexual orientation, especially for transgender people
	Healthcare providers educated about use of inclusive language
Changed health service practice and culture	Visual cues alerting patients that they can safely discuss same-sex and transgender issues are provided; brochures and posters, for example
	Targeted services and programmes for LGBTI populations
	Standards for clinically competent care of LGBTI populations are developed and implemented
	Standards for culturally competent care to LGBTI populations are developed and implemented
	LGBTI communities are involved in the development of standards

Improving the knowledge and behaviour of practitioners and enhancing the capacities of health services are important steps. A gendered perspective on health highlights the social influences on health status and healthcare access; however, an adequate response to social determinants requires services that respond to the complexity of patient's circumstances. The preponderance of mental health problems points to the difficulties of being members of highly stigmatized minority groups (Leonard, 2002; Sandfort et al., 2006). Feminists long ago complained that the convoluted problems women bought to practitioner's doors were all too often only treated with a prescription for medication (Lorber and Moore, 2002). Empirical investigation is needed on this point, but it is plausible that the complex psycho-social needs of non-heterosexuals and people of non-normative gender are treated in similarly reductionist ways.

An important factor likely to mitigate adequate health service response is the economics of healthcare in settings in which fee-for-service practice operate. Rogers and colleagues (2005) report from their Australian research that the long consultations needed to comprehensively respond to the complex needs of non-heterosexual men resulted in significantly lower income levels (about 35 per cent) for the practice concerned and its doctors. It is unlikely that most fee-for-service settings could absorb income reductions of this magnitude (Rogers et al., 2005). The overwhelming emphasis placed on efficiency and outputs under neoliberal-inspired governance make it unlikely that even publicly funded services could routinely provide the kind of comprehensive, yet expensive, care that responds adequately to the complex issues that many non-heterosexual and people of non-normative gender bring to practitioners. Improving the competency of practitioners and settings standards for practice are important initiatives that deserve to be enacted. Advocating for forms of service delivery that respond to the complex gendered needs of LGBTI people is likely to meet with less immediate success but should remain an integral part of the intellectual and political strategies directed at reforming health services.

Summary

- The health and healthcare needs of non-heterosexual people are profoundly influenced by a social order that, even in liberal settings, is heteronormative and heterosexist.
- Sexuality should not be an 'add-on' to gender; the interaction of gender and sexuality needs to be considered to ensure that the distinctive needs of non-heterosexuals are made visible.
- The LGBTI population is not a homogenous one. The existence of different groups with distinct needs must be acknowledged.
- Access to care is insufficient to address the needs of non-heterosexuals; services must also be appropriate and acceptable if the complex health needs of LGBTI people are satisfactorily to be addressed.

Key reading

Bakker, F. F, T. Sandfort, I. Vanwesenbeeck, H. Lindert and G. Westert (2006) 'Do Homosexual Persons Use Healthcare Services More Frequently than Heterosexual Persons: Findings from a Dutch Population Survey', *Social Science & Medicine*, 63 (8), 2022–30.

Edwards, J. and H. van Roekel (2009) 'Gender, Sexuality and Embodiment: Access to and Experience of Healthcare by Same-sex Attracted Women in Australia', *Current Sociology*, 57 (2), 193–210.

Hunt, R. and J. Fish (2008) *Prescription for Change: Lesbian and Bisexual Women's Health Check 2000*, at: www.stonewall.org.uk, accessed 22 March 2009.

Jillson, I. (2002) 'Opening Closed Doors: Improving Access to Quality Health Services for LGBT Populations', *Clinical Research and Regulatory Affairs*, 19 (2/3), 153–90.

References

Annandale, E. and K. Hunt (2000) 'Gender Inequalities in Health: Research at the Crossroads', in E. Annandale and K. Hunt (eds), *Gender Inequalities in Health* (Buckingham: Open University Press), 1–35.

Annandale, E. and E. Riska (2009) 'New Connections: Towards a Gender-inclusive Approach to Women's and Men's Health', *Current Sociology*, 57 (2), 123–33.

Bakker, F. F, T. Sandfort, I. Vanwesenbeeck, H. Lindert and G. Westert (2006) 'Do Homosexual Persons Use Healthcare Services More Frequently than Heterosexual Persons: Findings from a Dutch Population Survey', *Social Science & Medicine*, 63 (8), 2022–30.

Beehler, G. (2001) 'Confronting the Culture of Medicine: Gay Men's Experiences with Primary Care Physicians', *Journal of the Gay and Lesbian Medical Association*, 5 (4), 135–41.

Callahan, J., B. Mann and S. Ruddick (2007) 'Editors' Introduction to Writing against Heterosexism', *Hypatia*, 22 (1), V11–XV.

Cochran, S., V. Mays, D. Bowen, S. Gage, D. Bybee, S. Roberts, R. Goldstein, A. Robison et al. (2001) 'Cancer-related Risk Indicators and Preventive Screening Behaviours among Lesbians and Bisexual Women', *American Journal of Public Health*, 91 (4), 591–7.

Cochran, S. and V. Mays (2007) 'Physical Health Complaints among Lesbians, Gay Men and Bisexual and Homosexually Experienced Heterosexual Individuals: Results from the California Quality of Life Survey', *American Journal of Public Health*, 97 (11), 2048–55.

Commonwealth of Australia (1989) *National Women's Health Policy: Advancing Women's Health in Australia* (Canberra: Australian Government Publishing Service).

Diamant, A., C. Wold, K. Spritzer and L. Gelberg (2000) 'Health Behaviours, Health Status and Access to and Use of Health Services: A Population Based Study of Lesbian, Bisexual and Heterosexual Women', *Archive of Family Medicine*, 9 (10), 1043–51.

Diamant, A. and C. Wold (2003) 'Sexual Orientation and Variation in Physical and Mental Health Status among Women', *Journal of Women's Health*, 12 (1), 41–9.

Edwards, J. and H. van Roekel (2009) 'Gender, Sexuality and Embodiment: Access to and Experience of Healthcare by Same-sex Attracted Women in Australia', *Current Sociology*, 57 (2), 193–210.

Gay and Lesbian Medical Association and LGBT health experts (2001) *Healthy People 2010: Companion Document for Lesbian, Gay, Bisexual and Transgender (LGBT) Health* (San Francisco: Gay and Lesbian Medical Association), at: www.glma.org, accessed 19 March 2009.

Guy, R., A. McDonald, M. Bartlett, J. Murray, C. Geile, T. Davey, R. Appuhamy, P. Knibbs et al. (2007) 'HIV Diagnoses in Australia: Diverging Epidemics within a Low-prevalence Country', *Medical Journal of Australia*, 187 (8), 437–40.

Hayes, R. (2003) 'Promoting Men's Health: From Pathologies to Partnerships', in P. Liamputtong and H. Gardner (eds), *Health, Social Changes and Communities* (Melbourne: Oxford University Press), 142–62.

Hunt, R. and J. Fish (2008) *Prescription for Change: Lesbian and Bisexual Women's Health Check 2000*, at: www.stonewall.org.uk, accessed 22 March 2009.

Jillson, I. (2002) 'Opening Closed Doors: Improving Access to Quality Health Services for LGBT Populations', *Clinical Research and Regulatory Affairs*, 19 (2/3), 153–90.

Kuhlman, E. (2009) 'From Women's Health to Gender Mainstreaming and Back Again: Linking Feminist Agendas and New Governance in Healthcare', *Current Sociology*, 57 (2), 135–55.

Lacquer, T. (1990) *Making Sex: Body and Gender from the Greeks to Freud* (Cambridge: Harvard University Press).

Leonard, W. (2002) 'Developing a Framework for Understanding Patterns of Health and Illness Specific to Gay, Lesbian, Bisexual, Transgender and Intersex (GLBTI) People', in Department of Human Services (ed.), *What's the Difference? Health Issues of Major Concern to Gay, Lesbian, Bisexual, Transgender and Intersex (GLBTI) Victorians* (Melbourne: Department of Human Services), 3–8.

Lorber, J. (1994) *Paradoxes of Gender* (New Haven: Yale University Press).

Lorber, J. and L. Moore (2002) *Gender and the Social Construction of Illness*, Second Edition (Walnut Creek: Altamira Press).

McDonald, C., M. McIntyre and B. Anderson (2003) 'The View from Somewhere: Locating Lesbian Experience in Women's Health', *Healthcare Women International*, 24 (8), 697–711.

McNair, R. (2003) 'Lesbian Health Inequalities: A Cultural Minority Issue for Health Professionals', *Medical Journal of Australia*, 178 (12), 643–5.

McNair, R. (2008) 'Recognizing the Unique Health-care Needs of Sexual Minorities', *The Lancet*, 371, 377–8.

Mathieson, C., N. Bailey and M. Gurevich (2002) 'Health-care services for Lesbian and Bisexual Women', *Healthcare for Women International*, 23 (2), 185–96.

NHS Scotland (2003) *Towards a Healthier LGBT Scotland*, at: www.lgbthealthscotland. org.au, accessed 22 February 2009.

Pitts, M., A. Smith, A. Mitchell and S. Patel (2006) *Private Lives: A Report on the Health and Well-Being of GLBTI Australians* (Melbourne: Australian Research Centre in Sex, Health and Society, La Trobe University).

Rogers, G., C. Barton, B. Pekarsky, A. Lawless, J. Oddy, R. Hepworth and J. Beilby (2005) 'Caring for a Marginalised Community: The Costs of Engaging with Culture and Complexity', *Medical Journal of Australia*, 183 (10), S59–S63.

Sandfort, T., F. Bakker, F. Schellevis and I. Vanwesenbeeck (2006) 'Sexual Orientation and Mental and Physical Health Status: Findings from a Dutch Population Survey', *American Journal of Public Health*, 96 (6), 1119–25.

Scarce, M. (2000) 'The Second Wave of the Gay Men's Health Movement: Medicalisation and Cooptation as Pitfalls of Progress', *Journal of the Gay and Lesbian Medical Association*, 4 (1), 3–4.

Schofield, T. (2008) 'Gender and Health Inequalities: What Are They and What Can We Do about Them?', *Australian Journal of Social Issues*, 43 (1), 139–57.

Tjepkema, M. (2008) 'Health-care Use among Gay, Lesbian and Bisexual Canadians', *Health Reports*, 19 (1), 53–64.

Wang, J., M. Hausermann, P. Vounatsou, P. Aggleton and M. Weiss (2007) 'Health Status, Behaviour and Health-care Utilization in the Geneva Gay Men's Health Survey', *Preventive Medicine*, 44, (1), 70–5.

18
Mothers and Children: What Does Their Health Tell Us about Gender?

Tulsi Patel

Introduction

Significant advances in hygiene, medical science and technology have curtailed mortality and enhanced life expectancy over the world. Yet in the year 2000, the United Nations member states proposed eight Millennium Development Goals (MDG), including children's and women's health (MDG, 2000), in order to address persisting differences in health status across population groups. Recent statistics reveal the gendered dimensions of a circle of health inequality that will be the focus of this chapter. *The State of World Children's Report* (UNICEF, 2009) shows that children's health is intricately related with women's health and nutrition (see also Chapter 23 by Sandall et al.). But what else do the survey figures tell us about the trends and contexts of the health of people, especially about women and children?

This chapter begins with a general overview of maternal and child health inequalities, followed by a consideration of South Asia, and specifically India, which is the main focus of the chapter. The chapter then deals with inequalities in structural provisions of healthcare. Ethnographic data are presented to highlight the life-threatening gender inequalities that can arise due to problems in the provision of and access to healthcare.

The most unequal mortality rates: maternal and neonatal mortality

Over the world, every year more than half a million women die as a result of pregnancy or childbirth complications (UNICEF, 2009; World Bank, 2007). Based on 2005 data, UNICEF (2009) reports that nearly four million new-born babies die within 28 days of birth, and millions more suffer from disability, disease, infection and injury. Furthermore, women's risk of dying of pregnancy and childbirth related causes is 300 times higher in least developed countries than in developed countries; India and Nigeria together have a third of the world's maternal mortality rate (UNICEF, 2009). While differences between developed and developing countries are clearly relevant (see also Chapter 2 by Abdool et al. and Chapter 3 by Standing), economic indicators do not reveal the full story of gendered inequality in the health of mothers and children.

Table 18.1 draws on UNICEF (2009) data to compare health and income indicators of selected countries for 2007. Comparison shows that child mortality at different ages varies among the developed countries just as it does among the developing countries. For instance, Singapore stands out in health indicators, with the least mortality figures, lower than Denmark and Sweden which in turn show better life chances for children than those in the USA. Similarly, Indian infant and child mortality figures are higher than China's and Bangladesh's, the latter a country with a lower income than that of India.

The data in Table 18.1 exclude a direct unicausal link between income and health. Something more than income seems to influence health. For example, research reveals that as many as 80 per cent of maternal deaths are preventable if women take essential maternity and basic healthcare steps (UNICEF, 2009). Anaemia and complications in abortions each cause four per cent of maternal deaths; a further 34 per cent are caused by haemorrhage, 10 per cent by sepsis, and as many as 30 per cent of deaths are due to other causes. These clearly point to the question: 'Why do women not access the healthcare that they need to either help prevent or treat these life-threatening conditions?' Is lack of income or low income responsible for women's inability to access healthcare?

While the UNICEF Report (2009) deals with women's health across the world, specific data are available for South Asian countries as well. The World Bank Report *Sparing Lives: Better Reproductive Lives for Poor Women in South Asia*

Table 18.1 Child mortality rates in selected countries, 2005

Country	NnMR	IMR	< 5MR
Bangladesh	36	47	61
China	36	19	22
Denmark	4	4	–
Saudi Arabia	11	25	20
Singapore	1	1	3
Sweden	2	3	–
India	39	54	72
United States	11	7	8

NnMR: neonatal mortality rate (number of deaths during the first 28 completed days of life per 1000 live births).
IMR: infant mortality rate (number of deaths of infants under one year of age per 1000 live births).
<5MR: under five mortality rate (number of deaths of children under five years of age per 1000 live births).
Source: UNICEF (2009).

(World Bank, 2007) pertains to the 98 per cent of the South Asian population that lives in the five countries (Bangladesh, India, Nepal, Pakistan and Sri Lanka) which account for more than 50 per cent of low birth-weight babies. Except for Sri Lanka, maternal mortality ratios are two to four times higher than the United Nations' MDGs recommend. Again, with the exception of Sri Lanka, less than half of the women in these countries receive antenatal care and, in turn, the attendance of skilled practitioners at birth. Institutional births are 15 to 20 times higher among the richest and most educated quintile of women in four of the five countries. The fertility rate is no indicator of low maternal and infant mortality ratios in South Asia except in the case of Sri Lanka (World Bank, 2007). In other words, whether women have fewer than two children in all or more than three or four, their risks of dying in four of the South Asian countries are two to four times higher than those set for the MDGs. For example, the World Bank (2007) report shows that South Asian countries with higher maternal mortality, such as India and Bangladesh, have a lower fertility rate (2.7) than the fertility rate of 3.1 for Nepal and 4.1 children per woman for Pakistan.

Over two fifths of all children in South Asia are malnourished. The poorest economic quintile in Nepal has twice and India and Sri Lanka have three times as many malnourished children compared with the richest quintile in these countries. Malnourishment peaks in children between one and two years of age and remains higher until age five. Of the malnourished children up to five years of age, the numbers of girls are five to ten per cent higher compared to boys (World Bank, 2007).

Regional variations: paradoxes of health and cultural differences in gender disparities in India

What underlies the general vulnerability of mothers and children in any given population irrespective of per capita income, fertility rate or peak fertility years, and the level of institutional deliveries? This question will now be addressed through a case study of India (see also Claeson et al., 2000). Paradoxes of health exist in India. The country has seen impressive economic growth as well as progress in terms of human development since the mid-1990s. The Indian economy experienced growth rates as high as nine per cent in 2006–7 despite the widespread global turndown in developed country economies. Also, India is emerging as one of the favourite destinations for medical tourism not only for people from South Asian countries but also from western countries, such as Australia and Europe among others (Healthcare in India, 2009). Significant inequities are found in the Indian healthcare system which has a mix of state and private facilities. The poorest 20 per cent of the population get only ten per cent of the state subsidies, while the richest 20 per cent get 33 per cent (Sharma, 2004). In 1991, India, like many other low-public-spending Asian countries, had 10 beds and four medical practitioners per 10,000 inhabitants (UNICEF, 2009). In all, it had 22,400 Primary Health Centres (PHC), 11,200 hospitals and 27,400 clinics. Half of the total number of hospitals were run by central, federal state and local government, 25 per cent by charitable trusts with partial support from the government and the remaining 25 per cent were private. Asia has among the lowest levels of government spending in the world on healthcare as a share of total public spending. By 2008, Indian government spending on healthcare was increased from three to five per cent during 2005–7 to eight per cent of GDP, that is, $680 per capita (Healthcare in India, 2009).

Sharma (2004) maintains that the Indian healthcare system is characterized by a unique paradox: on the one hand, medical capacity in five-star private hospitals remains under-utilized because people in India cannot pay for this, forcing the healthcare industry and government to promote health tourism; on the other hand, Primary Health Centres in rural areas are suffering from lack of government support.

Despite health improvements over the past 30 years, one million people, mostly women and children, die in India every year due to inadequate healthcare. More than two million children die every year from preventable infections. Most infant deaths occur in the first month of life; up to 47 per cent die in the first month itself. Tetanus in the new-born remains high in some states, namely Uttar Pradesh, Madhya Pradesh, Rajasthan, West Bengal and Assam. Furthermore, polio has not yet been eradicated (Healthcare in India, 2009). Despite vast improvements in the country's economy, children in India continue to lose their life to vaccine-preventable diseases such as measles (which remains the biggest killer) and tetanus, which remains a problem in newborns in at least five Indian states. There are important differences between the states (provinces) in India, as data from the second and third rounds of National Family and Health Surveys conducted in 1998 and 2006 respectively reveal (NFHS, 1998; 2006). For example, Delhi, Uttar Pradesh and Rajasthan performed poorly in vaccination rates for preventable diseases and there were also high rates of childhood anaemia. While Himachal Pradesh did better than Kerala in vaccination, it had more anaemic children aged six to 35 months (NFHS, 1998). The vulnerability of homeless children, often called street children, and poorer migrants increases the size of the community that needs better healthcare.

Malnutrition also continues to be a problem in India. In 1998, the National Family Health Survey (NFHS, 1998) found that 47 per cent of all children under the age of three were underweight – a higher average prevalence than in sub-Saharan Africa. National Family Health Survey III (NFHS, 2006) data for 2006 show only a very small decline, with child malnutrition levels remaining around 45 per cent. In several states, such as Madhya Pradesh and Bihar, malnutrition levels have even increased. To combat malnutrition in young children, the Government of India (2000) relies largely on the Integrated Child Development Scheme (ICDS). Introduced in 1975, this scheme provides health and nutrition education for mothers of infants and young children, along with other services (NFHS, 2006).

Maternal deaths are also very high. Unsafe childbirth and post-partum care, poor nutrition and infections such as malaria, tuberculosis and HIV/AIDS are among the causes revealed in demographic and health surveys. Very few women have access to skilled birth attendants and fewer still to quality emergency obstetric care. Only 15 per cent of mothers receive complete antenatal care and only 58 per cent get iron or folate tablets or syrup (NFHS, 2006). Furthermore, women's health is also affected by 'wife bashing'; this form of intimate partner violence is deemed acceptable by 71 per cent of men and 41 per cent of women if women have disrespected their in-laws or have been lax about household chores or childcare (TNN, 2009).

The demographic and kinship differences between south and north India have been studied over some time and draw on anthropological research in these areas (see, for example, Basu, 1992; Dyson and Moore, 1983; Miller, 1981). The differences are not simply manifestations of socio-economic disparities, but reflect deep-seated customary gender norms in female seclusion, marriage, family, lineage and inheritance. The north Indian states, such as Delhi, Haryana, Himachal Pradesh, Punjab, Rajasthan and Uttar Pradesh, continue to show trends unfavourable to females, especially towards daughter discrimination, affecting health through high fertility, anaemia, maternal mortality, infant and child mortality compared to the south Indian states of Andhra Pradesh, Karnataka, Kerala and Tamil Nadu. For example, the National Family Health Survey in 2006 shows that Rajasthan accounts for 7.0 per cent of the total live births, but 9.2 per cent of the maternal deaths, while the states of Karnataka, Kerala, Andhra Pradesh and Tamil Nadu together have 18 per cent of live births and ten per cent of maternal deaths (NHFS, 2006).

National Family and Health Survey II data (NFHS, 1998) reveals geographic differences in health for women and children in India (see Table 18.2). More than 52 per cent of women, overall, were anaemic, and this was higher in some states in the north than the southern Indian states; the only exception was Himachal Pradesh. With a higher age at marriage and greater autonomy in healthcare decision-making, Punjab, a prosperous state in the north, is better for women on both of these counts than the rest of the north Indian states. Furthermore, in Uttar Pradesh a woman has a one in 42 lifetime risk of maternal death compared with a risk of just one in 500 for women in Kerala. In effect, while the states in the north and south Indian regions are strikingly different in terms of gender and health indicators, the health indicators also vary within a region and do not necessarily follow a uniform direction of north–south differences.

Table 18.2 Women and child health indicators in selected Indian states, 1998

State	IMR	< 5MR	Hospital delivery %	Babies born underweight %
Delhi	46.8	55.4	59	34.7
Himachal Pradesh	34.4	42.4	28.9	43.6
Kerala	16.3	18.8	93	26.9
Punjab	57.1	72.1	37.5	28.7
Rajasthan	80.4	114.9	21.5	50.6

IMR: infant mortality rate (number of deaths of infants under one year of age per 1000 live births).
<5MR: under five mortality rate (number of deaths of children under five years of age per 1000 live births).
Source: NHFS (1998).

In summary, data clearly highlight that north Indian states, in contrast to the south Indian states, continue to display cultural differences in their gender disparities.

Healthcare for women and children: provision and access

Just as underweight women are likely to have underweight babies, the poor health of mothers is likely to influence babies' and children's health. The UNICEF report (2009) highlights that babies whose mothers die during the first six weeks of their lives are far more likely to die in the first two years of life than babies whose mothers survive. In a study in Afghanistan, for example, about three quarters of infants born alive to mothers who died of maternal causes also subsequently died. A child born in a less developed country is almost 14 times more likely to die during the first 28 days of life than one born in a developed country (for an overview, see UNICEF, 2009). In India, scores of unexplainable infant deaths within 24 to 72 hours of birth have been reported several times from nurseries in prestigious government referral hospitals (such as in Kerala in May 2007, and in West Bengal in September 2001 and 2002 and December 2006).

In India, state-of-the-art diagnostic equipment is found in urban areas and, since 1991, in private medical facilities. Though government facilities are set up to provide services to the people free of charge, 80 per cent of health costs in India are met out of pocket. Further, with the rise of medical tourism, privatization of healthcare has been rapidly rising alongside overburdened staff and overcrowding at government facilities. The healthcare system fails to respond to cultural and economic inequalities. Most of the poor are employed in the unorganized sector, about half in self-employment with sub-optimal productivity. Privately employed workers are known to use private medical facilities in India to avoid loss of wages due to long waiting hours.

Furthermore, approximately one million people die each year due to inadequate healthcare (Healthcare in India, 2009). Access to specialty care is severely limited, particularly in rural areas, because 80 per cent of the specialists live in urban areas (see also Chapter 19 by Bourgeault and Sutherns). In this situation, one woman's enormous efforts to reach a city hospital and then return without managing to make it to the doctor after a full day's travelling long distances in the state of Tamil Nadu is an example of the reality for many in far-flung areas who can neither afford to pay nor have the time to access effective but inequitable healthcare (Zurbrigg, 1991).

In summary, the organization and provision of healthcare in India faces a number of serious problems, including regional variations and inequalities between public and private provision of healthcare. However, lack of efficiency may occur for additional reasons. The following example is indicative of the state of affairs at many of the government-run primary health centres and dispensaries in villages and towns. In 2004, in an interview reported in the *Hindustan Times* (2004), the Health Secretary recounted his experience, after taking charge of the Ministry of Health and Family Planning, of one of his visits to a health centre in Rai Bareily, a small city in Uttar Pradesh, north India. Rai Bareily has special significance because it happens to be the constituency of the Gandhi family (presently it is the constituency of Rahul Gandhi, and previously of his mother Sonia Gandhi and earlier of his father Rajiv Gandhi). The Health Secretary's visit was a mission to endeavour to improve the delivery of rural healthcare in states where little else works. He reported amazement at the quality of facilities at the Primary Health Centre (PHC). The unit had 27 beds instead of the required six, the place was clean and well-stocked with equipment, medicines and clean linen. There were two female and two male doctors. Still, to his surprise there were no patients. On inquiring, he was told that the place did not have enough nursing staff. '"Who will take care of the patients?," the doctors replied in interrogation' (*Hindustan Times*, 2004: 20). Obviously, the best facilities were available, but they were put to little use. There is no need to explain that the people went elsewhere even though they were covered for government-provided health according to state records (*Hindustan Times*, 2004).

A total contrast to the above example is the case of one of the prestigious research and training hospitals in Delhi, the All India Institute of Medical Sciences (AIIMS) (see Kumar, 2006). In October 2006, an outbreak of dengue fever left all government hospitals reeling under the pressure of 13,000 cases in Delhi and 30 deaths, with patients in long queues waiting to be screened. The most effective treatment was reportedly provided by AIIMS where the largest number of suspected patients (over 1000 every day) from all over Delhi and the outskirts were flocking. People were treated in corridors and tents outside the building. The shortage of doctors was so severe that patients were helping each other administer intravenous saline drips. The hospital started a

24-hour laboratory service to test blood samples from patients suffering from fever. Fifty medical interns were deployed in the paediatric casualty and medical wards to deal with the situation. Most other departments at AIIMS were requested by the administration to spare two doctors each to meet the crisis situation. During the crisis, one AIIMS doctor died due to dengue and several other staff were reported ill. Other government hospitals in Delhi were housing two to three patients per bed, and yet others did not disclose any clear plans of how to deal with the emergency situation. Despite fumigation and fogging drives, the situation did not come under control (Kumar, 2006). This example of the inability to control what is a relatively routine annual occurrence throws into harsh relief the crisis within the Indian health system. Furthermore, this hospital has recently come under attention for unethical drug trial research that led to the death of 49 children from unsuspecting poor families in the three years after 2006 (TimesOnline, 2008).

The examples stated here give an impression of an overall lack of systemic efficiency in India's healthcare system that has a negative impact on the health of women and children more generally, despite many high-quality facilities and increasing medical tourism. It also gives a picture of the enormous pressure in terms of the sheer numbers of health-seekers on the infrastructure in public-referral healthcare facilities. The next section highlights, however, that 'access' and 'provision' do not reveal the whole story of gendered healthcare.

Looking beyond provision and access to healthcare: excess female deaths and abortions

Aday and colleagues (2004) provide a model for analysing healthcare systems in terms of their effectiveness, efficiency and equity. This model defines the *effectiveness* of a healthcare system in terms of clinical effectiveness and population effectiveness; *efficiency* is measured in terms of both production efficiency – the combination of inputs that produce services at the lowest cost – and allocative efficiency, that is, the combination of inputs that produce maximum health improvements with available resources; finally, *equity* can be measured in terms of procedural equity – the maximization of fairness in the distribution of services across groups – and substantive equity – the minimization of disparities in the distribution of health across groups (Aday et al., 2004). But healthcare measurement also needs to incorporate the demand side of healthcare access, including the role of women as players who reproduce gender discrimination.

Indices of development, including the NFHS III (NFHS, 2006) data, show that India neglects the early care and development of its children. Only one per cent of the health budget is spent on children under six. The Working Group on Children under Six (2007) provides a comprehensive review of the situation and proposes social solutions to overcome child neglect in India. The child is the responsibility of the family in Indian society since the family is seen as emotionally best equipped for childcare. Though this is largely the case, especially when contrasted with homeless and orphaned children, the mortality and morbidity figures and healthcare access practices discussed below show that families are not gender neutral, even in regard to their own children.

Girls are 30 to 50 per cent more likely than boys to die between their first and fifth birthdays (Claeson et al., 2000). North India was notorious for its violence against women, especially for female infanticide, up to the early decades of the 20th century (Panigrahi, 1972; Vishwanath, 2000). The region is also infamous for female neglect (Das Gupta, 1987; Miller, 1981). Das Gupta's (1987) study in Punjab showed that during the first two years of a child's life, parents spent 2.3 times more on healthcare for sons than for daughters (see also Chatterjee, 1990).

Khanna and colleagues (2003) studied records of causes of infant and child deaths in three locations in Delhi among lower-class migrants for the five years from 1997 to 2001. The recall was recorded by auxiliary nurse midwives (ANMs) who had been working there for more than two decades. The sex ratio at birth was 869 females per 1000 males; the mean infant mortality was 1.3 times higher in females than in males (72 for females as against 55 for males per 1000 births). Diarrhoea was responsible for 22 per cent of deaths overall, though twice as many girls died from diarrhoea. There were no significant differences between girls and boys in the numbers of deaths from birth asphyxia, septicaemia, pre-maturity and congenital anomalies. But for infant and child deaths girls were clearly at a disadvantage; most sudden and unexplained deaths occurred largely among girls. Three out of every four such deaths were in girls with no preceding illness and no satisfactory explanation of cause of death. Khanna and colleagues (2003) conclude that the excess number of unexplained deaths and deaths due to treatable conditions, such as diarrhoeal disease in girls, may be because girls are treated less favourably. They found no difference between Hindus and Muslims in gender differences in child mortality. Furthermore, they did not find that sex discrimination was strongly related to poverty; in fact low female/male ratios are less common among the poor than among wealthy Indians, including the educated (Khanna et al., 2003).

Daughter dislike is a disease of the rich in India, who use healthcare services not only to the disadvantage of girl babies, but for preventing them being born in the first place. Booth and colleagues (1994) found in their Punjab study that foetal sex determination – ultrasonography-based foetal sex-testing – was more common among families with higher incomes. Those who have better access to medical facilities are more likely to use foetal sex identification technologies with the purpose of eliminating the female foetus. Sex ratio at birth by birth order reveals strikingly fewer births of daughters with every successive birth: 577 daughters to 1000 sons at fourth birth in Himachal Pradesh, and only 96 daughters to 1000 sons at fourth birth in Punjab (Bose and Shiva, 2003).

Gender discrimination via selective female elimination is an invisible form of heightened gender discrimination in the name of healthcare (see Agnihotri, 2000). The use of prenatal diagnostic technology to test the sex of the foetus with the intent of aborting a female foetus has been illegal in India since 1994 (Prenatal Diagnostic Techniques, Regulation and Prevention of Misuse Act). Yet the NFHS-II survey conducted in 1998–9 found that 13 per cent of pregnant women self-reported having gone for prenatal sex determination during their last pregnancy, amounting to about 3.6 million women having access to the technology (reported in Jha et al., 2006). The 1994 Act seemingly led to little difference in children's sex ratios. Instead, the test went undercover and became more costly. The Act now has been renamed the 'The Preconception and Prenatal Diagnostic Techniques (Prohibition of Sex Selection) Act'. The Act prohibits sex selection before and/or after conception, and the rules became more stringent after amendments in 2002 and 2003. But even after these amendments, which implicate the medical practitioner as well as the sex-test seeker, no more than a handful of doctors have lost their registration for this unlawful but highly financially lucrative practice (Chandran, 2005).

Gender discrimination and sex selection: women seen as active players

The following anecdote (based on an observation by the author) shows that even young children in north India know that daughters are not the preferred child in the family. A five-year-old boy with two older sisters sitting amidst a group of women interjected in a conversation at a neighbour's house in March 2007: 'Girls should not be born.' On being asked why he thought so, he replied: 'Because they have to be married off.' On asking how will he find a wife if girls should not be born, he replied: 'Girls born to others will be there for me to marry.' The tendency is not wanting to 'water another's garden' – a symbolically significant metaphor of the female representing the land whose reproductive capacity will provide heirs only to other families. Though the first daughter was tolerated, I discovered dislike for the second daughter's birth among aspiring middle-class and upper-class people in several districts in north India (Patel, 2007a). The mindset that views the daughter as a burden, who has to be raised with special care in the light of family honour, is related to the control and regulation of her sexuality and to arranging her marriage (Patel, 2007b). Many of these practices are connected with wider material and historical influences mediated through culture. Culture here implies the ideas and values by which people make sense of their social and personal lives. It also includes the material and technological resources they deploy in accordance with the social values they infuse into these resources.

The following examples, taken from my fieldwork (Patel, 2007c), reveal the role of women as active players within this scenario. But it needs to be clarified that women's role must be viewed in light of the material and historical contexts in which they live, which are mediated through culture. The examples further show how women contribute to a persistent practice of sex selection and devaluing of women, while securing their own personal position in the family.

Family, kin and friends are well-meaning in coming forward to provide support for sex identification tests to the pregnant woman. Maina, one of the participants in this study, a nurse working in a town in Rajasthan, was chided by her urban natal family for producing a second daughter, and her husband's rural family members also felt unhappy that she had produced another daughter. Maina had been hoping to have a son. Two of her sisters went to see Maina after her mother-in-law and her mother had been to help her out for a fortnight each after her daughter's birth. Besides looking after her, both sisters chided her. One of the sisters said:

> You are already so overburdened with work in the hospital and then have the house to look after. You also have blood pressure. And now you have to produce another baby (as you need to have a son at least). Why did you have to be so innocent? Had I been told about your pregnancy I would have suggested the test to you and you would have been more free today. It is such a burden to raise daughters in present times. And who gets two daughters these days? (Patel, 2007c: 254)

On having a second daughter in Jhansi, a town in Uttar Pradesh, Raj's sister was listless after visiting her in the hospital. Her husband and his family's dislike of the girl's birth was loud and clear. They did not see the baby, let alone ask after her well-being or that of the mother. Little was brought by way of food or medicine for the new mother. Instead her husband abused her verbally for producing another girl (a disaster for the family). That morning her husband's threat was too hard on the parturient mother. He made it clear that he did not want the girl [his daughter] in his house. The post-partum mother expressed her wish to her younger sister, 'I wish this girl were dead. She will not let me survive' (Patel, 2007c: 255). She felt guilty for having produced a second daughter. She had not fed or held the baby the previous night. Finally, Raj (confident of her NGO work experience) and her parents volunteered to raise the new-born girl on their own, making way for Raj's sister to regain her entry into the marital home. The neonate had to part with her mother and her parental family to be raised in her maternal grandmother's home.

Paradoxically, cases such as the above occurred in hospitals accessed for healthcare. During the fieldwork my respondents recalled newspaper reports where vigilant nurses had caught a couple of parturient mothers trying to kill their babies by stuffing their mouths with tobacco or thrusting jute into their throats (Patel, 2007a). Government health employees, such as ANMs who work at the ground level, are also expected to meet family planning targets such as sterilization as part of their job. ANMs share the culture and gender values of the community of which they are themselves members: 'How can I suggest to a woman that she gets sterilized unless one has at least a son,' they say (Patel, 2007d: 338–9). As part of the undercover network of sex detection testing, ANMs obliged women so they could have a son and then agree to get sterilized.

The micro politics of the family disadvantages its women, especially younger ones. It is with the birth of sons that women get a stronghold in the family. The household and the family in India, as elsewhere, is a cooperative-conflicting unit hinged along culturally unequal gender, age and kinship relations (Patel, 2005), as conceptualized by Scheper-Hughes and Lock (1987). Pregnancy, child-birth, abortion and healthcare have always been of public (in the sense of the body politic) as well as of private concern (in the sense of the individual and social body). In her study of infant and child deaths in Brazil, Scheper-Hughes (1997) found that mother love is provided judiciously, as spending more of the meagre economic and emotional resources especially on babies that show a spirit to survive is justified. Lesser care is provided to those babies that are seen as lacking the spirit to survive, whose death should not be mourned as they are 'angels' who are fated not to be in this world. While state-of-the-art availability, accessibility and equity of healthcare is no less critical, Indians may delay the use of medical technology for daughters' healthcare in comparison to sons' healthcare, but are eager to use healthcare to avoid a daughter's birth even if such an act means evading the law.

Conclusion

The health of women and mothers has close links with that of babies and children and this linkage has long-term consequences. While individual capacities, socio-economic status and efficient and effective healthcare provision are important, historical and socio-cultural gendered contexts are significant for health inequities. In everyday life, who gets healthcare access, and when and why, is related to preferences for sons over daughters, as revealed through skewed sex ratios (Patel, 2007a). In their desire to have small families, Indians will accept the birth of a daughter if a son comes by. The desire for sons over daughters is more accentuated in north than in south India. While the whole of north India is not identical, and there are differences between states in north India, gender disparities in health are not always found to be related to poverty. Among rich, middle-class and educated north Indians, the female/male child ratio is highly unfavourable for girls. Under the guise of accessing healthcare, pregnant women clandestinely incur expenses to avoid a second daughter's birth, as even one is considered too many.

Summary

- Children's health is closely related to and dependent on mothers' health; children's health is significantly related to the risks of women dying during or soon after childbirth.
- Of the two-fifth of children in South Asia who are malnourished, more girls than boys are malnourished.
- Women's and girls' ill-health is not simply correlated with poverty, and not exclusively dependent on the availability of state-of-the-art healthcare facilities. It is also dependent on how women and girls and their health are perceived.
- Mortality and morbidity rates of women and girls vary across regions in India, but the difference between north and south India is greater and can be understood in terms of differences in kinship and historical and material contexts.
- In India, familial politics of reproduction perpetuate selective dislike for daughters while cherishing the birth of at least one son through differential use of healthcare facilities. Though it appears that women are active in perpetuating dislike for daughters, other family members exert pressure on pregnant women to avoid having more than one daughter by clandestinely using new reproductive technologies.

Key reading

Claeson, M., R. Bose. T. Mawji and I. Pathmanathan (2000) 'Reducing Child Mortality in India in the New Millennium', *Bulletin of World Health Organization*, 78 (10), 1192–9.

Khanna, R., A. Kumar, J. F. Vaghela, V. Sreenivas and J. M. Puliyel (2003) 'Community Based Retrospective Study of Sex in Infant Mortality in India', *British Medical Journal*, 327, 126–8.

Patel, T. (ed.) (2007) *Sex Selective Abortion in India* (New Delhi: Sage).

UNICEF (2009) *The State of World's Children Report – 2009*, at: www.unicef.org/infoby country/indep.htm, accessed 20 May 2009.

Acknowledgements

I have benefited greatly from the support of Ellen Kuhlmann, Anjana Mangalagiri and Shikha Bedi in working towards this paper and thank them for all their help.

References

Aday, L. A., C. E. Begley, D. R. Lairson and R. Balkrishnan (2004) *Evaluating the Health Care System: Effectiveness, Efficiency, and Equity* (Washington, DC: Academy Health).

Agnihotri, S.B. (2000) *Sex Ratio: Patterns in the Indian Population, a Fresh Exploration* (New Delhi: Sage).

Basu, A.M. (1992) *Culture, the Status of Women, and Demographic Behaviour: Illustrated with the Case of India* (Oxford: Clarendon Press).

Booth, B. E., M. Verma and R. S. Beri (1994) 'Foetal Sex Determination in Infants in Punjab, India: Correlations and Implications', *British Medical Journal*, 309, 1259–61.

Bose, A. and M. Shiva (2003) *Darkness at Noon: Female Foeticide in India* (New Delhi: VHAI).

Chatterjee, M. (1990) *A Report on Indian Women from Birth to Twenty* (New Delhi: National Institute of Public Cooperation and Child Development).

Chandran, D. (2005) *InfoChange News and Features*, September, at: http://infochangeindia.org/20050907152/Women/Features/Sting-operation-to-find-missing-girl-child.html, accessed 14 September 2009.

Claeson, M., R. Bose, T. Mawji and I. Pathmanathan (2000) 'Reducing Child Mortality in India in the New Millennium', *Bulletin of World Health Organization*, 78 (10), 1192–9.

Das Gupta, M. (1987) 'Selective Discrimination against Female Children in Rural Punjab, India', *Population and Development Review*, 13 (1), 77–100.

Dyson, T. and M. Moore (1983) 'On Kinship Structure, Female Autonomy and Demographic Behaviour in India', *Population and Development Review*, 9 (1), 35–60.

Government of India (2000) *National Sample Survey Organization, Round 55*: July 1999–June 2000 (New Delhi: Ministry of Statistics and Programme Implementation).

Healthcare in India (2009) Entry in Wikipedia, the free Encyclopedia, at: http://en.wikipedia.org/w/index.php?title=Healthcare_in_India&oldid=299950211, accessed 2 July 2009.

Hindustan Times (2004) 'Private Role a Must in Rural Healthcare, an Interview', 13 December, 20.

Jha, P., R. Kumar, P. Vasa, N. Dhingra, D. Thiruchelvam and R. Moineddin (2006) 'Low Male-to-Female Sex-ratio of Children Born in India: National Survey on 1.1 Million Households', *The Lancet*, 367 (9506), 185–6.

Khanna, R., A. Kumar, J. F. Vaghela, V. Sreenivas and J. M. Puliyel (2003) 'Community Based Retrospective Study of Sex in Infant Mortality in India', *British Medical Journal*, 327, 126–8.

Kumar, P. (2006) 'Out of Control', *Sunday Pioneer*, Lucknow, 15 October 2006, 2.

MDG – Millennium Development Goals (2000) at: www.un.org/millenniumgoals, accessed 9 October 2009.

Miller, B. (1981[1991]) *The Endangered Sex. Neglect of Female Children in Rural North India* (Ithaca: Cornell University Press).

NFHS (1998) *National Family and Household Survey II* (Mumbai: International Institute of Population Sciences).

NFHS (2006) *National Family and Household Survey III* (Mumbai: International Institute of Population Sciences).

Panigrahi, L. (1972) *British Social Policy and Female Infanticide in India* (New Delhi: Munshiram Manoharlal).

Patel, T. (2005) *The Family in India: Structure and Practice* (New Delhi: Sage).

Patel, T. (2007a) (ed.) *Sex Selective Abortion in India* (New Delhi: Sage).

Patel, T. (2007b) 'The Mindset behind Eliminating the Female Fetus', in T. Patel (ed.), *Sex Selective Abortion in India* (New Delhi: Sage), 135–74.

Patel, T. (2007c) 'Informal Social Networks: Sonography and Female Foeticide in India', *Sociological Bulletin*, 56 (2), 243–62.

Patel, T. (2007d) 'Female Feticide, Family Planning and State-Society Interaction in India', in T. Patel (ed.), *Sex Selective Abortion in India* (New Delhi: Sage), 316–56.

Scheper-Hughes, N. and M. Lock (1987) 'The Mindful Body: A Prolegomenon to Future Work in Medical Anthropology', *Medical Anthropology Quarterly*, 42 (2), 6–41.

Scheper-Hughes, N. (1997) *Death without Weeping: The Violence of Everyday Life in Brazil* (Berkeley: University of California Press).

Sharma, D.C. (2004) 'Indian Health Groups Demand Right to Health', *The Lancet*, 363, 1044.

TimesOnline (2008) 'Drug Trials in India under Investigation after 49 Babies Die at Leading Hospital', at: www.timesonline.co.uk/tol/news/world/asia/article4568717.ece, accessed 3 September 2009.

TNN – Times News Network (2009) '13 Children Die Every Hour in Rajasthan', at: http://timesofindia.indiatimes.com/Cities/Delhi/13-children-die-every-hour-in-Rajasthan/articleshow/4019212.cms, accessed 3 September 2009.

UNICEF (2009) *The State of the World's Children Report – 2009*, at: www.unicef.org/infoby country/indep.htm, accessed 20 May 2009.

Vishwanath, L. S. (2000) *Social Structure and Female Infanticide in India* (Delhi: Hindustan).

Working Group on Children under Six (2007) 'Strategies for Children under Six', *Economic and Political Weekly*, XLII (52), 87–101.

World Bank (2007) *Sparing Lives: Better Reproductive Lives for Poor Women in South Asia* (New Delhi: World Bank).

Zurbrigg, S. (1991) *Rakku's Story: Structures of Ill Health and the Sources of Change* (Bangalore: Centre for Action).

19
Gender, Health, Care and Place: Living in Rural and Remote Communities

Ivy Lynn Bourgeault and Rebecca Sutherns

Introduction

The intersection between gender, health, care and place has garnered increasing attention in the international health services and policy literatures. This has largely been dominated by concerns about the provision of healthcare in rural and remote communities. In these discussions of how to provide equitable access to care, the consideration of gender and women's health in particular is necessary to complete the picture of health needs, service provision and utilization. It is also clear from a growing literature that rural/remote living is an important determinant of health in numerous ways. This not only includes limited access to healthcare services and information and limited community services and infrastructure, but also a lack of anonymity in rural/remote communities coupled with the invisibility of rural/remote women's concerns to researchers and policy-makers, limited employment options – for women in particular – low incomes and sometimes high costs for food and transportation, rural-specific occupational health effects, and a need for healthcare that is sensitive to diverse rural cultures and to women's particular needs (Sutherns et al., 2007). Very little, however, is written about the cumulative impact of and interplay between these various place-related determinants on women's and men's health.

The purpose of this chapter is to begin to address the gaps in our knowledge and to deepen our understanding of the health issues of living in rural and remote communities with a particular focus on women in Western countries. We draw upon an extensive review of the international literature (Sutherns et al., 2007) which is supplemented with data from a Canada-wide empirical study of health issues of women living in rural/remote communities. This study employed two primary modes of data collection to address these research questions. Qualitative data were derived from 34 in-person focus groups and 16 telephone interviews conducted with women living in rural and remote communities across

Canada. Responses to a closed-ended web-based survey mirroring the interview guide from 346 women supplemented these data (Bourgeault et al., 2005).

We begin our exploration of the intersection between gender, health, care and place with contextual information addressing who is living in rural and remote communities, how rural is defined, how demographics have shifted over time and the consequences of these shifts. We then address the range of ways that rural and remote living affects health, with a focus on the physical, social and built aspects of the environment. Typical work undertaken in rural and remote communities and its related health impacts is the focus of the section that follows. We next describe the influences upon access to health services by juxtaposing the situation of health service providers and those seeking care in rural and remote communities. Finally, we address the impact of health reform in Canada. The key insights from this overview are that both gender and geography matter.

Demographic context

Defining what is rural in western countries affects how health status is measured, how the magnitude of problems is perceived, and how areas and services are funded (Cox, 1999). There are numerous definitions and taxonomies of rurality, including those that focus on *spatial features* such as distance from an urban centre, land use, population density, demographic structure, environmental characteristics and population characteristics (Crosato and Leipert, 2006), on *service-related features* such as availability of specialist medical services, or on *cultural features* such as quality of life and work ethic (Leipert and Reutter, 1998). Rurality is often, although not always, defined in reference to the urban (Murdoch and Pratt, 1993). Although rural may often be contrasted to urban, rurality should be described on its own merits, as Murdoch and Pratt suggest, 'rather than trying to "pin down" a definition of rurality or the rural, we should explore the ways in which rurality is [selectively] constructed and deployed in a variety of contexts' (1993: 411). Understandings of rurality are not fixed but rather socially constructed, as evidenced by the variability within and the many myths surrounding the term. Definitions of rurality are negotiated, dynamic and context-specific. There is no unique and privileged vantage point from which the rural can be captured and assessed. It is constructed in varying ways with varying emphases in different settings (Murdoch and Pratt, 1993).

While the concept of rurality may be socially negotiated, that negotiation occurs in reference to an external reality that is spatial. Cloke (1994) describes this as different social spaces that overlap the same geographical space. It is common to refer, for example, to rural places, and although the understandings of those places may differ and change, the geographic foundation of the notion remains. But despite the enormous diversity within rurality, there are a few defining characteristics that still allow rurality to be discussed as a meaningful geographic and social category. In most western societies rural places tend, for instance, to be small and dispersed, with low population density, and usually peripheral to a regional core centre.

How small? Statistics Canada's official definition of rural and small town includes communities of fewer than 10,000 people outside of commuting distance to an urban centre. Using this definition, 22.2 per cent of Canadians live in rural areas. Using the OECD definition of predominantly rural areas, which focuses on population density, that figure rises to 31.4 per cent, putting Canada roughly in the middle of OECD countries in terms of rural population. This has decreased from 33.6 per cent in 1981 (Statistics Canada, 2001). Despite a decline in the proportion of Canada's population living rurally, the overall population of rural and small-town Canada is in fact growing. This growth is the result of birth rates outpacing death rates – particularly in rural Aboriginal communities, rural areas adjacent to metropolitan centres, and retirement destinations.

In terms of who makes up rural and remote communities in Canada, seniors, women, children and youth under the age of 20 years are over-represented (Johns and Havelock, 2006; Nagarajan, 2004). There is a current phenomenon of out-migration of young adults from rural areas for educational and job opportunities within larger urbanized areas which is contributing to this bifurcated demographic profile and the steady increase of elders – who are largely women – in rural settings (Crosato and Leipert, 2006). As Wong and Regan write, 'providing health services to an aging rural population will present increasing challenges to jurisdictions mandated to provide equitable health care' (2009: 8).

Rurality and remoteness as determinants of health

Living in rural and remote communities comes with specific health risks and benefits – both geographic and social – of which residents have little control (CIHI, 2006; Leipert and Reutter, 2005a). In general, however, as distance from an urban metropolitan area increases, health indicators decrease in quality (Nagarajan, 2004). In a large national study, it was found that in comparison to their urban counterparts, rural residents are more likely to report low income, higher unemployment and lower educational attainment, which together make significant and interdependent contributions to health outcomes (CIHI, 2006; Nagarajan, 2004). Those who live in these communities are also more likely to report high risk factors such as smoking and obesity (Pampalon, 2005) and to have higher overall mortality rates, particularly for men (CIHI, 2006). As Dolan and Thien succinctly state:

> … rural contexts pose distinct challenges that limit … access to multiple health determinants (e.g., education, employment, health care, healthy behaviours) and serve to create and exacerbate health inequalities. (2008: 38)

In our study of the health of women in rural and remote communities, we teased apart the broader environmental influences in three categories – the physical, social and built environments – and probed specifically both positive and negative aspects within each of these categories (Bourgeault et al., 2005). Some rural women spoke emphatically about the positive health effects of living rurally; these included the ability to get outdoors, natural physical features and fresh air/lack of pollution among the most important features keeping them feeling healthy. Leipert and Reutter similarly found that rural women in Canada took advantage of 'ready access to outdoor activities such as skiing, hiking, fishing and camping' (2005a: 58). Features of the social environment such as a sense of community and a safer place for families were also salient. Another health asset women derive from living rurally is a strong sense of social support. One woman described her community as being like 'one big family', while another said, 'Up here, ... there are times when it is like getting a big hug from the community'. This reported sense of community has emerged from similar studies (Richmond and Ross, 2009; Sutherns 2004). As Leipert and George explain:

> Because of the familiarity of rural residents with one another, they are often aware of particular needs and lack of resources. This awareness can lead rural communities to create a culture of support and capacity that can foster women's health. (2008: 215)

These features were considered relatively stable features of rural and remote living.

By way of contrast, the women spoke at great lengths of the negative health impacts of living in a rural or remote community and how this was getting worse as a result of healthcare and social service cutbacks. That is, the women identified their deprivation and lack of resources as important factors hindering their good health. This was particularly salient for elements of the built environment – housing, employment opportunities, transportation – or lack thereof, and presented the greatest challenges to those who were already disadvantaged. The lack of housing, housing affordability stress, general overcrowding, and unsanitary and unhealthy housing is felt most acutely in rural and remote Aboriginal communities (Whitzman, 2006). As one woman in our study stated, 'It's come to the point where it's not even a question of whether it's affordable or not; is there any housing period?' (Bourgeault et al., 2005: 35). Rural and remote communities are also more likely to experience economic difficulties which are linked to the population loss we described above as well as their dependence on single resource-based incomes that can be unstable, subject to the vagaries of weather, market demands, changes in the economy and international trade agreements (Leipert and Reutter, 2005a).

Despite the myth of the rural idyll, the women we spoke to also recognized the health risks directly related to living rurally, including concerns about air and water quality due to the presence of particular industries such as agriculture or limestone quarries. One woman described the result of an expansion of factory farms:

We have a lot of these big pig barns being built ... that, I'm afraid that's probably eventually going to damage our water. Cause last year we have a problem with our ... well water and there was a bacteria got in it. ... it must have been something [that] leaked into it because ... I think there [are] a lot of farms around us with the liquid manure tanks and they're kind of a hazard to our health. (Bourgeault et al., 2005: 33)

Similarly, Leipert and Reutter (2005a) noted how air pollution from resource-based industries can initiate and exacerbate physical health problems.

The geographic isolation experienced in rural and remote communities was another negative feature mentioned, often not just in physical but also in social terms. For some women in our study geographic isolation meant living with the inconvenience of having to drive everywhere, while for others it resulted in being unable to make contact with other people at all due to lack of transportation. Social isolation has significant mental health consequences in terms of boredom, loneliness and depression (Leipert and Reutter, 2005b). As one of the women in our study mentioned, 'The fact that you can't just hop on a plane or hop in a car and just drive somewhere ... there's that kind of mental challenge ... [that] sometimes is hard' (Bourgeault et al., 2005: 38). Isolation can also be significantly associated with increased risks to women in abusive relationships (Leipert and Reutter, 2005b).

Further, contrary to the common stereotype of small communities having strong social ties, women's social networks actually may be more limited in rural areas, resulting in fewer sources of support. As one of the women in our study said, 'If you didn't grow up here, people don't know you and they don't really want to know you' (Bourgeault et al., 2005: 39). Everybody knowing everybody can also mean that there is more at risk in rural communities from 'rocking the boat', since doing so can endanger one's entire social network. Indeed, a rural woman's ties to community can be more strongly constrained by their consistency with rural and gender ideologies (Dolan and Thien, 2008). Divorced and lesbian women face particular difficulties in the context of a more conservative climate in rural communities (Leipert and George, 2008).

In sum, despite some significant and relatively stable positive features of rural and remote living, both the women we interviewed and the literature speak eloquently of some of the inherent challenges of rural living and of how things are getting more difficult. This is not particular to the Canadian context, as Ryan-Nicholls emphasizes:

> Countless international rural communities encounter tremendous demographic, economic, social and ecological challenges associated with geographic isolation, depopulation, population aging, environmental decay and depletion of natural resources. (2004: 2)

The work that men and women do in these communities, its strict gendered division and its implications for their health and care, also needs examination.

Men and women's work in rural and remote communities

Differences in men's and women's relationships to natural resources, their educational backgrounds, the sexual division of labour at work and at home, the invisibility of women's work and the persistence of a male breadwinner model in resource-dependent areas ensure that the relationship between health and work is mediated by gender, in ways that often serve to make women more vulnerable. In this section we address the health effects of the work that predominates in rural and remote communities and how this affects men and women differently. Smith and colleagues (2008) alert us to how most of the differences found between rural and urban locations in terms of the incidence of disease and illness are most likely to result from occupational hazards. They note that:

> ... there are particular health risks associated with rural industries and their higher exposure to chemical, biological, physical and mechanical hazards. [...] Forestry and fishing have the highest death rates of all industry groups, and death rates in mining and agriculture are well above the workforce average. (2008: 57)

For example, Contant (2006) notes that in the province of British Columbia, more than 450 lives were lost due to forestry accidents in the years between 1984 and 2003. Beyond these physical and chemical exposures, the stress and uncertainty associated with precarious employment in single resource and/or agricultural communities take a toll. In the case of agriculture, farmers lurch from one crisis to another – whether market or weather-related – which causes stress and anxiety about finances, future livelihood and legacy in terms of the sustainability of their family farm (Arpalotai, 2005). As one of the women in our study noted:

> Between drought and BSE and some of the other problems [stress] is very high. And that can't really be alleviated until the policies which govern how

we market our product internationally and how we live, I mean that's not something you can [easily] fix. (Bourgeault et al., 2005: 40)

Although these occupational exposures are largely borne by the men who work in these industries, women and children are also exposed. Arpalotai, for example, has shown that 'a disproportionate number of farm accidents involve children and youth' (2005: 157) of which some are work-related, for example, when youth work on family farms. Women also express concern about the health impact of agricultural practices, including pesticide spraying and hog farming (Wathen and Harris, 2007). In cases of potential marital dissolution of farm couples that is either stress- or violence-related, although Canadian law provides some financial protection to the wife, in reality many women will feel pressured by their partner or family to stay in the relationship or to not exert their property rights in order to keep the family farm intact (Leipert and George, 2008).

Access to paid employment for women is also a concern in single-industry communities. As one of the women we interviewed explained, young women in particular are restricted if they wish to stay in the community:

It's not that easy because there is only one industry ... for the young girls, the only places they can work is probably in a restaurant, grocery store, or if you're career minded ... you have to leave the community to find employment and move away because you're not going to make a living here. You know. You could stay with your parents I guess or get married young. (Bourgeault et al., 2005: 34)

These challenges are exacerbated by strong social pressure in rural areas for women to get married very young, making them and their children more dependent on men for economic and social support (Leipert and Reutter, 2005b). If one opts to work outside of the community the high financial cost and negative health effects of commuting long distances become an issue.

Accessibility to healthcare

Clearly, geography matters when the provision of healthcare services is concerned, affecting accessibility for the population as well as the sustainability of the healthcare workforce. As Goerzten noted for Canada, 'our extreme weather conditions and diverse geography prove obstacles to travelling over the vast distances and difficult terrain between our scattered communities' (2005: 1181). In this section we juxtapose these two sometimes competing interests, with a specific focus on maternity and mental healthcare.

Canada is not a particularly special case in the challenges it faces in rural health human resources; data from Australia and the USA point to similar problems

(Australian Institute of Health and Welfare, 2004; US General Accounting Office, 2003). The sustainability of rural healthcare systems is challenged in many countries by the difficulties in recruiting and retaining family physicians and specialists (Curran and Rourke, 2004) and by the general maldistribution of health workers. Although more than 20 per cent of Canada's population lives in rural areas, less than 10 per cent of physicians (Giles and Giles, 2008) and less than 18 per cent of registered nurses practise in these communities (MacLeod et al., 2004). Although impressive, these overall numbers mask the impact that the movement of even a small number of practitioners has on local communities. As Rourke noted: 'The loss of a single physician from a rural community can change how the entire health care system is organized and run' (2008: 322). Research suggests that physicians leave rural and remote communities because of a combination of factors, including social and professional isolation, a lack of amenities, local poverty, and the hardships of rural work – long hours, frequent on-call shifts and low income (Donald et al., 2004).

This lack of health human resources in turn creates a lack of accessibility; this had two main consequences for the women we studied. In terms of control, in the words of one participant in our study, 'There are fewer specialists and [the] health care centre has moved out of the community to the interior so I feel we have less *control* of health in our community' (Bourgeault et al., 2005: 47). In terms of choice, another noted: 'I don't really have a *choice* with what's available for doctors'; she later expanded upon her lack of comfort with who was available (Bourgeault et al., 2005: 62). In several predominantly rural/remote provinces/territories the recruitment of international medical graduates to these underserviced areas has been an implicit policy, with some important negative consequences – including those for their country of origin. Many of the women we spoke to lamented the lack of retention of these physicians beyond past their return-of-service agreement, and how this translated into a lack of continuity of care. As one woman stated, 'The high turnover rate of physicians adversely affects consistency of care. It is easier for some patients to fall through the cracks' (Bourgeault et al., 2005: 66).

Another dimension of the lack of accessibility relates to distances travelled for healthcare when services are not locally available and the consequent problem of increased waiting times. It is here where we see the greatest impact of income, access to affordable transportation, or family or social networks on accessibility to care (Whitzman, 2006). Fuller and O'Leary (2008) found, for example, that 35 per cent of rural women in Canada are 'transportation poor'. This, as they noted, not only has implications for healthcare accessibility but also for employment opportunities. Although Canada has universal access to care, this often does not cover the costs for travelling to care. As one of the women in our study stated, 'Living in a rural community it is a given that I will have to pay for travel and accommodation expenses in order to see a specialist of any kind' (Bourgeault et al., 2005: 54). Another pointed out how 'it can be an all-day trip for a 15-minute doctor's appointment' (Bourgeault et al., 2005: 53). Because of these additional costs that some cannot pay, 'travel might need to be postponed, women might live with isolation and morbidity longer, their treatment and recovery may be more difficult, and their quality of life compromised' (Leipert and Reutter, 2005: 52). All in all, as Fuller and O'Leary argue, 'the quality of women's lives in rural areas is bound up in transportation access of one sort or another' (2008: 5). It is what Brown and colleagues call the 'tyranny of distance' (1999: 148).

A particularly vulnerable group of women are teenagers, whom Johnson (2004) studied in regards to access to abortion services in Canada. In addition to their concerns about the procedure, these teenagers also had to deal with the logistics of making an appointment and getting to it – assuming that they even knew what services were available. She described the potential difficulties:

If I were a pregnant teen with nowhere to turn, how would I get to a clinic? Any bus service is 30 kilometres from here, and runs only twice a day. I couldn't walk, and where would I get the $50 return cab fare to get to the bus stop? (Johnson, 2004: 14)

The costs of travelling long distances are not only economic but also social in terms of reliance on care by strangers and being separated from family and friends for extended periods of time (Allan et al., 2009). This was particularly salient for women from remote Aboriginal communities who were 'flown south' often weeks before delivering their babies in an unfamiliar environment with unfamiliar people, culture and language (Dooley et al., 2009). Although designed with the good intention to reduce the high perinatal mortality rates found in Canada's remote communities, numerous authors have documented the negative impact of these policies for the women, their families and their communities (Dooley et al., 2009; Kornelsen, 2009).

The case of maternity care

Maternity care in rural, non-remote communities is also under threat in Canada. As many acknowledge, the delivery of maternity care to rural and remote communities will always be challenging, in part because of the lack of consistent availability of the range of health professionals involved and the lack of predictability as to when care is needed. This difficult situation is, however, getting worse. Family doctors providing intrapartum care are in dwindling supply: In 1983, 68 per cent of Canadian family physicians attended births. Yet as of 2001, just 32 per cent of Alberta family physicians and 12 per cent in Ontario attended births (Reid et al., 2001). Reasons for this decline in attendance at births are that it interferes with personal and office life, there are low financial incentives and increasing disincentives, and there is inadequate specialist back-up due in part to the closure of local maternity units and a consequent declining confidence in skills (Reid et al., 2001).

As a result, women are forced to travel out of their home communities for care, despite growing evidence that giving birth locally is safer and less costly (Kornelson et al., 2009). As one of the women we interviewed told us:

> I would agree that health services particularly for women during the child-bearing years have really gone downhill in the last five years. [...] you can't get a doctor any more so you know, there you are pregnant and your doctor doesn't even know you and, you know, you're at the walk-in clinic and your doctor might not even have hospital privileges. But they're the only one available, and that's pretty disastrous for a lot of women. (Bourgeault et al., 2005: 50)

Some of the key areas of concern for women are en route deliveries and the inconvenience travel entails, especially in inclement weather (Kornelson et al., 2009; Sutherns and Bourgeault, 2008). Dooley and colleagues (2009) have also noted that the geographical challenges of rural maternity care and the centralization of obstetric services are among the multiple factors associated with Canada's rising induction rate.

Stigma, confidentiality and quality

In addition to the structural barriers to accessing care, there are some key social barriers as well. One of the primary issues hindering access to care for some of the Canadian women we interviewed is the concern about confidentiality and stigma, so even when services are available they are not accessed. This was particularly the case in relation to mental health issues. A sizeable proportion of women we interviewed reported that this sometimes or frequently prevented them from accessing care. The lack of a private place in the pharmacy where the pharmacist could confidentially advise and counsel women, as well as judgmental or condescending attitudes, often discouraged women from asking health-related questions (Leipert et al., 2008). Leipert and George (2008) made similar findings in relation to intimate partner violence; relationships with policy officers and rural healthcare providers could create barriers for women to disclose abuse. As Johnson puts it: 'Anonymity and confidentiality do not exist in places where everyone knows everyone else for miles around' (2004: 5).

As well as issues of confidentiality, a sizeable majority of the participants in our study were dissatisfied with the healthcare and medical services available to them. In many instances this focused on the variety of factors that influenced this, including burnout, and a lack of consistency and insensitivity among predominantly male medical staff to female health concerns. Access to female healthcare providers was also an issue, since most participants noted that having their healthcare provided by a woman was important to them. What was notable about living in rural and remote communities was that these women had few options when poor quality healthcare was all that was available.

The impact of reform

Restructuring of healthcare in Canada has resulted in changes in rural areas; there has been centralization of services through hospital, bed and clinic closures despite a rhetoric of decentralization, privatization of services, and shifting of responsibility for services to the community level without a matching shift in funding (Armstrong et al., 2002). This kind of restructuring and regionalization of services has significantly affected rural residents' access to healthcare services, both men and women (Crosato and Leipert, 2006). As Dolan and Thien assert:

> While infrequent, irregular and limited health services and lack of access to care locally is a reality for most rural Canadians, health care reforms are further exacerbating significant distances to travel for care, which is costly, inconvenient and even dangerous given precarious environmental conditions, especially in the north. (2008: 41)

Furthermore, healthcare reform has also created difficulties with recruiting and retaining healthcare professionals, adversely affecting access and waiting times (Ryan-Nicholls, 2004). As one of the women we interviewed said:

> [In] the area we were in ... they have closed hospitals there. We had a doctor for two hours, one day a week, who came into the community. There was no backup health unit. There was nothing. [It's] scary. (Bourgeault et al., 2005: 45)

Many of the concerns regarding access to care were linked directly to recent restructuring, cutbacks and closure of services.

Through the continuing debates on healthcare reforms, gender and the health of women have not had a clear or decisive place in the planning and definition of rural and remote health policies. There has been scant research about sex- and gender-specific health-determining influences on access to appropriate health services, experience of quality of care, environmental exposures and socio-economic factors particular to rural and remote regions of Canada (Armstrong et al., 2002). These changes in health services are occurring in a context of wider economic restructuring, which also has had profound effects on health.

Restructuring also affects women differently and often more severely than men, in part because of their roles as informal caregivers within families and because of women's experiences of economic vulnerability and disengagement from public decision-making. Rural women are particularly vulnerable. In rural contexts, women's roles as healthcare users, as formal and informal healthcare providers, and as citizens intersect with rural stereotypes where informal caregiving is seen as an extension of women's domestic role and as consistent with rural neighbourliness and intergenerational stability; this all creates additional burdens for women.

Conclusion

Goerzten succinctly summarizes some of the health and healthcare challenges facing rural communities in Canada:

> Rural communities suffer from a chronic shortage of family physicians who are challenged to provide primary and secondary medical care to patients who are older, poorer, less healthy, less well educated, and more likely to be obese and to smoke than Canadian patients in urban areas. (2005: 1181)

What he and many others fail to consider are the unique gendered aspects of these challenges. Women comprise the bulk of those who are older and poorer, while some of the services that are particularly limited are those women are most in need of, like maternity and mental healthcare.

Our empirical data relating to women in rural and remote communities and our review of the related literature on this topic reveal that although there are both positive and negative features of rural and remote living, when it comes to health and care, negative features predominate. Although there are positive aspects of the physical and social environment (open space, fresh air, community ties), negative aspects also exist. The built environment (housing, employment infrastructure, transportation, or lack thereof) in rural and remote communities presents great challenges, particularly to those who are already disadvantaged. In particular regard to healthcare, women were concerned not just with poor access but also poor quality. Many aspects of access were limited in ways particular to rural and remote settings, by far the most significant of which was the greater distances that women had to travel to seek treatment or care, and the cost incurred both in terms of time and money to do so.

Recent restructuring of healthcare services in these communities not only did not address these problems, it exacerbated them. Funding cuts often translated into units or entire hospitals closing or being threatened with closure, doctors moving away and services no longer being available in communities. Services located further away, creating longer distances to travel and greater inaccessibility, made things particularly difficult for women. An increasing proportion of women were paying out of pocket for healthcare services and for travel to those services. Women also expressed their frustration with the high turnover of medical personnel and the resulting inability to establish continuity in care – and with how things seemed to be getting worse.

While some of these findings are particular to the vast geography of rural and remote Canada, many of the themes raised resonate in the international literature (see for instance, Barnes and Bern-Klug, 1999; Harvey, 2007; Ryan-Nicholls, 2004). A metasynthesis of the international literature conducted by Harvey (2007) revealed themes similar to ours. Rural women experience a paradoxical sense of both isolation and belonging. The literature she reviewed also revealed a tension between 'adherence to a strong gendered rural identity which fosters a culture of stoicism and self reliance and feelings of resistance to societal expectations of coping with adversity' (Harvey, 2007: n.p.).

Therefore, in Canada and elsewhere, key areas for policy development and implementation would include those that address not only specific healthcare access and quality improvement issues that have been raised in previous research – more providers, particular female providers, sensitivity to women's health issues – but also broader social determinants of health, including better employment opportunities, improved transportation and enhanced childcare resources.

Summary

- Rural and remote healthcare is a neglected area of health policy; recent restructuring of healthcare may worsen the challenges.
- Healthcare in rural and remote areas has gendered effects; negative effects may be even stronger for women than for men.
- Contrary to the common stereotype of small communities having strong social ties, women's social networks may be more limited in rural areas, resulting in fewer sources of support.
- Policy development and implementation must move beyond specific healthcare access and availability and address broader social determinants of health, including better employment opportunities, transportation and childcare resources.

Key reading

Bourgeault, I. L., R. Sutherns, M. Haworth-Brockman, C. Dallaire and C. Neis (2006) 'Between a Rock and a Hard Place: Access, Quality and Satisfaction among Women

Living in Rural and Remote Communities in Canada', *Research in the Sociology of Health Care*, 24, 175–202.

Donald, E., M. D. Pathman, T. R. Konrad, R. Dann and G. Koch (2004) 'Retention of Primary Care Physicians in Rural Health Professional Shortage Areas', *American Journal of Public Health*, 94 (10), 1723–9.

Smith, K., J. Humphreys and M. Wilson (2008) 'Addressing the Health Disadvantage of Rural Populations: How Does Epidemiological Evidence Inform Rural Health Policies and Research?', *Australian Journal of Rural Health*, 16 (2), 56–66.

Wong, S.T. and Regan, S. (2009) 'Patient Perspectives on Primary Health Care in Rural Communities: Effects of Geography on Access, Continuity and Efficiency', *Journal of Rural Remote Health*, 9 (1), Project # 1189, 1–12.

References

Allan, D., S. Waskiewich, K. Stajduhar and D. Bidgood (2009) 'Use of Palliative Care Services in a Semirural Program in British Columbia', *Canadian Journal of Rural Medicine*, 14 (1), 10–15.

Arpalotai, A. (2005) 'A Web of Support for Rural Girls: A School/Community Healthcare Partnership', *Canadian Woman Studies*, 24 (4), 153–9.

Armstrong, P., C. Amaratunga, J. Bernier, K. Grant, A. Pederson and K. Willson (2002) *Exposing Privatization: Women and Health Care Reform in Canada* (Aurora: Garamond Press).

Australian Institute for Health and Welfare (2004) *Australia's Health: the Ninth Biennial Health Report of the Australian Institute of Health and Welfare* (Canberra: AIHW).

Barnes, N. D. and M. Bern-Klug (1999) 'Income Characteristics of Rural Older Women and Implications for Health Status', *Journal of Women & Aging*, 11 (1), 27–37.

Bourgeault, I. L., R. Sutherns, M. Haworth-Brockman, C. Dallaire, K. White and J. Winkup (2005) *The Impact of Restructuring on Rural, Remote and Northern Women's Health [2002–2004]* (Ottawa: National Research Steering Committee on Rural and Remote Women's Health [NRSC] and National Centres of Excellent in Women's Health [CEWH]), at: www.cewh-cesf.ca/en/resources/rural_remote/index.html, accessed 15 September 2009.

Bourgeault, I. L., R. Sutherns, M. Haworth-Brockman, C. Dallaire and C. Neis (2006) 'Between a Rock and a Hard Place: Access, Quality and Satisfaction among Women Living in Rural and Remote Communities in Canada', *Research in the Sociology of Health Care*, 24, 175–202.

Brown, W. J., A. F. Young and J. E. Byles (1999) 'Tyranny of Distance? The Health of Mid-age Women Living in Five Geographical Areas of Australia', *Australian Journal of Rural Health*, 7 (3), 148–54.

CIHI – Canadian Institute for Health Information (2006) *How Healthy are Rural Canadians? An Assessment of Their Health Status and Health Determinants* (Ottawa: Canadian Institute for Health Information).

Cloke, P. (1994) '(En)culturing Political Geography: A Life in the Day of a Rural Geographer', in P. Cloke, M. Doel, D. Matless, M. Phillips and N. Thrift (eds), *Writing the Rural: Five Cultural Geographies* (London: Paul Chapman), 149–90.

Contant, J. (2006) 'Safety Cuts', *Occupational Health and Safety Canada*, 22 (5), 30–2, 34–5.

Cox, J. (1999) 'Rural Poverty, Deprivation and Health', in J. Cox and I. Mungall (eds), *Rural Healthcare* (Oxford: Radcliffe Medical Press), 115–20.

Curran, V. and J. Rourke (2004) 'The Role of Medical Education in the Recruitment and Retention of Rural Physicians', *Medical Teacher*, 26 (3), 265–72.

Crosato, K. E and B. Leipert (2006) 'Rural Women Caregivers in Canada', *Rural and Remote Health,* 6, Project # 520, 1–11, at: www.rrh.org.au, accessed 2 June 2009.

Donald, E., M. D. Pathman, T. R. Konrad, R. Dann and G. Koch (2004) 'Retention of Primary Care Physicians in Rural Health Professional Shortage Areas', *American Journal of Public Health,* 94 (10), 1723–9.

Dolan, H. and D. Thien (2008) 'Relations of Care: A Framework for Placing Women and Health in Rural Communities', *Canadian Journal of Public Health,* 99, S38–S42.

Dooley, J., N. St Pierre-Hansen and J. Guilfoyle (2009) 'Rural and Remote Obstetric Care Close to Home: Program Description, Evaluation and Discussion of Sioux Lookout Meno Ya Win Health Centre Obstetrics', *Canadian Journal of Rural Medicine,* 14 (2), 75–9.

Fuller, T. and S. O'Leary (2008) 'The Impact of Access to Transportation on the Lives of Rural Women', RWMC Library, Rural Women Making Change, University of Guelph, 12 May 2009, at: www.rwmc.uoguelph.ca/document.php?d=181, accessed 19 May 2009.

Giles, S. and A. Giles (2008) 'Industrious, Submissive, and Free of Diseases: 156 Years of Physicians in Liidlii Kue/Fort Simpson, Northwest Territories', *Canadian Journal of Rural Medicine,* 13 (3), 111–20.

Goerzten, J. (2005) 'The Four-legged Kitchen Stool: Recruitment and Retention of Rural Family Physicians', *Canadian Family Physician,* 51 (Sep), 1181–3, 1184–6.

Harvey, D. J. (2007) 'Understanding Australian Rural Women's Ways of Achieving Health and Wellbeing – A Metasynthesis of the Literature', *Rural and Remote Health,* 7 (online), Project # 823, 1–12, at: www.rrh.org.au, accessed 22 June 2009.

Hunsberger, M., A. Baumann, J. Blythe and M. Crea (2009) 'Sustaining the Rural Workforce: Nursing Perspectives on Worklife Challenges', *Journal of Rural Health,* 25 (1), 17–25.

Johns, N. and J. Havelock (2006) 'Rural Women's Action Workshop: Carlyle, Saskatchewan', *Prairie Women's Health Centre of Excellence, Project #127,* at: www.uwinnipeg.ca/admin/vh_external/pwhce/pdf/ruralCarlyle.pdf, accessed 21 Feb 2010.

Johnson, N. (2004) '"What's Hot in Women's Health?" Reproductive Choice is Not a Reality in Rural and Remote Regions', *Canadian Women's Health Network,* 6/7 (4/1), 14–16.

Kobetz, E., M. Daniel and J. A. Earp (2003) 'Neighborhood Poverty and Self-reported Health among Low-income, Rural Women, 50 Years and Older', *Health & Place,* 95 (3), 264–271.

Kornelsen, J., S. Moola and S. Grzybowski (2009) 'Does Distance Matter? Increased Induction Rates for Rural Women Who Have to Travel for Intrapartum Care', *Journal of Obstetrics and Gynaecology Canada,* 31 (1), 21–7.

Leipert, B. D. and J. A. George (2008) 'Determinants of Rural Women's Health: A Qualitative Study in Southwestern Ontario', *The Journal of Rural Health,* 24 (2), 210–18.

Leipert, B. D., D. Matsui, J. Wagner and M. J. Rieder (2008) 'Rural Women and Pharmacologic Therapy: Needs and Issues in Rural Canada', *Canadian Journal of Rural Medicine,* 13 (4), 171–9.

Leipert, B. D. and L. Reutter (1998) 'Women's Health and Community Health Nursing Practice in Geographically Isolated Settings: A Canadian Perspective', *Health Care for Women International,* 19 (6), 575–88.

Leipert, B. D. and L. Reutter (2005a) 'Developing Resilience: How Women Maintain Their Health in Northern Geographically Isolated Settings', *Qualitative Health Research,* 15 (1), 49–65.

Leipert, B. D. and L. Reutter (2005b) 'Women's Health in Northern British Columbia: The Role of Geography and Gender', *Canadian Journal of Rural Medicine*, 10 (4), 241–54.

MacLeod, M. L. P., J. C. Kulig, N. J. Stewart, J. R. Pitblado and M. Knock (2004) 'The Nature of Nursing Practice in Rural, Remote Canada', *Canadian Health Services Research Foundation*, 100 (6), 7–31.

Murdoch, J. and A. C. Pratt (1993) 'Rural Studies: Modernism, Postmodernism and the Post-Rural', *The Journal of Rural Studies*, 9 (4), 411–27.

Nagarajan, K. V. (2004) 'Rural and Remote Community Health Care in Canada: Beyond the Kirby Panel Report, The Romanow Report and the Federal Budget Of 2003', *Canadian Journal of Rural Medicine*, 9 (4), 245–51.

Pampalon, R. (2005) 'Does Living in Rural Areas Make a Difference for Health in Québec?', *Health & Place*, 12 (4), 421–35.

Pong, R. W., M. DesMeules and C. Lagacé (2009) 'Rural-Urban Disparities in Health: How Does Canada Fare and How Does Canada Compare with Australia?', *Australian Journal of Rural Health*, 17 (1), 58–64.

Reid, A., I. Gravin-Gublins and I. Carroll (2001) *Results of the 2001 National Family Physician Workforce (Weighted Data), The Janus Project* (Mississauga, Ontario: College of Family Physicians of Canada).

Richmond, C. and N. Ross (2009) 'The Determinants of First Nation and Inuit Health: A Critical Population Health Approach', *Health & Place*, 15 (2), 403–11.

Ryan-Nicholls, K. D. (2004) 'Health and Sustainability of Rural Communities', *Rural and Remote Health*, 4, 1–11, at: www.rrh.org.au, accessed 3 July 2009.

Smith, K., J. Humphreys and M. Wilson (2008) 'Addressing the Health Disadvantage of Rural Populations: How Does Epidemiological Evidence Inform Rural Health Policies and Research?', *Australian Journal of Rural Health*, 16 (2), 56–66.

Statistics Canada (2001) Canada: Population Urban and Rural, by Province and Territory, at: www40.statcan.ca/l01/cst01/demo62a-eng.htm, accessed 20 July 2009.

Sutherns, R. (2004) 'Adding Women's Voices to the Call for Sustainable Rural Maternity Care', *Canadian Journal of Rural Medicine*, 9 (4), 239–44.

Sutherns, R. (2005) 'So Close Yet So Far: Rurality as a Determinant of Women's Health', *Canadian Women Studies*, 24 (4), 117–22.

Sutherns, R. and I. L. Bourgeault (2008) 'Accessing Maternity Care in Rural Canada: There's More to the Story than Distance to a Doctor', *Health Care for Women International*, 29 (8), 863–83.

Sutherns, R., M. McCallum and M. Haworth-Brockman (2007) 'A Thematic Bibliography and Literature Review of Rural, Remote and Northern Women's Health in Canada 2003–2006', *Resources for Feminist Research*, 32 (3/4), 142–78.

Wathen, N. and R. Harris (2007) '"I Try to Take Care of It Myself". How Rural Women Search for Health Information', *Qualitative Health Research*, 17 (5), 639–51.

Whitzman, C (2006) 'At the Intersection of Invisibilities: Canadian Women, Homelessness and Health Outside the "Big City"', *The Journal of Gender, Place and Culture*, 13 (4), 383–99.

Wong, S. T. and S. Regan (2009) 'Patient Perspectives on Primary Health Care in Rural Communities: Effects of Geography on Access, Continuity and Efficiency', *Journal of Rural Remote Health*, 9 (1), Project # 1189, 1–12.

Part IV
Gendering the Organization and Delivery of Healthcare

20
The New Management of Healthcare: 'Rational' Performance and Gendered Actors

Jim Barry, Elisabeth Berg and John Chandler

Introduction

In many countries across the world, and especially in Europe, we have seen an increasing concern with management as a key component of new governance and policy reforms in healthcare (Dent, 2003). In this chapter we focus on the new management of healthcare and the gendered actors who work to deliver the human services involved. By 'new' management, we are referring to what has been called New Public Management (NPM), thought to have developed in many countries around the world from the 1970s onwards with the purpose of reducing costs, increasing efficiencies and accountabilities, and generally enhancing the quality of human services and experience of users (see Chandler et al., 2002; Dent et al., 2004; McLaughlin et al., 2002). Accordingly, our focus is on the management and implementation of healthcare, and of those involved in its delivery. In the middle of these processes are the new managers, often professionals, charged with responsibility for delivery. This is not to suggest that healthcare, like other human services within the public realm, has not been managed and organized in the past. It is rather to point to the growth of a new group or cadre of workers involved in the implementation of the new work regimes who draw on private sector management techniques and mindsets in their attempt to achieve the desired ends. We consider these changes with particular reference to gender (Barry et al., 2003).

The chapter consequently aims to explore both the gendered nature of NPM and the gendered responses to it. It does so through a focus on a particular group of healthcare managers who often have a nursing background – a group where women are numerically dominant (see also Chapter 28 by Wrede). There are some obvious limitations of such a focus but we think it does raise some important issues on the gendered nature of new models of healthcare organization and delivery.

We start the chapter by outlining the development of NPM and the forms it has taken, focusing on the notion of performativity that has overseen the widespread introduction of performance indicators, targets and use of NPM-based practice across public sectors in different parts of the world. We then use case studies from Britain and Sweden to illustrate the way in which NPM and performativity operate and consider the implications for professional identities. Both these countries are forerunners in the implementation of NPM but differ with respect to both the regulatory structure of health and welfare provision, and gender regimes. We conclude by considering some challenges and opportunities in respect of the new management of healthcare for gender relations.

New Public Management in healthcare

Hood (1995) has outlined several elements of NPM which have been pressed into service to bring about change in the public sector. These include a focus on 'discipline and parsimony' in the use of resources, disaggregation, the use of performance measurement and 'pre-set output measures', and greater 'hands-on' management (Hood, 1995: 95–7), with surveillance and audit thrown in for good measure. Dent (2003) has argued that this has had a profound impact on the professions dominating healthcare – with medicine and nursing undergoing a shift from professional autonomy to responsible autonomy, whereby professionals are increasingly subject to management via rules and regulations and held accountable for their performance. Others have pointed to the declining importance of professional and bureaucratic models of control and increasing reliance on management and contracts (Clarke and Newman, 1997). Hood (1995) has referred to the development of these reforms as effectively a movement across OECD countries. Some early adopters such as New Zealand and the UK have embraced them enthusiastically whilst others, such as Germany with its more decentralized state system, seem less inclined. However, in different contexts it has taken somewhat different forms, leading to the suggestion that NPM is a kind of toolbox of techniques for interested parties to dip into according to taste (see also Pollitt and Bouckaert, 2000; Schedler and Proeller, 2002).

It is generally acknowledged in the academic literature that the development of NPM occurred from the late 1970s (see, for example, Hood, 1995), around the time that neoliberal influences were discerned worldwide (see Harvey, 2005). The timing is perhaps significant, with Clarke (2004a: 116–17) talking of 'managerialism' as, in effect, the 'organizational glue' of what has been called the dispersed state, remaking and holding together its 'vertical and horizontal relations of power, authority and control'. In the context of neoliberalism it is managerialism, drawing as it does on private sector managerial techniques and ideologies, which operationalizes policy and enables service delivery. But what background assumptions are associated with neoliberalism? Harvey (2005) has characterized neoliberalism as a theory of political-economic practices that sees human well-being as best promoted through the exercise of individual entrepreneurialism within an institutional context that provides strong private property rights, free markets and free trade. He argues that such ideas and policies have become so widespread since the 1970s that it has 'become hegemonic as a mode of discourse' (Harvey, 2005: 3).

We have thus seen the elevation of market ideologies, associated with the politics of choice, risk and uncertainty (Beck and Beck-Gernsheim, 2002), and an individualism that makes citizens and employees individually responsible and holds them to account. This chimes with the central tenets of NPM, designed to cut back public sector expenditure in favour of fiscal austerity and private sector market solutions, hold employees to account and intensify work regimes. As Pollitt and Bouckaert (2000: 1) explain, in somewhat dramatic terms, the development of NPM has been a pandemic, sweeping across much of the OECD, altering the working lives of millions of public service workers and leading to the premature termination of employment in tens of thousands of cases. They emphasize, too, that budgets and ways of managing public finance have been affected, with large claims made for efficiency gains. If, however, such reforms often rest upon a rhetoric of freedom, choice and entrepreneurialism, performance management seems to be at the heart of these reforms as the 'organizational glue' holding things together. We turn next, therefore, to an exploration of this phenomenon.

Performance management and the notion of performativity

In this chapter we will focus on the issue of performance in the public sector through the notion of performativity. There are a number of ways in which performativity can be understood but a useful starting point is that suggested by Dent and Whitehead (2002) who draw upon the work of Lyotard to emphasize that performativity requires the nurse, doctor or other public sector worker to perform and be judged according to external yardsticks of impersonal, objective criteria. It is no longer enough to internalize knowledge and practise skills as a competent performer, and account for this in narrative and subjective terms. Accordingly, the professional's account is no longer enough. Professional practice is subject to external scrutiny according to formal and supposedly cold, objective, value-neutral criteria. Increasingly the professional performs and is judged according to targets and evidence; it is through these mechanisms that their performance is 'managed'. But there is a gender dimension to such performativity, too, and before considering our case studies we wish to explore this in theoretical terms.

Gendering performativity

We consider gender as central to issues of performativity in health. Approaches to gender in studies of management and organization have traditionally focused on differences between women and men. Whilst perhaps implicit historically this was reinforced in the 1980s by the work of Gilligan (1982) who studied moral development in children, concluding that girls developed an 'ethic of care' and boys a 'logic of justice' in relation to abstract reasoning. Gilligan challenged conventional wisdom about boys' development being superior to girls', contending that they were simply different. In this way she moved analysis forward, but she nevertheless simultaneously confirmed to many readers that women and men really were different, feeding stereotypical assumptions about gender and inspiring or affirming a number of studies into areas where difference might play a part, such as organization, leadership and management (Ferguson, 1984; Rosener, 1990; Schein, 1973).

This was challenged by the poststructuralist and postmodern turn in the latter part of the 20th century that eschewed simplistic binaries such as those of female and male, women and men, and sought to decentre the difference agenda in favour of plural masculinities and femininities; reintroducing, some might argue, another binary. On this count, however, it was contended that women and men might engage in a variety of differing behavioural displays of both masculinity and femininity; and whilst there are studies that continue to count, for example, the numbers of women and men in management and recount differences between them, there has also been a tendency to embrace a multi-faceted approach to studies of gender.

There are, of course, many varieties of masculinity and femininity, with Collinson and Hearn (1994: 2; see also Connell, 1987), for example, identifying what they termed 'multiple masculinities' back in 1994. But our concern here is to locate masculinity and femininity within research on the healthcare sector. To begin with, the very term care itself evokes gendered images; and as we have seen, Gilligan (1982) argued quite specifically that girls develop an 'ethic of care' and boys a 'logic of justice', each of which reflects stereotypical ideas about gender difference. In examining the management of healthcare it is, however, also helpful to draw upon the work of Thomas and Davies (2002) who bring into perspective a number of elements of the new performance regimes that can be considered masculine; whilst their focus was higher education, their comments are indicative of the public sector more widely, including public healthcare. The elements include 'masculine discourses of competitiveness, instrumentality and individuality, which conflict[ed] with feminine discourses of empathy, supportiveness and nurturing' (Thomas and Davies, 2002: 390).

These writers are not alone in associating management with particular forms of masculinity. Clarke and Newman (1997: 70; see also, for a more recent analysis, Newman, 2005) argue that many public sector organizations 'have taken on images of competitive behaviour as involving hard, macho or "cowboy" styles of working', with Davies (1995: 27; see also Young, 2003) pointing to a shift in the British National Health Service (NHS) towards a more aggressive, harsh and confrontational approach. There are plenty of other studies, too, which point to a close association between management more generally (whether in the public or private sector) and particular forms of masculinity (see, for example, Collinson and Hearn, 1994; Kerfoot, 2002).

Of course such 'masculine' or patriarchal behaviours are not new in healthcare, with bureaucratic and professional organizational regimes also characterized by similar forms of masculine discourse, behaviour and relations (Davies, 1996; Ferguson, 1984; Savage and Witz, 1992). If there is a difference between the forms of masculinity adopted under the sway of managerialism and the style of earlier regimes perhaps it lies in a greater likelihood that bureaucracy and professionalism involve paternalistic behaviour (Burris, 1996). However, the detailed comparison of the forms of masculinity taken in different organizational forms is beyond the scope of this chapter; here, it is sufficient to note that managerialism is *not* gender-neutral.

If managerialism is gendered, however, the possibility of resistance to this character of contemporary work regimes instituted by advocates and implementers of NPM is something to be considered. This is because, despite the apparent strength of the neoliberal agenda and the managerial stickiness of an organizational glue that has promoted a 'business agenda', its dominance in many public sectors around the world cannot be assumed, since it remains an incomplete project, to which the economic turmoil experienced in world markets in 2008 and 2009 attests. As Clarke argues, dominant strategies do not have everything their way:

> Dominant strategies do not occupy an empty landscape. They have to overcome resistances, refusals and blockages. For many reasons the public realm (and the attachments that it mobilises) is part of the 'grit' that prevents the imagined neo-liberal world system functioning smoothly. (Clarke, 2004b: 44–5)

Resistance is something Thomas and Davies (2002), whom we referred to earlier, also explicitly consider, with a particular focus on micro-political processes. Seen in this way, resistance can take many forms. It might consist of distinct acts of refusal, or of insubordination, or misbehaviour (Ackroyd and Thompson, 1999), but it might also take the form of interpretive challenges such as Davies' (1995: 27) example of disparaging remarks towards 'men in suits'. Thus resistance is one of the issues illustrated in our cases.

New managerial regimes and professional identities: case studies

The two cases that we are going to focus on are located in Britain and Sweden, both countries, as indicated earlier, at the forefront of NPM reforms. The main differences between the two countries concern, first, a time lag in take-up of the new managerial regimes; second, the institutional structure of the welfare and healthcare state; and third, traditions of gender equity. Our cases have been selected from published academic sources as well as empirical studies carried out by ourselves. Before commencing, however, a few words are in order about the contexts for our cases.

In respect of timing, a social democratic political tradition has been stronger in Sweden, with neoliberal politics arriving only in the early 1990s in a short-lived right-wing coalition, revived in 2006 with the election of another right-of-centre neoliberal-inspired alliance. In Britain, by contrast, a neoliberal centrist government reined from 1979 to 1997, when a new Labour administration came to power bearing the legacy of a strident Thatcherite neoliberalism (see Pollitt and Bouckaert, 2000 for country overviews). In respect of gender, Britain has a liberal tradition that reflects a concern with equality of opportunity. Change is slow as a result and women remain under-represented in positions of power and decision-making (Dent, 2003; Glover and Kirton, 2006). In Britain, there has also been a shift from a concern with equal opportunities, often with a strong focus on gender equality, towards a concern with the management of diversity, with many forms of difference acknowledged. While in many ways this is an apparently progressive move which recognizes many forms of inequality and difference, it has also been seen as tending to individualize concerns and water down gender equity considerations (Liff and Wajcman, 1996). Sweden, by contrast, has been more concerned with outcomes than procedures, and has followed a 60/40 rule whereby attempts are made to ensure that women (and men) secure no less than 40 per cent of public sector appointments and political representation. This does not mean, however, that discrimination and inequality have been somehow eradicated, as we will see. Indeed, in Sweden as well as in Britain there are pronounced gender differences in the make-up of occupations providing healthcare (Dent 2003; Glover and Kirton, 2006; SCB, 2007).

Performing gender identity

The first case study concerns nurses in Britain's NHS, and is drawn from Halford (2003) who used a narrative methodology involving interviews. Her focus is organizational change and discourses on gender, with an 'emphasis on agency, resistance and personal politics', to show how performance at work, and related performative response, can impact on the shaping of identity through micropolitical processes (Halford, 2003: 286). Yet, whilst viewing the performative cultures of management in many work organizations as masculine, using her empirical research undertaken in the NHS, she argues that these cultures are not determinate, seeing them as interacting with 'older practices, informal practices and resistances' (Halford, 2003: 291).

Halford outlines recent organizational changes that have affected the NHS. These include the following: a growing credentialism in the nursing profession; the restructuring of senior nursing positions to embrace managerial functions, thereby opening up the nursing profession to candidates with professional and/or managerial expertise; and the intensification of work through the delegation of managerial tasks such as budgeting, human resource management and the monitoring of performance. It is clear in all this that the new managerialism has indeed arrived in the NHS. In all, Halford reports on in-depth interviews with five nurses from two hospitals, of whom three are women and two men. The women interviewees all talked of their identities as nurses and the recent shift to embrace management within the NHS. For instance, Fiona started her working life as a nurse, before gaining management qualifications that enabled her to secure a post as a senior general manager. As she explained, the two were complementary:

Women are expected, from the management perspective, probably to behave with the less feminine type of [identity] performing similar to the male masculine [sic] traits. Whereas within the nursing side of things there's an acceptance that there's a little bit of the feminine. (Halford, 2003: 295)

Sarah had some managerial responsibilities but also a nursing role as well. There was, however, a degree of ambivalence, with her expressing concern about incompatibility since management responsibilities made it difficult to meet the demands of 'staff, patients and, indeed, more senior managers'. She nonetheless enjoyed the status and authority that accompanied a management position:

It means you are becoming, you are becoming the person that you didn't want to become, I'm not a person who finds it easy, or had found it easy to say no. But I'm learning pretty quick. (Halford, 2003: 296)

Brenda, on the other hand, saw herself as a traditional nurse – an identity she maintained by working in a unit separate from the hospital – and bemoaned the loss of respect for nurses generally. This she attributed to managers: 'The senior managers are not nurses. Very few are nurses. And, as such, they don't have the same feelings' (Halford, 2003: 297).

The men interviewees, by contrast, distanced themselves from nursing, at least from its caring elements. Martin, for example, initially considered a career in army nursing, which he saw as embodying masculine elements, emphasizing notions of career strategy, status and authority when referring to himself. Douglas also distanced himself from nursing. Having changed occupation from engineering, he now found himself the only male nurse in his working area. He was initially unhappy. However, once he had become more settled, he was to follow what was considered an option open to men nurses: to transform caring into technical knowledge, something that was even encouraged by women nurses:

> They [male nurses] are put into positions where it's impossible for them to care, and it's deliberately done. I mean, I found when I was a student nurse I would be treated as the technical nurse. I would be put in situations where I was dealing with patients who had technical problems, not touchy-feely, whereas I'm quite good at that. (Halford, 2003: 299–300)

Douglas later offered a reason as to why he might be different from other male workers in this respect: he was gay. Halford comments that 'his sexuality may explain why he says "I've never met a male nurse I could model myself on (all are either techies or straight [at least closeted])"' (2003: 300).

Halford highlights the active construction involved in identity work, and its performative character within processes of organizational and managerial change. In these processes, notions of caring appear linked inextricably to ideas of femininity and management to masculinity, with women and men nurses variously aware of incompatibilities and contradictions, as well as complementarities and opportunities. Whilst actively engaged in the performance of identity, they are also negotiating the performative requirements of managerialism per se. There is no easy resolution for these nurses who adapt, resist and generally muddle through the everyday processes involved.

Gendered politics in the organization

Further examples of these processes, covering the 'everyday' (De Certeau, 1984) work of Britain's NHS nurses, can be found in Bolton's (2005) account of women gynaecology nurses who have a strong sense of collective identity, and one highly differentiated from those of the doctors they worked with, who are mainly men. Commenting on change in the organization, one of the nurses said:

> What hasn't changed is the fact that we are women doing an excellent job of looking after women and a lot of change has centred round our determination to continue with that. (Bolton, 2005: 180)

The nurses she reports on were critical of men operating within gynaecology – whether as nurses or doctors. Bolton describes how the nurses would sometimes humiliate junior doctors. One of the nurses is quoted as saying:

> Some of these doctors don't have a clue. They don't know what the hell is going on. Women's health? I'm sure they think it's about neutering cats or something. They rely on us to carry them and then try and lord it over us. They soon get the message. Most of them wouldn't get through this part of their training if it weren't for our knowledge in this area. If they get too big for their boots we'll sort them out and they're on their knees by the time we've finished with them. (Bolton, 2005: 180–1)

This is sexual politics of the rawest kind, involving the 'writing [of] expletives on doctor's backs, locking them in toilets, depriving them of various pieces of equipment, in addition to almost constant reprimands and put downs' (Bolton, 2005: 181). There is no evidence that these women see themselves as feminists, although possibly their awareness of gender issues and identification with women might justify the use of the term latent feminist, even if many feminists would be distinctly at odds with both the tactics and beliefs of these nurses with comments such as: '[...] generally I feel women make better nurses, we are just naturally more sensitive to the environment, to what people are feeling and how to deal with it' (Bolton, 2005: 173). Nevertheless, Bolton makes clear that:

> In the day-to-day lived reality of the women's world of gynaecology the multiple meanings of many symbolic universes and past experiences are simultaneously used as cultural resources. That is, gender is a dynamic and continuing process, a distinct social accomplishment that is achieved through the lived experiences of women and men ... Thinking about gender in this way displays the 'contradiction, opposition and dynamic' ... involved in carrying out women's work and dirty work *and* highlights how spaces are created where the status quo can be challenged and, however gradually, ultimately changed. (Bolton, 2005: 171)

If all this suggests that gendered symbolic and experiential orders are far from static or uncontested, the case considered in the following section points to uneasy accommodation and avoidance.

The 'hard work' of management

The study of the impact of managerialism on nurses in Britain by Wise (2003) was based on interviews with 40 nurses at a variety of levels of the organization in her study of one NHS Hospitals Trust employing 6766 nursing and midwifery staff over several sites. Her findings illustrate the dynamic nature of managerial change as well as changes in discourse. Thus she reports, for example, how the post of Clinical Nurse Manager was transformed into that of 'Ops Manager' (we assume this is an abbreviation for Operations Manager, although this is not made clear). Sometimes this role was occupied by people who were not qualified nurses. At a stroke this change of title seems to reflect a distancing of the position from the job of nursing and from its clinical or professional (and perhaps caring) nature. This was accompanied by a change of tasks where budgetary responsibilities increased as well as those for 'waiting time targets, bed management, complaint procedures, health and safety, clinical standards and service planning. Responsibility for personnel also widened to include junior doctors and other health professionals' (Wise, 2003: 99). Similarly, Charge Nurses were re-named Ward Managers and were responsible for the day-to-day running of hospital wards. These new positions seem to be associated with long working hours, with all Ops Managers and Ward Managers reporting that they worked in excess of contractual hours (see also Allen, 2001). As one Ward Manager put it:

> On a normal week you can add 2 extra hours onto every day but it can be worse. I used to note down extra hours but I gave up the ghost. It's a waste of time because you so rarely get it back. (Wise, 2003: 100)

Long hours seemed to be a recurring feature, with some nurses expressing considerable strain in coping. Even for men with no family responsibilities this seems to have made the jobs unattractive to many. One male staff nurse explained:

> I don't know if I want to go as high as that. [Our Ward Manager] has left because of the job. I saw what it did to her. I'd be happy staying at a [grade] F. (Wise, 2003: 101)

As Wise's study makes clear, the managerial position seems to be associated with long working hours that are difficult to reconcile with family life. Where men and women do take up these positions they seem required to behave as if they have supportive 'housewives' at home, something not available to most women. This is an example of how managerialism is associated with gendered substructures within organizations (Acker, 1990; 1998) whereby the manager, in particular, is expected to be an abstract person (Acker, 1998), able to give their all to the job and to fit other commitments around it. As Wise (2003) argues, this creates problems for people in such roles, and makes the job unattractive. As a consequence, many choose to avoid such roles or to exit from them.

Gendered positioning in the organization

Studies of women's working lives in Sweden (Berg, 2003; Gonäs and Karlsson, 2008) show that opportunities for women in secure paid employment are still limited and labour markets highly segregated. In health and social work, however, where women have a dominant numerical position (70–95 per cent), they are also in the majority in lower and middle management positions (SCB, 2007). These job positions have had a long tradition of being seen as women's work, and few men have challenged this segregated organization of the public sector.

Since the late 1980s and 1990s there have been organizational changes in the public sector that have led to a change in the kinds of knowledge required by staff working in management positions (Berg et al., 2008). Interviews with women and men working in social care in Sweden, with an educational background in nursing and social work, revealed how they presented their work in different ways depending on how they preferred to position themselves in their organizations (Berg, 2000; 2003; Berg et al., 2008). These middle managers described how they had started in lower positions, whilst continuing with their education to gain a nursing or professional social work degree. They were proud to explain that they knew their job thoroughly and that they were enjoying a job where they helped people. As a nurse or a social worker they have a management position, and they all find that challenging, but it also means more administration, including responsibility for the budget. One of the top managers explained how budgets have been crucial for the job they have today: 'It is totally about saving money, that is the policy and it is quite tough. In general terms it's all about finance, everything has a price' (Berg, 2000: 79).

With the introduction of NPM organizations have been changing, affecting the social welfare departments where the interviews for Berg's research took place. There was a clear division of labour: nurses worked with patients/users in institutional care and social workers with decisions about how much help the users needed. These changes have led to lack of clarity about middle managers' work conditions. As one middle manager said:

> Earlier I had an understanding of what happened. I knew all that concerned staff and when the other managers had problems they called me. They asked about how to take decisions about different matters and also asked for advice when they had problems with staff. I knew everything and I had also a responsibility for staff education and development. (Berg, 2000: 125)

This manager felt that the specialization and division of labour had led to a narrowing of her work as a professional social worker and middle manager. Social welfare departments have reorganized social and health work in local authorities in favour of a clear specialization and division of labour over the past 25 years (Berg, 2003). These changes have led to a more differentiated organizational structure, which has cemented the existing gender structure. In interviews with men and women in middle management positions, gender differences surfaced in how they presented their work. Men said that they identified themselves with the senior management group and that their job included responsibility for the budget, staff development and administration. Women presented their jobs in a similar way, with responsibility for budget and staff, but they also emphasized the importance of being in touch with the real social and health work undertaken by their subordinates. One female middle manager commented about men working in social care:

> It is luck that there are women who work with social care, men would never manage it ... You cannot just concentrate on one thing at the time; often it is several issues at the same time that have to be dealt with. (Berg, 2000: 108)

What this female middle manager was referring to was her belief that men were not as suitable as women in social and health work because they could not handle more than one thing at a time. This shows a stereotypical view of both women and men, assuming that health and social care is women's work. Several comments showed that women in this profession thought men acted differently to women. In one organization a middle manager, who had a male mentor from a technical department, pointed out how differently she felt this man acted in contrast to her female colleagues:

> There was a mentor from a 'hard department' [technical department] something that has been good because they think different and see things different. Men work differently, they are straighter than women are, we walk around and talk, well, a little chaotic to create order, and they just walk straight to the point, I believe, in certain issues. (Berg, 2000: 103)

This middle manager's view was that although men from this 'hard department' acted very tough and that this hurt some people, there was something positive about it for her since she felt it gave her new ideas about how to act as a manager. She felt she could model herself on the behaviour of such men, suggesting that these gender differences were not seen as essentially tied to the performance of men or women – that women could begin to manage like men. One senior manager made a comment about how a woman presented herself when she applied for a management position:

> The first thing she said [in the job interview] was that she would not be a manager, and instead be a part of the group, and I thought a man would never say something like that. (Berg, 2000: 105)

However, this still suggests that management is associated with masculine performances. This might explain why there is evidence that, in this female-dominated social care sector where few men were to be found, the men experienced positive discrimination. They found themselves encouraged by both female and male colleagues to take on more responsibility and therefore to rise in the organization (Berg, 2003).

Conclusion

The cases presented here indicate that managerialism is not a gender-neutral set of practices but is instead characterized by masculine performativity. Management is associated with masculine behaviours that, as Thomas and Davies (2002) have summed it up, involve competitiveness, instrumentality and individuality. Moreover, managerial positions are associated with long working hours and are seen as difficult to reconcile with other commitments. While there is no suggestion here that women cannot take on managerial positions and, indeed, manage like men, such a move always involves a particular form of gendered politics, an elevation of certain values and forms of power above others. This is where 'hard' objective rationality seems to dominate over caring. But if masculine forms of management are pervasive as the organizational glue of neoliberalism, we can also expect complex reactions to it as women and men resist and accommodate to them, and not always in expected ways.

The cases presented here deal with managerialism in areas of healthcare in which women are numerically dominant and where NPM reforms have offered some new opportunities for women to take on managerial roles. They suggest a number of complex interplays between people and dominant forms of masculinity – some are downright oppositional and conflictual, involving ridicule and humiliation, some represent more or less grudging accommodation to the changes. However, also represented are feelings that the managerial identity, when taken on, is hard to bear: this does not seem a very attractive proposition, despite the higher hierarchical position it implies. This analysis and the cases presented consequently suggest several pressing questions that need to be addressed by women and men of varying sexualities working in healthcare or concerned about how it is to be provided.

Summary

Opportunities

- New Public Management (NPM) offers new career opportunities for women prepared to take managerial roles, with relatively high income and power.
- NPM enables women to behave in ways that challenge gender stereotypes.

Challenges

- Do women and men have to manage 'like men'?
- What are the alternatives to masculinist managerialism?
- How might alternative forms of management and organization be formulated and fought for?

Key reading

Barry, J., M. Dent and M. O'Neal (eds) (2003) *Gender and the Public Sector* (London: Routledge).
Dent, M. and S. Whitehead (2002) 'Introduction', in M. Dent and S. Whitehead (eds), *Managing Professional Identities* (London: Routledge), 1–16.
McLaughlin, K., S. P. Osborne and E. Ferlie (eds) (2002) *New Public Management: Current Trends and Future Prospects* (London: Routledge).
Newman, J. (2005) 'Regendering Governance', in J. Newman (ed.), *Remaking Governance: People, Politics and the Public Sphere* (Bristol: Policy Press), 81–99.

References

Acker, J. (1990) 'Hierarchies, Jobs, Bodies: A Theory of Gendered Organizations', *Gender and Society*, 4 (2), 139–58.
Acker, J. (1998) 'The Future of "Gender and Organizations": Connections and Boundaries', *Gender, Work and Organization*, 5 (4), 195–206.
Ackroyd, S. and P. Thompson (1999) *Organizational Misbehaviour* (London: Sage).
Allen, I. (2001) *Stress among Ward Sisters and Charge Nurses* (London: Policy Studies Institute).
Barry, J., M. Dent and M. O'Neal (eds) (2003) *Gender and the Public Sector* (London: Routledge).
Beck, U. and E. Beck-Gernsheim (2002) *Individualization* (London: Sage).
Berg, E. (2000) *Kvinna och chef i offentlig förvaltning* (Lund: Liber).
Berg, E. (2003) 'Women's Positioning in a Bureaucratic Environment – Combining Employment and Mothering', in J. Barry, M. Dent and M. O'Neal (eds), *Gender and the Public Sector* (London: Routledge), 104–19.
Berg, E., J. Barry and J. Chandler (2008) 'New Public Management and Social Work in Sweden and England: Challenges and Opportunities for Staff and Predominantly Female Organizations', *International Journal of Sociology and Social Policy*, 28 (3/4), 114–28.
Bolton, S. (2005) 'Women's Work, Dirty Work: The Gynaecology Nurse as "Other"', *Gender, Work and Organization*, 12 (2), 169–86.
Burris, B.H. (1996) 'Technocracy, Patriarchy and Management', in D. L. Collinson and J. Hearn (eds), *Men as Managers, Managers as Men: Critical Perspectives on Men, Masculinities and Managements* (London: Sage), 61–77.
Chandler, J., J. Barry and H. Clark (2002) 'The Wear and Tear of the New Public Management', *Human Relations*, 55 (9), 1051–69.
Clarke, J. (2004a) *Changing Welfare, Changing States: New Directions in Social Policy* (London: Sage).

Clarke, J. (2004b) 'Dissolving the Public Realm? The Logics and Limits of Neo-Liberalism', *Journal of Social Policy*, 33 (1), 27–48.

Clarke, J. and J. Newman (1997) *The Managerial State: Power, Politics and Ideology in the Remaking of Social Welfare* (London: Sage).

Collinson, D. L. and J. Hearn (1994) 'Naming Men as Men: Implications for Work, Organization and Management', *Gender, Work and Organization*, 1 (1), 2–22.

Connell, R. W. (1987) *Gender and Power* (Cambridge: Polity Press).

Davies, C. (1995) 'Competence versus Care? Gender and Caring Work Revisited,' *Acta Sociologica*, 38 (1), 17–31.

Davies, C. (1996) 'The Sociology of the Professions and the Profession of Gender', *Sociology*, 30 (4), 661–78.

De Certeau, M. (1984) *The Practice of Everyday Life* (Berkeley: University of California Press).

Dent, M. (2003) *Remodelling Hospitals and Health Professions in Europe: Medicine, Nursing and the State* (Basingstoke: Palgrave Macmillan).

Dent, M. and S. Whitehead (2002) 'Introduction', in M. Dent and S. Whitehead (eds), *Managing Professional Identities* (London: Routledge), 1–16.

Dent, M., J. Chandler and J. Barry (eds) (2004) *Questioning the New Public Management* (Aldershot: Ashgate).

Ferguson, K. E. (1984) *The Feminist Case against Bureaucracy* (Philadelphia: Temple University Press).

Gilligan, C. (1982) *In a Different Voice: Psychological Theory and Women's Development* (Cambridge, MA: Harvard University Press).

Glover, J. and G. Kirton (2006) *Women, Employment and Organizations* (Abingdon: Routledge).

Gonäs, L. and J. C. H. Karlsson (eds) (2008) *Gender Segregation: Divisions of Work in Postindustrial Welfare States* (Aldershot: Ashgate).

Halford, S. (2003) 'Gender and Organisational Restructuring in the National Health Service', *Antipode*, 35 (2), 286–308.

Harvey, D. (2005) *A Brief History of Neoliberalism* (Oxford: Oxford University Press).

Hood C. (1995) 'The "New Public Management" in the 1980s: Variations on a Theme', *Accounting, Organizations and Society*, 20 (2/3), 93–109.

Kerfoot, D. (2002) 'Managing the "Professional" Man', in M. Dent and S. Whitehead (eds), *Managing Professional Identities: Knowledge, Performance and the 'New' Professional* (London: Routledge), 81–95.

Liff, S. and J. Wajcman (1996) '"Sameness" and "Difference" Revisited: Which Way Forward for Equal Opportunity Initiatives?', *Journal of Management Studies*, 33 (1), 79–94.

McLaughlin, K., S. P. Osborne and E. Ferlie (eds) (2002) *New Public Management: Current Trends and Future Prospects* (London: Routledge).

Newman, J. (2005) 'Regendering Governance', in J. Newman (ed.), *Remaking Governance: People, Politics and the Public Sphere* (Bristol: Policy Press), 81–99.

Pollitt, C. and G. Bouckaert (2000) *Public Management Reform: A Comparative Analysis* (Oxford: Oxford University Press).

Rosener, J. B. (1990) 'Ways Women Lead', *Harvard Business Review*, 68 (6), 119–25.

Savage, M. and A. Witz (1992) *Gender and Bureaucracy* (Oxford: Blackwell).

SCB (2007) *Yrkesstrukturen i Sverige* (Stockholm: SCB, Statistics Sweden), at: www.scb.se/statistik, accessed 13 August 2009.

Schedler, K and I. Proeller, I (2002) 'The New Public Management: A Perspective from Mainland Europe', in K. McLaughlin, S. P. Osborne and E. Ferlie (eds), *New Public Management: Current Trends and Future Prospects* (London: Routledge), 163–80.

Schein, V. (1973) 'The Relationship between Sex Role Stereotypes and Requisite Management Characteristics', *Journal of Applied Psychology*, 57 (2), 95–100.

Thomas, R. and A. Davies (2002) 'Gender and New Public Management: Reconstituting Academic Subjectivities', *Gender, Work and Organization*, 9 (4), 372–97.

Wise, S. (2003) 'Reconciling Career and Family Life in NHS Nursing and Midwifery: Dilemmas in Ward Management', in J. Radcliffe, M. Dent, S. Suckling and L. Morgan (eds), *Dilemmas for Human Services* (Stafford: Staffordshire University), 98–102.

Young, A. (2003) '"Hard Nosed or Pink and Fluffy?" An Examination of How Middle Managers in Health Care Use the Competing Metaphors of Business and Care to Achieve Desired Outcomes', in J. Barry, M. Dent and M. O'Neill (eds), *Gender and the Public Sector: Professionals and Managerial Change* (London: Routledge), 154–69.

21
Old Age Care Policies: Gendering Institutional Arrangements across Countries

Viola Burau, Hildegard Theobald and Robert H. Blank

Introduction

Demographic changes have put old age care on the political agenda in many healthcare states across industrialized countries. From a gender perspective this is interesting as women dominate caregiving in old age care. Further, the policy problem of old age care is characterized by strongly gendered framing and enactment, although there are interesting variations across countries. Old age care is a new and pressing issue in health policy with important gender implications, but which is neglected in the literature on health policy. This chapter focuses on old age care policies, which are situated between the public and the private sphere and between the worlds of formal and informal care. More specifically, the chapter adopts an institutionalist (see, for example, Thelen, 1999; 2003) and cross-country comparative perspective to analyse the policies and politics of organizational reform in old age care services. It examines the particular configurations of gendered institutions at play and how these configurations impact on the substance of organizational reform (see also Chapter 20 by Barry et al.).

Empirically, the chapter presents two case studies of reforms of old age care policies, namely Sweden and Japan, where reforms have taken place in response to the demographic challenges of ageing populations. Yet, the respective configurations of gendered institutions are quite different in these two countries which make them good case studies for our analysis. The two case studies are taken from a broader cross-country comparative study of the governance of home care (Burau et al., 2007), and rely on secondary literature together with selected primary sources (only those in English in the case of Japan).

The chapter begins by discussing the policy challenges posed by old age care and how to conceptualize gendered institutions in theoretical terms. The next section operationalizes the conception of gendered institutional configurations, which provides a springboard for the two case studies. The chapter concludes with a comparative analysis and an outline of the broader implications for the study of gender in healthcare.

Policy challenges of old age care

Old age care is becoming a higher priority on the health policy agenda in many countries and this reflects a combination of policy pressures, especially ageing populations, cost containment, and women's increasing labour market participation. All industrialized countries will experience significant ageing of their populations over the next 30 years (for an overview see Burau et al., 2007). Although the ageing process is taking place earlier and more rapidly in some countries than others, all are expected to experience the ageing process that began in the 1970s and is now accelerating. The primary cause of the ageing of western societies is the precipitous decline in fertility rates that has naturally increased the proportion of elderly. As the number of older people increases so does the need for long-term care. However, this comes at a time of intense concerns about costs and efforts to contain public spending on healthcare (for an overview see Blank and Burau, 2007). For many observers, home care promises to square the circle, based on the assumption that care in the home is much less costly than care provided in high-tech hospitals and labour-intensive nursing homes. Moreover, home care settings make it easier to combine formal and informal care arrangements.

Yet the pool of informal carers is becoming smaller. Besides falling birth rates, this reflects the increasing labour market participation of women (for an overview see Burau et al., 2007). Substantial social transformations in modern societies associated with individualization have begun to undermine traditional, largely informal and family-based care and, in combination with social movements towards equality, this means that more women today seek fulfilment through a career. Within this new cultural milieu women are less likely than in the past to be willing or able to forgo paid employment to serve as a caregiver. Importantly, while old age care policies are pushed by universal policy challenges, they are shaped by country-specific factors. This raises questions about how to conceptualize such gendered contexts from a comparative perspective.

Studying institutional configurations in old age care policy

The analysis presented in this chapter looks at configurations of gendered social and political institutions. Drawing on feminist studies, especially in political science, we suggest that a good way forward is to build on recent contributions to the emerging field of feminist institutionalism. In political science, feminist analyses have been extensively used to study institutions. Studies are characterized not only by an explicit interest in power in institutions but also by a broad understanding of institutions that encompasses both social and private institutions, and political and state institutions (Kenny, 2007; Krook, 2009; Mackay and Meier, 2003; Randall, 2000). Importantly, the private–public nexus has led to the study of the interrelations between different types of institutions.

Against this background and more specifically, we define the configurations of *gendered* social and political institutions underpinning policies of old age care as follows. To capture the relevant social institutions we use the typology of different care models or care regimes developed by Antonnen and Sipilä (1996) as a starting point and combine this with Pfau-Effinger's (2004) notion of gender orders. This describes the existing structures of the gendered division of labour and allows for analysing the prerequisites of such care regimes in terms of the gendered structures of the family, the labour market and the welfare state. More specifically we distinguish between the extent to which the state supports the delivery of formal care services and informal caregiving on the one hand and the labour market participation of women on the other.

This leads us to propose four models: the public service, the family care, the means-tested, and the subsidiarity model; the first and the last models are particularly relevant for the analysis in this chapter. In the public service model the state supports both care services and female employment; as a result, formal care services are universally available and women's participation in the labour market is high. Under the subsidiarity model, state support for formal care services is secondary to other forms of support, especially support for informal care, and state support for women's labour market participation is limited. In this model publicly funded services are limited and meant to support family care and the labour market participation of women mainly takes the form of part-time employment.

In terms of the political institutions underpinning policies of old age care, the analysis focuses on the institutions related to the political power over old age care. Here, feminist writing on public policy points to the importance of the interplay between women's agency and the state (see, for example, Lovenduski and Randall, 1993). In the present context, old age interest groups are in principle particularly relevant although these are confronted with the paradox of 'large numbers but small influence'. Instead, although pursuing different interests, proxy actors, and especially the state, offer important sources for potential alliance and political exchange (Bonoli, 2005). The following analysis therefore examines the structure of the state and its resources in relation to care services as the key formal political institutions for policies of old age care.

We follow Alber (1995) who defines the resources of the state as consisting of two dimensions. The first dimension is the relative vertical centralization of political power. Here, policies of old age care have traditionally been local but are now firmly positioned in the context of central–local relations. This puts tensions over issues of control and funding, where central and local levels have different interests and resources, at the centre of the analysis of this dimension. The second dimension of political power is horizontal cohesiveness, and this is related to the ways in which care services are organized. Specifically, this captures the relative integration of health and social care services in terms of funding and regulation and the importance of public sector provision.

Gendered institutional configurations in policies of old age care

This part of the analysis outlines the gendered configurations of social, welfare and political institutions in Sweden and Japan. As such, it provides the background for the analysis of the trajectories of reforms of old age care policies in the subsequent part of the chapter.

Sweden

In Sweden the institutional configurations in relation to policies of old age care combine a care regime based on the public service model with highly decentralized and cohesive political power over care services. The care regime gives preference to formal care services and both health and social care services are available largely on a universal basis. This applies fully to healthcare where access to services is needs-based, whereas in the area of social care there is some means-testing. The organization of care services underpins the universality of access: the delivery of both health and social services is predominantly in the hands of public providers; and this is an almost unique feature when compared to other non-Nordic countries; funding comes from a combination of various local and regional taxes together with some national funds. In sum, the care regime emerges as strongly publicly integrated and care services are an integral part of the welfare state. This reflects a gender order that combines ideas of individualism and universalism, whereby universal access to formal care services is seen as the central means to secure the independence of individual citizens both as older people and as women in paid employment. Not surprisingly, the other side of the care regime is that the state extensively supports female labour market participation, which is high in Sweden (Burau et al., 2007).

In terms of the political power over care services, it is significant that care services have long been part of the fabric of the welfare state and formal care services were already established in the 1950s. This has provided the state with a platform for developing extensive resources for governing and, not surprisingly, political power over care services is highly cohesive. Public authorities have power over both the funding and the regulation of old age care, and even the provision of services is in public hands. However, opening up the care sector for private providers within the current framework of an emerging ideology of welfare-mix has put the existing system under pressure. The number of non-public providers delivering home care for municipalities increased by

146 per cent between 1995 and 1998 (National Board of Health and Welfare, 2000), although the overall number remains small. In terms of the relative integration of different services, half of the counties have delegated the responsibility for home nursing to local municipalities (National Board for Health and Welfare, 2000). This is significant since municipalities also provide social care-oriented home-help services.

At the same time, political power over care services is characterized by a high degree of decentralization and some observers even suggest that the large differences at local level make it more appropriate to talk about a multitude of *welfare municipalities* rather than a single welfare state (Trydegard and Thorslund, 2001). In terms of regulation, the national government defines the framework for policies by setting basic norms for public responsibility for home nursing and social care services, while it is up to local/regional authorities to decide on specific goals and rules for implementation. Significantly, this not only applies to the organization of services, but also to the accessibility of services. The Swedish municipalities enjoy considerable freedom in relation to defining the scope and the volume of services as well as over the definition of eligibility criteria and the charges for services. This has led to unequal access to services, as discussed in more detail below (Trydegard, 2003). Further, funding is almost exclusively determined at local/regional levels.

Japan

In Japan, the institutional configurations of old age care policies combine a care regime based on the subsidiarity model with moderately cohesive and recently decentralized political power over care services. The care regime is based on the principle of subsidiarity and this is embedded in a gender order that has traditionally been very strongly based on the ideas of family care and women as housewives or part-time employees (see, for example, Peng, 2002). This gives primacy to care by the family in the first instance and by civil society in the second instance. State support for female labour market participation continues to be low and focuses on increasing the general employment rate to offset the ageing population. Together with underlying changes in gender relations (see Boling, 1998), this has been the prime motor for extending state support for formal care services and for introducing public schemes dedicated to long-term care. In 1989, the government instituted the so-called 'Gold Plan' to expand and thereby to facilitate access to care services (for an overview see Adachi et al., n.d.). The underlying idea was to support women in their informal caregiving and to shift resources from hospitals to social support services, such as home nursing and social care. Under the new scheme, access to care services continues to be means tested, taking into consideration both financial means and the availability of informal support. Although local authorities are generally responsible for the organization of care services, the expanded provision of care services is largely in the hands of non-profit providers. These providers tend to be different types of self-help organizations (Adachi et al., n.d.). Some have emerged from grassroots initiatives of volunteers, but which now charge fees and which offer care staff the possibility of earning eligibility for formal care services, when retired staff are no longer able to care for themselves. Others have been set up and are managed by municipalities. Beyond voluntary work and user fees, local and national taxes are the main source of funding of care services.

Compared to Sweden the cohesion of political power over care services is moderate. While public authorities, especially at local and to some extent at national levels, have power over funding and regulation, the provision of care services is largely not in public hands and instead different types of non-profit self-help organizations are mainly responsible for the expansion of formal care services. Further, political power remains split between health and social care, as the government scheme, the so-called Gold Plan (for details, see below), covers only home help services.

At the same time, political power over care services is decentralized, although compared to Sweden this is a relatively new phenomenon and a direct result of the introduction of the Gold Plan (Aratame, 2007). This particularly applies to the regulation of care services. As part of the Gold Plan, the government defines the overall framework for the development of care services and also sets broad policy targets, for example, those relating to the number of home helps, day centres and providers of home-based care services. In contrast, municipalities are responsible for the developing and implementing of specific programmes; this includes the organization of care services and the specification of eligibility criteria. In contrast, political power over funding is less highly decentralized than in Sweden. Funding comes from a combination of local and national taxes, but local authorities do not enjoy independent tax-raising powers. This is significant because the expansion of the responsibilities of municipalities for care services occurred without sufficient funding from central government (Peng, 2002). The Gold Plan therefore put considerable strains on municipalities. This is especially problematic as the municipalities are also responsible for the development of care services at the local level (Boling, 1998).

Trajectories of institutional change: reforms of old age care policies

In the analysis above Sweden and Japan emerge as countries with two very different institutional configurations. How does this impact on trajectories of institutional change and more specifically on reforms of old age care policies? This is the focus of the next part of the chapter.

Sweden: challenging universality in the context of multi-level politics

In Sweden public home help services were already established in the 1950s and further expanded during the 1960s and 1970s. Although the overall idea of public responsibility for care services has remained unchanged, since the 1980s the proportion among the elderly receiving services has fallen (Rauch, 2005). This reflects changes in care policies at the national level and corresponding policies of service targeting and user fees at the local level, specifically the implementation of ambitious national policies under a regime of cost containment, a form of national legislation which specifies basic goals only, together with the freedom of municipalities to make their own policies concerning access to care services.

Public home help services were already introduced in the 1950s and quickly became an important part of the Swedish universal welfare state. The access to social care services emerged as a social right for all citizens based on needs and was therefore to be paid for and organized publicly. The changing gender relations since the 1960s further pushed the expansion of home help services, as care services enable the simultaneous participation in paid and unpaid work for both women and men. The development of public care services peaked in the 1970s when more than 30 per cent of the population 65 years and older received services mainly delivered at home (Brodin, 2005).

Importantly, home help services and their expansion were only loosely regulated within the relevant legislation. In response, a Social Commission was set up to analyse the public responsibility for care. This provided the basis for the Social Service Act, which came into effect in 1982 and which still forms the basis for the delivery of home-based care services. In its report the Social Commission described the statutory responsibilities of the municipalities for care services; the Commission confirmed the idea of public responsibility but saw only a limited need for regulation. Further, the subsequent legislation required the reallocation of financial resources within municipalities, but crucially the national government did not offer any additional financial support. Instead, the municipalities were left to their own devices. As a result, and despite the ambitious goals of the legislation, the proportion of the elderly receiving services decreased, particularly in relation to housework duties (Szebehely, 2000).

In response, a parliamentary committee was set up to evaluate the developments (see Brodin, 2005) and the proposals of the Committee provided the basis for a new law. The report of the Committee envisaged opening up of parts of the service provision to private and non-profit provider organizations as well as de-hospitalization under the unified responsibility of municipalities. As previously, the municipalities were given no additional funds from the national government to support the implementation of the new legislation.

Subsequently, another parliamentary commission was set up to make more specific suggestions for the re-regulation and reorganization of elderly care services under the leadership of the municipalities. The Commission envisaged that the municipalities should take on the statutory responsibility for all forms of care services, both health and social care. In addition to nursing homes, this included all medical services relating to the elderly excluding medical treatment provided by doctors and home-based care for hospital patients ready for discharge. Crucially, the responsibility for the implementation of the reform lay in the hands of the municipalities and county councils, as did the reallocation of financial resources. Later legislation also increased the possibility for involving private providers and introduced a loose regulation of fees; under this, fees should not exceed the costs incurred by the municipalities and should leave the individual with an income for basic personal needs (Feltenius, 2004).

None of the reforms changed the public financial responsibility for elderly care provision, yet during the 1990s the number of elderly people receiving services fell dramatically. Instead, the municipalities introduced policies of service targeting, whereby home-help services focus on very frail elderly people (those most in need) and public services often no longer cover those elderly people who only need help with basic household tasks (those less in need). This reflects strong financial incentives for municipalities to offer home-based care services for often frail patients discharged from hospitals as well as demographic changes leading to a rising proportion of elderly people over 80 years of age (Trydegard, 2003). Policies of service targeting were complemented by policies of user fees and this further contributed to a fall in the number of potential care recipients (Szebehely, 2000).

The possibility for municipalities to introduce policies which restrict care services in a time of financial constraint is closely related to the loose nature of the provisions in the Social Service Act (see Rauch, 2005). Social services entitlements are defined as individual rights but this has been weakened in two respects. First, the content and scope of care rights remain unspecified, with the only requirements being that individuals have a reasonable standard of living and that public services support independent living. Second, public social care services are granted on the condition that the needs cannot be met *in other ways*. As this may include family care or sufficient financial means, entitlements remain unclear.

Japan: long-term care insurance and changing welfare politics

The introduction of long-term care insurance with its provision of comprehensive coverage for home-based care services in Japan is an example of wide-ranging institutional change. Indeed, in the context of a traditional gender order with filial care for the elderly, the insurance and the central role of government in the funding (and regulation) of care services presents a case of institutional innovation. Societal pressures together with multiple problem pressures opened up a window of opportunity which allowed the inclusion of new political actors and coalitions with inside political actors.

By the mid-1990s pressure was building for concerted governmental action to deal with the problems emerging from the confluence of demographic and social forces, which also reflected changes in underlying gender relations. A combination of the world's highest longevity and a decline in fertility acceler-ated the speed of societal ageing (Campbell and Ikegami, 2003). Complicating these demographic trends was a shift in the structure and function of Japanese families. There had been a rise in independent living and in the number of elderly-only households. Moreover the pool of family carers was shrinking partly because of women increasingly joining the labour market for paid work (Burau et al., 2007).

In addition, the end of the economic boom and the subsequent recession led to a decline in tax revenue, making it increasingly difficult for the govern-ment to achieve the expected increase in social security expenditure of an ageing society. Growing deficits in medical insurance were especially problematic as most institutional long-term care has been provided in hospitals (Izuhara, 2003). Healthcare costs were not capped and the number of elderly inpatients increased dramatically (Ikegami et al., 2003). The inappropriate and expensive social admissions to hospitals together with the inadequate supply of home-based care services were seen as an urgent problem, not least in the light of the trends above.

Finally, there were also problems with the Gold Plan introduced in the late 1980s. The scheme turned out to be expensive at a time when the Japanese electorate appeared to be opposed to tax increases. At the same time, the admin-istrative procedures for deciding eligibility and providing services were still essentially the same as those for public assistance and unsuited for large-scale services to many people. The accumulated pressures provided a window of opportunity for change that was strengthened by extensive lobbying from outside together with an alliance with resourceful actors from within that made for a strong coalition for reform. For Eto (2001: 33), it was an issue 'outside the established political system' where the conventional policy community of social welfare was destabilized, thereby allowing non-established political players to emerge. Typically, the process for making Japanese welfare policy begins with welfare ministry bureaucrats drafting a bill and forwarding it to the appropriate advisory council to allocate benefits among groups that have interests in the bill (Eto, 2001). After council approval, the bill is sent to the ruling party caucus and then presented to the parliament.

The advisory council in charge of welfare for elderly people largely reflected the views of those who resisted the introduction of the insurance.

On the other side were emerging forces who demanded a more open process which acknowledged the failure of existing policy to address the problem of caring for the middle-class elderly. During the process of drafting reform new political players, including women's groups, ordinary citizens and a group of mayors, emerged as important players and became actively involved (Hrebenar et al., 1998).

Further, by the late 1980s it became clear that taking care of the disabled elderly was a problem that could no longer be solved by families on their own. In Japanese society, according to the traditional gender division of labour, caring for the elderly has usually been carried out by women (Japan Ministry of Health, Labour and Welfare, 1999: 39). Faced with a situation where they were forced to resign from work and/or give up their lives outside the home entirely, women became active. With the creation of the Women's Association for Improving an Ageing Society in 1986 came an advocacy force for socializing care. In the mid-1990s the Women's Association was joined by a new citizens' action group that championed approval of long-term care insurance. In 1996 influential Japanese who were worried about the diminishing prospects of this insurance, despite its widespread public support, urged the parliament to approve the legislation (Eto, 2001). In response to the looming insurance problem, they organized a citizens' action group. Although only few of the proposals of the Citizens' Committee were incorporated into the final legislation, this was the first time that voters had succeeded in having part of a bill revised (Eto, 2001).

In contrast, smaller municipalities in particular were hesitant to assume responsibility for managing the new system and came out against it. This led to a public perception that all municipalities were opposed to the insurance system despite their key role in implementing it. In order to counter this perception, a group of mayors established the Mayors' Association to Promote Welfare Administration for their Residents (Welfare Mayors) in November 1997. They supported the insurance believing that it would provide them with a good opportunity to promote municipal welfare policy and demonstrate their leadership. Their stance stood in strong contrast to that of mayors opposed to the long-term care insurance. However, in cooperation with the Women's Association and the Citizens' Committee, the Welfare Mayors were able to protect long-term care insurance from forces that intended to derail it (Eto, 2001).

Some of the organizational features of the insurance built on the earlier Gold Plan. The insurance further strengthens the role of the municipalities, which have taken on the role of insurers and as such are also responsible for promoting the health and welfare of the elderly at home. Yet, in contrast to previous arrangements, the national government, prefectures and medical-care insurers provide multiple layers of support to prevent excessive administrative financial burdens on the municipalities (Japan Ministry of Health, Labour and Welfare, 1999). Indeed, the ratio of the share of public funds among the national government, prefectures and local municipalities is fixed at 2:1:1. Also, as under the Gold Plan, the municipalities contract with a wide variety of providers, including private, for-profit organizations. This corresponds to a specific design feature of the insurance. Care users access services based on an individual care plan; individuals are free to choose among different types of services and among different providers as well as being able to choose the mix of services between health and social services (Ikegami et al., 2003). Crucially, however, the insurance also marks a radical departure. Long-term care is no longer expected from the family or allocated by the state on the basis of need. Instead, long-term care is embedded in a social contract based on a system of mandatory contributions, uniform entitlements and consumer choice (Izuhara, 2003). This redefines care of the elderly from being a filial to being a social function and as such represents a radical departure from the traditional gender culture based on the primacy of the family.

Conclusion

Old age care is a new and pressing issue in health policy with important gender implications. Policy challenges consist of a combination of ageing populations, cost pressures and the increasing labour market participation of women. The analysis of the case studies in this chapter takes its starting point in the quite different institutional configurations in Japan and Sweden and subsequently shows how the respective gendered institutional configurations filter recent reforms to old age care policies (Table 21.1).

In Sweden, the highly decentralized nature of political power over care services means that regional/local authorities are largely responsible for the funding and regulation of care services, whereas the national government sets overall policy frameworks. This also applies to policies of de-hospitalization which are the key lever for recent reforms of old age care policies. The policy framework of the national government emerges as part of a series of reform initiatives which combine de-hospitalization with strong financial incentives as well as further decentralization; this also strengthens the cohesiveness of political power over care services. Importantly, however, this does not include more detailed regulation of the scope of care services or additional funding. This means that the financial room for expanding home-based care services is limited and therefore local authorities adapt by redefining the specific terms of service provision. It is against this background that local policies of service targeting and user fees emerge. Yet it is indicative that the overall commitment to public responsibility for old age care remains intact and this is testimony to the strength of the set of social and welfare

Table 21.1 Institutional configurations and trajectories of institutional change in old age care policies

		Sweden	Japan
Institutional configurations	Care regime	public service model	subsidiarity model
	Political power over care services	highly cohesive, highly decentralized	moderately cohesive, recently decentralized
Trajectories of institutional change	Type of institutional change	incremental change through institutional conversion	radical change through institutional innovation;
		policies of service targeting and user fees weaken role of state in old age care	long-term care insurance increases role of state in old age care
	Process of institutional change	national government opens window of opportunity by setting policy framework for de-hospitalization	demographic/ societal changes challenge care regime and this opens window of opportunity for new, civil society actors
		regional/local authorities design implementation based on their responsibility for funding and regulation	group of municipalities drives national policy change as inside advocate of reform and coalition partner of civil society actors
		loose national regulation coupled with cost containment makes for local policies which reduce access to formal care	strategies of decentralization and welfare-mix build on earlier reform

institutions that make up the Swedish care regime. In analytical terms, the policies represent a case of institutional conversion, where the existing institution of decentralized responsibility for care services remains intact, but is used for a different purpose, namely to redefine rather than to safeguard the specific terms of service provision. This has problematic implications for women, as the elderly are pushed to rely on informal care to an increasing extent.

In Japan, by contrast, the social and welfare institutions which make up the care regime are more in flux, and demographic developments, together with changes in gender relations, fundamentally challenge the traditional reliance on informal care by women. Together with specific financial pressures and the perceived failure of the Gold Plan, this weakens the established policy community around the government ministry and at the same time opens up a window of opportunity for new, civil society actors. These include women's groups which have been lobbying for the socialization of old age care for some years, and more ad hoc citizen groups which form specifically in response to proposals for long-term care insurance. The earlier Gold Plan initiated a significant decentralization of political power over care services and the municipalities held key responsibility for both the funding and the regulation of care services. Building on this, as part of the process of institutional change, a group of municipalities emerges as inside advocates for the introduction of the insurance. Importantly, this group also forms a coalition with the civil society actors, which helps to deflect opposition to the reform. The introduction of the long-term care insurance represents a radical change through institutional innovation and substantially increases the role of the state in old age care. Nevertheless, some of the substantive strategies used as part of the process of institutional change, such as the decentralization of political power and a strong welfare mix in the provision of services, build on earlier reforms and as such help to pave the way towards change.

In sum, the analysis above suggests the specific type of policy reform cannot simply be read off from, for example, the type of care regime in each country. On that basis Sweden would be an unlikely candidate for any reform which weakens the universalist orientation of care policies, in the same way as Japan would be an unlikely candidate for reform which substantially expands the role of the state in old age care. Instead, the reform of old age care emerged as the result of specific configurations of different gendered institutions and associated dynamics among political actors.

Summary

What are the challenges of and opportunities for including gender in the study of institutions and institutional configurations in old age care?

Challenges

- to identify the specific and multiple interrelations between different gendered institutions, especially the family and the state, and assess effects on policy reform;
- to review tools for comparing health policy across different countries, as existing approaches are gender-blind.

Opportunities

- to capture the dynamics of old age care as an emerging gendered field of health policy; to identify the gendered selectivity of institutions and the gendered power relations embedded in them;
- to arrive at a more thorough understanding of organizational change in healthcare, as the specific type of change cannot simply be read off from institutional contexts; instead gendered power relations and informal care arrangements also matter.

Key reading

Anttonen, A. and J. Sipilä (1996) 'European Social Care Services: Is It Possible to Identify Models?', *Journal of European Social Policy*, 6 (2), 87–100.

Blank, R. H. and V. Burau (2007) *Comparative Health Policy*, Second Edition (Basingstoke: Palgrave Macmillan).

Burau, V., H. Theobald and R. H. Blank (2007) *Governing Home Care: A Cross-national Comparison* (Cheltenham: Edward Elgar).

Kenny, Merry (2007) 'Gender, Institutions and Power: A Critical Review', *Politics*, 27 (2), 91–100.

Acknowledgements

We presented earlier versions of the analysis at several conferences. On all occasions we received detailed and constructive feedback, for which we would like to thank our colleagues.

References

Adachi, K., J. E. Lubben, N. Tsukada (n.d.) 'Expansion of Formalized In-home Services for Japan's Aged', manuscript, at: www.lit.kyushu-u.ac.jp/~adachi/ucla.htm, accessed 28 August 2007.

Alber, J. (1995) 'A Framework for the Comparative Study of Social Services', *Journal of European Social Policy*, 5 (2), 131–50.

Anttonen, A. and J. Sipilä (1996) 'European Social Care Services: Is It Possible to Identify Models?', *Journal of European Social Policy*, 6 (2), 87–100.

Aratame, N. (2007) 'Japan's Community-oriented Welfare for the Elderly: Its Implications for Asian Developing Countries', paper prepared for the Global Development Network Annual Conference, Beijing, January 2007.

Blank, R. H. and V. Burau (2007) *Comparative Health Policy*, Second Edition (Basingstoke: Palgrave Macmillan).

Boling, P. (1998) 'Family Policy in Japan', *Journal of Social Policy*, 27 (2), 173–90.

Bonoli, G. (2005) 'The Politics of the New Social Policies: Providing Coverage against New Social Risks in Mature Welfare States', *Policy and Politics*, 33 (3), 431–49.

Brodin, H. (2005) *Does Anybody Care? Public and Private Responsibilities in Swedish Eldercare 1940–2000*, doctoral thesis, University of Umeå.

Burau, V. and R. H. Blank (2006) 'Comparing Health Policy: An Assessment of Typologies of Health Systems', *Journal of Comparative Policy Analysis*, 8 (1), 63–76.

Burau, V., H. Theobald and R. H. Blank (2007) *Governing Home Care: A Cross-national Comparison* (Cheltenham: Edward Elgar).

Campbell, J. C. and N. Ikegami (2003) 'Japan's Radical Reform of Long-term Care', *Social Policy and Administration*, 37 (1), 21–34.

Eto, M. (2001) 'Public Involvement in Social Policy Reform: Seen from the Perspective of Japan's Elderly-care Insurance Scheme', *Journal of Social Policy*, 30 (1), 17–36.

Feltenius, D. (2004) *En Pluralistisk Maktordning? Om Pensionärsorganisationerna Politiska Inflyttande*, doctoral thesis, University of Umeå.

Hrebenar, R. J., A. Nakainura and A. Nakamura (1998) 'Lobby Regulation in the Japanese Diet', *Parliamentary Affairs*, 51, 551–8.

Ikegami, N., K. Yamauchi and Y. Yamada (2003) 'The Long Term Care Insurance Law in Japan: Impact on Institutional Care Facilities', *International Journal of Geriatric Psychiatry*, 18 (3), 217–21.

Izuhara, M. (2003) 'Social Inequality under a New Social Contract: Long-term Care in Japan', *Social Policy and Administration*, 37 (4), 395–410.

Japan Ministry of Health, Labour and Welfare (1999) *Annual Report on Health and Welfare: Social Security and National Life* (Tokyo: Ministry of Health, Labour and Welfare).

Kenny, M. (2007) 'Gender, Institutions and Power: A Critical Review', *Politics*, 27 (2), 91–100.

Krook, M. L. (2009) *Quotas for Women in Politics: Gender and Candidate Selection Reform Worldwide* (New York: Oxford University Press).

Lovenduski, J. and V. Randall (1993) *Contemporary Feminist Politics. Women and Power in Britain* (Oxford: Oxford University Press).

Mackay, F. and P. Meier. (2003) 'Institutions, Change and Gender-relations: Towards a Feminist New Institutionalism', paper presented at the workshop 'Changing Constitutions, Building Institutions and (Re)defining Gender Relations', at the Joint Sessions of the European Consortium of Political Research, Edinburgh, 28 March–2 April 2003.

National Board of Health and Welfare (2000) *Social Services in Sweden in 1999. Needs – Intervention – Development* (Stockholm: National Board of Health and Welfare).

Peng, I. (2002) 'Social Care in Crisis: Gender, Demography, and Welfare Restructuring in Japan', *Social Politics*, 9 (3), 411–43.

Pfau-Effinger, B. (2004) *Development of Culture, Welfare State and Women's Employment in Europe* (Aldershot: Ashgate).

Randall, V. (2000) *The Politics of Child Daycare in Britain* (Oxford: Oxford University Press).

Rauch, D. (2005) *Institutional Fragmentation and Social Service Variations: A Scandinavian Comparison*, doctoral thesis, University of Umeå.

Szebehely, M. (2000) 'Ældreomsorg i förändring – knappare resurser och nya organisationsformer', in SOU (ed.), *Välfärd, vård och och omsorg*, Antologi/Kommitten Välfärdsbokslut (Stockholm: Social Departement), 171–223.

Thelen, K. (1999) 'Historical Institutionalism in Comparative Politics', *Annual Review of Political Science*, (2), 369–404.

Thelen, K. (2003) 'How Institutions Evolve: Insights from Comparative Historical Analysis', in J. Mahoney and D. Rueschemeyer (eds), *Comparative Historical Analysis in Social Sciences* (Cambridge: Cambridge University Press), 208–40.

Trydegard, G. B. (2003) 'Swedish Elderly Care in Transition: Unchanged National Policy but Substantial Changes in Practice', paper presented at the ESPAnet Conference, Copenhagen, Denmark, 13–15 November 2003.

Trydegard, G. B. and M. Thorslund (2001) 'Inequality in the Welfare State? Local Variation in Care of the Elderly: The Case of Sweden', *International Journal of Social Welfare*, 10 (3), 174–84.

22
Primary Prevention and Health Promotion: Towards Gender-sensitive Interventions

Petra Kolip

Introduction

Health promotion and the primary prevention of illness are increasingly central to healthcare provision and are integral to New Public Health strategies as chronic and degenerative diseases rather than infectious diseases have become the most important cause of morbidity and mortality. For example, cardiovascular disease is the most significant cause of death worldwide. The World Health Organization estimates that 80 per cent of premature deaths could be avoided by healthy nutrition, physical activity and abstinence from tobacco (WHO, 2008). Hence, increasing attention is being paid to health-related behaviour and to illness prevention, not only in a bid to reduce morbidity and mortality but also to reduce escalating healthcare costs.

This chapter explores the gender aspects of health-related interventions. In doing so it draws a distinction between primary prevention and health promotion. While both concepts are concerned with improving population health, they take different starting points and pursue different intervention strategies. Primary prevention is based on an epidemiological risk factor model; it has its starting point in diseases and health impairments, identifies underlying risk factors, and attempts to prevent or reduce these risks. Typical examples of interventions of this type are vaccinations, safer sex campaigns and smoking prevention programmes. Primary prevention looks for instance at infectious diseases, sexually transmitted diseases, lung cancer and other smoking-related diseases and seeks to influence the most relevant risk factors for these diseases (Ewles, 2005).

By contrast, health promotion adopts a salutogenetic perspective (Antonovsky, 1987). From this perspective, the concern is less with what causes disease (pathogenesis) and more with what causes health (salutogenesis) (Lindstrom and Eriksson, 2006). Thus the focus is on resources for health and factors which are protective for health. The main goals of health promotion are to influence health and well-being directly (direct effect) and/or soften the impact of risk factors (moderating effect). Protective factors and resources can be located at the personal level, like coping strategies, self-esteem, self-efficacy, the immune system, as well as on a social level, such as through social support from family members, friends and colleagues, and social welfare systems. It aims to enhance and foster these personal and/or social resources. This includes initiatives to increase personal skills as well as the creation of supportive environments (see, for example, Pencheon et al., 2006).

This chapter begins by introducing the Public Health Action Cycle (Institute of Medicine, 1988) as a framework for intervention and explores the opportunities for a systematic inclusion of gender issues at all stages (gender mainstreaming); namely, assessment, policy development, assurance, and evaluation. This is followed by two case studies – smoking prevention and cessation, and drink-driving – that will illustrate how gender-sensitive intervention planning can increase the efficacy of primary prevention. A third case study turns our attention towards workplace health promotion and highlights a need for a complex approach that goes beyond gendered working conditions to take account, for instance, of work–life balance and the interaction between paid and unpaid work for both men and women. The chapter concludes by highlighting the need for gender-sensitive public health interventions to pursue the goal of equal opportunities with regard to health.

The Public Health Action Cycle as a framework for intervention

In many cases health promotion interventions follow the logic of the Public Health Action Cycle (PHAC) as defined by the Institute of Medicine (1988). This model suggests starting with carrying out a problem analysis (or assessment) that explores the health problem on the basis of epidemiological findings and theoretical analyses; this is followed by policy development and planning of intervention measures and programmes with reference to the available scientific evidence. The identified interventions are subsequently implemented (assurance) and, finally, evaluated to assess their impact (evaluation). This framework is used in this chapter to illustrate how a systematic linkage with gender mainstreaming may help to improve the quality of the interventions. The PHAC model has some weaknesses as it does not adequately capture the barriers to successful interventions. However, as an established and widely acknowledged model in public health planning (see Institute of Medicine, 1988) it provides a springboard for gender mainstreaming approaches in primary prevention and health promotion. I therefore introduce a systematic linkage arguing that gender mainstreaming has the capacity to enhance health, since a larger population group can be reached through target group measure planning. This view is strongly supported by WHO Europe (2001), as formulated in the Madrid Statement:

> The factors that determine health and ill health are not the same for men and women. Gender interacts with biological differences and social factors. Women and men play different roles in different social contexts. [...] This affects the degree to which women and men have access to, and control over, the resources and decision making needed to protect their health. (WHO Euro, 2001: 3)

WHO defines gender mainstreaming as a key strategy to reduce gender inequity in health and invites all member states to participate in the implementation of this strategy:

> To achieve the highest standard of health, health policies have to recognize that women and men, owing to their biological differences and their gender roles, have different needs, obstacles and opportunities. (WHO Euro, 2001: 2; see also Chapter 2 by Abdool et al.)

A gender perspective is meaningful primarily when the identification of gender-specific needs for action is important, such as, for instance, seeing accidents as mainly a male health problem, and domestic violence as mainly a female health problem, and in the analysis of whether interventions are planned in a gender-sensitive way to reach males and females, when this is relevant. The different steps of the Public Health Action Cycle are explored in greater detail in the following sections.

Assessment

In most countries men and women differ in their life expectancy and mortality; Table 22.1 gives some examples of life expectancy (see also WHO, 2008). Premature deaths are interesting for the analysis of the potential of gender-specific prevention measures. The indicator 'potential years of life lost' (PYLL) is an estimate of the average years a person would have lived if he or she had not died prematurely; that is before the age of 70. As international data reveal, men lose many more years due to premature deaths than women do (Table 22.1). Data on life expectancy and potential years of life lost reflect health risk behaviours in men (tobacco smoking, alcohol consumption, unsafe sex, reckless driving) which are related to avoidable deaths such as lung cancer, cirrhosis of the liver, myocardial infarction, HIV/AIDS and accidents. This initially leads to the conclusion that the prevention potential

Table 22.1 Life expectancy at birth and potential years of life lost (PYLL) in selected countries, 2005

	Life expectancy at birth			PYLL* (< 70 years)	
	Men	Women	Difference	Men	Women
Germany	76.7	82.0	5.3	4,244	2,302
France	76.7	83.7	7.0	4,805	2,292
Japan	78.5	85.5	7.0	3,617	1,912
UK	77.1	81.1	4.0	4,326	2,649
USA	75.2	80.4	5.2	6,291	3,633

* PYLL: per 100,000 men and women under 70 years of age.
Source: OECD Health Data, 2008.

is higher in the male population compared to women and prevention strategies should therefore be targeted towards men in order to encourage healthier lifestyles.

A closer look at the statistics on causes of death brings into perspective that female-specific problem areas do exist. Internationally 1.9 per cent of all women die during or after childbirth, primarily due to inadequate perinatal and postnatal care (see also Chapter 23 by Sandall et al.). Furthermore, women are more frequently affected by violence; according to international data intentional injuries make up 2.8 per cent of all deaths (1.4 per cent self-inflicted, 1.0 per cent by violence, and 0.3 per cent by war and civil conflict). The male population shows higher rates than women of self-inflicted injuries (62.6 per cent) and war-related mortality (84.3 per cent), while women are more frequently affected by physical violence (80.9 per cent). Therefore, WHO declared in 1996 that violence is a major and growing public health problem and advocated an evidence-based plan of action for its prevention (WHA, 1996). Programmes for the prevention of domestic violence have been applied in numerous countries and the US Centers for Disease Control and Prevention developed systematic strategies for primary prevention (CDC, 2009; see also Chapter 2 by Abdool et al.). Furthermore, interventions are increasingly also targeted to women in areas like tobacco control, where consumption rates in men have been higher but are rapidly increasing in women in many countries (see, for example, Bauld, 2009; Payne, 2004; USPSTF, 2009).

An analysis of the statistics on causes of death initially indicates the potential for gender-specific prevention initiatives, but further steps need to be taken. Such steps include the assessment of additional data sources – for instance, on morbidity, on disabilities and on need of care – and an in-depth analysis of complex social differences. While gender is an important dimension of inequality it intersects with other social differences, like age, ethnicity, socio-economic position and sexual orientation, that are all important when it comes to designing policy interventions (Burke and Eichler, 2009; Lademann and Kolip, 2005).

Although this chapter focuses on gender differences in health and health-risk behaviour, it is important to keep in mind that in many health areas gender differences are very small compared to other differences such as differences by income or age. Furthermore, differences are also important within the group of men and women. This is especially important when it comes to identifying vulnerable groups as target groups for prevention and health promotion. This can be exemplified through research on gender-sensitive health monitoring and health reporting in Germany (Lademann and Kolip, 2005), drawing on national health survey data including gender, occupational status and living conditions (with or without partner, with or without children) as social determinants of health and using (among other indictors) a cumulated index of 42 illnesses and disorders (lifetime prevalence, as an indicator of health). Taking 30- to 44-year-olds as an example, this research was able to demonstrate that women's health was worse than men's health. Furthermore, single parents had the highest rates of illnesses, and men and women living together with a partner and a child or several children had the lowest rates (Lademann and Kolip, 2005). In terms of family and living circumstances, a similar picture occurs when looking at smoking. As Lampert and Burger (2005) reveal, the proportion of smokers amongst 30- to 44-year-old German women ranges from 32 per cent (women living together with a partner and at least one child) to 62 per cent in the group of single mothers.

Overall, existing research suggests that single parents are an important target group for intervention. But this does not automatically answer questions about what interventions should actually be and how they should be focused. A large body of existing research has made clear that interventions which focus on individual behaviour meet with little success, if basic social conditions of life – such as economic conditions – are not also taken into account (Marmot and Wilkinson, 2006). Complex approaches to health promotion for single parents are therefore needed that take account of social conditions (Misra et al., 2007). For example, German data show that poverty among single mothers is significantly higher compared to any other group. Taking 60 per cent of median equivalized income, 34 per cent of single parents with one child are at risk of poverty, whereas only 10 per cent of households with two adults and one child are at risk (Eurostat, 2009).

Gender-sensitive health monitoring and health reporting extends beyond the mere documentation of data by sex to include data analysis informed by theory (Annandale, 2009; Bird and Rieker, 2008; Kuhlmann, 2009). Social constructionist approaches which emphasize gender as an ongoing accomplishment in everyday interaction may help us to better understand health-risk behaviour. As West and Zimmerman (1987: 127) argue, gender is 'the activity of managing situated conduct in light of normative conceptions of attitudes and activities appropriate for one's sex category'. From this approach, gender is an expression of what is perceived and evaluated as 'male' and 'female' behaviour, and not simply an individual characteristic. So gender is connected to social situations and 'done' in social interactions. Consequently, gender differences in health behaviour can be explained both as attempts to present oneself as man or woman, boy or girl by means of behaviour – such as smoking and tobacco consumption, eating behaviour, risky behaviours in street traffic – and as a desire to behave in accordance with dominant norms of femininity and masculinity (Courtenay, 2000; see also Chapter 16 by Schofield).

Policy development

The Public Health Action Cycle suggests developing policies that are based on epidemiological studies and theories. To enhance gender equity in health the most important question at this stage of the cycle is whether a gender-specific strategy is needed, either because the health problem addressed is sex-specific, like breast cancer or gender-specific, like domestic violence, or because the factors that determine health and illness are similar for men and women but vary in their degree, like smoking. As meaningful and consistent as the available data on the differences between women and men in health-risk behaviour are, they have barely been considered in the planning and setting of priorities in interventions. There are presently few health promotion interventions that have been explicitly developed from a gender perspective, for example, by taking gender differences in health behaviour as their main focus in intervention planning.

Assurance

A number of methodological questions need to be posed in order to ensure that interventions appropriately address both men and women. Are the methods adequate to reach women, men or both? In recent years feminist researchers have drawn attention to the impact of gender bias in health research and practice. Gender bias occurs if similarities between men and women are assumed in situations where they do not exist and/or where differences are suspected without convincing empirical evidence (Eichler et al., 1992). According to Eichler and colleagues, gender bias tends to show up in three main forms: gender insensitivity (ignoring gender which is seen as irrelevant), androcentrism (taking the male as the norm), and double standards (identical behaviours or situations are evaluated, treated, or measured by different criteria). In the past two decades or so several tools have been developed to raise awareness of the importance of social differentiation in programme implementation.

These tools take gender as a starting point for sensitization. For example, the Swiss Foundation for Health Promotion aims to sensitize health promotion professionals to the importance of gender-sensitive intervention planning and implementation (Health Promotion Switzerland, 2009; Kolip et al., 2003). In Switzerland every health professional applying for financial support is obliged to indicate whether gender is relevant in the specific intervention (and if yes, in what ways). To assist applicants, a catalogue of questions has been developed covering four main areas: namely policy; participation of gender experts in project planning; theoretical background; and methods (see also Chapter 6 by Klinge). For example, questions such as the following need to be asked in order to identify and reduce gender bias (for details, see Kolip et al., 2003):

- Policies: Does the planned intervention promote health equity between girls/women and boys/men?
- Participation: Are male and female representatives of the target group(s) involved in the project? Are both women and men adequately represented in the project organization (project team, advisory/steering groups)?
- Sex/gender and theoretical background: Are the gender needs of both sexes adequately considered when planning the implementation?
- Methods: When planning the procedure, has a possible need for gender-specific interventions been considered?

Recently these questions have been implemented in a tool for quality assurance called 'quint-essenz.ch', thus making gender issues an integrated part of quality assurance (Health Promotion Switzerland, 2009).

Evaluation

Finally, gender mainstreaming is important in programme evaluation. Methods and indicators must be selected in such a way that they, firstly, are applicable to males and females and, secondly, that they can identify differential effects in men and women, if there are any. In recent years a scholarly debate on gender bias in health research has emerged (see, for instance, Eichler et al., 1992; see also Chapter 6 by Klinge). Numerous studies have identified research designs that lack adequate tools to identify gender differences, for instance, where gendered power relations are neglected and where there is gender bias in the survey instruments. An example of bias in survey instruments is questionnaires used to assess physical activity (Abel et al., 2001; Sallis and Saelens, 2000). If physical activity is assessed via sports and exercise, a higher degree of physical activity is usually documented in males. If everyday exercise is also recorded (for instance, walking and biking), the degree of exercise in the female population typically is higher compared to the male population.

Gender-sensitive interventions: case studies

The following case studies illustrate how gender-sensitive intervention planning can increase the efficacy of primary prevention and health promotion. The cases selected are taken from three different areas of intervention and reflect both men and women as target groups.

Smoking prevention and smoking cessation

Smoking prevention and smoking cessation are interesting because they highlight the need for different methods in order to reach young men and women, since their motives for smoking often differ. To begin with lung cancer, this is the most common cancer worldwide, accounting for 17.8 per cent of all cancer deaths (WHO, 2008; Toh, 2009). Here, the female:male ratio of premature deaths is 1:2.7. It is well known that smoking counts for the main risk factor for lung cancer; here, the prevalence of smoking is higher in developed countries, but it is increasing in developing countries, especially amongst women (Toh, 2009).

An analysis of smoking in Germany (Figure 22.1) reveals that prevalence rates are still higher in the male population. However, while smoking in males has decreased in the past 15 years, it has increased in females. Apparently, to date tobacco prevention programmes in Germany have not been able to reach women in general and young women in particular. Lung cancer mortality has developed accordingly: it has decreased in males and increased in

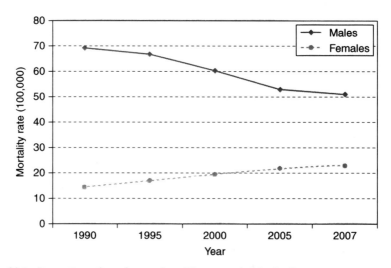

Figure 22.1 Proportion of regular smokers 15 years and older in Germany
Source: Statistisches Bundesamt (2009a).

females (see Figure 22.2). Among other things, this is presumed to be a major reason for the narrowing of the gender gap in life expectancy (Luy, 2003; Pampel, 2002).

Based on comparable observations in different countries, Payne (2004) analyses the influence of sex and gender and their interplay. She highlights that women and men differ not only in tobacco consumption patterns, but also become ill with different forms of lung cancer. Women more often suffer from small cell cancer which constitutes about 25 per cent of all lung cancers and which is seen as the more dangerous type of cancer; diagnosis of adenocarcinoma also is more frequent in women. In addition, the risk of cancer in women is greater at every level of smoking. In her analysis Payne explores the interaction of biological factors and socially shaped factors that contribute to gender differences in lung cancer risk. Sex-linked risk factors stem from biological differences between men and women, with women's pulmonary tissue more vulnerable to the carcinogens in tobacco smoke. By contrast, gender refers to behavioural differences associated with social and cultural constructions of femininity and masculinity. Here, women (in the UK) more often smoke cigarettes with a lower tar and nicotine yield, that are inhaled more deeply thus causing more damage to pulmonary tissue. When smokers change tobacco brands from high to low tar cigarettes – which is more common in women than in men – they often compensate for the decrease

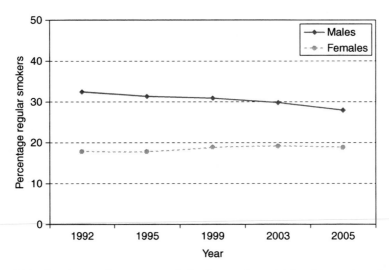

Figure 22.2 Death rate for cancer of the lungs, bronchial tubes and trachea in Germany*
* recently age standardized to European population.
Source: Statistisches Bundesamt (2009b).

in nicotine yield by increasing the depth of inhalation (for an overview, see Payne, 2004).

While there is still a lack of gender-sensitive interventions, attempts to take gender differences into account in smoking cessation intervention planning are now on the increase in several countries (see Doyal, 2005), as, for instance, in the UK in the European context. Such interventions often focus on pregnant women as a target group (see, for example, Bauld, 2009). While pregnancy intervention strategies are important, they do not adequately respond to the increase in female smokers referred to above. Establishing gender-sensitive tobacco smoking intervention and smoking cessation programmes beyond pregnancy-related interventions is more complicated, as motives and consumption patterns specific to women and men must be identified. For example, women smoke more often to buffer negative feelings, whereas men more often use cigarettes to increase positive feelings (Payne, 2004). In addition, many women are in fear of weight gain and therefore prefer to continue smoking (US Department of Health and Human Services, 2001); weight control is also frequently a reason to begin smoking (Honjo and Siegel, 2003). This makes smoking cessation more difficult for women than for men (Payne, 2004).

The example of smoking makes it clear that knowledge of gender-specific prevalence rates in itself offers no starting points for interventions; motives and consumption patterns specific to men and women must also be identified; and here we can observe an overall lack of gender-sensitive research and strategies. Similar to the prevention of substance use and misuse (Kumpfer et al., 2008), so far there are hardly any gender-sensitive prevention programmes that would allow for the different smoking patterns and consumption motives of women and men (USPSTF, 2009).

Drink-driving

Findings on alcohol use in Germany reveal a gendered pattern: more men than women drink alcohol in general, and men consume more alcohol and prefer harder, stronger and more bitter types of alcohol (spirits, beer); more men than women are alcoholics; and men demonstrate risk behaviour associated with alcohol, such as driving under the influence of alcohol, more often than women (Robert Koch Institut, 2006). This pattern is replicated in other countries and indeed frequently described, but it is rarely explained. The social constructionist theories already mentioned previously can help interpret these gender differences. Gender-specific consumption patterns and preferences are suited to the enactment of masculinity (Courtenay, 2000) and are especially appealing to men with 'traditional' gender identities (Mahalik et al., 2007). Specific types of alcohol, such as beer and 'hard' liquors, are typically considered to be male; others, such as sparkling wine and liqueurs, are considered feminine. Specific consumption patterns – such as binge drinking – may also serve as signifiers of masculinity. Consequently, risky drinking in males can only be modified if gender identity and attempts to express masculinity are taken into consideration (Lee and Owens, 2002).

The need for gender-sensitive intervention programmes is especially obvious when looking at alcohol-associated road traffic accidents, which are often caused by young adults. An analysis for Germany shows that these accidents are particularly frequent on weekend nights. Vehicles involved in accidents are often fully occupied and the driver is usually male, even when female passengers have not drunk as much alcohol (and therefore might be considered more appropriate drivers). Characteristically, in these situations the male sense of responsibility (taking the group home) is linked with the man's overestimation of his safe capacity for alcohol consumption (Linkenbach and Perkins, 2006).

The most effective strategies for prevention of alcohol-associated traffic accidents are measures directed at the social or environmental level such as the lowering of legal blood alcohol limits (particularly for young and inexperienced drivers) and sobriety checkpoints or intervention training programmes for servers of alcoholic beverages (Community Guide Preventive Services, 2009). The impact of such strategies is clearly documented, for example, in the *Community Guide* (2009) developed by the US Task Force and widely acknowledged as the evidence-based guideline for interventions. Consequently, these strategies are often in the focus of interventions. However, they must be supplemented by measures related to individual behaviour, and this is more challenging than defining, for instance, blood alcohol limits. One example is an intervention in which students drive a test course in a driver training area, initially sober, then with a little alcohol, and then with a blood alcohol content with which the young men believe that they are still able to drive the car safely (Wüst, 2006). The driving is video-recorded, analysed and subsequently shown to the men so they can observe that they make many driving mistakes even though they perceived themselves as capable of driving safely. However, this intervention is an exception rather than the rule, despite the fact that, in the area of drinking and driving, the significance of gender identity and stereotyped gender roles is common, everyday knowledge. The development of prevention measures that are able to identity the role of gender identity constructions in health-risk behaviour in men and in women are still to a large extent lacking. Rigorous implementation of the concept of gender mainstreaming in the area of prevention and health promotion could significantly contribute to improvements in health for women and men.

Workplace health promotion

Workplace health promotion is strongly informed by WHO policies. WHO has emphasized the creation of supportive environments for health as a key issue of health promotion and has developed the concept of the 'health-promoting setting'. Next to cities and regions, small-scale settings such as schools, hospitals or businesses/workplaces are the focus of this programme:

> Changing patterns of life, work and leisure have a significant impact on health. Work and leisure should be a source of health for people. The way society organizes work should help create a healthy society. Health promotion generates living and working conditions that are safe, stimulating, satisfying and enjoyable. (WHO, 1986: 2)

In Europe, the Luxembourg Declaration on Workplace Health Promotion in the European Union serves as a guideline for workplace health promotion (WHO Euro, 1997). Many measures are related to health protection (occupational health and safety legislation), and aimed at the avoidance of accidents and the prevention of occupational diseases. Leaving aside specific measures for pregnant and breast-feeding mothers, most are designed to be gender-neutral, but in reality primarily result in an improvement of the health of men. The reason for this is the gendered division of labour; for example, the risk of men suffering an accident at work is clearly higher since men more often work in areas connected to physical risks, such as the construction industry (for further examples, see Östlin, 2002). However, workplace health promotion (WHP) stretches far beyond safety at the workplace. Following the Luxembourg Declaration:

> WHP contributes to a wide range of work factors that improve employees' health. These include:
>
> - management principles and methods which recognize that employees are a necessary success factor for the organization instead of a mere cost factor;
> - a culture and corresponding leadership principles which include participation of the employees and encourage motivation and responsibility of all employees;
> - work organization principles which provide the employees with an appropriate balance between job demands, control over their own work, level of skills and social support;
> - a personnel policy which actively incorporates health promotion issues;
> - an integrated occupational health and safety service. (WHO Euro, 1997: 2)

The Declaration clearly has pioneered new healthy workplace promotion policies in Europe, but do women benefit from these attempts in the same way than men? The gender-neutral language totally ignores the gender segregation of the labour market and the gendered nature of both work and the organization within which it takes place. This occurs despite a large body of existing research which clearly highlights the persistent differences between men and women in areas such as control over work, skills, position in the organization and balancing different demands (Burchell et al., 2007). Although WHO has a strong commitment to gender mainstreaming, this does not adequately inform its framework for health workplace promotion. This arena therefore also highlights that many hurdles exist for gender mainstreaming when applied to practice; it is generally absent even when the existence of gender differences is well documented and gender equality increasingly monitored in public sector organizations and beyond.

Existing research reveals that the gendered division of labour affects the health of men and women in various ways. For example, a German study has shown that women working as bank employees more often suffer from monotony, while men more often report stress and work pressure (Koppelin and Müller, 2004). Another example is gendered opportunities for, and obstacles to, a healthy work-life balance; women are more often responsible for care – for children, older relatives and in the community – and have therefore less opportunity for recreation, which in turn may have negative effects on their health (Berntsson et al., 2006, for an overview, see Östlin, 2002).

We can conclude from these examples that planning and intervention of health promotion initiatives in the workplace need to adopt a gender mainstreaming approach in order to increase their sensitivity and to identify the interplay of complex gendered work conditions that may impact on the health of men and women. Health promotion at the workplace stretches far beyond the provision of healthy food in the staff canteen and the establishment of exercise and sports groups. Indeed, promoting workplace health for men and women includes a wide span of interventions into the organizations – such as, for instance, career support, new work-time models and the provision of easily accessible childcare facilities – that must all be designed in gender-sensitive ways as 'career', 'work hours' and 'childcare' embody different opportunities and barriers for men and women.

Conclusion

This chapter has highlighted the gendered dimensions of primary prevention and health promotion, arguing the need for gender-sensitive intervention strategies. Following a gender mainstreaming approach, it has suggested that the Public Health Action Cycle should be used as a framework for gender-sensitive planning and intervention strategies. This framework is useful for two reasons; it allows for a systematic analysis of gender issues from a public health perspective and for a systematic linkage with the concept of gender mainstreaming. Existing research highlights significant gender differences in health and health behaviour, in the resources for health and well-being, and the conditions of health and illness. It also highlights that planning and intervention do not adequately reflect the complex meaning of gender and often reduce 'gender' to the category of 'sex', although some examples of 'good practice' do exist and some methodological tools for gender-sensitive interventions have been developed. Overall, the systematic failure to pay attention to gender differences in the prevalence of risk factors, in the potentials and resources for the health and well-being of men and women, and the various gendered effects of intervention strategies, calls for an equally systematic, comprehensive strategy of bringing gender sensitivity to the heart of primary prevention and health promotion.

Within the context of prevention and health promotion, gender mainstreaming has the goal of producing horizontal and vertical equal opportunities with regard to health. If women and men have the same (horizontal) health needs, they should also receive the same service; if their health needs are different, (vertical) differentiated services should be developed to enable both sexes to exploit their health potential (see also Chapter 1 by Payne and Doyal). In doing so, it is important to understand the intersections of gender with other social factors and conditions of life. Consequently, health-related planning and intervention need to consider how gender intersects with, for instance, age, ethnicity, sexual orientation, education and occupational status in a specific area of investigation. Here, we can either start with a specific gender approach or monitor the significance of gender at a later stage in the planning process. One example is to choose migrants as a target group of an intervention and then move on to explore whether and how the health needs of male or female migrants should be addressed in different ways. However, an intersectional analysis of healthcare needs and the related planning and interventions are in the very early stages and pose many challenges for researchers and practitioners.

In summary, primary prevention and health promotion are gaining significance in healthcare as responses to changing patterns of illnesses. Within this context gender mainstreaming is especially relevant because both health-related behaviours and social conditions are heavily shaped by gender differences and may thus affect the health of men and women in different ways. Furthermore, health promotion moves beyond the promotion of healthy lifestyles and looks at the social and environmental factors that affect health as it aims to shape the environment 'to make the healthier choice the easier choice' (WHO, 1986: 2). Viewed through the lens of an environmental (or system) approach, power relations in society – gender as well as other dimensions of power differences – come into perspective, making health-related interventions fundamentally a political issue. This connectedness to power, policy and politics may help us to understand both the challenges and the opportunities of bringing mainstreaming gender into public health interventions in general and health promotion in particular.

Summary

- The model of the Public Health Action Cycle (PHAC), if linked to gender mainstreaming, is a useful framework for developing gender-sensitive primary prevention and health promotion.
- Gender differences in life expectancy and potential years of life lost reflect the more risky health behaviour of men, including smoking and alcohol consumption, in developed countries.
- Factors influencing health and health behaviour are, in many areas, different for men and women; they include work conditions as well as attitudes to health-risk behaviour.
- Intervention planning and implementation informed by gender theories may improve the quality and efficiency of health promotion and primary prevention.
- Tools have been developed to facilitate gender-sensitive approaches, but planning and intervention lack systematic gender approaches.

Key reading

Doyal, L. (2000) 'Gender Equity in Health: Debates and Dilemmas', *Social Science & Medicine*, 51 (6), 931–9.

Kumpfer, K. L., P. Smith and J. Franklin Summerhays (2008) 'A Wakeup Call to the Prevention Field: Are Prevention Programs for Substance Use Effective for Girls?', *Substance Use & Misuse*, 43 (8–9), 978–1001.

Mahalik, J. R., S. M. Burns and M. Syzdek (2007) 'Masculinity and Perceived Normative Health Behaviors as Predictors of Men's Health Behaviors', *Social Science & Medicine*, 64 (11), 2201–9.

Payne, S. (2004) *Gender in Lung Cancer and Smoking Research*, Gender and Health Research Series (Geneva: WHO).

References

Abel, T., N. Graf and S. Niemann (2001) 'Gender Bias in the Assessment of Physical Activity in Population Studies', *Sozial- und Präventivmedizin*, 46, 268–72.

Annandale, E. (2009) *Women's Health and Social Change* (London: Routledge).

Antonovsky, A. (1987) *Unravelling the Mystery of Health. How People Manage Stress and Stay Well* (San Francisco: Jossey Bass).

Bauld, L. (2009) 'Smoking during Pregnancy and Smoking Cessation Services', *Journal of Smoking Cessation*, 4 (Supplement 1), 2–6.

Berntsson, L., U. Lundberg and G. Krantz (2006) 'Gender Differences in Work-home Interplay and Symptom Perception among Swedish White-collar Employees', *Journal of Epidemiology and Community Health*, 60 (12), 1060–70.

Bird, C. E. and P. P. Rieker (2008) *Gender and Health. The Effects of Constrained Choices and Social Policies* (Cambridge: Cambridge University Press).

Burchell, B., C. Fagan, C. O'Brien and M. Smith (2007) *Working Conditions in the European Union: The Gender Perspective* (Dublin: European Foundation for the Improvement of Living and Working Conditions), at: www.eurofound.europa.eu/pubdocs/2007/108/en/1/ef07108en.pdf, accessed 5 August 2009.

Burke, M. A. and M. Eichler (2006) *The BIAS FREE Framework. A Practical Tool for Identifying and Eliminating Social Biases in Health Research* (Geneva: Global Forum for Health Research), at: www.globalforumhealth.org/Media-Publications/Publications/The-BIAS-FREE-Framework-A-practical-tool-for-identifying-and-eliminating-social-biases-in-health-research, accessed 5 August 2009.

CDC – Centers for Disease Control and Prevention, National Center for Injury Prevention and Control (2009) *Intimate Partner Violence Prevention, Preventing Violence Against Women: Program Activities Guide*, at: www.cdc.gov/ViolencePrevention/pub/PreventingVAW.html, accessed 21 May 2009.

Community Guide Preventive Services (2009) *Motor Vehicle-related Injury Prevention: Reducing Alcohol-impaired Driving*, at: www.thecommunityguide.org/mvoi/AID/index.html, accessed 18 May 2009.

Courtenay, W. H. (2000) 'Constructions of Masculinity and Their Influence on Men's Well-being: A Theory of Gender and Health', *Social Science & Medicine*, 50 (10), 1385–1401.

Doyal, L. (2000) 'Gender Equity in Health: Debates and Dilemmas', *Social Science & Medicine*, 51 (6), 931–9.

Eichler, M., A. L. Reisman and E. M. Broins (1992) 'Gender-bias in Medical Research', *Women & Therapy*, 12 (4), 61–70.

Eurostat (2009) *At Risk of Poverty Rates by Household Type in 2007*, at: http://epp.eurostat.ec.europa.eu, accessed 24 June 2009.

Ewles, L. (2005) *Key Topics in Public Health. Essential Briefings on Prevention and Health Promotion* (Edinburgh: Elsevier).

Health Promotion Switzerland (2009) *Checklist Gender Perspective*, at: www.quint-essenz.ch/en/files/Checklist_gender_10.pdf, accessed 5 July 2009.

Honjo, K. and M. Siegel (2003) 'Perceived Importance of Being Thin and Smoking Initiation among Young Girls', *Tobacco Control*, 12 (3), 1–7.

Institute of Medicine (1988) *The Future of Public Health* (Washington, DC: National Academy Press).

Kolip, P., I. Jahn and D. Summermatter (2003) 'Geschlechtergerechte Gesundheitsförderungspraxis. Die Kategorie Geschlecht als Kriterium für die Projektförderung von Gesundheitsförderung Schweiz', *Prävention*, 26, 107–10.

Koppelin, F. and R. Müller (2004) 'Macht Arbeit Männer krank? Arbeitsbelastungen und arbeitsbedingte Erkrankungen bei Männern und Frauen', in T. Altgeld (ed.), *Männergesundheit. Neue Herausforderungen für Gesundheitsförderung und Prävention* (Weinheim: Juventa), 121–34.

Kuhlmann, E. (2009) 'From Women's Health to Gender Mainstreaming and Back Again: Linking Feminist Agendas and Health Policy', *Current Sociology*, 57 (2), 135–54.

Kumpfer, K. L., P. Smith and J. Franklin Summerhays (2008) 'A Wakeup Call to the Prevention Field: Are Prevention Programs for Substance Use Effective for Girls?', *Substance Use & Misuse*, 43 (8–9), 978–1001.

Lademann, J. and P. Kolip (2005). *Gesundheit von Frauen und Männern im mittleren Lebensalter. Schwerpunktbericht der Gesundheitsberichterstattung des Bundes* (Berlin: Robert Koch-Institut).

Lampert, T. and M. Burger (2005) 'Verbreitung und Strukturen des Tabakkonsums in Deutschland', *Bundesgesundheitsblatt*, 48, 1231–41.

Lee, C. and R. G. Owens (2002) *The Psychology of Men's Health* (Buckingham: Open University Press).

Lindstrom, B. and M. Eriksson (2006) 'Contextualizing Salutogenesis and Antonovsky in Public Health Debate', *Health Promotion International*, 21 (3), 238–44.

Linkenbach, J. and H. W. Perkins (2006) *'Montana's MOST of Us Don't Drink and Drive Campaign: A Social Norms Strategy to Reduce Impaired Driving among 21–34 Year Olds*, National Highway Traffic Safety Admission Publication: DOT HS 809 869.

Luy, M. (2003) 'Causes of Male Excess Mortality: Insights from Cloistered Populations', *Population and Development Review*, 29 (4), 647–76.

Mahalik, J. R., S. M. Burns and M. Syzdek (2007) 'Masculinity and Perceived Normative Health Behaviors as Predictors of Men's Health Behaviors', *Social Science & Medicine*, 64 (11), 2201–9.

Marmot, M. and R. Wilkinson (eds) (2006) *Social Determinants of Health,* Second Edition (Oxford: Oxford University Press).

Miranda, J. J., S. Kinra, J. P. Casas, G. Davey Smith and S. Ebrahim (2008) 'Non-communicable Diseases in Low- and Middle-income Countries: Context, Determinants and Health Policy', *Tropical Medicine and International Health*, 13 (10), 1225–34.

Misra, J., S. Moller and M. Budig (2007) 'Work-family Policies and Poverty for Partnered and Single Women in Europe and North America', *Gender & Society*, 21 (6), 804–27.

OECD Health Data (2008) *Statistics and Indicators for 30 Countries*, at: www.gbe-bund.de, accessed 14 January 2009.

Östlin, P. (2002) 'Examining Work and Its Effects on Health', in G. Sen, A. George and P. Östlin (eds), *Engendering International Health: The Challenge of Equity* (Cambridge, MA: MIT Press), 63–81.

Pampel, F. C. (2002) 'Cigarette Use and the Narrowing Sex Differential in Mortality', *Population and Development Review*, 28 (1), 77–104.

Payne, S. (2004) *Gender in Lung Cancer and Smoking Research,* Gender and Health Research Series (Geneva: WHO).

Pencheon, D., D. Melzer, M. Gray and C. Guest (eds) (2006) *Oxford Handbook of Public Health Practice* (Oxford: Oxford University Press).

Robert Koch-Institut (2006*) Gesundheitsbericht für Deutschland* (Berlin: Robert Koch-Institut).

Sallis, J. F. and B. E. Saelens (2000) 'Assessment of Physical Activity by Self-report: Status, Limitations, and Future Directions', *Research Quarterly for Exercise and Sport*, 71 (Supplement 2), S1–S14.

Statistisches Bundesamt (2009a) *Verteilung der Bevölkerung nach ihrem Rauchverhalten*, at: www.gbe-bund.de, accessed 30 June 2009.

Statistisches Bundesamt (2009b) *Sterbeziffer ab 1980*, at: www.gbe-bund.de, accessed 15 May 2009.

Toh, C.-K. (2009) 'The Changing Epidemiology of Lung Cancer', in M. Verma (ed.), *Cancer Epidemiology, Vol 2, Modifiable Factors* (New York: Humana Press), 397–411.

US Department of Health and Human Services (2001) *Women and Smoking: A Report of the Surgeon General* (Washington, DC: US Department of Health and Human Services).

USPSTF – US Preventive Services Task Force (2009) *Counselling and Interventions to Prevent Tobacco Use and Tobacco-caused Disease in Adults and Pregnant Women,* at: www.ahrq. gov/clinic/uspstf09/tobacco/tobaccors2.htm, accessed 20 May 2009.

West, C. and D. Zimmerman (1987) 'Doing Gender', *Gender and Society*, 1 (2), 125–51.

WHA – World Health Assembly (1996) *Prevention of Violence: Public Health Priority*, Resolution No. WHA49.25 (Geneva: World Health Organization).

WHO (1986) *Ottawa Charter for Health Promotion*, at: www.who.int/hpr/NPH/docs/ottawa_charter_hp.pdf, accessed 20 June 2009.

WHO (2008) *Global Burden of Diseases. 2004 Update* (Geneva: Health Statistics and Informatics Department, World Health Organization), at: www.who.int/evidence/bod, accessed 13 May 2009.

WHO Euro (1997) *Luxembourg Declaration on Workplace Health Promotion in the European Union*, at: www.enwhp.org/fileadmin/downloads/luxembourg_declaration.pdf, accessed 21 May 2009.

WHO Euro (2001) *Mainstreaming Gender Equity in Health*, at: www.euro.who.int/document/a75328.pdf, accessed 1 July 2009.

Wüst, M. (2006) 'Don't Drink and Drive' – nur für Jungen ein Problem?', in P. Kolip and T. Altgeld (eds), *Geschlechtergerechte Gesundheitsförderung und Prävention* (Weinheim: Juventa), 89–102.

23

Gender and Maternal Healthcare

Jane Sandall, Cecilia Benoit, Edwin van Teijlingen, Sirpa Wrede,
Eugene Declercq and Raymond De Vries

Introduction

This chapter addresses some key issues in maternal healthcare which have
resonance in the international arena. In many middle and high-income countries, a key policy focus is on addressing disparities or inequities in healthcare
recently highlighted by the revisiting of work on the social determinants of
health by the WHO (CSDH, 2008). The report argues that social determinants
of health are the conditions in which people are born, grow, live, work and age,
including the health system. These circumstances are shaped by the distribution of money, power and resources at global, national and local levels, which
are themselves influenced by policy choices. The social determinants of health
are seen as mostly responsible for health inequities – the unfair and avoidable
differences in health status seen within and between countries, with ongoing
debate about the effective contribution that health services can make to mitigate the impact the these social determinants on health and well-being.

As a healthcare activity concerned with childbearing and the emergence of
families, maternity care is marked by a very specific set of gender relations.
In addition to the linkage to intimate relations in the family, maternity care
is structured by gendered power relations in healthcare. Policies regarding
maternity care quality improvement include notions of 'family-centred care'
in some countries, with an increased focus on fathers and 'woman-centred
care' in others. We will address the issue of gender relations in maternity care
in a comparative 'decentred approach' (see Wrede et al., 2006: 2986) drawing
on case studies of middle-income countries in North America (Canada and
the USA) and northern Europe (the UK and Finland). Each country provides
a different contextual framework concerning health system financing, workforce and professional regulation, the role of user groups, policy agendas and
the framing and solutions put forward to solve the problem of inequities in
maternity care.

This chapter explores the different ways in which disparities/inequities are conceptualized across different countries, and provides a gendered analysis of how health and social care systems attempt to address them in the context of maternal healthcare. The chapter starts with the recent healthcare reforms in Canada with its collective health insurance approach, it then moves on to the United States where the debates about gender inequality within the healthcare system appear to be overshadowed by race and ethnicity issues, and finishing off in the UK and Finland where gender inequality is overshadowed by the social inequality debate.

Redesigning maternal healthcare in Canada's health system

Universal health insurance arrived in Canada with the passing of the federal Medical Care Act of 1966. The new plan, known as Medicare, covered physician fees as well as hospital services. This plan teamed provincial administration with five national principles: universality (available to all Canadians), portability (between the provinces and territories), comprehensiveness (all medically necessary procedures provided free of charge), accessibility (not based on health status or ability to pay), and public (rather than private) administration (Badgley and Wolfe, 1967). Further specification of the principles of Medicare accompanied the Canada Health Act of 1984. This Act stated that:

> [t]he primary objective of Canadian health care policy is to protect, promote and restore the physical and mental well being of residents of Canada, and facilitate reasonable access to health services without financial or other barriers. (Canada Health Act, 1984: 6, 3)

Canada's Medicare system was a concerted attempt by federal and provincial governments to address inequities in access to physician and hospital services around the country (Mhatre and Derber, 1992). It meant that pregnant women had free access to physician and hospital services (Strong-Boag and McPherson, 1986). For women facing obstetrical complications and without the economic means to pay for hospital and physician fees, Medicare opened up access to core services that were hitherto available only to the privileged (CPSS, 2003). However, Medicare established the hospital as the core of the maternity care system, while at the same time assuring medical dominance over maternity care (only physicians were eligible for reimbursement of their services through Medicare). The result was 'medicalization' of pregnancy and childbirth, which for most women are uncomplicated and natural processes (Van Teijlingen, 2005). This centralization of childbirth in large urban hospitals generated restricted access to maternity services for vulnerable populations such as lower-income and Aboriginal women, and those living outside of large urban centres (Benoit et al., 2007a).

Recent healthcare reforms and maternal outcomes

Political pressure throughout the 1980s and early 1990s from an assortment of organizations, combined with efforts by government to control healthcare costs, resulted in legislative changes for the inclusion of formally trained midwives in the public healthcare systems of some provinces. Currently, six provinces – Ontario, British Columbia, Alberta, Quebec, Manitoba and Saskatchewan – and one territory – the Northwest Territories – have certification procedures in place for midwives (Sandall et al., 2009). Ontario, British Columbia, Quebec, Manitoba, the Northwest Territories and, most recently, Alberta, also fund midwifery services through provincial and territorial health insurance plans. Midwifery services are not publicly covered elsewhere in the country where pregnant women and their families can pay up to C$2500 per course of care (Hawkins and Knox, 2003), an out-of-pocket expense most lower-income pregnant women are unable to pay.

Research conducted by Benoit and colleagues (2007b) shows that, in British Columbia, where midwifery services are publicly funded, lower-income women are as likely to choose professional midwives as their primary care provider than better-off women. Both lower-lower income and better-off women reported high overall levels of satisfaction with the midwifery care they received, as has been found to be the case in other areas of Canada. However, despite these significant changes in the availability of midwifery care in some areas of Canada, the size of the change is still relatively small, with less than five per cent of births attended by a midwife. Some estimates suggest that as many as 40 per cent of women who want to see a midwife in Ontario are currently unable to find one and other provinces are also experiencing a situation where demand far outstrips supply (Canadian Institute for Health Information, 2004). Poor access to midwives is especially acute for Aboriginal women and those residing in rural and remote areas of the country (Kornelsen, 2000; see also Chapter 19 by Bourgeault and Sutherns).

At the same time, there is a shortage of doctors willing to provide maternity care. While family physicians are still the most common provider of prenatal care and the primary attendants at childbirth, their proportion of service provision has declined over the decades. In addition, they are less likely to deliver multiple births or perform caesarean sections (CS). Instead, obstetricians, trained to take care of 'abnormal' births, are increasingly under pressure to serve as women's primary attendants, despite a general lack of training and preparation for this role (Canadian Institute of Health Information, 2004).

These various changes in maternity human resources have been accompanied by a number of negative maternity-related outcomes. In 1990, Canada had an international ranking of second in maternal mortality and 12th in perinatal mortality rates. By 2002, however, it had dropped to 11th in maternal mortality and to 14th in perinatal mortality rates. Maternity care has at the same time become increasingly medicalized (OECD, 2005). As shown in Table 23.1, the proportion of women whose babies were delivered by CS, for example, increased from just less than 24 per cent in 2000–1, to just over 26 per cent in 2005 (Canadian Institute of Health Information, 2007; see also Chapter 8 by Ettorre and Kingdon). The data also show that the proportion of Canadian women who have a repeat CS is increasing and, conversely, the rates of vaginal birth after CS (VBAC) are decreasing (Canadian Institute of Health Information, 2007). The CS and VBAC rates are, moreover, not uniform across social groups and geographic areas. While there is a clear social gradient in CS rates – age-adjusted rates are significantly higher among women in low-income neighbourhoods than women in high-income neighbourhoods – the rates also vary among the country's various provinces and territories, and even among health authorities in the same province.

Nearly half of all vaginal deliveries in Canada in 2002–3 were accompanied by an epidural, and by 2005–6, the rate of epidural use among both vaginal and all deliveries increased (see Table 23.1). Although lower than the US rate (59 per cent), the Canadian rate was more than four times that of England (12 per cent) (Canadian Institute of Health Information, 2004). In 2005–6, there was an eight-fold variation in the rates of epidural use among vaginal deliveries across the country, with the highest provincial rates observed in Quebec and Ontario. On a positive note, there was a decrease in vacuum extractions and forceps rates between 2002–3 and 2005–6, as well as in the use of episiotomies. This last procedure was performed in half of all vaginal births in 1991–2, but by 2000–1 the rate had dropped to less than a quarter of all births (Canadian Institute of Health Information 2004). The recent drop in the episiotomy rate is attributed by some to changes in obstetric practice that are likely connected to scientific evidence that routine use of episiotomy increases maternal morbidity (Canadian Institute for Health Information, 2007).

In conclusion, recent healthcare reforms in Canada have had a mixed impact on maternal outcomes. A shortage of primary care providers has resulted in

Table 23.1   Maternity morbidity data, Canada, 2002–3; 2005–6

	2002–3	2005–6
Total C-section	23.8	26.3
Epidurals (all deliveries)	44.6	47.9
Vacuum extractions	10.5	9.8
Forceps	4.5	3.7

Source: CIHI (2007).

inadequate maternity care for certain populations, including lower-income women, those of Aboriginal background and those residing in rural and remote areas. Certified midwives have in a small way filled the void in some regions. However, their numbers still remain small, and less than half of the provincial/ territorial health plans cover midwifery services. With regard to efficiency, it should be noted that pregnancy and childbirth remain the leading causes of hospitalization among Canadian women, accounting for 24 per cent of acute care stays in 2001–2 (Canadian Institute of Health Information, 2007). The proportional increase of obstetricians providing primary care to pregnant women without medical complications, the continuously rising CS rates, and the rise of hospital readmission after this procedure have increased inequities in maternity care in Canada, despite the fact that lower-income women in many parts of the country have free access to midwifery care which hitherto was not available to them.

The race and ethnicity disparities lens in the United States of America

When Americans think about inequality they are less likely to think about income inequality than about disparities based on race, ethnicity and gender. The emphasis on racial and ethnic – rather than income – disparities in the USA is the result of three features of American society. First, most Americans believe that their country is a land of opportunity, a place where poor immigrants can 'pull themselves by their bootstraps', and make a better life for their children. Poverty is thus seen as just a (temporary) step on the way towards success and financial security (Waters et al., 2005). Second, and in spite of the fact that the United States Declaration of Independence declares equality for all, the country has a long history of discrimination against ethnic minorities and women. This history frames American inequality as a civil rights (not an economic) issue, appropriately handled by legislation or in the courts. Finally, the defining feature of US culture, noticed by many social scientists (see, for example, Bellah et al., 1985), is its individualistic orientation, which leads to the widely shared idea that individuals rather than systems are responsible for economic success and failure.

The historic emphasis on race in considering disparities in the USA has of late been substantially refined and two major adjustments are worth noting here. The first is the reporting of disparities by a combination of race and ethnicity – reflecting the rapidly growing Hispanic population in the USA. Hispanics accounted for almost one in four (24 per cent) of births in the USA in 2006, up from 15 per cent in 1990 (Martin et al., 2009). Data are typically not just reported for blacks and whites but according to the following categories: White non-Hispanic; Black non-Hispanic and Hispanic, with some jurisdictions also reporting data for Asian/Pacific Islanders. The second major change has been an effort to reflect the complexity in the racial make-up of the USA by allowing individuals to identify themselves as any combination of race and ethnicity they see as appropriate. The result was that in the 2000 census, almost seven million people (2.4 per cent of the population) self-identified as being of two or more races, while another 15 million (5.5 per cent) said they did not belong in any of the five racial categories (white, black, American Indian, Asian, Hawaiian Pacific Islander) available to them. These changes reflect the heightened sensitivity in US society – at least among census respondents – to racial/ethnic differences.

Research on disparities in maternal and infant health in the USA follows both the tendency to look at race and ethnic differences and the recent refinements. As early as 1921, Dr Raymond Pearl, an epidemiologist from Johns Hopkins University, noticed significant variation in birth outcomes between racial groups. His examination of biometric data on infant mortality (taken from the United States Birth Registration Area for the years 1915 to 1918) led him to conclude:

> The mean rates of infant mortality are, roughly speaking, something like twice as high for the colored population in each of the demographic units considered ... we have the precise figures on the point, which show definitely how tremendously poorer the negro baby's chances of surviving are than the white baby's. (Pearl, 1921: 420)

Nearly 90 years later, despite public health initiatives and resulting declines in mortality rates, infant mortality rates remain consistently higher for African-American babies than for white babies. In 1990, the infant mortality rate for black infants was 2.4 times that of white infants (18.0 per 1000 births compared to 7.6/1000). In 2005, both rates were lower, but the ratio remained exactly 2.4 (13.7 to 5.7) (Kung et al., 2008). The mortality rate for Hispanic infants has generally been very comparable to that of white non-Hispanic infants. Even more pronounced are disparities in maternal mortality, with the rate for black non-Hispanic mothers (39 per 100,000 births) more than three times higher than that of non-Hispanic white (12/100,000) or Hispanic (10/100,000) mothers. There is no national reporting of such outcomes by standard social class measures such as income or occupational status, though some data, as seen below, are presented by education.

The intuition that the health of mothers and babies is related to ethnicity, and not just to income level, is borne out by data. Factors typically related to health disparities, including income or health insurance coverage, do not account for all the race/ethnic differences in maternal/infant health. After adjusting for socio-economic differences, disparities in preterm birth, birth weight and infant mortality between African-American and white women persist (Behrman and Butler, 2006; Hogue and Bremner, 2005). In fact, infants born to black mothers with a college degree or more education have higher mortality rates than infants born to white, Hispanic or Asian women who are high school dropouts (Matthews and MacDorman, 2006; Pamuk et al., 1998). In a similar vein the ratio between white non-Hispanic and black non-Hispanic infant mortality rates and preterm birth rates is higher for college-educated mothers across racial/ethnic groupings than it is for those with eight or fewer years of education (Matthews and MacDorman, 2006).

With respect to the organization and delivery of services, the privatized, fragmented (non)-system in the USA provides an opportunity for racial/ethnic disparities to manifest in the provision of maternity care services as well as in health outcomes. In 2004, the rate of first-time mothers having late (after the sixth month) or no prenatal care was more than twice as high for black non-Hispanic mothers (4.3 per cent) than white non-Hispanic mothers (1.8 per cent). Interestingly, first-time Hispanic mothers reported even higher rates (5 per cent) of late/no prenatal care, yet generally had better outcomes than black non-Hispanic mothers (CDC, 2009). Black non-Hispanic mothers have the highest caesarean rates of any race/ethnicity group, seemingly a reflection of their higher risk status, except that these disparities persist even among the lowest-risk mothers (Declercq et al., 2007).

The inclination in the USA to focus on disparities not as a matter of income or social class, but as a matter of more immutable traits such as race and ethnicity, may reflect a profound reluctance to share personal economic data with researchers as well as a belief that individuals can change their social standing. It does not rule out substantial differences in services and outcomes based on economic status.

Social exclusion and maternity care in the UK: from woman-centred to family-centred care

In the UK, there has been general focus on improving inequalities in health outcomes with a more recent emphasis in government policy on the 'socially excluded'. It is increasingly recognized that pregnancy and the early parenting period can have a marked effect on the child's healthy development, on resilience to health problems encountered later in life, and on the woman's health and experience of motherhood (CSDH, 2009). Disadvantaged women are more likely to die in childbirth, or shortly afterwards, and their babies are more likely to be born with low birth weights. Disadvantaged women are also less likely to initiate and sustain breastfeeding, which helps to perpetuate health inequalities (House of Commons Health Committee, 2003). The main inequalities in health recognized in the UK are: a) socio-economic; b) regional; c) ethnic; and

d) gendered. Of these main inequalities in health, the focus has been more on social class, region and ethnicity than on gender and, as in Finland (discussed below), maternity service provision has largely been seen as gender-neutral.

Social class

Since the *Black Report* in 1980 (Townsend and Davidson, 1982) the focus on inequalities has been on social class with an increasing interest in ethnicity from the 1990s. Through most of the 1990s, neoliberal governments focused on 'variations in health', a concept narrowly focused on population health behaviour and lifestyle changes, and the contributions the National Health Service (NHS) could make to reduce this variation. There was little government enthusiasm for addressing structural determinants affecting health and well-being. However, more recent government-commissioned work has recognized that wide differentials are noted in the rates of low birth weight, premature birth and perinatal and maternal mortality between high and low-income groups (D'Souza and Garcia, 2004). In maternity care we find that women from lower socio-economic backgrounds are more likely to become pregnant as teenagers and have low-birth-weight babies. Young mothers in low-income groups, and who have fewer years of education, are least likely to initiate and to continue breastfeeding (Sikorski et al., 2003).

In 2004, the NHS published the National Service Framework for Children, Young People and Maternity Services (DH, 2004); this included policies to reduce socio-economic inequality within and between regions in England and Wales, and later extended to Scotland. Midwives were encouraged to deliver care in community settings in poor localities such as Sure Start centres. Sure Start is a government initiative aimed at poorer communities where local people, parents and health and social care providers work together to direct local integrated services in one geographical setting. More recently in England, a range of policies based on reviews of effective interventions have targeted the socially excluded with a view to reducing inequalities in infant mortality. Such proposals are focused on broader areas than maternity services, and have used modelling techniques to estimate the impact on infant mortality. These include reducing overcrowding and child poverty, maternal obesity, smoking, under-18 teenage pregnancy and bed-sharing, and increasing early access to maternity care and breastfeeding (DH, 2007a; 2007b).

From women-centred care to family-centred care

Men (as partners of pregnant women) have been relative outsiders in the maternity services, although this has changed over the past decades. Kiernan and Smith (2003) estimate that 86 per cent of fathers now attend the birth of their children. Jeremy Davies (2009) of the Fatherhood Institute, itself a fairly recently established UK organization, highlights that the maternity services ask only two formal questions about fathers: 1) their genetic stock; and 2) whether they are violent. It would be fair to say that community midwives will discuss during antenatal visits the support (or lack of it) a pregnant woman receives from her partner.

In the UK the 'problem' of young single mothers and concerns regarding delinquent children have been coupled with the concept of a one-to-one intervention in the shape of a model of intensive, nurse-led home visiting for vulnerable, first-time, young parents (Cabinet Office, 2009). The Family-Nurse-Partnership programme (FNP) consists of a programme of structured regular visits by nurses/midwives to low-income first-time mothers, both while the mothers are pregnant and for the first two years following birth. It focuses on teaching parenthood and encouraging mothers back into education and/or into employment. Although the FNP marks a considerable discontinuity with previous approaches to family health, which were more focused on individual behavioural change, it is congruent with an emerging new approach to social exclusion. This new approach maintains that the most important task of social policy is to identify quickly the most 'at-risk' households, individuals and children so that interventions can be targeted more effectively at those 'at risk', either to themselves or to others.

Dodds (2009) illustrates this new approach by analysing a succession of reports by the Social Exclusion Unit, highlighting that there is a considerable amount of ambiguity about the relationship between specific risk-factors and being at risk of social exclusion. Given this context, it is legitimate to ask why the FNP has been given such prominence as a new policy programme to help tackle social exclusion. The answer is that the FNP fits with the Social Exclusion Unit's new focus on enabling individuals to become 'resilient' to the risks that they face, not necessarily through providing extra resources or tackling structural barriers, but through the exhortation and encouragement of professionals, such as nurses and midwives. In the USA, instead of acknowledging the need for increased support for those living on low incomes, the welfare services have increasingly become entwined with moral aspirations to manufacture 'better' clients and citizens (Soss, 2005). The Social Exclusion Unit's focus on individually based, therapeutic approaches, exemplified by the FNP, suggests that welfare policy in the UK may be leaning in the same direction.

The Finnish welfare state as a comprehensive, state-centred project

In Finland, there is a strong tradition in health policy focusing on socio-economic differences in health that builds on the idea of the welfare state as a comprehensive, state-centred project. The history of maternity care is more complex, however, building on early pronatalist policies aimed at securing the future of the nation. The primary rationale for making access to free preventive healthcare available to all women and children was not their individual welfare, but that of the nation (Wrede, 2001). In the 1960s, the tone of the health policy discourse changed and social equality was the core value underpinning the 1972 Primary Health Care Act. The expanding welfare state provided all women access to basic maternity care and specialized services were made available on the basis of need. The position of maternity care was less straightforward, as the special emphasis previously given to the service was withdrawn. Ante- and postnatal care activities became incorporated into newly established municipal primary care centres (PHCs) (Wrede, 2001). The PHCs coordinated the care of women facing complicated pregnancies with hospital maternity units, where outpatient clinics emerged. Antenatal care within primary care, by way of contrast, became framed primarily by family policy, geared at diminishing social inequalities and with the emphasis on the well-being of the child.

The equality discourse that framed health policy was explicitly gender-neutral, an emphasis that in the case of maternity care created an odd mix with the practical focus on women. The policy has been criticized for highlighting the needs of the coming child at the cost of those of the pregnant woman (Wrede, 2001). On the other hand, the social democratic orientation underlying the country's maternity care system resonated with what Henriksson and her colleagues (2006) identify as an overall orientation towards social service professionalism in the Finnish welfare state. Within maternity care this approach to professionalism can be seen as 'women-friendly' in that it was premised on egalitarian relationships between medical and other health professionals and partnership with knowledgeable clients (Wrede et al., 2008).

However, the tradition of social service professionalism has become fragmented. A series of neoliberal healthcare reforms in Finland the early 1990s prodded the municipalities to devise more 'flexible' practice patterns for the primary care workforce. The policy emphasized that 'generalist' orientations were expected from public health nurses and primary care doctors, reflecting the attention to cost-consciousness and effectiveness that were central values underlying the new health policy. The policy was also in line with the efforts to streamline public management that included dissolution of central elements of state steering (Sandall et al., 2009).

Paradoxically, the new flexible programs have been paralleled with continued growth in the use of services. Until 2002, PHC antenatal visits increased for all pregnant women, regardless of age and the number of previous pregnancies. At the same time, visits to hospital outpatient clinics increased even more rapidly for all categories of pregnant women (Finnish Ministry of Social Affairs and Health, 2007). In addition, while maternal health outcomes remain among the best in the world, there are concerns related to maternity care practice. Increasing criticism has focused particularly on the fragmented work pattern of public health nurses and the unnecessary medicalization of antenatal care. Fragmented work patterns have been seen to hinder the provision of equitable antenatal care, whereas medicalization impairs the experience of the woman and elevates the risk of unnecessary interventions. Furthermore, regional inequalities related to service fragmentation and increasing differences in the antenatal packages offered by different municipalities are also recognized as policy concerns (Finnish Ministry of Social Affairs and Health, 2007).

In the current decade Finnish policy emphasis has shifted from efficiency back to primary prevention of inequalities in health, paving the way for maternity-care-related policy initiatives. In 2005, antenatal care was reaffirmed as the key instrument for securing equity in perinatal health (the Law on the Changes of the Public Health Act). In 2007, a new policy instrument, a national action programme for the promotion of sexual and reproductive health, was created. Maternity care was reinforced as a core universal public health area and the service package was mandated to be unitary in character (Finnish Ministry of Social Affairs and Health, 2007). This policy instrument is linked to a revised Health Care Act that aims to restructure the entire public provision of health services. According to plans, the legislation affirms the mandate for the government to steer the content and style of key preventive health services provided by the municipalities. Particular emphasis is put on 'specific health promotion missions', including antenatal care, that are considered to be of vital importance from the perspective of health equity (Finnish Ministry of Social Affairs and Health, 2008a: 16). The new act rejects the long-term generalist emphasis in Finnish primary care, as 'basic-level' specialized medical care is planned to be made available in the community (Finnish Ministry of Social Affairs and Health, 2008a: 16).

At the moment two possible directions of change can be discerned for maternity care. The action programme for sexual and reproductive health proposes midwife services that when first raised onto the agenda were referred to as 'women's centres' that would be able to take care of, for instance, the many women who are afraid of childbirth, allowing hospital outpatient clinics to concentrate on particular groups, including, for example, pregnant women with addiction problems (Finnish Ministry of Social Affairs and Health, 2007). The second model for reorganizing municipal antenatal services is linked to family policy that aims at developing 'family centres', sometimes also referred to as 'welfare centres'. The plan is to coordinate all the publicly provided services available for families with children into a universally available, low-threshold service (Finnish Ministry of Social Affairs and Health, 2008b). As the planned new Health Care Act incorporates both models, it thus anchors antenatal care into two competing policy areas. In policy discourse women's centres and welfare centres have been placed into opposition with each other and treated as alternatives.

In sum, Finnish health policy has regained much of its political clout, and public service provision continues to be its key instrument. This does not mean a simple return to the old. Rather, new models of service provision are emerging, where both effective public management and new types of partnerships with NGOs are sought. For antenatal care it is likely that the policy process will result in a settlement that is a hybrid of the two models described above. In terms of championing unnecessary medicalization of maternity care, as well as equitable service provision, the situation holds promise. From a gender perspective it is important to note that maternal healthcare in the Finnish welfare state became incorporated into a larger health political framework of family policy rather than in a women's health framework (Wrede, 2001). In current policies, attention to care needs as gendered needs is more evident, but mainly this concerns the need to include fathers. Accordingly, a women-centred model threatens the articulation of maternity care as family-centred care.

Conclusion

To conclude, in Canada, a shortage of primary care providers has resulted in inadequate maternity care for certain populations, including lower-income women, those of Aboriginal background and those residing in rural and remote areas. The proportional increase of obstetricians providing primary care to pregnant women without medical complications, the continuously rising CS rates, and the rise in hospital readmission after this procedure have increased inequities in maternity care in Canada, despite the fact that lower-income women in many parts of the country have free access to midwifery care which hitherto was not available to them. In the USA, instead of acknowledging the need for increased support for those living on low incomes, the welfare services have increasingly become entwined with moral aspirations to manufacture 'better' clients and citizens (Soss, 2005). In both Finland and the UK, there is an increasing emphasis on family-centred care and the role of fathers; however, the Social Exclusion Unit's focus on individually based, therapeutic approaches, exemplified by the FNP in the UK, suggests that welfare policy in the UK may be leaning in the same direction as in the USA.

In all four countries, inequalities in maternal and infant healthcare have risen up the policy agenda for a range of reasons, such as evidence from the field of foetal programming that events in pregnancy and early infancy can have a lifelong impact on future health, and from the field of neurosciences that early parenting experiences can affect ongoing social, cognitive and emotional development. What is rarely done, however, is to pull together data from a range of fields and conduct analyses that take into account a range of factors, rather than the single variable analysis that is predominant, whether it is a focus on social class, ethnicity or age. Nevertheless, the focus on the 'socially excluded' is not new and was a dominant theme in family policy in high-income countries to a greater or lesser extent over the 20th century, when the prime focus was on improving the health of the nation (Koven and Michel, 1993).

However, the solutions being put forward to reduce inequalities and the evidence base that is drawn upon ranges widely from a rhetorical attempt to reduce structural disparities and determinants to restructuring services and changing health behaviours and family culture. In essence the field suffers from poor theorizing, poor research and politically driven interventions that say more about the way that 'undesirable behaviours and family formation' are socially constructed within a society than they constitute a concerted attempt to improve health outcomes and reduce inequity.

Summary

- Gender as a key social issue is often secondary to other 'big' social issues such as, for example, social class or ethnicity.
- The focus on the 'socially excluded' has been a dominant theme in family policy over the 20th century, as part of policies to improve the health of the nation.
- Solutions being put forward to reduce inequalities range from a rhetorical attempt to reduce structural disparities and determinants, to restructuring services and changing health behaviours and family culture.
- Solutions say more about the way that 'undesirable behaviours and family formation' are socially constructed within a society than they constitute a concerted attempt to improve health outcomes and reduce inequity.

Key reading

De Vries, R., C. Benoit, E. van Teijlingen and S. Wrede (2001) *Birth by Design* (New York: Routledge).

Sandall, J., C. Benoit, S. Wrede, S. F. Murray, E. van Teijlingen and R. Westfall (2009) 'Social Service Professional or Market Expert? Maternity Care Relations under Neoliberal Healthcare Reform', *Current Sociology*, 57 (4), 529–53.

Wrede, S., C. Benoit and T. Einarsdottir (2008) 'Equity and Dignity in Maternity Care Provision in Canada, Finland and Iceland', *Canadian Journal of Public Health*, 99 (Supplement 2), S16–S21.

References

Badgley, R. and S. Wolfe (1967) *Doctors' Strike: Medical Care and Conflict in Saskatchewan* (Toronto: Macmillan).

Behrman, R. and A. Butler (2006) *Preterm Birth: Causes, Consequences and Prevention*, Committee on Understanding Premature Birth and Assuring Health Outcomes,

Institute of Medicine of the National Academies (Washington, DC: National Academies Press).

Bellah, R., R. Madsen, W. M. Sullivan, A. Swidler and S. M. Tipton (1985) *Habits of the Heart: Individualism and Commitment in American Life* (Berkeley: University of California Press).

Benoit, C., D. Carroll and R. Westfall (2007a) 'Women's Access to Maternity Services in Canada: Historical Developments and Contemporary Challenges', in C. Varcoe, O. Hankivsky and M. Morrow (eds), *Women's Health in Canada: Critical Theory, Policy and Practice* (Toronto: University of Toronto Press), 507–27.

Benoit, C., R. Westfall, A. Treloar, R. Phillips and S. M. Jansson (2007b) 'Social Factors Linked with Postpartum Depression', *Journal of Mental Health*, 16 (6), 719–30.

Cabinet Office, (2009) Family-Nurse-Partnership website, at: www.cabinetoffice.gov.uk/social_exclusion_task_force/family_nurse_partnership.aspx, accessed 16 July 2009.

Canada Health Act (1984) at: www.hc-sc.gc.ca/hcs-sss/medi-assur/cha-lcs/index-eng.php, accessed 27 August 2009.

Canadian Institute for Health Information (2004) *Giving Birth in Canada: A Regional Profile* (Ottawa: CIHI).

Canadian Institute for Health Information (2007) *Giving Birth in Canada: Regional Trends from 2001–2002 to 2005–2006* (Ottawa: CIHI).

CDC – Centers for Disease Control and Prevention (2009) *National Center for Health Statistics*, VitalStats, at: www.cdc.gov/nchs/vitalstats.htm, accessed 28 June 2009.

CPSS – Canadian Perinatal Service System (2003) *Canadian Perinatal Health Report* (Ottawa: Health Canada).

CSDH – Commission on Social Determinants of Health (2008) *Closing the Gap in a Generation: Health Equity through Action on the Social Determinants of Health*, Final Report of the Commission on Social Determinants of Health (Geneva: World Health Organization).

Davies, J. (2009) 'Involving Fathers in Maternity Care: Best Practice', *Midwives: The Official Magazine of the RCM*, February/March, 32–3.

Declercq, E. R., M. Barger, H. Cabral, S. Evans, M. Kotelchuck, C. Simon, J. Weiss and L. Heffner (2007) 'Maternal Outcomes Associated with Planned Primary Cesareans Compared to Planned Vaginal Births', *Obstetrics and Gynecology*, 109, 669–77

DH – Department of Health (2004) *National Service Framework for Children, Young People and Maternity Services* (London: Department of Health).

DH – Department of Health (2007a) *Review of the Health Inequalities Infant Mortality PSA Target* (London: Department of Health).

DH – Department of Health (2007b) *Implementation Plan for Reducing Health Inequalities in Infant Mortality: A Good Practice Guide* (London: Department of Health).

Dodds, A. (2009) 'Families "at Risk" and the Family Nurse Partnership: The Intrusion of Risk into Social Exclusion Policy', *Journal of Social Policy*, 38, 499–514.

D'Souza, L. and J. Garcia (2004) 'Improving Services for Disadvantaged Childbearing Women', *Child: Care, Health and Development*, 30 (6), 599–611.

Finnish Ministry of Social Affairs and Health (2007) Seksuaali – ja lisääntymisterveyden edistäminen, Toimintaohjelma 2007–2011, Helsinki.

Finnish Ministry of Social Affairs and Health (2008a) *The New Health Care Act*, Memorandum of the Working Group Preparing the Health Care Act, 16 June 2008, Helsinki.

Finnish Ministry of Social Affairs and Health (2008b) *Development of Family Centre Services*, final report of the FAMILY project, Helsinki.

Hawkins, M. and S. Knox (2003) *The Midwifery Option: A Canadian Guide to the Birth Experience* (Toronto: HarperCollins).

Henriksson, L., S. Wrede and V. Burau (2006) 'Understanding Professional Projects in Welfare Service Work', *Gender, Work and Organization,* 14 (2), 174–92.

Hogue, C. J. and J. D. Bremner (2005) 'Stress Model for Research into Preterm Delivery among Black Women', *American Journal of Obstetrics and Gynecology,* 192 (5), Supplement 1, S47–S55.

House of Commons Health Committee (2003) *Inequalities in Access to Maternity Services, Eighth Report of Session 2002–03,* Volume 1 (London: The Stationery Office).

Kiernan, K. and K. Smith (2003) 'Unmarried Parenthood: New Insight from the Millennium Cohort Study', *Population Trends,* 114, 26–33.

Kornelsen, J. (2000) *Pushing for Change: Challenges of Integrating Midwifery into the Health Care System* (Vancouver: BCCEWH), at: www.bccewh.bc.ca/publications-resources/documents/pushingforchange.pdf, accessed 4 June 2009.

Koven, S. and S. Michel (1993) *Mothers of a New World: Maternalist Politics and the Origins of Welfare States* (New York: Routledge).

Kung, H. C., D. L. Hoyert, J. Q. Xu and S. L. Murphy (2008) 'Deaths: Final Data for 2005', *National Vital Statistics Reports,* 56 (10) (Hyattsville: National Center for Health Statistics).

Martin, J. A., B. E. Hamilton, P. D. Sutton, S. J. Ventura, F. Menacker, S. Kirmeyer and T. J. Mathews (2009) 'Births: Final Data for 2006', *National Vital Statistics Reports,* 57 (7) (Hyattsville: National Center for Health Statistics), at: www.cdc.gov/nchs/data/nvsr/nvsr57/nvsr57_07.pdf, accessed 4 June 2009.

Mathews, T. J. and M. F. MacDorman (2006) 'Infant Mortality Statistics from the 2003 Period Linked Birth/Infant Death Data Set', *National Vital Statistics Reports,* 54 (16) (Hyattsville: National Center for Health Statistics).

Mhatre, S. and R. Derber (1992) 'From Equal Access to Health Care to Equitable Access to Health', *International Journal of Health Services,* 22 (4), 645–68.

OECD Annual Report (2005) 45th Anniversary (Paris: Public Affairs Division, Public Affairs and Communications Directorate, OECD).

Pamuk, E., D. Makuk, K. Heck and C. Reuben (1998) *Health United States* (Hyattsville: National Center for Health Statistics).

Pearl, R. (1921) 'Biometric Data on Infant Mortality in the United States Birth Registration Area, 1915–1918', *The American Journal of Hygiene,* 1, 419–39.

Sandall, J., C. Benoit, S. Wrede, S. F. Murray, E. van Teijlingen and R. Westfall (2009) 'Social Service Professional or Market Expert? Maternity Care Relations under Neoliberal Healthcare Reform', *Current Sociology,* 57 (4), 529–53.

Sikorski, J., M. Renfrew, S. Pindoria and A. Wade (2003) 'Support for Breastfeeding Mothers; A Systematic Review', *Paediatric & Perinatal Epidemiology,* 17 (4), 407–17.

Soss, J. (2005) 'Making Clients and Citizens: Welfare Policy as a Source of Status, Belief, and Action', in A. L. Schneider and H. M. Ingram (eds), *Deserving and Entitled: Social Constructions and Public Policy* (Albany: State University of New York Press), 291–328.

Strong-Boag, V. and K. McPherson (1986) 'The Confinement of Women, Childbirth and Hospitalization in Vancouver 1919–1939, *BC Studies,* 69/70, 142–74.

Townsend, P. and N. Davidson (1982) *Inequalities in Health* (London: Penguin).

Van Teijlingen, E. (2005) 'A Critical Analysis of the Medical Model as Used in the Study of Pregnancy and Childbirth', *Sociological Research Online,* 10, at: www.socresonline.org.uk/10/2/teijlingen.html, accessed 27 August 2009.

Waters, M., C. Jiménez and R. Tomás (2005) 'Assessing Immigrant Assimilation: New Empirical and Theoretical Challenges', *Annual Review of Sociology*, 31 (1), 105–25.

Wrede, S. (2001) *Decentering Care for Mothers. The Politics of Midwifery and the Design of Finnish Maternity Services* (Turku: Abo Akademi University Press).

Wrede, S., C. Benoit, I. L. Bourgeault, E. R. van Teijlingen, J. Sandall and R. De Vries (2006) 'Decentered Comparative Research: Context Sensitive Analysis of Health Care', *Social Science & Medicine*, 63 (11), 2986–97.

Wrede, S., C. Benoit and T. Einarsdottir (2008) 'Equity and Dignity in Maternity Care Provision in Canada, Finland and Iceland', *Canadian Journal of Public Health*, 99 (Supplement 2), S16–S21.

24
Women's Health Centres: Creating Spaces and Institutional Support

Pat Armstrong

Introduction

The Canadian women's health movement learned with and from movements in other countries, and like them had roots stretching back long before second wave feminism (Vickers, 1992). Nevertheless, Canadian feminists have carved their own path and even taken the lead in some areas. Like other western activists (Kuhlmann, 2009), they were concerned about what Sherwin and her colleagues (1998; see also Sherwin, 1992) called agency and autonomy. But the Canadian women's health movement from the 1960s also addressed the structural and institutional supports that promote or undermine women's health (Feldberg et al., 2003). Like their European counterparts who fought for gender mainstreaming, the movement demanded gender-based analysis in research, policy and practices (see Chapter 26 by Lagro-Janssen and Chapter 6 by Klinge). However, it also sought to create and maintain separate women's centres for research and action on women's health, centres that are connected to the movement (Johnson et al., 2009). The differences are explained by multiple factors, including the small population that encouraged interchange among various factions within the feminist movements, by resistance to influences from what were often defined as colonial powers and by welfare state traditions that meant there was some faith held in appeals to state intervention and institutions (Black, 1992).

Using the specific case of the Women's Health Contribution Program at Health Canada, this chapter analyses the factors that have contributed to the development and maintenance of Centres of Excellence for Women's Health and the related Working Groups for a dozen years. They offer one example of the continuing space for women's health in Canada, one that explicitly acknowledges that it is *for* women's health not *on* women's health, as is the case in many countries. Mandated to develop action-oriented and policy-relevant research and education through citizen engagement, these federally funded organizations have provided an institutional base for research, popular materials and action on women's health and healthcare issues. They have provided links for and with communities, as well as evidence that is useful in efforts to change policies and practices in women's health. In spite of relatively low levels of funding and continual efforts needed for survival, the Program has managed to produce a large body of research used by governments and community groups in making changes. It has established a presence for women's health issues and helped extend gender-based analysis to men. This chapter describes the development and structure of the Program before going on to outline the contributions and the forces that have sustained it, focusing primarily on one Working Group, Women and Health Care Reform. It concludes with a discussion of current threats and lessons learned.

Locating the Women's Health Contribution Program: historical factors

The women's movement has long insisted that context matters, and this is no less the case for women's health than it is for other women's issues (see, for the UK, Doyal, 1994; for the USA, Clarke and Olesen, 1999; Morgen, 2002). Although there are certainly global pressures and shared efforts across borders, understanding the forces leading to the establishment of the national Women's Health Contribution Program requires the exploration of a little Canadian history and some Canadian political economy.

Canada emerged from the Second World War with an expanded state and an active citizenry that insisted on the extension of social services and attention to human rights. Canadian government representatives, for example, played a central role in the development of the United Nations' Universal Declaration on Human Rights. Within Canada, traditional women's organizations, such as the farm women's institutes, were active in growing demands for public healthcare. Their focus was on access, on getting into care. By the end of the 1950s, such efforts resulted in a universal hospital insurance plan and later, in public payment for doctors' care. Access to health services improved significantly, especially for women. There was a downside, however. Both because Canadian Medicare was focused on hospitals and doctors and because doctors were successful in retaining their power to define what was medically necessary care and thus covered under the public plan, accessible services were increasingly medical ones (Armstrong and Armstrong, 2003). With doctors paid fee-for-service, and paid higher fees for more complicated care, there was a financial incentive to do more, and more invasive, care. With medical practice still male-dominated, this care seldom took women's interests into account and, worse, often served to reinforce inequities between women and men (Sherwin, 1998).

During the same period, other kinds of women's organizations were emerging in response to rising expectations and government failures (Backhouse and Flaherty, 1992). While Canadian women were certainly not alone in making such demands, their struggles were uniquely Canadian even as their actions were taking place in tandem with women in other countries. Groups from the French-speaking province of Quebec and from the rest of Canada came together to demand a traditional Canadian approach, a Royal Commission. When it reported in 1970, the Royal Commission on the Status of Women focused only five of its 167 recommendations on women's health. Although far from radical, it did lead to significant money for research on women's issues, legitimated many demands and resulted in a federal government office responsible for women's issues. Equally important, the National Action Committee on the Status of Women (NAC) was formed in its wake and received full funding from the federal government as a result. Explicitly committed to equity and social justice, NAC followed in the pattern of the National Council of Women, an organization established in 1893 by Canada's first woman doctor, to bring together women's groups for political action.

Many of these groups were devoted to improving women's health. Strong links and partnerships amongst groups with different primary interests were forged, including groups not specifically focused on women's issues. For example, in 1968 the students' council at McGill University, with support from other student councils across Canada, flaunted the law banning the distribution of information on birth control by writing and distributing a handbook on the issue; 'Packed with information about birth control, the Handbook also contained controversial editorial commentary on women's liberation and population control' (Sethna, 2006: 90). It preceded the more famous Boston Women's Health Book Collective's *Our Bodies Ourselves* (BWHBC, 1973), and the Canadian handbook was distributed for free to thousands. The law on birth control that it challenged was changed in 1969. The Montreal Women's Health Press, established to continue the work begun at McGill and supported primarily by government money, went on not only to publish a new version of the *Handbook* but also companion handbooks on a range of women's health issues.

Similarly, a wide range of women's organizations joined in the 1970 Abortion Caravan, a cross-Canada trek that led to Canada's capital and eventually to the legalization of abortion. Violence against women was taken up as a health as well as a social issue, indicating the growing emphasis within the movement on the social determinants of health. Women academics began writing about the care they received in a wide range of services. The collection, *Women Look at Psychiatry* (Smith and David, 1975), is just one example, albeit one that indicates such writing was still mainly in the alternative press. Reflecting on their experiences, activists in the movement during the 1960s and 1970s concluded that:

> ... the women's health movement has focused on three main issues: the healthcare delivery system, the development and analysis of the social determinants of health, and a commitment to increase the participation of women in all aspects of health care. (Boscoe et al., 2006: 8)

In short, a women's health movement emerged in Canada between 1960 and 1990 with a strong community foundation and links among organizations (for an overview, see Armstrong and Deadman, 2009; Morrow et al., 2007). Some laws were changed as a result, and women's centres of various sorts emerged. An institutional base for women's issues was established within government, with many feminists taking on government work and with networks formed between elected officials and community groups. At the same time, a significant number of feminist organizations received federal financial support. Pressured by women's organizations and their own members, the federal government made commitments to equity internationally through the UN *Convention on the Elimination of All Forms of Discrimination Against Women* (CEDAW) and nationally through the *Charter of Rights and Freedoms* (Greaves, 2009). Although women's groups remained critical of governments and their services, and committed to a social justice agenda, they were willing to lobby and even work within governments for change, in part because they had enjoyed some success in these strategies.

By the end of the 1980s, however, a new Conservative government began shifting the terrain, withdrawing support for women's organizations both within and outside government. With their established networks, women's organizations successfully resisted some of these efforts but funding disappeared for many organizations, and along with it their programmes. Meanwhile, a flurry of government and medical reports in the early 1990s pointed to the gaps in, and need for research on, women's health (Morrow, 2007).

Establishing the Women's Health Contribution Program

It was in this context that the federal government's Women's Health Bureau was established in 1993. With a mandate 'to address how sex and gender affect women's health across the lifespan, determine the health and healthcare issues pertinent to women and to carry forward the gender-based analysis policy of Health Canada' (Greaves, 2009: 5), the Bureau reflected not only the pressure from women's groups and Canada's international commitments but also a narrower focus on fewer areas, even though health was broadly defined and the goal was help 'ensure the Canadian health system recognizes and responds to women's health needs' (Tudiver, 2009: 21). It nevertheless provided a place for women to work within government to promote women's health issues and some significant support for work outside, mainly through a funding plan called the Women's Health Contribution Program.

Led by Abby Hoffman, a former Olympic athlete and a feminist who promoted women in sport, the Bureau, under her guidance, called for proposals to establish centres of excellence for women's health. As she explained in an interview at the time:

> ... the purpose of a centre is to bring people and organizations together that are interested in and have expertise in women's health. The program and centres individually and collectively will hopefully generate significant new knowledge about women's health which could be applied to improving the health of Canadian women. (CWHN, 1996: 1)

The centres were intended to do policy-based non-clinical research and to provide policy advice to both government and other organizations, with research reflecting community as well as academic concerns (CWHN, 1996).

Hoffman stressed that expertise was not understood as exclusively academic research and that both advocacy and communications were part of the purpose. She also specifically mentioned that this meant employing a wide variety of research methods going well beyond quantitative approaches and double-blind, randomized trials. Centres were intended to legitimate new methods and to work for change. The Bureau funded five of the 25 proposals submitted, with approximately C$2 million each initially for six years (1993–9) (Centres of Excellence for Women's Health, 1997). Each had a different structure and focus. All had a governing structure, a workplan for research, policy and communications, and a means of ensuring community involvement. One way that the Centres connected to communities was through advisory boards; another was through joint research projects and a third was through the appointment of co-directors, with one from the academic world and the other from the community. One was hosted by a hospital, another by a health centre and three by universities, although directors did not necessarily have university appointments. The university, hospital and health centre connections were intended to provide a shelter, a formal structure to receive and monitor the funding.

Hoffman recognized that making the system responsive to the needs of women and women's health was no easy task, especially given the dramatic cutbacks, amalgamations and privatization strategies under way in health services (Armstrong and Armstrong, 2003). 'The challenge is to ensure women's health is part of the process of renewal and modernization' (Centres of Excellence for Women's Health, 1997: 1). More specifically, the Centres were separately and together to contribute to the improvement of women's health

Box 24.1   Centres of Excellence for Women's Health – what do they contribute?

- identify key women's health issues and do research on them;
- produce health data that is sensitive to gender issues;
- communicate the knowledge they generate;
- build local, national networks that bring together researchers, community and policy partners working to improve the health of women;
- provide analysis, advice and information to governments, agencies and individuals involved in health and policy;
- help define a women's health research agenda for Canada.

through a range of initiatives (Box 24.1; see Centres of Excellence for Women's Health, 1997: 2).

Institutional structure of the Centres

Bringing together three provinces in Atlantic Canada, the Maritime Centre (now the Atlantic Centre) of Excellence for Women's Health initially concentrated on women's perceptions of health determinants and on health determinants for women living in poverty. It quickly added unpaid caregiving and other issues for marginalized women to this agenda. Representatives from governments, women's organizations and academic groups were all part of the plan. The Centre in Quebec (le Centre d'excellence pour la santé des femmes – Consortium Université de Montréal) was particularly concerned with issues facing immigrant and Aboriginal women, and set up groups representing these women. Based in two provinces, the Prairie Women's Health Centre of Excellence had five themes: gender analysis of population health, consumer input in health policy, the impact of social support on health, the effects of health reform, and gender-specific programming. It too planned to develop working relationships with a wide variety of communities, including service providers.

The British Columbia Centre was a partnership among health institutions, community organizations, universities and government designed to foster multidisciplinary research and action-oriented approaches to three main theme areas: health determinants and status, healthy women in healthy communities, and women-centred care. The fifth Centre, located in Ontario, was also a partnership but one that was intended to operate across the country. This National Network on Environments and Women's Health (NNEWH) had academic and community partners from many provinces. The plan was to begin with a series of conceptual papers on issues such as research methods, risk, alternative therapies and work restructuring, as well as with a number of pilot studies on areas such as breast cancer support groups (Centres of Excellence for Women's Health, 1997).

In addition, the Bureau funded the Canadian Women's Health Network (CWHN). Providing communications among the various components of the Women's Health Contribution Program, the CWHN was also mandated to develop user-friendly information and forums for critical debate, to advocate for community-based research models and to alert communities to emerging issues in women's health. The CWHN Newsletter and website were soon complemented by the *Research Bulletin* that produced summaries of the research conducted through the Program (see www.cwhn.ca). While CWHN, like the Centres, received a significant amount of money from the federal government for both infrastructure and research, this money was understood to be seed money that would help establish an infrastructure for attracting additional funding. And while each Centre had considerable independence in following its own path, reports were submitted to and finances monitored by the Bureau. The Bureau also convened meetings that involved all the Centres (Tudiver, 2009).

It took a while to create the infrastructure, form advisory boards and begin producing research as well as networks that could promote women's health. The process was far from simple or easy. There were differences in understandings within, among and between Centres and the Bureau about how exactly to fulfill the work plans. Tensions arose in part because this was a new kind of funding that required the details to be worked out. Tensions also arose because the Centres were intended to bring together diverse groups with different ways of practising that necessarily involved conflicts over ways of seeing and doing. Equally important, the work of Centres necessarily and frequently involved critiques of the very hand that fed them, given their lobbying role and their mandate to address issues in women's health services. To a large extent these, or at least similar, debates continue, often with a healthy resolution or at least recognition of the need for multiple forms of intervention (Majury, 1999).

Women's health and healthcare reform

It became obvious that there were some critical gaps in programming and some need to bring together issues across Centres. One missing area was pharmaceuticals. In 1998, a group initially organized over concerns related to the drug Diethystilbestrol (DES) brought together various organizations to consider proposed federal legislation on health protection. Out of this meeting came a Working Group on Women and Health Protection:

> [A] coalition of community groups, researchers, journalists and activists concerned about the safety of pharmaceutical drugs. The group keeps a close watch over ongoing changes in the federal health protection legislation and examines the impact of those changes on women's health. (www.whp-apsf. ca/en/index.html)

This Group, renamed Women and Health Protection in 2002, received their main financial support from the Women's Health Contribution Program. In addition to commissioning papers on issues such as Selective Serotonin Reuptake Inhibiters (SSRIs) and Depo Provera, the group actively intervenes to promote access to things such as emergency contraception and to limit access in areas such as direct-to-consumer advertising. As well, in 1998, the National Coordinating Group on Women and Health Care Reform (later just Women and Health Care Reform) was formed to coordinate research on healthcare reform and to translate this research into policies and practices. This collaborative group includes a member from each of the Centres and from CWHN. It investigates and advises on how health systems and healthcare reforms affect women as providers, decision-makers and users of healthcare systems (see www.womenandhealthcarereform.ca). The Group's work is centred around three questions:

1. Why is this a woman's issue?
2. What are the issues for women?
3. For which women?

Women and Health Care Reform began by bringing together available research to develop a picture of what healthcare reforms mean to women. The commissioned papers were published in *Exposing Privatization: Women and Health Care Reform in Canada* (Armstrong et al., 2002), a book that was assigned in numerous university courses and distributed in government circles. Indeed, the book became the basis of submissions to and appearances before the Royal Commission on the Future of Health Care in 2001 and the Senate Committee on Health Science and Technology in 2000. The Bureau facilitated these appearances and supported the presentation of the materials. All of the papers were also available online through the Centres and CWHN. At the core of Women and Health Care Reform's subsequent activities was an annual workshop organized in cooperation with a Centre, and building on their expertise. The first of these provided a template for subsequent ones, although the format and structure shifted with the topics. It covered homecare and unpaid caregiving, and it is worthwhile describing it in more detail because it illustrates the range of activities involved in the overall programme.

In 2001, the Maritime Centre began a multi-year project, using the infrastructure to develop successfully an innovative proposal. *A Healthy Balance: A Community Alliance for Health Research on Women's Unpaid Caregiving* 'brought together more than 25 researchers from universities, the public policy domain, health practitioners, communications professionals and the wider community to examine the ways in which women's work, both as paid workers and unpaid caregivers, affects health status' (www.acewh.dal.ca/e). In the same year, the Centre and Women and Health Care Reform cooperated to organize the

National Think Tank on Unpaid Caregiving, building on work of the Maritime Centre and of the Reform Group. With core funding from the Bureau, additional financial support from other government and research funding agencies helped ensure these other organizations had a stake in the proceedings while still providing an open space for discussion (see Grant et al., 2004). The unique combination of participants, made possible by networks, combined with an innovative agenda, opened the way for new strategies.

Institutional infrastructure, networking and knowledge-sharing

Committed to sharing with all communities, the Think Tank began with a public forum. With experts from the three constituencies, the panel also offered a grounding for the subsequent strategy sessions involving only invited participants. The following intense days avoided formal presentations and instead created a flexible forum for discussion and debate (Pederson and Huggan, 2001). One immediate result was the spontaneous, collective production of the *Charlottetown Declaration on the Right to Care* (Women and Health Care Reform, 2001), a document that set out the principles for an equitable approach to a national programme for home care, taking diversity as well as the rights of patients and providers into account. It reflected the range of expertise among participants and the strong feeling that we know enough now to move towards action, although we also identified issues for further research. Indeed, new research projects were made possible by the links established at the Think Tank. Available through CWHN and Centre websites, the *Declaration* was included on the websites of many community groups and was downloaded in countries around the world.

In addition, the group built on the workshop to produce what became the first in a series of plain-language documents or what we call popular pieces. *Women and Home Care* (www.womenandhealthcarereform.ca/en/work_homecare.html), like the eight others that followed, was printed on glossy paper and distributed for free in hard copy as well as online. It included cartoons and various other means to ensure the material was attractive and accessible. It worked as a format, at least if the demand on the web and for hard copies is any indication. Indeed, there have been requests from other countries not only to translate and distribute this material but also to use it as a template for their own work. The materials were in turn used by the Women and Health Care Reform Group, as well as by a wide variety of other organizations, as the basis for policy discussions on home care with governments and local communities. Here, too, the Bureau often facilitated these discussions by, for example, organizing policy forums with senior bureaucrats.

These workshops provide just one example of the varied and innovative activities in the Program and of the ways in which the Bureau provided not only financial but also other forms of support. In 2000, the Bureau identified Aboriginal women's health as a priority, creating the Women's Health Research Synthesis Group, composed of representatives from each Centre, the Canadian Women's Health Network and Health Canada's Women's Health Bureau (www.cewh-cesf. ca/en/resources/synthesis/index.html). Here, too the Bureau was taking a policy lead in supporting an area where demand was growing while allowing considerable independence for those conducting the work.

Policy interventions

The expertise in the Centres and the infrastructure provided by them established a basis for a wide range of interventions at all levels of government and policy (Majury, 1999). One significant early example of direct impact relates to the reorganization of research funding in Canada. When a set of interdisciplinary institutes for health research were proposed in the late 1990s, there was no indication that women, sex or gender would be taken into account. In response, the Executive Director of BCCEWH served as principal investigator for a research project intended as an intervention in the development of the institutes. Although the team also received funding from other granting agencies, the principal investigator thanked the Bureau 'for its support in creating the climate for input and networking addressing the issues of sex, gender and women's health research in Canada' (Greaves et al., 1999: n.p.).

The report demonstrated the need for further research on women's health, described the current capacity and concluded that 'the establishment of a Women's Health Research Institute with an enhanced gender mainstreaming capacity is the most effective operational mechanism for Canada, particularly given the then federal Health Minister's stated commitment to promoting women's health' (Greaves et al., 1999: 23). The intensive lobbying that accompanied the report built on Program networks, with somewhat limited success. The new body was an Institute of Gender and Health (IGH), rather than of women's health alone. Nevertheless, IGH was a victory, given that it

> supports research excellence regarding the influence of gender and sex on the health of women and men throughout life and the application of these research findings to identifying and addressing pressing health challenges. (www.cihr-irsc.gc.ca/e/8673.html)

In sum, by the end of the first six years significant progress had been made in developing an infrastructure to support research, networking inside and outside governments, and knowledge-sharing across communities. Program members worked with and for other forms of support, leveraging new money, and creating new research and new methods. The Bureau, largely staffed by those with strong connections to women's health issues, provided important links to governments as well as some additional financial support for new initiatives, while allowing the Centres considerable independence. The Program was not without internal tensions and external critics. But there can be no question that significant progress was made in providing a research base for policy development on women's health.

Sustaining development*

There were no guarantees that funding would be renewed after the initial mandate to the Program. Indeed, there were those who argued that the initial contribution was seed money and that the Centres should be able to survive on their own. The Centre in Quebec decided to close its doors at the end of the initial funding period, having completed its initial workplan. But the rest of the Program members began what has become a continuing struggle to maintain the infrastructure and linkage support from the Bureau.

The formal review of the Progam conducted by the Bureau in 2003 was very positive, recommending that the government establish multi-year funding agreements in order to provide a stable base for the Program. There were, of course, suggestions for improvements. Most of these suggestions, however, were challenged by the Program members on the grounds that the evaluators missed critical evidence. Nevertheless, new approaches were developed and delivered to address these recommendations.

A cross-Program Communications Committee was established, monthly meetings were held with Program members to hammer out joint projects and a special meeting organized with parliamentarians from all parties to highlight research and policy issues. Réseau québécois d'action pour la santé des femmes (RQASF), an organization in the Province of Quebec long involved in francophone women's health issues, received funding, as did a group concerned with Aboriginal women's health, the Aboriginal Women's Health and Healing Research Group (AWHHRG). But a number of factors combined to shift the focus, at least at the Bureau level, from development to survival. There was considerable and continual turnover in staff at the Bureau, with fewer of the new personnel coming out of the women's health movement or with connections to it. With less expertise in women's health, and fewer contacts inside and outside the government, the Bureau was less able to provide the kinds of links between policy-makers and Program members that it had provided in the past.

In 2005, the Bureau changed its name to Women's Health and Gender Analysis as a means of signalling a broadening of its mandate beyond women's issues to one of 'enhancing equitable outcomes for women and men, boys and girls', a more politically acceptable goal (Tudiver, 2009: 21). Although this could be interpreted as a way of moving into new areas, it could also be understood as a move away from a focus on women's health. The new emphasis on accountability in government increased the emphasis on counting and on making contributions visible. While it is relatively easy to demonstrate research outputs and successful grant applications, it is not easy to make policy impact visible and countable. As Program members (WHCP) put it in response to the 2007 evaluation, the mandate 'includes providing policy advice, but the WHCP members cannot be held accountable for matters beyond their control, i.e. whether that advice is acted upon' (WHCP Members, 2007: 5). Equally important, the election of a minority Conservative government at the federal level in 2006 shifted the terrain. Support for women's programmes was slashed. Projects had to demonstrate how their agendas fitted with government priorities. No programmes with funding could lobby, contradicting the original mandate. This new notion of accountability challenged both the independence of the Program and created a moving, as well as a not very clearly defined, target for programmes.

Members responded pragmatically, but in ways consistent with their own agendas. One example is waiting times for health services. The federal government made the reduction of waiting times in specified surgical and testing areas a priority, appointing a federal advisor on the issue. Using their contact with the policy-makers, the Women and Health Care Reform Group managed to have an appendix on gender included in the final report (Jackson et al., 2006). This in turn provided a legitimate base for the Program as a whole to develop a workshop on timely access to care designed to expand policy debate and analysis on the evolving issue of waiting times in ways that take the determinants of health and especially gender into account. Through the use of concrete examples from the entire Program,

> the workshop illustrated how consideration of the unique needs and realities of diverse groups among women and men with particular attention to marginalized groups adds value to policy, research and program development on wait times and to the broader issue of timely access to care. The workshop also demonstrated how gender based analysis can strengthen health planning and service delivery for governments at all levels to the 60 policy researchers and analysts from the federal, provincial and regional sectors who participated. (Women and Health Care Reform, 2007: 1)

It thus simultaneously addressed government priorities, conducted policy analysis, expanded beyond women to gender and pushed the agenda to include larger policy issues.

In spite of making these kinds of adjustments, the Program remained under threat. Members not only wrote long reports demonstrating their significant contributions (a matter confirmed by the external summative evaluation conducted in 2007) but also approached parliamentarians from all parties seeking support for continuation. These lobbying efforts were successful, in part because the Program had established critical networks. The fact that the minority Conservative government was under threat may also have been a factor. The funding was renewed. However, the terms changed. In the past, the Contribution Program funded Centres and Groups which had submitted workplans indicating the kinds of projects and 'deliverables' determined by the members. Now, only projects are funded, with projects individually approved by the Bureau. This means the end of overall infrastructure money, and transforms the Program members into contractors, albeit ones with considerable leeway, on the basis of projects determined by the Bureau. No projects that involved lobbying were approved, indicating the dramatic shift in decision-making and priority-setting. Meanwhile, the Bureau itself was significantly downsized and demoted.

In short, the Women's Health Contribution Program began with a commitment to provide infrastructure support for developing policy-based research focused on change, through work with governments and communities to improve women's health. When the time came to renew the Program, crucial networks as well as significant contributions helped sustain funding. But changes within and outside the Bureau made it harder to maintain independence of Program members while more time was devoted to justifying and accounting as opposed to project development. Bureau personnel changed and so did its name, both reflecting new approaches in government. There was continuing pressure to produce quantitative work, rather than the wide spectrum of methods promoted initially, and growing pressure to focus primarily on areas defined by the government.

Conclusion

Institutional supports are neither necessary nor sufficient conditions for developing and integrating gender- and diversity-sensitive organizations and practices in healthcare. However, the specific case of the Canadian Women's Health Contribution Program, and the Centres of Excellence and the working groups it funds, show how an institutional base can:

- promote sustained research and policy-directed strategies that develop significant expertise in both research and knowledge-sharing with policy and other decision-makers;
- encourage networks with community organizations as well as with government actors;
- develop capacity in conducting and applying gender-based analysis that takes other social locations into account;
- influence policy and practices in and outside the public sector; and
- establish a presence that is hard to ignore or dismiss.

But an institutional base is difficult to create and even harder to sustain over the long term, even though long-term supports can be the most effective in making significant change. In times of cutbacks, women's health research centres may be seen as easily expendable and even as a threat. New notions of accountability defined in terms of visible, countable results can also make it difficult to demonstrate contributions and create pressure to shift priorities. Equally importantly, there is always the risk that more energy will be directed at maintaining the base than at transforming care and that this base will become institutionalized in ways that undermine the goals of the women's health movement.

Summary

- The Canadian Women's Health Centres highlight the significance of institutional support in order to create spaces for women's health.
- The Women's Health Centres were able to promote sustained research and policy-directed strategies that develop significant expertise in both research and knowledge sharing with policy and other decision-makers.
- Gender-based analysis can strengthen health planning and service delivery for governments at all levels; but broadening the mandate towards gender issues may also provoke tensions with women's healthcare.
- Institutional support and financial resources have been increasingly slimmed down and new health policies emphasizing accountability in government have created further challenges for Women's Health Centres.

Key reading

Armstrong, P. and J. Deadman (eds) (2009) *Women's Health. Intersections of Policy, Research, and Practice* (Toronto: Women's Press).

Health Canada (1999) *Women's Health Strategy*, at: www.cwhn.ca/resources/cwhn/strategy.html, accessed 22 June 2009.

Johnson, J. L., L. Greaves and R. Repta (2009) 'Better Science with Sex and Gender: Facilitating the Use of a Sex and Gender-Based Analysis in Health Research', *International Journal for Equity in Health*, 8 (4), 1–38.

Women and Health Care Reform (2001) *Charlottetown Declaration on the Right to Care*, at: www.womenandhealthcarereform.ca/publications/charlottetownen.pdf, accessed 20 June 2009.

Note

* This section is based on materials I received as Chair of Women and Health Care Reform. They are internal – but not confidential – documents not available on any website.

References

Armstrong, P. and H. Armstrong (2003) *Wasting Away: The Undermining of Canadian Health Care* (Toronto: Oxford University Press).

Armstrong, P., C. Amaratunga, J. Bernier, K. Grant, A. Pederson and K. Willson (eds) (2002) *Exposing Privatization: Women and Health Care Reform in Canada* (Aurora: Garamond Press).

Armstrong, P. and J. Deadman (eds) (2009) *Women's Health. Intersections of Policy, Research, and Practice* (Toronto: Women's Press).

Backhouse, C. and D. K. Flaherty (eds) (1992) *Challenging Times: The Women's Movement in Canada and the United States* (Montreal: McGill University Press).

Black, N (1992) 'Ripples in the Second Wave: Comparing the Contemporary Women's Movement in Canada and the United States', in C. Backhouse and D. K. Flaherty (eds), *Challenging Times: The Women's Movement in Canada and the United States* (Montreal: McGill University Press), 94–109.

Boscoe, M., G. Basen, G. Alleyne, B. Bourrier-Lacroix and C. White of the Canadian Women's Health Network (2006) 'The Women's Health Movement in Canada', *Canadian Woman's Studies*, 24 (1), 7–13.

BWHBC – The Boston Women's Health Book Collective (1973) *Our Bodies, Ourselves* (New York: Simon and Schuster).

Centres of Excellence for Women's Health (1997) *Update Summer* (Winnipeg: Canadian Women's Health Network).

Clarke, A. E. and V. L. Olesen (eds) (1999) *Revisioning Women, Health, and Healing* (New York: Routledge).

CWHN – Canadian Women's Health Network (n.d.) 'An Interview with Abby Hoffman. Director General, Women's Health Bureau', at: www.rcsf.ca/network-reseau/network/network_sept96/intrview.html, accessed 21 June 2009.

Doyal, L. (1994) 'Women, Health, and the Sexual Division of Labour: A Case Study of the Women's Health Movement in Britain', in F. Fee and N. Krieger (eds), *Women's Health, Politics, and Power* (New York: Baywood), 931–9.

Feldberg, G., M. L. Taylor, K. McPherson and A. Li (eds) (2003) *Health and Nation: American and Canadian Perspectives* (Montreal: McGill-Queen's University Press).

Grant, K., C. Amaratunga, P. Armstrong, M. Boscoe, A. Pederson and K. Willson (2004) *Caring for/Caring About. Women, Home Care and Unpaid Caregiving* (Aurora: Garamond Press).

Greaves, L. (2009) 'Women, Gender and Health Research', in P. Armstrong and J. Deadman (eds), *Women's Health Intersections of Policy, Research, and Practice* (Toronto: Women's Press), 3-20.

Greaves, L., O. Hankivsky, C. Aramatunga, P. Ballem, D. Chow, M. De Koninck, K. Grant, A. Lippman et al. (1999) *CIHR 2000: Sex, Gender and Women's Health* (Vancouver: BCCEWH).

Health Canada (1999) *Women's Health Strategy*, at: www.cwhn.ca/resources/cwhn/strategy.html, accessed 22 June 2009.

Jackson, B., A. Pederson and M. Boscoe (2006) 'Gender-based Analysis and Wait Times. New Questions, New Knowledge', Discussion Paper produced for, and published in, *The Final Report of the Federal Advisor on Wait Times*, Brian Postl, at: www.womenandhealthcarereform.ca/publications/genderwaittimesen.pdf, accessed 20 June 2009.

Johnson, J. L., L. Greaves and R. Repta (2009) 'Better Science with Sex and Gender: Facilitating the Use of a Sex and Gender-based Analysis in Health Research', *International Journal for Equity in Health*, 8 (4), 1–38.

Kuhlmann, E. (2009) 'From Women's Health to Gender Mainstreaming and Back Again: Linking Feminist Agendas and New Governance in Healthcare', *Current Sociology*, 57 (2), 135–54.

Majury, D. (1999) *Promoting Women's Health: Making Inroads into Canadian Health Policy* (Ottawa: Women's Health Bureau, Health Canada).

Morgen, S. (2002) *Into our Own Hands. The Women's Health Movement in the United States, 1969–1999* (New Brunswick: Rutgers University Press).

Morrow, M. (2007) 'Our Bodies, Ourselves. Reflections on the Women's Movement in Canada', in M. Morrow, O. Hankivsky and C. Varcoe (eds), *Women's Health in Canada. Critical Perspectives on Theory and Policy* (Toronto: University of Toronto Press), 33–63.

Pederson, A. and B. P. Huggan (2001) *The Objective Is Care: Proceedings of the National Think Tank on Gender and Unpaid Caregiving*, Charlottetown, Prince Edward Island, at: www.womenandhealthcarereform.ca/publications/guc-think-tanken.pdf, accessed 24 February 2010.

Sethna, C. (2006) 'The Evolution of the *Birth Control Handbook*: From Student Peer-education Manual to Feminist Self-empowerment Text, 1968–1975', *Canadian Bulletin of Medical History*, 23 (1), 89–118.

Sherwin, S. (1992) *No Longer Patient. Feminist Ethics and Health Care* (Philadelphia: Temple University Press).

Sherwin, S. (1998) *The Politics of Women's Health: Exploring Agency and Autonomy* (Philadelphia: Temple University Press).

Smith, D. E. and S. David (eds) (1975) *Women Look at Psychiatry* (Vancouver: Press Gang).

Status of Women (1970) *Royal Commission on the Status of Women. Report* (Ottawa: Information Canada).

Tudiver, S. (2009) 'Integrating Women's Health and Gender Analysis in a Government Context: Reflections on a Work in Progress', in P. Armstrong and J. Deadman (eds), *Women's Health Intersections of Policy, Research, and Practice* (Toronto: Women's Press), 21–34.

Vickers, J. (1992) 'The Intellectual Origins of the Women's Movement in Canada', in C. Backhouse and D. K. Flaherty (eds), *Challenging Times. The Women's Movement in Canada and the United States* (Montreal: McGill-Queen's University Press), 39–60.

WHCP – Women's Health Contribution Plan Members (2007) 'Comments on the Draft Evaluation of the Women's Health Contribution Program Summary Report', internal document.

Women and Health Care Reform (2001) *Charlottetown Declaration on the Right to Care*, at: www.womenandhealthcarereform.ca/publications/charlottetownen.pdf, accessed 2 June 2009.

Women and Health Care Reform (2007) 'Workshop on Women and Timely Access to Care', Ottawa, 2007, at: www.womenandhealthcarereform.ca, accessed 2 June 2009.

Part V
The Professions as Catalyst of Gender-sensitive Healthcare

25

Women in the Medical Profession: International Trends

Elianne Riska

Introduction

The position of women doctors has continued to draw the attention of feminists, women's health advocates and policy-makers as the number of women doctors has increased markedly since the 1970s in most western societies. Despite the remarkable inroads made by women doctors the persistence of gender segregation in the practice of medicine and the existence of a glass ceiling in the careers of women doctors have become signs of the persistence of gender inequality in healthcare and of barriers to the advance of women's health.

Women's position in the medical profession is currently debated and examined in both the sociology of professions and research on medical education. This chapter will draw on research in these two areas and examine two issues. First, the purpose is to explore the international trends in women's position in the medical profession and women's representation in various medical specialties. Second, the changes in the gender composition of medicine have resulted in the question: Are women practising medicine differently from men? A number of recent meta-analyses of studies on this topic will be reviewed. The argument of this chapter is that the changing position of women doctors has provided a context for identifying and interpreting the structural and cultural changes taking place in medicine, although some of those changes are not necessarily related to women at all.

This chapter is divided into four parts. The first part reviews the debate about the importance of promoting women's health and women doctors' role in achieving gender equality in health. The second part looks at the representation of women doctors in the medical profession in OECD countries. The third part examines the distribution of women doctors in various specialties in five societies – Finland, Sweden, Lithuania, the United Kingdom and the United States – and the character of horizontal and vertical gender segregation of medical practice that has evolved. The fourth part addresses the question whether it makes any difference if the doctor is a man or a woman for the promotion of quality of care and women's health issues.

Women doctors and women's health

The women's health movement in the 1970s was an outgrowth of second-wave feminism in the USA and in Europe. It addressed the issues of gender equality in healthcare and brought up concern over access and quality of healthcare for women. Feminists asked a number of new questions: Why were women so sparsely represented among doctors?; How could women's health concerns be promoted?; and Could women receive proper care if the knowledge of their bodies was based on knowledge of men's bodies? (Boston Women's Health Collective, 1973; Oakley, 1984). For radical feminists, the answer was readily at hand: medicine was a patriarchal enterprise headed by men to maintain women in a subordinate position both as patients and as a group in the gender order. Furthermore, they argued that medical knowledge was gender-biased and women's own experiences should guide the search for a new kind of knowledge about women's health (Ehrenreich and English, 1978).

But there was another branch of feminism that followed a more reformist agenda. This was a voice stemming from the first wave of feminism in the mid-to-late 19th century that had demanded women's right to enter medical schools and to practise medicine. More than a hundred years later, the quest is still for gender equality but with the added demand for an increase of women doctors in all fields and at all levels of medicine, for example, in surgery and academic medicine, two heavily male-dominated areas, both in numbers and values (for example, see More, 1999; RCP, 2009). The existence of horizontal and vertical gender segregation in the practice of medicine has been a reminder of the deficient integration of women doctors in the medical profession.

But the story about women doctors is not merely about the history of feminism, women's rights and women's health. It is also about a gender aspect of health and healthcare that medical sociologists neglected for a long time, despite the feminist health advocacy occurring in society. Recent reminiscences of medical sociologists, who tell the story about the early years of medical sociology, tend to be free of any acknowledgements of the on-going vibrant feminist discussions and academic writings about women's health and critiques of the male-dominated medical profession that went on in the discipline from 1970 onwards (for example, Bloom, 2002; Elling, 2007).

In the early writings in medical sociology the character of the medical profession and its tasks were analysed by means of the theoretical framework set forth by the American sociologist Talcott Parsons (1951) in the early 1950s. This theoretical model on the values guiding the behaviour of doctors presents the medical professions in gender-neutral terms. This view derives from the functionalist perspective on professions that delegated the notion of gender to the particularistic character of the family and considered the world of professional work to be guided by other (gender-neutral) norms. Two classics on professional socialization conducted in the late 1950s in the USA – *The Student-Physician* and *Boys in White* – solidified this tradition by depicting the process of medical education of doctors as mainly an enterprise of training (white) male students and thereby made gender, race and ethnicity invisible. For example, *The Student-Physician* (Merton et al., 1957) presented medical students in gender-neutral or in masculine terms and did not mention women as medical students, nor even whether they were included in the study. The authors of *Boys in White* (Becker et al., 1961) confessed that women were not included in that study because of the overwhelmingly male composition of the medical profession. The authors concluded, therefore, that 'we shall talk mainly of boys becoming medical men' (Becker et al., 1961: 3).

The feminist perspective on health professions has therefore pointed out that the major theoretical perspectives on professions have since their inception been unmarked by gender, although the very behaviour depicted as professional is not gender-neutral but male-gendered (Beagan, 2000; Davies, 1996). The early feminist writings on the medical profession pointed to the gendered character of the attitudes and behaviour of doctors (Ehrenreich and English, 1978) and challenged the existing medical knowledge about women's health (Boston Women's Health Collective, 1973). The first sociological analyses of women's position in the medical profession were represented in the USA by Judith Lorber's (1984) pioneering study *Women Physicians* and in the UK by Anne Witz's (1992) *Professions and Patriarchy*, which also included an analysis of other healthcare professions, such as midwifery. These works documented and theorized how different structural mechanisms (Lorber, 1984) and discursive strategies and social closures (Witz, 1992) had prevented women from entering into and advancing in the medical profession on equal terms with men and how other subordinate health professions – nursing, midwifery – had become women's work (see Chapter 28 by Wrede).

Women in the medical profession: international trends

During the past decade research on women's position in the medical profession has been conducted in various countries (for example, Boulis and Jacobs, 2008; Elston 2009; More, 1999; Riska, 2001a). In some countries women constitute almost half or even a majority of doctors; in others a third. In most western countries the major numerical increase happened after 1970. The variations in the proportion of women among doctors and their status before this date are related to the history of women in the higher educational system and in the labour force in general. The organizing principles of the healthcare system and the expansion of the healthcare sector after the Second World War have also influenced the proportion and status of women doctors.

Some regional characteristics seem to suggest common historical and cultural features that have influenced women's entry and later opportunities in the medical profession. The OECD countries can in this respect be divided into four areas: Post-Soviet societies, Scandinavia, Central Europe and non-European countries. As Table 25.1 illustrates, women constitute a majority of the practising doctors in post-Soviet countries. In the Baltic region, the rate was as high as 77 per cent in Estonia in 1991 (Barr, 1995) and was still 70 per cent in 2009 (EMA, 2009). In another post-Soviet Baltic country, Lithuania, women made up 71 per cent of licensed medical doctors in 2007 to 2008 (see Table 25.1).

The Scandinavian societies also have a high proportion of women physicians, around 40 per cent, but in the case of Finland over 50 per cent. Central Europe is a third region that has about 35 to 40 per cent women among practising

Table 25.1   Women in the medical profession in selected OECD countries in 2006

Region	Female doctors (as %) of practising doctors
Post-Soviet countries	
Czech Republic	52
Hungary	52
Poland	55
Scandinavia	
Denmark	43
Finland	54
Norway	38
Sweden	44
Central Europe	
Austria	38
Belgium	36
France	38
Germany	39
Ireland	38
Italy	35
Netherlands	39
Spain	43
Switzerland	34
United Kingdom	39
Non-European countries	
Canada	36
Japan	17
New Zealand	37
United States	29

Sources: OECD Health Data (2009); Nordic Medical Associations (2006).

physicians. A separate and quite diverse region is composed of non-European OECD countries, where one finds a range from a very low proportion, as in Japan (17 per cent), to something more like the Central European pattern, as in Canada and New Zealand. The United States seems to differ from most of the listed regions because of its low proportion, although the increase in women's proportion has been rapid, from a low base. For example, women constituted a mere eight per cent of physicians in the USA in 1970 but the rate increased to 12 per cent in 1980 and to 24 per cent by 2000 (AMA, 2009; Boulis and Jacobs, 2008). In 2005, 49 per cent of medical students and 42 per cent of the residents in the USA were women and the medical profession is expected to be gender-balanced within a decade or two (Carnes et al., 2008).

In their analysis of the increase of women physicians in the USA, Boulis and Jacobs (2008) examine why and how women's representation in American medicine has grown so rapidly since 1970. They test the so-called the 'male-flight' hypothesis: Has women's entry into medicine implied a declining status of American medicine, with the result that men are leaving the profession and women are taking over? Boulis and Jacobs (2008) show convincingly that women's entry into American medicine is not related to any loss of its status. Instead, broader changes in women's position in society and increased opportunities in medicine explain the inroads of women. Yet, each decade has had its own dynamics: the 1970s was influenced by affirmative action legislation and the growth of US medical schools. The 1980s is the only decade that could in any way be characterized by male flight: the number of male applicants to US medical schools fell, and more lucrative fields, such as business and finance, lured male students. The 1990s witnessed an increase in the entry both of women and men because both were interested in medicine as a high-income career.

The Scandinavian and the Soviet/post-Soviet countries have had a relatively high proportion of women doctors over the past 50 years, but for different reasons. The current high proportion of women doctors in post-Soviet societies, such as the Czech Republic, Hungary, Poland, Estonia and Lithuania, is related to the status of doctors during the Soviet period. In Soviet society the character of the medical profession changed in two respects. First, the medical profession lost its traditional professional status because medicine was no longer a prestigious occupation in a state economy that gave priority to the industrial sector and its occupations. Second, doctors became just one group of state employees among others in the state economy of the Soviet Union. These two conditions resulted not only in the loss of the academic status and professional autonomy of doctors but also in doctors having a lower salary level than industrial workers. It has been noted that medicine became one of the few professional jobs available to women as they encountered restricted choices in the labour market, because jobs in the industrial sector were high-status and highly paid and became a male-dominated sector of the economy (Harden, 2001). Under these economic and political conditions, medical work became a female occupation. Hence, in 1950, 77 per cent of medical doctors in the Soviet Union were women (Riska, 2001a).

The fall of the Soviet Union resulted in a gradual inclusion of social insurance mechanisms and opportunities for private practice in healthcare, but also in efforts to re-establish the academic and professional status of the medical profession. The medical profession has strived to regain its professional autonomy but it is still part of the hierarchical structure of the state in most of post-Soviet societies (Field, 1991; Rivkin-Fish, 2005). Furthermore, the medical profession has remained female-dominated in Russia and in other post-Soviet societies.

In Scandinavia healthcare sector growth became part of the construction of the modern Scandinavian welfare state. The expansion of the public sector created a female-dominated labour market, especially in healthcare. The expansion of medical schools was initiated to provide doctors with improved access to the public primary care system and women became an increasing part of the new entrants. Furthermore, in Scandinavia, official gender equality policy, especially family and labour market legislation, has supported women's capacity to balance the demands set by work and family (Mayer and Tikka, 2008). Women's high proportion among doctors is therefore not an isolated phenomenon, but rather a reflection of women's participation in working life in general and their majority among enrolled and graduated university students in particular (Riska, 2001a).

In the early literature on the sudden increase of women doctors in the 1970s and onwards, the term 'feminization' was often used to allude to the loss of power that a medical profession will experience when its composition becomes increasingly female. As 'evidence' of the inevitability of professional decline with the increase of women in a previously high-status profession, the case of Soviet Union was often used. Even today some medical journals tend to use the term in this way (Riska, 2008). This kind of discourse on feminization reproduces notions of the organization of healthcare, medical knowledge and medical practice as being gender-neutral in the past and that it is currently women doctors as a category that have brought gender into the previously neutral character of medicine. But the term feminization has also been given a mainly numerical meaning and is used to describe the global trend in the growing proportion of women in the medical profession. Used in this way, the term feminization portrays the medical profession as a homogeneous and united body and it is assumed that any changes will affect its members equally. Nevertheless, the gender-segregated character of medical work implies that the changes will have a different impact on female and male doctors (Riska, 2001b). The ambiguous and multiple meanings of the term feminization is a reason why it should be avoided when describing the process and effects of the increased proportion of women in the medical profession.

Gender segregation of medical specialties

Most studies on women doctors have found that women's status in the medical profession is still not equivalent to men's status. Some have suggested that the fact that female physicians now tend to occupy lower positions in medical work is merely a lag phenomenon, because when the current cohort of women advance in their career, the figures will be self-corrective and result in a gender-balanced structure. It is assumed that the current pattern of horizontal and vertical gender segregation will wither away as the number of women increases. The female majority of first-year medical students is often used as an indicator of the future majority of women at all levels in the profession (Riska, 2008).

The pessimists suggest that women will be channelled to work in highly segregated niches within the profession that are characterized by lower status and pay, while the high-status specialties and the organizational leadership of the profession will remain in the hands of male doctors (Lorber, 1984). This interpretation has been further developed by feminist scholars, who have argued that organizations (Acker, 2006; Britton, 2000) and professions (Witz, 1992; Davies, 1996) are male-gendered: the workings of these institutions valorize masculine values, such as, for instance, efficiency, professional authority and autonomy. More recently the term inequality regimes (Acker, 2006) has been introduced as a way of understanding the reproduction of gender, race and class in organizations and of shedding light on why efforts to change organizations have failed or have had a minor impact.

Current statistics on the distribution of women doctors among and within various specialties show a remarkably similar pattern among the medical professions in the five countries examined here (Table 25.2). The countries represent different organizing principles of providing healthcare: a market-driven system like that of the USA; a welfare state provision of health and social services like Sweden and Finland; a neoliberal system of public and private healthcare like the UK; and post-Soviet, transitional healthcare systems like Lithuania.

Although women have a high presence in the medical profession in Scandinavia and post-Soviet societies, they are not evenly distributed in the existing medical specialties. In all the countries examined here, women doctors are relatively well represented in specialties that confirm gender-essentialist notions of women's task, such as child and adolescent psychiatry, geriatrics and paediatrics. For example, women constitute 88 per cent of the practitioners in child and adolescent psychiatry in Finland; they are relatively well represented in this specialty also in Sweden (66 per cent) and the USA (46 per cent) compared to their representation in the profession (Table 25.2). Furthermore,

Table 25.2   Proportion (%) of women doctors in selected medical specialties in Finland, Sweden, Lithuania, the United States, and the United Kingdom

Specialty	Finland 2009	Sweden 2009	Lithuania* 2008	USA 2007	UK 2007
Anaesthesiology	45	32	48	23	29
Child/adolescent psychiatry	88	67	–	46	–
General medicine	57	44	85	35	25
Geriatrics	69	63	50	–	26
Internal medicine	43	34	84	32	19
Pathology	40	40	75	35	39
Paediatrics	64	49	91	55	44
Psychiatry	61	52	72	34	38
Obstetrics/Gynaecology	72	63	84	45	33
General surgery	21	19	22	16	8
% women of all doctors	52	46	71	28	40

* The figures in Lithuania represent those who were licensed in 2007–8.
Sources: FMA (2009); SMA (2009); MHRL (2008); AMA (2009); RCP (2009).

women are the majority of the practitioners in geriatrics in Finland, Sweden and Lithuania. Similarly, women are markedly overrepresented in paediatrics in Lithuania (91 per cent), Finland (64 per cent) and the USA (55 per cent) (Table 25.2). US figures show that women are highly underrepresented in 10 of the existing 37 specialties, and overrepresented only in child psychiatry, obstetrics/gynaecology and paediatrics. For example, 26 per cent of all women doctors in the USA practise mainly in two specialties: paediatrics and family medicine (AMA, 2009: 416).

Obstetrics and gynaecology is a specialty that has previously been male-dominated and it was therefore the primary target of feminist criticism of medicine in the 1970s and 1980s (Boston Women's Health Collective, 1973; Ehrenreich and English, 1978; Oakley, 1984). Today this specialty has a high proportion of women practitioners (Table 25.2): 72 per cent in Finland, 84 per cent in Lithuania, 63 per cent in Sweden, 45 per cent in the USA. The US figure is expected to rise significantly over the next decade. For example, women constituted 15 per cent of the residents in obstetrics and gynaecology in US medical schools in 1975, but they made up 70 per cent of the residents in this specialty in 2000. Hence, women are expected to make up 60 per cent of the obstetrics and gynaecology practitioners in the USA in 2020 (Emmons et al., 2004: 331).

This trend is further explained by a recent study of the development of obstetrics/gynaecology as a specialty in the USA (Zetka 2008a; 2008b). The study points to the integration of new knowledge – psychopathology – in the 1960s and 1970s into the core knowledge of the specialty. During these decades the mastery of psychopathology as a skill required of practitioners of obstetrics and gynaecology was seen as important in order to understand the assumed high prevalence of psychosomatic symptoms among women. The annexation of this approach was one way in which obstetricians and gynaecologists could claim that they possessed a special kind of knowledge of women's health *vis-à-vis* their main rivals, surgeons, who were criticized for failing success rates in their surgical interventions (Zetka, 2008a). During the past two decades, claiming a special knowledge of women's health and acting as managers of those concerns have paved the way for an increase of female practitioners in obstetrics and gynaecology in the USA (Zetka, 2008b).

Surgery continues to be a markedly male-dominated area in the five countries examined. The lowest proportion is found in the UK, where women comprise only eight per cent of surgeons, while women surgeons constitute between 16 and 22 per cent in the other countries (Table 25.2). The change has been slow in all the countries. For example, in 1999 there were only 21 per cent women in surgery residencies in the USA, while the proportion of female residents was already 47 per cent in family practice, 65 per cent in paediatrics and 67 per cent in obstetrics and gynaecology (Bickel, 2001: 264).

A post-Soviet society, Lithuania, confirms the anomaly of surgery: while women constituted 71 per cent of doctors who were licensed in Lithuania in 2007 to 2008, only 22 per cent of the licensed surgeons were women. A recent study of male and female surgeons and paediatricians in Lithuania showed that practice in these specialties was influenced by gender discourses on women's nature and tasks in reproduction. Women were perceived both by themselves and by their male colleagues as particularly fit for the caring and nurturing tasks in medicine, like paediatrics, but not very good at what was described as the physically and mentally taxing tasks of surgery (Riska and Novelskaite, 2008). Hence, as several studies of post-Soviet medicine have shown, the culture of medicine has remained male-dominated although women have constituted the majority of doctors during the past 50 years. Although the financing and organization of healthcare in these societies are in transition, the gendered values and gendered structures of medicine seem to persist (Harden, 2001; Riska and Novelskaite, 2008; Rivkin-Fish, 2005).

How has this almost universal pattern of gender segregation of medicine emerged? Boulis and Jacobs (2008) offer three interpretative frameworks: the personal choice/different voice perspective; the institutional discrimination thesis; and the social change perspective. In their analysis of women doctors in the USA the second and especially the third explanation found empirical support. For example, they show that differences in work schedules across specialties have been quite modest and career decisions would seem therefore not to be based on women choosing to keep their work-week hours low. By contrast, preferences for part-time work and regular working hours have been shown to be the two major factors affecting the selection of specialty and work-setting for British women doctors (RCP, 2009: 9). For example, 49 per cent of women GPs worked part-time compared to 12 per cent of male GPs in 2007. Furthermore, 30 per cent of the female doctors in paediatrics worked part-time compared to 16 per cent of the female surgeons. Instead of individual preferences and choices as the explanation for women's career patterns in medicine, Boulis and Jacobs (2008) suggest that experiences of gender stereotyping and discrimination in medical school and the expansion of some specialty fields have been the most important factors in influencing women doctors' career patterns in the USA.

Will women doctors change medicine?

The ongoing changes in the gender composition of the medical profession have resulted in new questions: Does it make any difference whether there are more women doctors today? Is medicine practised differently if the doctor is a woman and not a man? To what extent do women physicians represent a vanguard within the profession, which will head the rest of the profession towards a substantial change in the way medicine is practised? Feminists have also asked: What kind of impact will the increased proportion of women doctors have on women's health issues (for example, Boulis and Jacobs, 2008; More, 1999; Riska, 2001a)?

The first question about whether female and male physicians relate to patients in different ways has been addressed in several recent reviews that have compiled meta-analyses of the results of studies. These reviews have not been able to come up with clear-cut answers. Although studies tend to confirm that women doctors have a more patient-centred and empathetic style of communicating with patients than their male colleagues, there is conflicting or no evidence that women would otherwise practice medicine differently (Bertakis and Azari, 2007; Heru, 2005; Kilminster et al., 2007; Roter and Hall, 2004).

The second issue that has been researched is what impact women doctors will have on medical practice. There is more optimism in countries where women doctors have recently increased in numbers than in countries with a long tradition of women in the profession. For example, women doctors in post-Soviet societies do not provide any specific practice patterns or practice styles to be emulated in other healthcare systems. Women doctors' work is based on a gender-essentialist and maternalist discourse that legitimates not only the gender segregation of medical work but also women's subordinated position at work and in the family (Harden, 2001; Rivkin-Fish, 2005). Furthermore, analysing the question in the US context, Boulis and Jacobs (2008) remain sceptical that women doctors would have any special impact. They point to the increasing specialization of physicians and the decline of primary care in American medicine, a trend which will give remaining primary care practitioners little time and occupational space for humanizing patient care, regardless of their gender.

Boulis and Jacobs also point to the current economic and structural constraints in the organization of healthcare which hamper any specific impact of uniquely female leadership styles (see also Chapter 20 by Barry et al.). Instead of women doctors being the saviours of the spirit of primary care, neoliberal healthcare policies and broader structural and technological changes in healthcare have created constraints for a return of the 'old time' family doctor system (McKinlay and Marceau, 2008). In Canada and Europe, the doctor-focused provision of healthcare delivery has been changed to a coalition of other healthcare professionals who provide primary care. These changes have been initiated by political leaders who are concerned about health costs, and by organized health professions. Political leaders have had cost efficiency in mind, while the new health professions have used the new health policy as a way to promote their own professional projects (Bourgeault, 2005; Wrede, 2008; see also Chapter 28 by Wrede).

More recently the term 'glass ceiling' has been used to refer to the interconnection between the lack of advancement of female doctors into leadership positions in academic medicine and of the advancement of women's health (Carnes et al., 2008). The importance of promoting women's health in the medical curriculum and in health policy has in particular been raised in the Netherlands, Sweden and the USA. For example, in Sweden and the Netherlands medical schools have taken initiatives to include gender-related medical knowledge in the medical curriculum (Hammarström, 2003; Verdonk et al., 2006; 2008). The Dutch approach has been to introduce gender-specific topics to the curriculum. This approach is defined as bringing into medical education the knowledge of the meaning of sex and gender for health and illness and its application to practice (Verdonk et al., 2006; see also Chapter 26 by Lagro-Janssen). These gender-specific topics include gender differences in symptoms and morbidity of coronary heart disease, sexual violence, falling accidents in elderly female patients, and men's lifestyle-related health risks.

A survey of all US medical schools in 2004 found that courses or topics related to gender differences in health and illness and women's health issues were sparsely represented in the curriculum (Henrich and Viscoli, 2006). For example, only nine schools of a total of 126 offered a women's health course. In general there was little gender-specific information in the curriculum about many conditions that cause the greatest morbidity and mortality in women (Henrich and Viscoli, 2006). A noteworthy finding was that the presence of a female medical school dean was positively associated with the range of topics taught on gender. This confirms the importance of having women in top positions in academic medicine if the culture and attitudes to gender in medical education are to change.

Conclusion

Women's marked increase among doctors is a worldwide trend and signals two global changes. One change is the high proportion of women in university-level education to the point that women have become a majority of university graduates in many western countries. Another change is the expansion of the healthcare system in most western societies, a change that has resulted in a growth of medical schools to meet the need for more healthcare professionals. This development has increased the number of entrants to medical schools and women have become an increasing part of the students accepted to medical school. Hence, rather than a flight away of men from medicine as an explanation for women's increase in medicine, the expansion of the healthcare sector has offered women new professional careers as doctors (Boulis and Jacobs, 2008; Riska, 2008).

Women's increasing proportion among doctors has resulted in optimism about the impact that women will have in changing the values and practice of medicine. This point of view has arisen in the public and research discourse during the past two decades and it still seems to attract optimistic followers. The topic addresses an important issue – how to change medicine to a more patient-centred and humanistic enterprise. Some give women doctors a special mission to change medicine and expect this to automatically take place when women's numbers increase in medicine. This sociology-of-numbers reasoning, which derives from Kanter's (1977) optimistic thesis about the impact of the proportion of women in corporations, has been challenged. The pessimists have pointed to the persistence of certain universal features in organizations generally, because of embedded gendered values and gendered structures (Acker, 2006; Britton, 2000).

Furthermore, the character of the professional socialization of doctors seems to change slowly. First, the current criteria for admitting students to medical school result in both a self-selection and formal selection of certain types of students, regardless of gender. The current admissions criteria reproduce a certain profile of students who are admitted to medical schools based on their proficiencies in natural sciences rather than in emotional skills or caring. The specific character of education in biomedicine and the self-selection of students to medicine have resulted in doctors not being particularly empathetic. Instead, emotional and caring work has been delegated to be the expected tasks of nurses and other healthcare professionals. Second, as studies have shown, current training in medicine and medical knowledge are far from gender-neutral; current medical curricula inculcate gendered medical knowledge and reproduce gendered career paths for both male and female students and residents (Beagan, 2000).

Women doctors have in media and public discourse often been singled out as the primary reason for some major changes occurring in medicine and healthcare. Meanwhile the assumption seems to be that male doctors have remained unchanged and they have nothing to do with the current changes in medicine. The continuing interests in female-specific practice styles points, however, to the existence and importance of different styles of doctoring. The quest for improvements in the doctor–patient relationship should, however, be addressed in the education of doctors rather than being derived from notions of gender-essentialist competence in this area of women, who have so far been located in subordinate tasks in the medical division of labour – be it as doctors or nurses. Furthermore, if improvements in social equity in access to healthcare and gender equality in health are the primary goals, then such issues are in most countries less related to the number of women doctors than to improvements in the financing and organization of healthcare in general.

Summary

- Women constitute from a third to a majority of practising doctors in most western societies.
- Gender segregation of specialties is a universal pattern in healthcare and this pattern refutes the homogenization argument of the 'feminization of medicine' view.
- Women doctors have a more empathetic practising style than their male colleagues but no or only minor gender differences have been found in clinical decision-making.
- The presence of more women doctors has revitalized concerns for women's health.

Key reading

Boulis, A. K. and J. A. Jacobs (2008) *The Changing Face of Medicine: Women Doctors and the Evolution of Health Care in America* (Ithaca: Cornell University Press).

Kilminster S., J. Downes, B. Gough, D. Murdoch-Eaton and T. Roberts (2007) 'Women in Medicine – Is there a Problem? A Literature Review of the Changing Gender Composition, Structures and Occupational Cultures in Medicine', *Medical Education*, 41 (1), 39–49.

Riska, E. (2001) *Medical Careers and Feminist Agendas: American, Scandinavian and Russian Women Physicians* (New York: Aldine de Gruyter).

References

Acker, J. (2006) 'Inequality Regimes: Gender, Class, and Race in Organizations,' *Gender and Society*, 20 (4), 441–64.

AMA – American Medical Association (2009) *Physician Characteristics in the US, 2009 edition* (Chicago: AMA).

Barr, D. A. (1995) 'The Professional Structure of Soviet Medical Care: The Relationship between Personal Characteristics, Medical Education and Occupational Setting for Estonian Physicians,' *American Journal of Public Health,* 85 (3), 373–8.

Beagan, B.L. (2000) 'Neutralizing Differences: Producing Neutral Doctors for (Almost) Neutral Patients', *Social Science & Medicine,* 51 (8), 1253–65.

Becker, H. S., B. Geer, E. C. Hughes and A. L. Strauss (1961) *Boys in White: Student Culture in Medical School* (Chicago: University of Chicago Press).

Bickel, J. (2001) 'Gender Equity in Undergraduate Medical Education: A Status Report', *Journal of Women's Health and Gender-Based Medicine,* 10 (3), 261–70.

Bertakis, K. D. and R. Azari (2007) 'Patient Gender and Physician Practice Style', *Journal of Women's Health,* 16 (6), 859–68.

Bloom, S. W. (2002) *The Word as Scalpel: A History of Medical Sociology* (New York: Oxford University Press).

Boston Women's Health Collective (1973) *Our Bodies, Ourselves: A Book by and for Women* (New York: Simon and Schuster).

Boulis, A. K. and J. A. Jacobs (2008) *The Changing Face of Medicine: Women Doctors and the Evolution of Health Care in America* (Ithaca: Cornell University Press).

Bourgeault, I. L. (2005) 'Rationalization of Health Care and Female Professional Projects: Reconceptualizing the Role of Medicine, the State and Health Care Institutions from a Gendered Perspective', *Knowledge, Work and Society,* 3 (1), 25–52.

Britton, D. M. (2000) 'The Epistemology of the Gendered Organization', *Gender and Society,* 14 (3), 418–34.

Carnes, M., C. Morrissey and S. E. Geller (2008) 'Women's Health and Women's Leadership in Academic Medicine: Hitting the Same Glass Ceiling', *Journal of Women's Health,* 17 (9), 1453–62.

Davies, C. (1996) 'The Sociology of Professions and the Profession of Gender', *Sociology,* 30 (4), 661–78.

Ehrenreich, B. and D. English (1978) *For Her Own Good: 150 Years of Experts' Advice to Women* (New York: Anchor Press).

Elling, R. (2007) 'Reflections on the Health Social Sciences – Then and Now', *International Journal of Health Services,* 37 (4), 601–17.

Elston, M. A. (2009) *Women and Medicine: The Future* (London: Royal College of Physicians).

Emmons, S. L., K. E. Adams, M. Nichols and J. Cain (2004) 'The Impact of Perceived Gender Bias on Obstetrics and Gynecology Skills Acquisition by Third-Year Medical Students', *Academic Medicine,* 79 (4), 326–32.

EMA – Estonian Medical Association (2009) Unpublished data, information provided by Katrin Rehemaa via e-mail on 9 January 2009.

Field, M. (1991) 'The Hybrid Profession: Soviet Medicine', in A. Jones (ed.), *Professions and the State: Expertise and Autonomy in the Soviet Union and Eastern Europe* (Philadelphia: Temple University Press), 43–62.

FMA – Finnish Medical Association (FMA) (2009) *Statistics on Physicians 2009,* at: www.laakariliitto.fi/tilastot/laakaritilastot/erikoislaakarit.html, accessed 30 June 2009.

Harden, J. (2001) '"Mother Russia" at Work: Gender Divisions in the Medical Profession', *The European Journal of Women's Studies,* 8 (2), 181–99.

Hammarström, A. (2003) 'The Integration of Gender in Medical Research and Education: Obstacles and Possibilities from a Nordic Perspective', *Women and Health,* 37 (4), 121–33.

Heru, A. M. (2005) 'Pink-collar Medicine: Women and the Future of Medicine', *Gender Issues,* 22 (1), 20–34.

Henrich, J. B. and C. M. Viscoli (2006) 'What Do Medical Schools Teach about Women's Health and Gender Differences?', *Academic Medicine*, 81 (5), 476–82.

Kanter, R. M. (1977) *Men and Women of the Corporation* (New York: Basic Books).

Kilminster S., J. Downes, B. Gough, D. Murdoch-Eaton and T. Roberts (2007) 'Women in Medicine – Is There a Problem? A Literature Review of the Changing Gender Composition, Structures and Occupational Cultures in Medicine', *Medical Education*, 41 (1), 39–49.

Lorber, J. (1984) *Women Physicians* (London: Tavistock).

Mayer, A. L. and P. M. Tikka (2008) 'Family-friendly Policies and Gender Bias in Academia', *Journal of Higher Education Policy and Management*, 30 (4), 363–74.

Merton, R. K., G. G. Reader and P. L. Kendall (eds) (1957) *The Student-Physician: Introductory Studies in the Sociology of Medical Education* (Cambridge, MA: Harvard University Press).

MHRL – Ministry of Health of Republic of Lithuania (2008) *Data of Physician License Registry* (2007–2008) (Vilnius: Ministry of Health).

McKinlay, J. B. and L. D. Marceau (2008) 'When There Is No Doctor: Reasons for the Disappearance of Primary Care Physicians in the US During the Early 21st Century', *Social Science & Medicine*, 67 (10), 1481–91.

More, E. S. (1999) *Restoring the Balance: Women Physicians in the Profession of Medicine, 1850–1995* (Cambridge, MA: Harvard University Press).

Nordic Medical Associations (2006) *Physicians in the Nordic Countries 2006*, at: www.legeforeningen.no.asset/32194/1/32194_1.pdf, accessed 24 June 2009.

Oakley, A. (1984) *The Captured Womb* (Oxford: Blackwell).

OECD Health Data (2009) *Statistics and Indicators*, version December 2008, at: www.ecosante.org/affmultiphp?base=OECDE&valeur=&langh=Eng&langs=EN, accessed 24 June 2009.

Parsons, T. (1951) *The Social System* (New York: Free Press).

Riska, E. (2001a) *Medical Careers and Feminist Agendas: American, Scandinavian and Russian Women Physicians* (New York: Aldine de Gruyter).

Riska, E. (2001b) 'Towards Gender Balance: But Will Women Physicians Have an Impact on Medicine?', *Social Science & Medicine*, 52 (2), 179–87.

Riska, E. (2008) 'The Feminization Thesis: Discourses on Gender and Medicine', *NORA*, 16 (1), 3–18.

Riska, E. and A. Novelskaite (2008) 'Gendered Careers in Post-Soviet Society: Views on Professional Qualifications in Surgery and Pediatrics', *Gender Issues*, 25 (4), 229–45.

Rivkin-Fish, M. (2005) *Women's Health in Post-Soviet Russia: The Politics of Intervention* (Bloomington: Indiana University Press).

Roter, D. L. and J. A. Hall (2004) 'Physician Gender and Patient-centered Communication: A Critical Review of Empirical Research', *Annual Review of Public Health*, 25, 497–519.

RCP – Royal College of Physicians (2009) *Women and Medicine: The Future* (Summary of Findings from Royal College of Physicians Research) (Suffolk: Lavenham Press).

SMA – Swedish Medical Association (2009) *Läkarfakta 2009* (Statistics on Physicians), at: www.lakarforbundet.se, accessed 24 June 2009.

Verdonk, P., L. J. L. Mans and T. L. M. Lagro-Janssen (2006) 'How Is Gender Integrated in Curricula of Dutch Medical Schools? A Quick Scan on Gender Issues as an Instrument for Change', *Gender and Education*, 18 (4), 399–412.

Verdonk, P., Y. W. M. Benschop, H. C. J. de Haes and T. L. M. Lagro-Janssen (2008) 'From Gender Bias to Gender Awareness in Medical Education', *Advances in Health Sciences Education*, 14 (1), 135–52.

Witz, A. (1992) *Professions and Patriarchy* (London: Routledge).

Wrede, S. (2008) 'Educating Generalists: The Flexibilisation of Finnish Auxiliary Nursing and the Dilemma of Professional Identity', in E. Kuhlmann and M. Saks (eds), *Rethinking Professional Governance: International Directions in Healthcare* (Bristol: Policy Press), 127–40.

Zetka, J. R. (2008a) 'Radical Logics and Their Carriers in Medicine: The Case of Psychopathology and American Obstetricians and Gynecologists', *Social Problems*, 55 (1), 95–116.

Zetka, J. R. (2008b) 'The Making of the "Women's Physician" in American Obstetrics and Gynecology: Re-forging an Occupational Identity and a Division of Labor', *Journal of Health and Social Behavior*, 49 (3), 335–51.

26
Sex, Gender and Health: Developments in Medical Research

Toine Lagro-Janssen

Introduction

Over the past decade, three major developments have taken place in the discipline of women's health studies. First, the concept of women and health has shifted into the concept of gender and health, which explicitly includes men and the social construction of masculinity. Women's health studies has widened its scope to include the health of men, not only because men generally have lower life expectancy than women, but also because alcohol abuse, traffic accidents, suicides and drug addiction in men are largely attributed to traditional gender-role patterns and social conceptions of masculinity (Mansfield et al., 2003; see also Chapter 14 by Hunt et al. and Chapter 16 by Schofield).

Secondly, increasing attention is now being paid to how biological differences between men and women may serve as possible explanations for differences in risk factors, symptoms and disease course, whereby the genetic information in the sex chromosomes can be expressed differently between men and women owing to a wide range of environmental factors (Wizemann and Pardue, 2001; see also Chapter 6 by Klinge). A compelling aspect in this upsurge of the primacy of biology in medical gender discourse is the tremendous increase in possibilities for visualizing processes in the brain by means of imaging techniques, such as functional Magnetic Resonance Imaging (MRI) and, hence, for visualizing possible differences between men and women. It is a major challenge for women's health studies, therefore, to establish connections between the currently dominant biological concepts in the medical sciences with concepts dominant in the humanities and social sciences to help explain differences between men and women. The importance of interdisciplinary collaboration between fundamental medico-scientific research, epidemiology, the social sciences and clinical research is therefore greater than ever (Lagro-Janssen, 1999; see also Bird and Rieker, 2002; Doyal, 2000).

Thirdly and finally, we have witnessed the introduction of the concept of diversity, which is mainly used to refer to ethnic and cultural differences (see, for example, Ahmad and Bradby, 2008). It is clear that gender and culture do not operate in isolation but that differences other than gender, such as ethnicity, age, socio-economic status (SES) and sexual orientation interact with gender differences and impact in health (Lagro-Janssen et al., 2008). Although the impact of differences in ethnicity or SES should not be underestimated, out of all these social characteristics gender is the most crucially important difference. Moreover, biological aspects play a much more prominent part in male–female differences than in ethnic differences.

All these changes have boosted research interest in gender differences in medical research (Lagro-Janssen, 2007). And yet, despite all of this, the theme of gender in illness and health has not managed to secure a permanent position on research agendas in the medical sciences. To explain this peculiarity, we need to scrutinize three claims that doggedly persist in medicine: the principle of *neutrality*, which says that medicine is about *people* rather than about men and women; the principle of *uniformity*, which says that what goes for one human being also goes for all others; and the *biomedical concept of illness*, which dominates our understanding of illness and therefore assumes a top priority in the medical hierarchy of importance. These three claims currently are the principal causes of gender bias in medicine and in medical research.

In this chapter, I elaborate these principles in terms of their consequences for the consideration of gender in medical research. By presenting some case studies, I illustrate how breaking through gender bias may help to produce a new understanding of the health of men and women. In so doing, I also discuss the importance of gender for medical education. The examples presented here mainly draw on research carried out by the author and her colleagues and, together with other studies, mainly concern developments in the Netherlands. However, many of the issues are relevant to medical research in other countries. Finally, where gender and health hold out development opportunities, areas for future research are indicated.

The principle of neutrality

It is a persistent misconception in medical research that medicine is about people rather than about men and women. By extension, the principle of neutrality implies there is also a biological principle of equality between men and women. In the medical model, the organism is commonly studied as a generalized human organism that is the same for men and women, excepting some sex-specific hormonal and anatomical differences. After all, men and women are differently fitted out with a view to reproduction, which is why medicine has no difficulty acknowledging anatomical, genetic and hormonal differences to explain differences between them. Medical interests, consequently, also by and large focus on the well-demarcated domain of specific sex-related disorders of reproductive functions, such as pregnancy, infertility, contraception, menstrual disorders and prostate disorders. Sex-specific disorders, in other words, get priority in medical research and gender differences in health and illness do not.

In all this, we should bear in mind that a biological system or organism cannot be considered a static given of nature. On the contrary, biological systems are open systems, susceptible to evolutionary and environmental influences. The biological principle of equality between men and women, therefore, is a premise that is open to discussion. This failure to recognize or acknowledge the importance of gender is called gender blindness. One consequence of gender blindness is that the effects of medicines that have been tested in men are assumed to be the same in women. In major intervention studies on medicines, women are greatly underrepresented. If researchers and clinicians do not manage to produce gendered analyses and reports, the delivery of evidence-based care for men, women and children will certainly come under pressure (Correa-de-Araujo, 2006; Grant, 2002), with overtreatment or undertreatment being one consequence of missing data or hidden information and sub-optimal effectiveness and treatment safety (side-effects) being another risk involved here. It has only recently become known, for instance, that important preventive measures in the field of heart and vascular diseases, such as cholesterol-lowering drugs and salicylates, produce different effects in men and women.

Of course, there are plausible reasons for excluding women from drug trials such as these, but these are precisely the reasons that run parallel with crucial biological differences: men and women may show different responses to an intervention in terms of effectiveness and tolerance; the intervention may have an effect on the foetus; the particular stage of the menstrual cycle may cause response variation; pre- and post-menopausal women respond differently to therapy; and oral contraception and oestrogen treatments interfere with the intervention (Soldin and Mattison, 2009). All these reasons contradict the propriety of the biological equality principle because, if you expect response patterns to be the same, sex can never serve as a valid exclusion criterion. This approach, therefore, leads to overgeneralization, involving the exclusive study of either sex (either the male or female sex), with the results being generalized to both sexes (human beings).

The principle of neutrality, therefore, leads to gender blindness: it causes people to neglect gender differences in domains other than that of reproduction. Heart and vascular diseases, meanwhile, are prime examples of a field in which, until recently, men were the only subjects of research, but where an abundance of studies has now demonstrated differences between men and women (see Chapter 10 by Riska on coronary heart disease). In disorders and complaints that mainly occur in women, such as eating disorders, being victims of sexual abuse, or depressive disorders, we see quite the reverse trend, namely that what applies for women is also considered applicable to men (Sweet, 2006). Research into gender bias in medical textbooks, finally, has shown that gender-specific information is scarce or altogether absent and hardly retrievable through indexes or layout pointers (Dijkstra et al., 2008). The scarce gender-specific information that is available mainly pertains to epidemiological data and reproductive items. Textbooks also lack somatic and psychosocial information that is relevant to good medical practice. Contemporary medical textbooks, therefore, still show a great deal of gender bias (see also Hammarström, 2003; Phillips, 1997). This will be explained in greater detail in the following section, using depressive disorders as an example.

Gender differences in coping with depressive disorders

Depressive complaints, defined according to the Diagnostic and Statistical Manual of Mental Disorders IV (DSM–IV – APA, 1994), are twice as prevalent in women as in men (Angst et al., 2002). The criteria of the DSM–IV for diagnosing depression are the core symptoms 'depressed mood' and 'decrease in interest' (at least one of the core symptoms is obligatory) and at least four of the following: suicidal thoughts, indecisiveness, worthlessness/sense of guilt, insomnia, psychomotor agitation or retardation, hypersomnia, change in appetite, loss of energy, concentration problems (APA, 1994). Research into depressions tends to focus on women and on the effectiveness of medication and tends to disregard patients' experiences and feelings induced by their depressive complaints and the influence of gender. A recent study, therefore, used interviews to investigate whether there were any differences between Dutch men and women in the way they perceived and thought about depression and its treatment (Van den Berg and Lagro-Janssen, 2009). In this study, 20 patients with depression (nine men and 11 women between the ages of 19 and 72) were interviewed, participating through their general practitioners (GPs). These interviews were recorded on audiotape, fully transcribed, and further analysed by three researchers in conformity with grounded theory methods.

The study showed clear gender differences in the way depression was experienced. The men mainly described their depression as an activation issue and were more inclined to solve this problem in the present without lingering over their emotional experience of the depression. They mainly situated problems in their work environment, since this was where great demands were made upon them within the confines of time constraints. The women mentioned negative thoughts as the main component of their depression: they rather tended to dwell on their negative emotions and to feel guilty. Besides negative thoughts about themselves, almost half the women indicated that fear was also a feature of their depression. The men had greater difficulty talking openly about their depressive complaints because they were ashamed of potential loss of face; the women were also ashamed, but they were ashamed of their personal failure as mothers or partners. A striking finding was that the men had a more positive idea than the women did about the future course of their depression and the possible occurrence of relapse. The men in this study also believed they personally had a greater influence on the recovery process than women did.

This study suggests that the DSM–IV criteria for diagnosing depression are better suited to 'female' than to 'male' depression because females tend to emphasize despondency and negative feelings. The DSM–IV thus both reflects and creates gender blindness for the experience of depression in men, which impedes its recognition by healthcare professionals.

The principle of uniformity

The principal of uniformity proclaims that all people are equal and that what goes for one human being also goes for everyone else. This assumption gives rise to gender bias of a different kind than gender blindness: 'andronormativity' or male bias. Andronormativity signifies a state of affairs whereby male values are regarded as normal (Hølge-Hazelton and Malterud, 2009), with the male serving as the standard or the frame of reference for analysing females and female characteristics. This phenomenon causes men to appear as normal human beings and women to appear as deviating from the standard.

The question that arises, of course, is what we should consider normal and whether we should consider everything outside the boundaries of such normality as a disease or as abnormal. To define the concept of normality, medicine uses different parameters: statistical normality (that which is most prevalent in a normal distribution); medical normality (that which is non-pathological); and cultural normality (that which is proper or right). Interpreting deviations from what is normal is conditional upon standards and values and may also have different results in men and women, even if it is within the boundaries of statistical normality. You might think, for example, of the fact that growth hormones are prescribed much more frequently in boys than in girls of below-average expected height, and, conversely, that growth-inhibiting hormones are chiefly used in girls who are expected to grow 'too tall' (see also Conrad, 2007; and Chapter 7 by Bell and Figert).

Gender is like a hushed and subtle intruder in all sorts of phenomena that we tend to take for granted. Medicine, for instance, often tends to take for granted that intimate partner violence (IPV) is a family matter and, hence, is a relationship issue rather than a gender-related power issue. The next section turns our attention towards the important role of family physicians in recognizing IPV.

Intimate partner violence and the role of family physicians

Research into IPV and the role played by family physicians clearly highlights how influential gender is for GPs interpreting medical complaints of women presenting with IPV at their consultation (Lo Fo Wong, 2006; Lo Fo Wong et al., 2006). The aim of the study by Lo Fo Wong and colleagues (2006) was to explore gender differences in family doctors' views, attitudes, experiences and practices regarding sexual abuse of women. The focus group method was used, consisting of three male and three female groups of general practitioners from Rotterdam. The conversations were recorded on audiotape and fully transcribed; two independent researchers analysed the transcripts.

There were marked differences between the male and female family physician groups in their discussion of IPV. There proved to be major divergence of opinion, first, on the role of sexuality: some of the male family physicians declared that, if female spouses denied sexual relations to their male partners, this was a contributing and eliciting cause of male aggression; all female physicians, on the contrary, unanimously emphasized the humiliation of sexual coercion, a woman's right to set limits in a sexual relationship and the dangers involved in denying sexual relations. Moreover, the female group held that children witnessing IPV was a major issue to be taken into consideration, whereas this issue did not come up in the male groups. Female physicians also remembered many more actual cases of IPV than their male colleagues. Finally, female physicians viewed women leaving an abusive partner as process – women could learn from their experiences although it would sometimes take time, and the observation that repeated experiences of IPV do not denote failure was heard only in the female doctors' group. Male doctors, on the other hand, did not view leaving a partner in these terms. Male physicians in particular revealed views of sexuality that held women responsible for their own abuse because they denied their spouse access to sex. This represents cultural values about masculinity and andronormativity that may be harmful to female victims. Gender-related differences between doctors, therefore, may affect care and healthcare for abused women.

In the medical sciences, the principle of uniformity often causes the male to be considered normal and the female to be neglected. Another trend now perceptible in medicine is the tendency to consider pathological what formerly used to be considered normal physiological events in the female life-cycle, and involves thrusting a medical diagnosis on something that is not a disease. Women's lives are particularly prone to this happening, as women in the present day almost universally end up treated by hormonal, endocrinological medicine: from the contraceptive pill in the menarche, infertility treatments, pregnancy and delivery, to oestrogen treatments during and after menopause, women's lives have become susceptible to hormonal management and so are subject to routine medical intervention of this kind.

In obstetrics, for instance, such medicalization has caused the supine position in delivery to be the most common one because it is convenient for healthcare professionals rather than based on scientific evidence or on women's preference (De Jonge et al., 2004). The supine position, meanwhile, has become so common that neither healthcare professionals nor mothers-to-be regard this as an intervention. Even if healthcare professionals do not tell women to take a recumbent position, they will simply do so because they assume that this is what is expected of them. Therefore, the next section examines the advantages and disadvantages of the routine use of the supine position in the second stage of labour and those factors that prejudice the use of birthing positions.

Birthing positions and women's views

The aim of the research by De Jonge and colleagues (De Jonge, 2008; De Jonge et al., 2004) was to question the routine use of the supine position, and a variety of study designs were used to answer this question. In a meta-analytical review of the benefits of the routine use of the supine position compared to other positions, the authors found no evidence to support the superiority of the supine position versus other positions and hence there was no evidence for the continuation of this routine use.

A large randomized controlled trial conducted in obstetric clinics in primary care in the Netherlands assessed whether the risk of severe blood loss was increased in semi-sitting and sitting positions and whether women's position at the time of birth had an influence on perineal damage. No differences were found in blood loss or in intact perineum rates between women in recumbent, semi-sitting and sitting positions. In conclusion, these findings do not recommend any particular birthing position (De Jonge et al., 2004). Moreover the routine use of the supine position can be considered an intervention in the normal course of labour. Finally, women were interviewed about their views and preferences based on the experiences with the position they had used when they gave birth. The main finding was that women benefited from having the autonomy to choose the positions that were most useful to them. Advice given by midwives proved to be the most influential factor in their choice. From this study we can conclude that midwives should empower women to choose positions that are the most suitable to them (De Jonge et al., 2004).

Women's lack of voice in medical science and practice also plays a role in the discussion of andronormativity, as scientific interest and experience affect what is considered interesting as a research topic. What counts as interesting is different for female and male physicians, but it is the men who are the main movers and shakers in the scientific domain in medicine (Simon, 2005).

The primacy of the biomedical concept

In medicine, there is no general agreement as to what constitutes a disease. There is a range of concepts, which, to aid the clarity of my argument, I will represent as two extremes (Lagro-Janssen, 1997). At one extreme, the biomedical concept assumes that a disease is an entity that happens to people. Each disease has its own phenomena and runs its own course: the disease is unique. The biomedical concept seeks to generalize and reproduce diseases and, consequently, acts in the tradition of the physical sciences. The disease is independent of the patient.

At the other extreme, we have an integrated concept which underlines the coherence and interaction between the biological (organism–body), the psychological (perception–experience) and the socio-historical (the life-course) and undertakes to interpret these aspects in their coherence. Here a disease springs from the concerted action of internal and external factors and manifests itself in each individual in an individual way: the patient is unique. The disease is dependent on the patient's life-course, social context and system of meaning.

As the biomedical concept dominates medical discourse, sex and gender differences are largely downgraded. While this was the focus of women's health activism decades ago (see, for example, Ruzek, 1978), the problem still persists (Annandale, 2009; Correa-de-Araujo, 2006). I am expressly referring to sex and gender here because both sex and gender matter in health and healthcare. Sex plays a major role in the aetiology, onset, complications and course of diseases. Gender influences risk factors, symptom detection, seriousness, coping strategies and compliance with medical treatment. It is of the essence, therefore, that biomedical research on sex and socio-scientific research on gender be integrated in order to be able to learn how gender inequality in healthcare can be prevented precisely by paying due attention to differences between men and women.

Gender awareness in medical education

Gender awareness means that healthcare professionals have a gender-sensitive attitude as well as knowledge and understanding of the full significance of gender in illness and health (Lagro-Janssen, 2007). Besides this attitude, healthcare professionals must have the skills to apply their understanding to medical practice. Gender needs to be recognized as an essential determinant of illness and health. As medical education plays a pivotal role in closing the gap between gender bias and gender awareness in medicine, gender-sensitive healthcare also requires gender-sensitive medical education (see also Chapter 27 by Cheng et al.). Medical education, however, has a lot of catching up to do. The medical curriculum largely bypasses the question of whether it matters for patients to be male or female (gender neutrality, gender bias) and whether major risks for women, such as sexual abuse and violence, are disregarded due to a dominant male perspective (uniformity, male bias) (Risberg et al., 2003).

There also appears to be a gradient on the legitimacy of different diagnoses. Disorders in which the majority of patients are women, such as rheumatoid arthritis, anxiety, fibromyalgia and eating disorders, are at the bottom of the list in the medical status hierarchy and are less often taught (Album and Westin, 2008). Owing to the primacy of the biomedical model of illness, the question of whether an integrated bio-psycho-social concept of illness is a more appropriate framework for interpreting complaints than the biomedical model of illness is not raised systematically. Gender stereotypes that play a role in treatment by doctors and that negatively impact medical treatment must be discouraged (Scheper-Hughes, 1991). Therefore, it is important to investigate which criteria make a medical curriculum gender-specific and how a gender-neutral curriculum can be implemented in medical education. This approach assumes that gender differences are an underexposed subject in medical education, that knowledge of gender differences in illness and health is relevant for medical practice, and that such knowledge helps to improve quality of care and to promote greater equality between men and women.

In what follows in this section I introduce a model for improving gender awareness and implementing gender-sensitive curricula in medicine that was developed at Radboud University Nijmegen Medical Centre in the Netherlands (see also Chapter 24 by Armstrong for examples from Canada). This project proceeded by first screening the medical curriculum at the Radboud University Nijmegen Medical Centre for its content (which subjects were and were not taught in the curriculum), context (the context in which male and female patients were presented) and language. This screening showed that gender-specific issues were dealt with only haphazardly and that there were gaps in the field of knowledge and attitude formation (Lagro-Janssen, 2002). In order to make sure that gender-specific aspects of illness and health in medical education received the professional attention and thoroughness they deserved, we took two roads. On the one hand, we decided to take the road of the interdisciplinary integration of gender-specific aspects in compulsory basic courses, linking up with the practice-centred themes that prevail in the disciplines concerned. On the other hand, we decided to take the road of raising the profile of the discipline of Gender Studies as a topic in its own right in optional courses and scientific internships in medicine, focusing on the theoretical exploration of the concepts of sex and gender in healthcare.

Implementing gender in medical education: a long way to go

A stepping stone in implementing gender in medical education was the establishment of a Knowledge Centre for gender-specific education in medicine at Radboud University Nijmegen Medical Centre that was based on available academic expertise and experience with gender-specific research and education (Mans et al., 2006). The main tasks of this Centre, which was accommodated with the Women's Studies in Medicine Department at the University, are to translate research-generated knowledge into concrete medical learning objectives; to develop core educational modules on the theme of gender differences in illness and health; to apply contemporary educational materials and teaching methods; to develop teacher training courses; and to develop gender-specific testing and assessment procedures. The Knowledge Centre also serves as a centre for continuous stocktaking, documentation, and lending of materials to and consultation with teachers and policy-makers. Taking the literature into account and having consulted gender experts, we formulated criteria that a gender-specific curriculum should meet (see Box 26.1).

Second, we used a phased, step-by-step approach to implementing gender-specific aspects in education nationwide at all eight medical faculties in the Netherlands. Meanwhile, the recommendations of the paradigm project at Radboud University Nijmegen Medical Centre have been evaluated, including the

Box 26.1 Integration of gender into the basic medical curriculum

1. Medical students are able to recognize and explain gender differences with regard to the following issues: transitional phases such as menopause and adolescence; pharmacotherapy; cardiovascular diseases; urinary tract infections and other micturition complaints; urinary incontinence; reproduction, particularly contraception, sexually transmitted diseases, and infertility; eating disorders and obesity; addiction to alcohol or benzodiazepines; depression and anxiety disorders; sexual abuse and violence, child abuse and intimate partner violence; post-traumatic stress disorders; sexuality, sexual problems and sexual identity; communication; gender and culture; gender-specific healthcare and quality of care;
2. These gender differences are included in the learning objectives of the education received by students;
3. Students have received education that focused on both biomedical and socio-cultural differences;
4. Students have received education on gender differences over the course of several studies (two years minimum);
5. In at least six to eight teaching units of two to four weeks each in the central curriculum, students have received education in which specific attention was paid to gender differences;
6. Students have been given the opportunity to take one extra optional unit on sex or gender, whether or not combined with ethnicity.

strong and weak points of the project implementation: Had its recommendations been applied? If not, why not? Had its objectives been achieved? What were teachers' and students' evaluations? What were their problems and needs? The major facilitating factors for a successful implementation of gender into the medical curriculum proved to be: practicable recommendations; an insightful translation of gender differences into patient care; the motivation and commitment of coordinators; the presence of an advocate in the medical faculty; its embedding in existing curricula; and practical support. These outcomes have subsequently been used in implementation procedures at other medical faculties.

In addition, we evaluated the gender-specific education on offer in the basic curricula of other medical faculties in various stages of innovation, and we collected information on the content, appreciation, wishes and problems of teachers and students. Future plans were also evaluated, and we particularly looked at which year and which module in the curriculum would present opportunities for integrating gender-specific aspects (Verdonk et al., 2006).

We then proceeded to conduct interviews with several influential individuals, such as education directors, coordinators, deans, education management teams, students and gender experts, on how to integrate gender-specific aspects into the curriculum. The aim of this procedure was to gain broad-based support for integrating new gender-specific components into the curriculum (Verdonk et al., 2009). Evaluation and monitoring of the introduction of new gender-specific components into education was also high on the agenda. Finally, we formulated relevant topics and themes for an optional four-week course on gender, possibly combined with aspects of culture. We also actively involved those teachers and disciplines that championed the integration of gender-specific and cultural aspects into education. In addition to a teacher training course developed by the Knowledge Centre, which was offered to teachers and student teachers with a view to building an expert pool of teachers, we also staged two invitational conferences, primarily aiming to exchange experiences, inform interested innovators and policy-makers, and gain broad-based support. In summary, this strategy was based on the assumption that a bottom-up as well a top-down approach would prove to be successful.

The incorporation of gender perspectives at eight medical faculties

An important question is, whether, and if so, how the incorporation of gender issues into medical education is capable of challenging dominant systems of thought (see, for example, Benshop and Verloo, 2006; Hammarström, 2003; Phillips, 1997; Risberg et al., 2003). To answer this question, we conducted 18 semi-structured interviews with education directors and agents of change (Verdonk et al., 2009). Antagonism and obstacles to mainstreaming gender into medical education proved to be implicit in four areas.

First, biomedical knowledge was perceived to be gender-neutral, and it was felt that knowledge of women could be added to this body of biomedical knowledge either with or without framing it as a gender issue. Second, the relevance of gender was informally denied by downplaying this concern, particularly in comparison with culture and ethnicity. Third, the social accountability of medical education was hardly ever mentioned, and gender inequalities in health were framed as feminist political issues rather than as medical issues. And fourth, we were urged to be cautious in our communications so as to increase acceptance and avoid overt resistance, situating gender inequalities outside the medical domain. Recommendations for changing educational materials were widely discussed, but specific gender features were easily lost among them. This was especially true for considerations of power differences between men and women. Nevertheless, we did succeed in challenging dominant systems of thought. Our experiences confirm that there is a widespread assumption that a feminist perspective produces biased knowledge, and this assumption consequently biases the consideration of gender issues (Risberg et al., 2003). Our results indicate that a gender perspective in medicine is considered to be merely a feminist opinion, and thus contrary to objective biomedical knowledge. Our findings stress the need to spend more money and time on research into gender and health and to underline the importance of strong cooperation between gender research and education, and vice versa (Celik et al., 2008).

Conclusion

By focusing on three persistent principles operative in medicine, this chapter has demonstrated why the topic of gender has difficulty securing a place for itself in scientific medical research. First of all, there is the principle of neutrality, which causes gender differences to be ignored (gender blindness). Second, there is the principle of uniformity, with the male perspective being dominant and being considered the standard and the female perspective being neglected and being considered deviant (andronormativity). Norms in medicine, like those involved in pathologizing physiological phenomena, are also the products of the dominant male perspective. Third, the prevailing concept of illness is of a predominantly biomedical kind, which is an impediment to the study of gender because an integrated concept of illness would be much better positioned to study bio-psycho-social aspects of gender and health in a coherent, mutually reinforcing manner. An integrated concept of illness also provides a better match with doctors' and patients' stories, some of which I have cited as examples in this chapter.

I have indicated how integrating gender-specific knowledge, heightening gender awareness, and breaking through gender stereotyping are important preconditions for establishing gender-specific medicine. It is of the utmost importance to make clear to medical students that, on the one hand, medicine neutralizes gender differences by narrowing them down to sex differences, where biological explanations for differences between men and women are presented as self-evident and natural. On the other hand, appealing to the biomedical concept, medicine heightens differences between men and women by pathologizing women's bodies and subjecting them to gender stereotyping. Differences between men and women, however, are not mutually exclusive categories. The difference between both sexes is not statically given but actively made and framed in the signification system of a culture. In this sense, research in women's health not only qualifies and complements medicine but operates as a critique of it (Lagro-Janssen, 1997).

The examples given here, which exemplify gender bias in medicine, have led me to conclude this chapter with some suggestions for future research. The case studies that have been discussed indicate that, first of all, attention needs to be paid to gender differences in patients' presentation of complaints, perceived meaning, the course and complications involved in diseases, and the effects of treatment of disorders. Chronic diseases should be given priority in studies on gender differences in issues such as co-morbidity and precautionary measures. Men and their health also need to be involved in these processes, as the depression case study illustrated so markedly. In doing all this, we should not overlook medical research into reproductive aspects for women who do not have easy access to healthcare or find themselves in socially deprived situations. Health-threatening risks such as abuse and violence also need to be prioritized on the research agenda.

Second, andronormativity in medical research should remain an object of critical examination, exposure and avoidance. The need for this was well illustrated in the case studies on the naturalness of birthing positions and on family doctors' opinions on intimate partner violence. Third, interdisciplinary research that takes on board an integrated concept of illness is of the utmost importance in helping us understand the relations between sex, gender and health. Research into the implementation of gender in medical education is crucial here, as is making space for gender in the professional development of physicians and physicians-to-be.

Summary

- Three persistent principles in medicine act as barriers to the introduction of gender in scientific medical research, namely gender blindness, andronormativity and the predominantly biomedical concept of illness.
- Attention needs to be paid to gender differences in the diagnostic process and treatment; andronormativity in medical research should remain an object of critical examination.

- Interdisciplinary research, including an integrated concept of illness, is vital in understanding the relation between sex, gender and health.
- Gender-sensitive healthcare requires gender-sensitive medical education. It is of the utmost importance to make space for gender in the professional development and to explore 'good practices' of implementing gender-sensitive curricula in medicine.

Key reading

Album, D. and S. Westin (2008) 'Do Diseases Have a Prestige Hierarchy? A Survey among Physicians and Medical Students', *Social Science & Medicine*, 66 (1), 182–8.

Correa-de-Aruajo, R. (2006) 'Serious Gaps: How the Lack of Sex/Gender Based Research Impairs Health', *Journal of Women's Health*, 34 (10), 1116–21.

Lagro-Janssen, A. L. M. (2007) 'Sex, Gender and Health Developments in Research', *European Journal of Women's Studies*, 14 (1), 9–20.

Verdonk, P., Y. Benschop, H. de Haes, L. J. L. Mans and A. L. M. Lagro-Janssen (2009) '"Should You Turn This into a Complete Gender Matter?" Gender Mainstreaming in Medical Education', *Gender and Education*, 21, 1–17.

References

Ahmad, W. I. U. and H. Bradby (eds) (2008) *Ethnicity, Health and Health Care* (Special Issue of *Sociology of Health and Illness*) (Oxford: Blackwell).

Album, D. and S. Westin (2008) 'Do Diseases Have a Prestige Hierarchy? A Survey among Physicians and Medical Students', *Social Science & Medicine*, 66 (1), 182–8.

APA – American Psychiatric Association (1994) *Diagnostic and Statistical Manual of Mental Disorders (DSM–IV)* (Washington, DC: American Psychiatric Association).

Angst, J., A. Gamma, M. Gastpar, J. P. Lépine, J. Mendlewicz and A. Tylee (2002) 'Gender Differences in Depression: Epidemiological Findings from the European DEPRES I and II Studies', *European Archives of Psychiatry and Clinical Neuroscience*, 252 (5), 201–9.

Annandale, E. (2009) *Women's Health and Social Change* (London: Routledge).

Benshop, Y. W. M. and M. Verloo (2006) 'Sisyphus' Sister. Can Gender Mainstreaming Escape the Genderedness of Organizations?', *Journal of Gender Studies*, 15 (1), 19–34.

Bird, C. E. and P. P. Rieker (2002) 'Integrating Social and Biological Research to Improve Men's and Women's Health', *Women's Health Issues*, 12 (3), 113–15.

Celik, H. I., I. Klinge, T. Weijden, G. van der Widdershoven and A. L. M. Lagro-Janssen (2008) 'Gender Sensitivity among General Practitioners: Results of a Training Programme', *BMC Medical Education*, 8, 36, at: www.biomedcentral.com/1472-6920/8/36, accessed 26 June 2009.

Conrad, P. (2007) *The Medicalization of Society* (Baltimore: John Hopkins University Press).

Correa-de-Araujo, R. (2006) 'Serious Gaps: How the Lack of Sex/Gender Based Research Impairs Health', *Journal of Women's Health*, 34 (10), 1116–21.

De Jonge, A. (2008) *Birthing Positions Revisited: Examining the Evidence of a Routine Practice*, PhD thesis, Radboud University Nijmegen.

De Jonge, A., D. A. M. Teunissen and A. L. M. Lagro-Janssen, (2004) 'Supine Position during the Second Stage of Labour: A Meta-analytic Review', *Journal of Psychosomatic Obstetric Gynecology*, 25 (1), 35–45.

Dijkstra, A. F., P. Verdonk and A. L. M. Lagro-Janssen (2008) 'Gender Bias in Medical Textbooks: Examples from Coronary Heart Disease, Depression, Alcohol Abuse and Pharmacology', *Medical Education*, 42 (10), 1021–8.

Doyal, L. (2000) 'Gender Equity in Health: Debates and Dilemmas', *Social Science & Medicine*, 51 (6), 931–9.

Grant, K. (2002) 'Gender-based Analysis: Beyond the Red Queen Syndrome', *Research Bulletin of the Centres of Excellence for Women's Health*, 2 (3), 16–20.

Hammarström, A. (2003) 'The Integration of Gender in Medical Research and Education – Obstacles and Possibilities from a Nordic Perspective', in L. Manderson (ed.), *Teaching Gender, Teaching Women's Health* (New York: Haworth Medical Press), 121–33.

Hølge-Hazelton, B. and K. Malterud (2009) 'Gender in Medicine – Does It Matter?', *Scandinavian Journal of Public Health*, 37 (2), 139–45.

Lagro-Janssen, A. L. M. (1997) *The Ambivalence of the Difference* (Nijmegen: SUN).

Lagro-Janssen, A. L. M. (1999) 'State of the Art: Developments in the Field of Women's Studies Medicine', *European Journal of Women's Studies*, 6 (4), 487–500.

Lagro-Janssen, A. L. M. (2002) 'The Implementation of Sex within the Medical Education', *Tijdschrift voor Gezondheidswetenschappen*, 4, 269–71.

Lagro-Janssen, A. L. M. (2007) 'Sex, Gender and Health Developments in Research', *European Journal of Women's Studies*, 14 (1), 9–20.

Lagro-Janssen, T., S. Lo Fo Wong and M. van den Muijsenbergh (2008) 'The Importance of Gender in Health Problems', *European Journal of General Practice*, 14 (S1), 33–7.

Lo Fo Wong, S. (2006) *The Doctor and the Woman "Who Fell down the Stairs". Family Doctors' Role in Recognizing and Responding to Intimate Partner Abuse*, PhD thesis, Radboud University Nijmegen.

Lo Fo Wong, S., A. De Jonge, F. Wester, S. S. L. Mol, R. K. Römkens and A. L. M. Lagro-Janssen (2006) 'Discussing Partner Abuse: Does Doctors' Gender Really Matter?', *Family Practice*, 23 (5), 578–86.

Mans, L. J. L., P. Verdonk and A. L. M. Lagro-Janssen (2006) 'The Role of the Digital Knowledge Centre for Medical Education in Integrating Gender in Medical Education', *Journal of Medical Education*, 25, 66–74.

Mansfield, A. K., M. E. Addis and J. R. Mahalin (2003) '"Why Won't He Go to the Doctor"? The Psychology of Men's Help Seeking', *International Journal of Men's Health*, 2 (2), 93–110.

Phillips, S. P. (1997) 'Problem Based Learning in Medicine: New Curricula, Old Stereotypes. Personal View', *Social Science & Medicine*, 45, 497–9.

Risberg, G., K. Hamberg and E. E. Johansson (2003) 'Gender Awareness among Physicians – The Effect of Specialty and Gender. A Study of Teachers at a Swedish Medical School', *BMC Medical Education*, 3 (8) at: www.biomedcentral.com/1472-6920/3/8, accessed 27 October 2008.

Ruzek, S. B. (1978) *The Women's Health Movement: Feminist Alternatives to Medical Control* (New York: Praeger).

Scheper-Hughes, N. (1991) 'Virgin Territory: The Male Discovery of the Clitoris', *Medical Anthropology Quarterly*, 5 (1), 25–9.

Simon V. (2005) 'Wanted: Women in Clinical Trials', *Science*, 308, 1517.

Soldin, O. P. and D. R. Mattison (2009) 'Sex Differences in Pharmacokinetics and Pharmacodynamics', *Clinical Pharmacokinetics*, 48 (3), 143–54.

Sweet, H. (2006) *Couples Counselling with Sad or Silent Men: Implications for Practice* (New Orleans: APA).

Van den Berg, F. and A. L. M. Lagro-Janssen (2009) 'Differences in the Views and Feelings among Male and Female Patients with a Depressive Disorder in General Practice', unpublished paper, Radboud University Nijmegen.

Verdonk, P., Y. Benschop, H. de Haes, L. J. L Mans and A. L. M. Lagro-Janssen (2009) '"Should You Turn This into a Complete Gender Matter?" Gender Mainstreaming in Medical Education', *Gender and Education*, 21 (6), 1–17.

Verdonk, P., L. J. L Mans and A. L. M. Lagro-Janssen (2006) 'How Is Gender Integrated in the Curricula of Dutch Medical Schools? A Quick Scan of Gender Issues as an Instrument for Change', *Gender and Education*, 18 (4), 399–412.

Wizemann, T. M. and M. L. Pardue (2001) *Exploring the Biological Contribution to Human Health: Does Sex Matter?* (Washington, DC: National Academy Press).

27
Gender Mainstreaming at the Cross-roads of Eastern-Western Healthcare

Ling-fang Cheng, Ellen Kuhlmann and Ellen Annandale

Introduction

Gender has long been ignored in the education and practice of health professionals in many developing societies. Recently, the wheels have begun to turn and gender issues are now more visible and acknowledged in health policy and practice as a result of both feminist struggle and political change in many developing countries. Indeed, change may even be more radical and rapid than in western countries (see Chapter 24 by Armstrong and Chapter 26 by Lagro-Janssen), bringing into force legal, institutional and educational reforms, including the introduction of gender studies and gender-sensitive professional education in healthcare.

This chapter explores the windows of opportunity for gender mainstreaming in the health professions at the crossroads of western and eastern healthcare using the illustrative case of Taiwan. Here, we find the interesting situation of rapid change towards gender mainstreaming approaches alongside strong and persistent sex segregation of the health professional workforce. The predominantly male medical profession embraces western medicine with its masculinist underpinnings. By contrast, Traditional Chinese Medicine (TCM) has a strong appeal to women and an image of providing 'holistic', and thus more gender-sensitive, healthcare (for an overview see Flesch, 2007), but is rooted in eastern patriarchal society and a tradition of male healers. The illustrative case of Taiwan helps to better understand context-dependency and the variety of gender mainstreaming approaches and how they create different windows of opportunity for change. Drawing a contextualized map of gender policies also highlights how institutions – like the family, the law and state regulation, and professional bodies – shape the gendered landscape of healthcare (see also Chapter 21 by Burau et al.).

The chapter begins in historical perspective by exploring the coexistence of two health systems, TCM and western or biomedicine, and then provides an overview of the present-day gendered landscape of the health professions in Taiwan. The focus then turns to the driving forces towards, and implementation of, gender equality policies and gender-sensitive healthcare. These developments are analysed by focusing on gender-sensitive approaches to the education and training of health professionals. The conclusion highlights novel contributions to the discourse of gender mainstreaming which to date has been dominated by western perspectives.

The meeting of western and eastern healthcare systems

Taiwan's healthcare system is heavily shaped by two institutionally and culturally different approaches on health and healing – biomedicine and TCM – that embody competing logics of western and eastern medicine (Chi, 1994; Chi et al., 1996). Two other approaches with limited contemporary relevance are not included in our analysis: aboriginal medicine, which has now almost disappeared (Hsu, 2006), and the Chinese Han peoples' folk medicine, which is still practised in some communities (Chang, 2006). Although TCM is more integrated in medical care in Taiwan than in western countries (see, for example, Saks, 1997), the two systems of TCM and biomedicine have been struggling against each other in Taiwan for a century or so. This situation has created specific opportunities for gender mainstreaming. In order to explore this, it is important to briefly outline the historical context.

Prior to the arrival of the Japanese in 1895, the vast majority of doctors in Taiwan practiced TCM. Japanese records show that in 1897 there were 1046 traditional practitioners but only 24 western-trained missionary doctors (Chen, 1992). TCM is not only a medical treatment but also a philosophy emphasizing the harmony of the human being and the universe. Since illness is seen to result from a disruption in the balance of Yin and Yang in the body, the body should be treated from a holistic perspective. Practised for over one thousand years in China, TCM followed Chinese migrants to Taiwan. It was discouraged under Japanese colonial rule (1895–1945), which promoted western medicine as part of a modernist crusade. Adopting a policy of 'withering away naturally', the colonial government no longer issued licences to TCM practitioners after 1901. As a consequence, the number of practitioners fell from nearly 1000 at the turn of the 20th century to fewer than a 100 in 1942 (Chen, 1992).

In line with the hostile policy towards TCM practitioners, the Japanese colonial government fuelled the rise of the biomedical profession. The first Taipei Hospital and the Medical Training Institute (later upgraded to a Medical College) were established in 1895 and 1897 respectively in order to promote western medicine. So westernization and the professionalization of medicine were closely linked with colonialism, and subsequently with racial discrimination. For instance, during the colonial period, very few Taiwanese biomedical doctors were selected to hold posts in public hospitals; these posts enjoyed higher social status than solo practice. Overall, however, the supportive politics of Japanese colonial rule fuelled the rise of the medical profession as the most prestigious group amongst healthcare providers in Taiwan; biomedical doctors usually had better financial opportunities than the TCM practitioners (Cheng, 1998).

However, the modernist vision of the Japanese regime did not include the modernization of gender relations; indeed, traditional patriarchal gender arrangements were perpetuated. During the period of Japanese rule, both TCM and biomedicine were practised in a gendered social-cultural context that encouraged men to take educational and career paths and women to be 'good' mothers and wives. Men were privileged in both TCM and biomedicine, while women were perceived as suitable only for midwifery and nursing. Only in exceptional cases did fortunate middle-class women have the chance to follow the steps of their brothers to Japan for medical and nursing education (Cheng, 1998).

After the end of the Second World War in 1945, Japan had to cede Taiwan to the rule of the Chinese Nationalist Government (KMT) that was then defeated a few years later, in 1949, by forces of the Chinese Communist Party. Despite many differences, the Japanese colonial regime and its KMT successor shared some common ground when it came to the governance of the healthcare professions. Both followed a modernist vision of prioritizing biomedicine over TCM as well as an authoritarian style of governance and policy-making. As a consequence, state control and hierarchical governance were reinforced. In stark contrast to western healthcare systems where health professions had self-governing bodies, the state had, for instance, oversight of professional licenses (Cheng, 1998).

The KMT government promoted co-education for boys and girls. To some extent, for the first time, male and female students of middle-class background had equal opportunities, including to be trained as a TCM practitioner or biomedical doctor via the national examination system (Cheng, 1998). But despite the 'softening' of women's exclusion from higher education and medicine, the wider gendered division of labour in healthcare remained inviolate; the nursing profession was regarded suitable for women, but not for men (Yang et al., 2004). The following section highlights the gendered implications of the differing roads taken towards the professionalization of TCM, biomedicine and nursing.

Roads towards professionalization and their gendered implications

TCM was gradually revitalized after the Second World War following the more integrated and less hostile health policies of the KMT compared to those of the colonial government. In 1958, a number of prominent TCM practitioners established the China Medical College (which was upgraded to university status in 2003) that aimed to make TCM more 'scientific'. But overall, these efforts did not meet with much success since until the mid-1980s there was a lack of qualified teachers as well as interested students, and the government allocated only minimal resources to TCM (Chi, 1994). However, the advance of a more 'scientific' TCM opened the door to different educational pathways, and this had gendered effects.

In the 1990s, the group of TCM practitioners who had passed the state examination and held a licence comprised doctors with two types of professional backgrounds. One group had an academic education but little experience in clinical practice; the other group were traditionally trained apprentices without an academic education, but experienced in clinical practice (Chi et al., 1996). Consequently, the professionalization of TCM and associated academic training brought more diversity into the educational system, and this in turn, may to some extent have weakened the gendered knowledge track of an eastern patriarchal society that passed knowledge to sons or sons-in-law but not to daughters (Cheng, 1998).

Next to academic training and upgrading, the introduction of public insurance policies was indicative of the professionalization of TCM. Beginning in 1975, the new policies included TCM services in their coverage. Finally, in 1995 the National Health Insurance, a low-cost compulsory scheme, was implemented, with healthcare coverage including TCM (Chi et al., 1996; for an overview, see Lu and Hsiao, 2003). In summary, the profession of TCM is now more integrated into the healthcare system and the once much more strongly patriarchal form of knowledge is being challenged from all sides. This may be one of the reasons why women's access to the profession of TCM has improved.

Biomedical doctors, though highly regarded as the core of the Taiwanese healthcare system and promoted by health policies, also experienced a difficult route to professionalization (Cheng, 1998). Importantly, they have never achieved complete control of the healthcare market due to their co-existence with TCM practitioners. It is also important to keep in mind the configuration of the state–profession relationship in Taiwan where state power is strong and clearly overrides professional interests. This is in contrast to most western countries where health professions usually enjoy high levels of self-governing power (for an overview, see Kuhlmann and Saks, 2008).

Viewed through the lens of western professionalization theories (see, for example, Freidson, 2001), biomedical doctors in Taiwan have not achieved the status of a fully fledged profession controlling the market and the point of entry to healthcare, due largely to the co-existence of eastern and western medicine. However, within the context of more integrated eastern–western medical approaches, Taiwanese biomedicine enjoys the highest socio-economic status among the health professions. Unsurprisingly, it is the most appealing career track for middle-class men (Cheng, 1998).

The final group to consider in relation to gendered routes to professional status is the nursing profession. This group has faced a number of radical institutional reforms and educational expansion. Prior to their recognition as a profession in the mid-1960s, nurses were required to do ward cleaning and trivial clerical jobs (Chen, 2008). Professionalization has brought the expansion of educational institutes and the upgrading of nursing courses from Bachelors to Masters and later to PhD level. From the late 1980s onwards, well-trained graduates entered the profession, and training in specialty areas of nursing also increased (Chen, 2008). At the same time, heavy workloads and lower income and status compared to medicine have driven many qualified nurses out of the profession; this has been the main concern of the profession's leaders from the 1980s to the present (Chen, 2008).

Professionalization and academic training also changed the social class composition of nursing. While the nursing profession had previously been the mobility track for working-class daughters, since the late 1980s it has attracted more middle-class daughters – and even some sons. Changes in recruitment policy partly mirror a general trend in the western world, and partly a new need for nurses in emergency and psychiatric units where physically strong males are regarded as more capable of dealing with violent patients than are women. Professionalization was thus not only a facilitator for women's upward social mobility, but also a door-opener for male nurses (Chen, 2008; Yang et al., 2004).

In summary, professionalization had gendered implications for TCMs, biomedical doctors and nurses but the effects have been different. Professionalization opened the door for women in TCM, strengthened the appeal of a career in biomedicine to men, and opened the door to nursing for men, but also made nursing more acceptable as a career for middle-class women. The next section considers contemporary statistics in order to explore how men and women used these opportunities.

Variations on a theme: gendered health professions in an eastern patriarchal society in transition

Health workforce statistics reveal specifics of an eastern patriarchal society with strong ideas on the sex segregation of labour and male dominance. In our analysis we focus on medical doctors, TCM practitioners and nurses who make up the lion's share of the health professional workforce (Table 27.1). In terms of numbers, the health workforce appears to be predominantly the domain of women with men constituting no more than 22 per cent of the workforce. This gender composition is closely linked with the occupational structure: nurses

Table 27.1 Composition of the medical and nursing workforce in Taiwan, 2008

	Medical doctors	TCM practitioners	Nurses	Total
Total	37,148	5,166	126,692	169,006
% women	15.0	24.6	99.1	78.0
% health workforce	22	3	75	
per 1000 inhabitants	1.6	0.2	5.5	7.3

Source: Department of Health (2009).

are the biggest group (75 per cent), followed by biomedicine (22 per cent) and TCM (3 per cent). By comparison, the figures from selected European countries combined reveal a doctor/nurse relationship in the range of roughly 1:2 up to 1:2.5, but the proportion of nurses to doctors in the British National Health Services is even higher than in Taiwan (see Bourgeault et al., 2008). While the ratio of doctors to population (1.6 for medical doctors and 1.8 if TCM is included) is significantly lower in Taiwan than in most western countries, it is nevertheless in the range of Japan and Britain and higher than in Singapore (see Blank and Burau, 2007: 125).

The picture of healthcare as a female terrain is turned on its head when we look at the hierarchical order. Data show very strong sex segregation with a predominantly male medical profession (15 per cent women), only 25 per cent women in TCM and a (nearly) all-female nursing profession (for comparison with western figures, see Chapter 25 by Riska on the medical profession). Despite its image as holistic and more 'female'-oriented, women count for just one quarter of the total numbers of TCM practitioners in Taiwan. Consequently, the (western) image of TCM as 'women-friendly' does not easily fit with the occupational structure of healthcare providers at the eastern-western cross-roads of medicine. Further, given the overall small contribution of TCM practitioners to the provision of healthcare as a whole (3 per cent), we should not expect TCM to act as an agent for change when it comes to gender equality and more gender-sensitive healthcare.

The educational structure reveals contemporary trends in the sex segregation of the health professional workforce. Table 27.2 provides information for the three professional groups using the percentage of women among students in 1997 and 2008 as an indicator for change. In 2008, 31 per cent of students in biomedicine were women, compared to almost 40 per cent in TCM and 95 per cent in nursing. Compared to the figures of the occupational structure in 1997, all three groups show a trend towards a less sex-segregated work-force. This trend cannot be estimated accurately for nursing, but a 99 per cent nursing workforce in 2008 (see Table 27.1) compared to 95 per cent female students in the same year clearly signals the likelihood of an increase in men

Table 27.2   Students of healthcare by percentage of women, 1997 and 2008

	Medical doctors	TCM practitioners	Nurses
1997	24.8	26.5	not available
2008	31.0	39.6	95.0
Increase %	+5.3	+13.1	not available

Source: Ministry of Education, Department of Statistics (2009).

in the future. Given that nurses make up roughly three quarters of the health professional workforce, it may well be the case that, in absolute numbers the increase of men in nursing contributes to the 'softening' of the gendered boundaries of the health professions and society at large.

It is interesting to note the differences in the pace of change in biomedicine and TCM. In biomedicine, the percentage of men is higher and the influx of women slower than in TCM; there was an increase of 5.3 per cent in women in biomedicine compared to 13.1 per cent in TCM over the 11 years between 1997 and 2008. One reason for the more rapid influx of women into TCM compared to biomedicine might be the gendered image of TCM as holistic, close to the people and close to nature (Flesch, 2007), while the image of biomedicine is masculine, fragmented and artificial. As mentioned previously, the more diverse educational pathways of these professions may also contribute to this trend. Yet, despite its more 'female' image, still more men than women took up studies in TCM in both time periods.

In summary, data highlight persistent sex segregation of the health workforce – notably, both women and men overall are 'slow movers' in the gendered landscape of biomedicine and nursing, whereas TCM appears to be the most dynamic segment.

Why are there not more women doctors in Taiwan?

How can we explain that barriers towards women in the medical profession seem to be stronger in Taiwan compared to western countries that increasingly are showing a more balanced ratio of men and women, provoking debates about the 'feminization' of medicine (see, for example, Paik, 2000; for a critical discussion, Kuhlmann and Bourgeault, 2008; Riska, 2001)? Clearly, co-educational and equal opportunity laws have paved the way for women in Taiwan's medical profession, but social and cultural barriers have been strong in the profession and in society alike. This may explain the overall slower influx of women doctors in Taiwan than elsewhere and also the persistence of stronger sex segregation in the healthcare workforce compared to many other countries (see, for example, Bourgeault et al., 2008; Elston, 2009; Chapter 25 by Riska on women doctors).

Two factors may be important. First, parents depend on their sons' support in older age and, consequently, invest primarily in the education and skills of their sons. Women born into families with the resources to spare for educating daughters and sons may well have the opportunity to study medicine (Parish and Willis, 1993), but things are somewhat different for young women in less affluent families who are unlikely to have the chance of achieving a level of education equal to that of their brothers. Furthermore, men demonstrate hegemonic masculinity through their ability to earn money and thereby gain social status. Therefore, the medical profession is the number one aspiration for young men as well as their parents. These social and cultural traditions shape the agency of men and women even if gender arrangements are now becoming more flexible.

Second, the Taiwanese medical system is characterized by a strong hierarchy, with men occupying its upper reaches (Cheng, 1998). While hierarchy is a serious barrier to women's career chances in all countries, it is especially strong in Taiwan. Here, a tradition of Confucian patriarchal society spills over into medicine, where many powerful male leaders have tended to form their own 'family clan' with junior male fellows and probably are also joined by their doctor wives. So in medicine, valuable information and other resources are passed around within the 'families'. Occasionally, women reach the top, but they cannot simply emulate the successful networking patterns of their male colleagues (Cheng, 1998).

It is important to keep in mind the combination of social, cultural and occupational barriers and overall low proportion of women in the medical profession in the early 21st century in order to understand the context of the gender mainstreaming policies that are theme of the next section.

The wheels turn: gender mainstreaming policies in healthcare

Unequal gender relations in all health professions and gender insensitivity in the Professional–User relationship were the targets of reform when the wave of gender mainstreaming reached Taiwan in early 2000. Gender policies developed at the international level (for example, United Nations, 1999) met with national drivers for political renewal and new health policies (see Lu and Hsiao, 2003); these configurations created windows of opportunity for mainstreaming gender into healthcare.

In 2000, the Democratic Progressive Party (DPP) came to power following a general election that marked the end of half a century of the Nationalist Party (KMT) regime. The DPP was re-elected in 2004 but replaced again by the KMT in 2008. Prior to the governmental change in 2000, feminist activists contributed to the launch of White Papers on education, health and social welfare as part of the DPP election campaign. During the DPP era, many feminists were invited to take official posts in the ministries. Some Legislative Yuan members (equivalent to Members of Parliament in western countries) with liberal views collaborated with women's NGOs and feminist scholars pushing for the revision of laws and legal regulations in order to change the overriding patriarchal power structure within society (for an overview, see Chen, 2004; Yang, 2006).

From the early 1980s to the mid-1990s, feminist movements focused on raising women's consciousness for gender equality and bringing feminist discourses to public awareness. After the mid-1990s feminist movements turned grassroots forces into legal and policy-making powers, thus paving the way for the implementation of gender mainstreaming from 2000 onwards. The success of feminist activism was manifest in several important legal Acts. While the first step of the legal reform – prior to 2000 – was mainly concerned with violence against women, the subsequent reform Acts expanded the focus towards reshaping the three important pillars of the patriarchal–capitalist temple in Taiwan: employment, family kinship and education (Yang, 2006). Most important were the Gender Equality in Employment Act and the Revision of the Kinship and Relations in the Family of the Civil Law (both in 2002), that were followed by the Child and Youth Welfare Act in 2003, the Gender Equity Education Act in 2004, and the Sexual Harassment Prevention Act in 2005.

In healthcare, the Gender Equality in Employment Act of 2002 and the Gender Equity Education Act were key to the implementation of gender mainstreaming policies (Cheng, 2008). While the aims of the Gender Equity Education Act were broadly similar to gender mainstreaming policies in many other countries (see, for instance, Chapter 24 by Armstrong and Chapter 2 by Abdool et al.), there are also important differences. The policy processes and outcomes will be explored using continuing education for medical doctors and textbooks/training programmes for medical lecturers as illustrative examples. In our analysis we draw on document analysis and other literature together with the observations of one of the authors (Cheng) who has been involved in the education of health professionals.

Gender-sensitive training and education of health professionals

Article 15 of the Gender Equity Education Act (2004) introduced strategies towards gender equity in all stages of the education and training of all health professions. The actions covered pre-service training of staff, induction of new staff, continuing professional education programmes, and preparation programmes for educational administrators. Furthermore, gender training of teachers in the field of health was required and universities and colleges were obliged to offer a wide range of courses in gender studies. In summary, the Act attempted to introduce gender-sensitive education and training for medical, nursing and TCM students, practitioners and teachers. In a few years, the new legal requirements made their way into practice (Chen, 2008).

Implementation started with continuing medical education targeted at an easily accessible cohort; namely, obedient junior medical doctors in pre-service training who were now obliged to take a two-hour course on 'gender issues'. From practical experience it is apparent that while these efforts can be an eye-opener for some doctors who begin to realize the relevance of gender-sensitive approaches in healthcare, others perceive it simply as a have-to-do course. However, overall, there have been no signs of overt conflict and resistance.

The next step was the implementation of gender mainstreaming into the continuing professional education programme for doctors, which is compulsory for the renewal of their licences. This has turned out to be a more challenging enterprise. In 2007, gender equity education was added to the 18 components of the basic requirements for continuing education. It was met with strong resistance from some senior doctors and was even debated in the media. For example, a medical professor strongly criticized 'The Department of Health Harassing Doctors' law, attempting to deny a need for the new gender equity course (Hsieh, 2008). In a media comment, this professor reduced the intention of the gender equity course to the prevention of sexual harassment, and subsequently argued that sexual harassment is only a problem among a minority of doctors, so there is no need for other doctors to take such courses. Some female doctors argued that they expect to be exempted from the course because – as women – they are bound to practising gender equity.

The media protests of doctors against the gender equity course made the lack of gender sensitivity in healthcare visible, and as a consequence, rang the alarm bells of regulators. As we will see from the following example, resistance of some health professionals was able to delay, but not to stop, the implementation of gender mainstreaming approaches. It should be mentioned here that, in common with other countries, for some years now Taiwanese higher education has faced a series of evaluations of teaching and research performance as well as administrative efficiency. Most important for medicine and nursing were the evaluations of the Taiwan Medical Accreditation Committee (TMAC) starting in 2001 (see TMAC, 2009) and followed in 2006 by the Taiwan Nursing Accreditation Council (TNAC) (see TNAC, 2009). The results of these evaluations were relevant for the allocation of grants to higher education institutions by the Ministry of Education. So every institute busily collected data and rehearsed self-evaluations – with both male and female members keen to contribute to data collection – in order to be prepared for the evaluation. By 2006, gender equality was an indicator of the performance and accountability of nurses as defined by TNAC. Thus, nurses were the forerunners of mainstreaming gender into healthcare. It is interesting to note here that feminist professors held some of the key positions in the Nursing Accreditation Council. By contrast, barriers towards promoting gender sensitivity were stronger when it came to medical education; here, the Medical Accreditation Council (TMAC) delayed an assessment of gender-sensitive education of doctors until 2011.

In 2008, TNAC (2008a; 2008b) distributed handbooks to all nursing departments and graduate institutes containing instructions for the implementation of gender issues in accordance with the Employment and Education Acts. Amongst other things, the institutions were obliged to provide evidence-based data on the following issues:

- a general statement on the work on gender equality undertaken in the department/graduate institute;
- the regulation of student recruitment in relation to the principles of multicultural and gender equality;
- the provision of students with the resources and environment according to the principles of gender equality in order to assist in the management of their academic and daily life, as well as clinical practice and career planning;
- activities for students to promote gender equality;
- courses in gender studies and their relevance as an assessment criterion.

The Taiwan Joint Commission on Hospital Accreditation Council (TJCHAC), which came into being in 1998, was not initially concerned with gender issues, but introduced gender mainstreaming procedures in its 2006 handbook (TJCHAC, 2006) (these procedures are similar to what has been introduced by TNAC [2008a; 2008b]). By contrast, according to an interview with an officer by one of the authors (Cheng) in 2009, the Hospital Accreditation Handbook for TCM still does not include strategies towards gender-sensitive healthcare, and does not even promise future efforts such as TMAC did for medical doctors. This is especially interesting against the backdrop of a more 'female' image and higher ratio of women practising TCM compared to biomedicine. There are two different explanations for this seeming paradox: first, TCM has a marginal position in the healthcare system and thus failed to catch the attention of gender mainstreaming policy-makers; second, the knowledge perspective of TCM practitioners is limited to a balanced relationship of Yin-Yang in the body rather than being focused on power relationships between men and women in society.

In conclusion, the trajectories of gender mainstreaming policies into the practice of healthcare reveal the significance of top-down hierarchical implementation connected to general evaluations and performance indicators and measurements. Gender policies have clearly entered the key regulatory bodies and reached the vast majority of health professionals. This is interesting because Taiwan's health workforce is strongly sex-segregated and the proportion of women (biomedical) doctors is much lower than in western countries (see, for example, Elston, 2009; Chapter 25 by Riska on medical doctors). Thus the findings challenge assumptions of a straightforward relationship between numbers of women in the profession and opportunities for improving gender sensitivity in the provision of healthcare. We cannot accurately predict from gender mainstreaming policies the change in the actual practice of healthcare, but the uneven progress at the level of policy and the structure of the workforce at least calls for greater caution in relation to any simple assumptions about the relationship between the 'structure' and 'content' of healthcare.

Textbooks and teachers' training

While gender issues have long been invisible in the knowledge creation of both biomedicine and TCM in Taiwan, the evaluations of the Taiwan Medical Accreditation Committee (TMAC) and the Taiwan Nursing Accreditation Council (TNAC) brought, for the first time, the lack of gender-sensitive teaching material into perspective. In response to these deficits, Article 18 of the Gender Equity Education Act of 2004 stated that the compilation, composition, review and selection of course materials should comply with the principles of gender equity education. The content of teaching materials is expected to fairly reflect the historical contributions and life experiences of both sexes and of diverse gender perspectives. The Taiwan Joint Commission on Hospital Accreditation (TJCHA) was the first to take action in 2006 when a team of 10 authors (most with a medical background and two from medical sociology) developed a handbook. Entitled *Teacher's Guidebook for Gender and Health,* this handbook provides a user-friendly manual for biomedical doctors (Cheng et al., 2007). Case study material presented in this book includes domestic violence, breast-feeding, chronic and gynaecological diseases, masculinity and men's health, gendered mental health, menopause and women-centred healthcare, abortion, and pregnancy prevention, as well as advice on writing patients' medical records using gender-sensitive language.

In 2008, two other important books were published and are now widely used. One, entitled *A Dialogue between Medicine and Society* (Cheng et al., 2008), is edited from the perspectives of gender in the sociology of health and illness, and in science and technology studies (STS), and focuses on higher education, especially general education courses. The other publication is a special issue on gender and medicine published by *Gender Equity Education Quarterly,* an official journal supported by the Ministry of Education and edited by Cheng (2008). This issue contains 12 articles mainly written by highly regarded biomedical professors, doctors and feminist sociologists. It was made available in a run of 10,000 copies and distributed by the Ministry of Education free of charge to all educational institutes. This support from leading professionals and government was a clear 'green light' for the integration of gender issues into medical education.

Publication of gender-sensitive textbooks has been accompanied by several workshops organized by the Medical Education Committee of the Ministry of Education from 2007 onwards that aim to train teachers in medical and nursing departments on gender sensitivity. These initiatives are regulated by Article 19 of the Gender Equity Education Act that says that, when using teaching materials and engaging in educational activities, teachers shall maintain gender equity consciousness, eliminate gender stereotypes, and avoid gender prejudice and discrimination. The training programmes also include issues around gender sensitivity in the interaction between healthcare professionals and users. This is important because research has highlighted the poor quality of user–professional relationships; for example, on average, consultations last only three minutes and some doctors have expressed strong prejudices against and negative attitudes towards unmarried pregnant women and homosexual health service users (Cheng, 2002).

It is too early to draw conclusions about whether and how these efforts will improve the quality of teaching. However, younger members of staff in medical and nursing departments especially seem to be encouraged and are increasingly interested in gender-sensitive teaching material and attending workshops. Within this context the critical issue of how to apply the sex/gender distinction in healthcare and the controversial agenda of gender-specific medicine are also becoming relevant in Taiwan (Lau, 2008; for a general overview, see Annandale, 2009).

Conclusion

This chapter has set out to contextualize the mainstreaming of gender into the education and practice of health professions at the crossroads of eastern-western medicine using Taiwan as an illustrative case. We have argued that this example adds new knowledge to our understanding of gendered professions and gender-sensitive healthcare. The analysis has revealed windows of opportunity for implementing gender policies and trajectories of change that are different from the experiences in western countries. On top of this, in Taiwan, gender mainstreaming policies have been implemented more rapidly in the education of professionals, while at the same time the sex segregation of the health professional workforce has been more resistant to change compared to many western countries; this holds true for both 'male' medicine and 'female' nursing. In the conclusion we would like to highlight two issues that are relevant across countries for those who design, implement and research gender mainstreaming policies.

First and foremost, the findings suggest that the 'structure' and 'content' dimensions of healthcare – as well as the sex category and the gender category – need to be unpacked. Efforts towards gender-sensitive healthcare do not necessarily march in step with changes in the sex composition of the health workforce; and gendered stereotypes of a professional segment, like TCM's female image, should not lead us to predict particular attitudes towards gender mainstreaming. The findings challenge a discourse of the so-called 'feminization' of healthcare and the hopes (or fears) that women are the change agents. It also calls for rethinking the taken-for-granted linkage between more holistic approaches in healthcare – now in demand in many countries (see, for example, Flesch, 2007; Saks, 2003) – and the improvement of gender sensitivity and 'women friendly' healthcare.

Second, the findings highlight the significance of legal action and the top-down implementation of gender mainstreaming, where integration of gender into general evaluations and performance indicators and measurements is most efficient. Clearly, the hierarchical trajectories of Taiwan's gender policies are different from those in western countries with more plural policy-making tiers, a more participatory democratic culture of decision-making and stronger powers of self-governing professions that shape the practice of healthcare in complex ways. However, we can learn from this example that the new managerialist governance procedures, increasingly relevant across countries (see Chapter 20 by Barry et al.), may create windows of opportunity for gender-sensitive healthcare when linked with feminist action and wider modernization processes in health systems.

Summary

- The composition of the workforce by sex does not predict opportunities for gender mainstreaming and gender sensitivity.
- There is a need to unpack the structure and content of healthcare as well as the sex and gender categories in order to understand how they intersect.
- Linking gender mainstreaming to performance indicators and measurements can be a highly efficient strategy of implementation.
- Context-sensitive analysis of gender mainstreaming approaches highlights how institutions matter and creates windows of opportunity for feminists and other players in favour of gender equality.

Key reading

Cheng, L.-F., D.-W. Fu and Y.-P. Lin (eds) (2008) *A Dialogue between Medicine and Society* (Taipei: Socio Publishing Co.).

Chi, C.-H., J.-L. Lee, J.-S. Lai, C.-Y. Chen, S.-K. Chang and S.-C. Chen (1996) 'The Practice of Chinese Medicine in Taiwan', *Social Science & Medicine*, 43 (9), 1329–48.

Lau, Y.-T. (2008) 'Integrating Gender-specific Perspectives into Basic Medicine', *Gender Equity Education Quarterly*, 43, 36–9.
Yang, W.-Y. (2006) 'A Comparative Analysis of the Process of Gendered Law-making in Taiwan', *Political Science Review*, 29, 49–81.

References

Annandale, E. (2009) *Women's Health and Social Change* (London: Routledge).
Blank, R. H. and V. Burau (2007) *Comparative Health Policy*, Second Edition (Basingstoke: Palgrave).
Bourgeault. I. L., E. Kuhlmann, E. Neiterman and S. Wrede (2008) 'How to Effectively Implement Optimal Skill-mix and Why', *Policy Brief Series, Health Evidence Network* – WHO Europe, at: www.euro.who.int/document/hsm/8_hsc08_ePB_11.pdf, accessed 20 August 2009.
Chang, H. (2006) 'The Practice of Folk Remedy: A Study of Baoan Temple in Taipei City', in Classic Magazine (ed.), *Taiwan Medicine 400 Years* (Taipei: Classic Magazine), 42–9.
Chen, C.-K. (1992) *A Study of Social Status of Taiwanese Doctors under Japanese Rule* (Taipei: Institute of History, National Taiwan Normal University).
Chen, P. (2004) *Acting Otherwise: The Institutionalization of Women's/Gender Studies in Taiwan's Universities* (New York: Routledge).
Chen, Y.-C. (2008) 'Development and Change in the Nursing Profession', in L.-F. Cheng, D.-W. Fu and Y.-P. Lin (eds), *A Dialogue between Medicine and Society* (Taipei: Socio Publishing Co.), 82–92.
Cheng, L.-F. (1998) *En/Gendering Doctors: Gender Relations in the Medical Profession in Taiwan 1945–1995*, unpublished PhD thesis, Department of Sociology, University of Essex.
Cheng, L.-F. (2002) 'Knowledge/Power in Professional–User Relationship', *Taiwanese Sociology*, 3, 11–71.
Cheng, L.-F. (ed.) (2008) 'Gender and Medical Education', *Gender Equity Education Quarterly*, 43 (Special Issue), 8–68.
Cheng, L.-F., T.-Y. Chen and H.-W. Deng (eds) (2007) *Teacher's Guidebook for Gender and Health* (Taipei: Taiwan Joint Commission on Hospital Accreditation).
Cheng, L.-F., D.-W. Fu and Y.-P. Lin (eds) (2008) *A Dialogue between Medicine and Society* (Taipei: Socio Publishing Co.).
Chi, C.-H. (1994) 'Integrating Traditional Medicine into Modern Health Care Systems: Examining the Role of Chinese Medicine in Taiwan', *Social Science & Medicine*, 39 (3), 307–21.
Chi, C.-H., J.-L. Lee, J.-S. Lai, C.-Y. Chen, S.-K. Chang and S.-C. Chen (1996) 'The Practice of Chinese Medicine in Taiwan', *Social Science & Medicine*, 43 (9), 1329–48.
Department of Health (2009) *Statistics*, Executive Yuan, Taiwan, at: www.doh.gov.tw/Medical_Personnel/Index.aspx, accessed 11 May 2009.
Elston, M. A. (2009) *Women and Medicine: The Future*. Report on behalf of the Royal College of Physicians (London: Royal College of Physicians).
Flesch, H. (2007) 'Silent Voices: Women, Complementary Medicine, and the Co-optation of Change', *Complementary Therapies in Clinical Practice*, 13 (3), 166–73.
Freidson, E. (2001) *Professionalism: The Third Logic* (Oxford: Polity Press).
Hsieh, Y.-Y. (2008) 'The Department of Health Harassing Doctors', *Liberty News*, 9 January 2008.

Hsu, M.-T. (2006) 'Invisible and Visible: Two Remedies of Taiwanese Aborigines', in Classic Magazine (ed.), *Taiwan Medicine 400 Years* (Taipei: Classic Magazine), 20–5.

Kuhlmann, E. and I. L. Bourgeault (2008) 'Gender, Professions and Public Policy: New Directions', *Equal Opportunities International*, 27 (1), 5–18.

Kuhlmann, E. and M. Saks (eds) (2008) *Rethinking Professional Governance: International Direction in Healthcare* (Bristol: Policy Press).

Lau, Y.-T. (2008) 'Integrating Gender-specific Perspectives into Basic Medicine', *Gender Equity Education Quarterly*, 43, 36–9.

Lu, J. R. and W. C. Hsiao (2003) 'Does Universal Health Insurance Make Health Care Unaffordable? Lessons from Taiwan', *Health Affairs*, 22 (3), 77–88.

Ministry of Education (2009) *Statistics* (Taipei: Department of Statistics).

Paik, J. L. (2001) 'Editorial. The Feminization of Medicine', *Journal of the American Medical Association*, 283 (5), 666.

Parish, W. L. and R. J. Willis (1993) 'Daughters, Education and Family Budgets: Taiwan Experiences', *Journal of Human Resources*, 28 (4), 863–98.

Riska, E. (2001) 'Towards Gender Balance: But Will Women Physicians Have an Impact on Medicine?', *Social Science & Medicine*, 52 (2), 179–87.

Saks, M. (1997) 'East Meets West: The Emergence of a Holistic Tradition', in R. Porter (ed.), *Medicine: A History of Healing* (London: Ivy Press), 196–219.

Saks, M. (2003) *Orthodox and Alternative Medicine. Politics, Professionalization and Health Care* (London: Sage).

TJCHA – Taiwan Joint Commission on Hospital Accreditation (2006) *Self-Evaluation Handbook for Hospital Accreditation* (Taipei: TJCHA).

TMAC – Taiwan Medical Accreditation Council (2009), at: www.heeact.edu.tw/mp.asp?mp=3, accessed 4 September 2009.

TNAC – Taiwan Nursing Accreditation Council (2008a) *Self-Evaluation Handbook for the Department of Nursing*, revised edition (Taipei: TNAC).

TNAC – Taiwan Nursing Accreditation Council (2008b) *Self-Evaluation Handbook for the Graduate Program in Nursing*, revised edition (Taipei: TNAC).

TNAC – Taiwan Nursing Accreditation Council (2009) at: www.heeact.edu.tw/ct.asp?xItem=1087&CtNode=356&mp=5, accessed 4 September 2009.

United Nations (1999) *Women and Health. Mainstreaming the Gender Perspective into the Health Sector* (New York: UN Publication Sales No 99.IV.4).

Yang, C.-I., M.-L. Gau, S.-J. Shiau, W.-H. Hu and F.-J. Shih (2004) 'Nursing and Health Care Management and Policy Professional Career Development for Male Nurses', *Journal of Advanced Nursing*, 48 (6), 642–50.

Yang, W.-Y. (2006) 'A Comparative Analysis of the Process of Gendered Law-making in Taiwan', *Political Science Review*, 29, 49–81.

28

Nursing: Globalization of a Female-gendered Profession

Sirpa Wrede

Introduction

Governments, health managers and the general public in high-income countries invoke nurses as a central resource for achieving health political aims (Davies, 2007). This is hardly surprising, as nurses are the largest group of workers holding formal qualifications in healthcare. In OECD countries nurses usually outnumber doctors three to one (OECD, 2008: 14–15). Recent research suggests, however, that even though policies in high-income countries recognize nurses as important healthcare workers, the quality of nursing work from the point of view of the nurses as workers has been neglected. Recent health reforms have pushed for cuts in healthcare spending, resulting in deteriorating working conditions for nurses (Folbre, 2006). Neoliberal economic restructuring has emerged as a global force that has steered nation-states to explicitly create and reinforce the redistribution and internationalization of care work, including nursing (Misra et al., 2006). For instance, recent research evidence from the United States, the country that employs the largest number of foreign nurses, demonstrates that dissatisfaction with the nursing workplace is the key reason cited by nurses working outside of nursing employment (Black et al., 2008).

The emerging interconnections of the global political economy are expressed in global care chains, as neoliberalism shapes policies in both sending and receiving countries (Yeates, 2005; 2008). Also, in 2000 when the total number of foreign-born nurses in the OECD countries was estimated to be 710,000, nurses outnumbered doctors nearly two to one in the international migration of skilled health workers (OECD, 2008: 33). From a global development perspective the growing flows of nurses from low-income countries to high-income countries are problematic. Poverty boosts a brain drain when nurses and doctors trained by poorer countries benefit the health systems of affluent countries.

This chapter examines the cultural ideas underlying the globalization of nursing as female-gendered work on the one hand and as a profession on the other hand. Globalization of nursing refers here to the complex cultural and socio-economic dynamics that reorganize both professional ideologies and social orders among nurses. Nursing in the UK, Finland and the Philippines serve as critical points of reference in the consideration of key themes in the social shaping of the nursing profession. The UK constitutes the site where the foundation of modern nursing ideology was laid in the mid-19th century, an age when the British Empire provided an infrastructure for both exporting nursing ideology and importing migrant nurses. Finland offers an example of a welfare state context of a country that for many years served as a sending region in terms of nurse migration. Recently, and with a rapid pace, Finland has turned into a receiving region. Nursing in the Philippines, the third reference-point country, has been tailored according to western standards; for more than half a century Filipino nurses have emigrated to high-income countries serving as a global reserve of nursing labour. This selection of countries as reference points of globalization dynamics in nursing offers a means of demonstrating the complex interconnectedness of national settings as well as the continued transformative potential that globalization holds for nursing as a profession. More generally, the analysis of nursing also sheds light on the gendering of globalization.

The chapter begins by considering the feminist literature analysing the professional ideologies that shape nursing, arguing that transnational linkages and knowledge transfers are a permanent element in nursing professionalism. Second, the chapter further investigates how, in the mid-20th century, the welfare state provided the context for the rearticulation of nursing professionalism. The third theme is the global restructuring of welfare states, occurring internationally since the 1970s, that has increasingly opened the provision of healthcare to market mechanisms and efficiency campaigns and contributed to the further reframing of nursing work. The final part of the chapter explores the impact of these developments on nursing. The argument is that the complex social changes associated with the globalization of economy, politics and culture reorder the very foundation of professions and the arenas in which the professional organizations that represent professions act (see, for example, Allsop et al., 2009).

The making of moral boundaries of nursing: a gendered white and western project

Recent scholarship posits professionalism as a discourse consisting of a set of normative values and identities that both discipline and enable the social actors concerned by it (Fournier, 1999). The normative professional identities that contribute to the discursive government of professional fields are products of professional ideologies influenced by both internal and external claims-making (Evetts, 2003). Arguing in this vein, this chapter holds that the Anglo-American understanding of professions as occupations occupying central roles in core societal activities forms an important cultural resource for the present globalization of healthcare work (Mortimer, 2005). Furthermore, these ideas can be identified as both historically important and as a potent influence internationally at the present time, even though the development of occupations in different national settings has followed divergent paths (Mortimer and McGann, 2005; Rafferty et al., 1997). It is important here to recall that ideas about nursing have in essence also been ideas about femininity and the value of women's work (Davies, 1995; Witz, 1992). The present reshaping of nursing as work and as an occupation further demonstrates how the gendered notions associated with nursing have been rearticulated to fit the increasing globalization of healthcare and associated labour markets.

There is a vast literature to demonstrate how the British notion of nursing as a profession has influenced the shaping of the occupation in other countries (see, for example, Choy, 2003; Henriksson, 1998). While the production of this disciplining professional identity may have followed different paths in different countries, it nevertheless has been everywhere influenced by the complex international exchanges and transfer of ideas instigated in the late 19th century by the founders of international nursing organizations. To the early internationalizers, who were primarily internationally minded social movement activists from the UK and the USA, British nursing represented the yardstick for nursing as a profession. This particularly holds true for the development of nursing education. In the long-term, US nursing came to take a more diverse shape, reflecting the diverse pressures of a healthcare system based on the dominance of private market actors rather than the state (Davies, 1980; Mortimer, 2005).

Given the dominant role of British nursing, the critical analysis of nursing history and of the position of nursing in healthcare examines the complex cultural merging of the influences of Victorian womanhood and family ideas, militarism, charity as well as religious calling into a professional ideology. In the exchanges between nursing professionalizers from different countries and the transfers of the British model of nursing education to other countries the professional nurse was embodied in the image of Florence Nightingale. The idea of nurses as ideal women was discriminatory in that it empowered a particular type of woman – representing the emerging middle class – to become nursing leaders be it in the nursing organizations or in professional settings (Wildman and Hewison, 2009). The rank and file nurse, by way of contrast, was conceptualized as a disciplined worker who embodied feminine virtues (Davies, 1980; Hallam, 2000; Rafferty et al., 1997). The feminist literature in the 1980s and early 1990s attributed the failure of the earlier professionalizers to their unsuccessful attempt to distinguish British nursing and midwifery from medicine by interpreting it as care work which, as 'women's work', is devalued in society in general and in the family in particular. Authors such as Davies (1992) and Witz (1992) pointed out that such patriarchal cultural ideas make it possible to treat rank and file nurses as a disposable labour force.

Addressing the socio-cultural context of nursing in mid-19th century England, Davies (1995) argued that the professionalization of medicine was an identity project for middle-class men who did not own land. Their ambition was to constitute medicine as a learned profession, which not only provided them with a respectable way of earning a living, but a way of acquiring social recognition. This project positioned nursing as an adjunct to the medical profession, leaving nurses in a deeply contradictory position when trying to pursue a professional project of their own. Patriarchal social relations supported medical dominance, at the same time that the organization of healthcare was becoming increasingly complex and formalized and created a foundation for more advanced nursing competencies.

Late 19th-century ideology of how the nursing profession should be organized was premised on the supremacy of western culture in general and British culture in particular. Florence Nightingale's project of nursing served the very aims of the British Empire to civilize the colonies (Hallam, 2000). The Finnish case provides an example of how these British ideas travelled. The Finnish nursing pioneer Baroness Sophie Mannerheim was trained in London at the turn of the 20th century and brought home the Nightingale tradition of nursing that served as a standard for the early nursing programmes in Finland (Henriksson, 1998). Similarly, the Nightingale tradition of recruiting gentlewomen to nursing was transferred to the Philippines by the US colonial rule that sought to Americanize the country's nurse training in the early 1900s (Choy, 2003).

For the leaders of the British Empire, a British nurse constituted a civilizing agent that could transform the colonies (Hallam, 2000; Mortimer, 2005); but for nurse leaders internationally, the reform of the occupation opened doors to political action within their respective national settings. The International Council of Nurses was established in 1899 by largely Anglophone middle-class women eager to reform nursing into an occupation suitable for middle-class women (Mortimer, 2005). International collaboration offered useful strategies for the advancement of professional projects and arenas for knowledge transfers. The Nightingale project of nursing reform incorporated Victorian ideas about motherly 'true womanhood', at the same time as the role of the head nurse particularly was associated with efficiency and authority (Hallam, 2000: 20). These seemingly conflicting values justified an internal hierarchy within nursing; they supported the authority of nursing leaders and the subservience of the rank and file both towards matrons and doctors (Davies, 1995; Witz, 1992).

With reference to the true womanhood of 'moral' women, Tronto (1993) argues that this discourse excluded women of colour, immigrant women, poor women, lesbians and other women who were not considered fit for the roles that 'true women' play in society.

Summing up, recent research into nursing history demonstrates that the professional ideology shaping early British nursing associated with the larger projects of colonization has evident transnational consequences that are still relevant today (see, for example, Hallam, 2000; Mortimer and McGann, 2005). The British Empire, with its civilizing activities in the colonies, created a demand for a new type of nurse who could act both as civilizing agent and as leader of rank and file nurses by securing their input as disciplined workers. For the middle-class activists, the reform of the lowly occupation offered an avenue for defining nursing as a profession suitable for women of their own social standing (Hallam, 2000). The most central legacy concerns ideas about the internal organization of nursing. Accordingly, professionalizers of nursing outlined a class-based hierarchy for nursing that built on an internal division of labour. The professional nurse was portrayed as either a disciplined but caring 'angel' or a more militant agent of moral reform who embodied a more privileged femininity. Both images are essentially white and western (Hallam, 2000).

Nursing in the welfare state: ambiguous legacies

In the UK, the gender-sensitive literature on nursing has not assigned the welfare state of the 1960s and 1970s any particular empowering potential *vis-à-vis* nursing. Rather, researchers have concluded that a managerial view of the occupation has largely dominated over a professional view (Davies, 1995; Dingwall et al., 1988). Furthermore, the literature has remained critical of professionalism as an occupational ideology, arguing that its yardstick for 'true' professionalism is the hegemonic masculinity of privileged middle-class men, entailing devaluation of feminine qualities (Davies, 1996). Accordingly, the criticism holds that in the context of the welfare state too the professionalizers of nursing in the UK focused on the interests of particular segments within the occupation rather than the interests of all groups, aiming to protect or enlarge nursing's share of the market for well-qualified, middle-class girl school-leavers (Dingwall et al., 1988). This professional ideology persisted and remained largely untouched even in the 1980s as the managerial pressures boosted the demand for foreign healthcare workers who provided a cheap and flexible workforce in the British NHS (Hallam, 2000).

Experiences of the professional projects of female-gendered professions from the context of the Nordic welfare states have been interpreted in a somewhat different light. Indeed, Finnish scholars have argued that the social-democratic welfare state at the peak of its investment in social services in the 1980s provided an institutional matrix that was friendly to the professional projects of female-gendered professional occupations in social care and healthcare, but also steered them in specific directions (Henriksson et al., 2006). By issuing specific mandates, the state bound female professions to the state and to specific styles of practice (Wrede, 2001). The Nordic welfare state is identified as favouring egalitarian social service professionalism over elitist professionalism. The latter refers to the idea that the professional practice of certain key professions is based on universal knowledge and therefore the neutrality of these elite groups should be protected from state intervention. Furthermore, as guardians of neutral knowledge, elite professions are outlined as groups whose social authority goes beyond the context in which individual professionals practice – the idea of medical dominance over healthcare and healthcare professions is the classic example. From a critical perspective, elitist professionalism fuels 'tribalism', self-interest and social exclusion within and between professional groups. Social service professionalism, in contrast, emphasizes the role of professions as 'servants of the public' thus furthering a more egalitarian notion of professional knowledge when it forms the basis of a state-defined social service. Within this model the state not only has a democratic mandate to hold professions accountable for their styles of practice but commonly defines the boundaries within which professions provide their services (Wrede, 2008b).

It is evident, nevertheless, that in a way similar to the UK, professions in the Finnish context evolved in the early 20th century as hierarchical social orders where 'true' professionalism and social privilege overlapped, reflecting the ideological potency of dominant masculinities as well as femininities (Wrede, 2008a; 2008b). Reminiscent of the ideological connections between professional projects and British imperialism, the professional projects of early nursing in the early 20th century were part and parcel of the building of the Finnish nation-state (Henriksson, 1998; Yrjälä, 2005). Nationalism remained a core element of the ideological projects underpinning the so-called Nordic welfare-state model and the associated professional projects that took shape from the 1960s onwards (Wrede 2008b). The social recognition of the value of nursing was ambiguous, however, as nursing remained women's work with comparatively low salaries. This persistent disadvantage is reflected in the fact that at least temporary employment in other countries, particularly within the Nordic region, has remained an employment strategy for many young Finnish nurses since the 1960s (Bourgeault and Wrede, 2008). Furthermore, even in the 1970s and the 1980s many professionalizers favoured elitist professionalizing strategies that contributed to a stratification and segmentation of the nursing workforce (Henriksson et al., 2006).

From a Filipino perspective, nurse professionalism and the welfare state have an even more ambiguous history. Unlike in Finland where domestic activists played the central roles in importing the Anglo-American model of professional nursing to the country, Filipino nursing appeared in the early 20th century as a result of the vigorous efforts of the American Rockefeller Foundation to establish nursing in the Philippines. The philanthropic efforts were a part of a global public health agenda, within which nursing education all over the world was developed according to US standards (Brush, 1997; Davies, 1980; Healey, 2008; Yrjälä, 2005). In the Philippines, US-style nursing was intended to contribute to improving the public health in the islands (Brush, 1997). In the context of the US domination of the Philippines, however, the shaping of the nursing profession came to follow an imperialist logic; US nurse recruiters soon discovered that Filipino nurses could constitute a ready-made workforce for the US health system (Choy, 2003). The activities that eventually established Filipino nurses as the key group within the growing army of international migrant nurses from low-income countries was built on the footings laid by the Rockefeller Foundation. Since the 1960s, Filipino nurses, primarily trained by the private sector and at a cost to the trainees themselves, emerged as an 'export product' for the country.

The Filipino government has both supported and facilitated the export of nurses, as the country has benefited from the remittance income sent home by the migrant nurses. With an estimated 85 per cent of Filipino nurses working abroad, and with rapidly growing international demand, nurse emigration currently threatens the efforts to sustain healthcare provision in the Philippines (Aiken et al., 2004). In the mid-20th century, the Rockefeller Foundation followed a similar strategy of also investing in educating a nursing elite according to US standards in India, where this strategy had little success in lifting the social standing of nursing, an occupation traditionally stigmatized in wider Indian society due to the taboos associated with many nursing tasks (Healey, 2008). In the 2000s, as the number of educated Indian nurses has increased, a 'brain drain' has occurred (Hawkes et al., 2009).

The migration flows of Filipino nurses, which have constantly grown during the past 50 years, are part of a larger movement of nurses across continents and national borders. The demand for a large number of nurses is related to the creation of large hospitals that boomed after the Second World War. The European countries that remained outside the war – Switzerland and Sweden – soon emerged as destination countries for migrant nurses. In the growing economy of the post-war years, the demand for immigrant nurses also soon grew in many other western European countries, as well as in the wealthy new-world countries. The United States emerged as the largest importer of nurses; in the past 50 years the US has steadily imported nurses from all over the globe. The biggest group has been Filipino nurses, with other major source countries being Canada, the UK, India, Korea and Nigeria (Brush et al., 2004). Since the 1940s, UK healthcare has also relied on 'overseas' recruits and other migrant nurses whose recruitment was facilitated by governments that have defined the training of nurses from former colonies as 'overseas aid', securing the availability of a growing number of primarily female black nursing trainees from former colonies (Hallam, 2000; Mortimer, 2005). The availability of overseas nurses may have contributed to the continued treatment of nurses as disposable labour (Davies, 1992). Such a management style serves to explain why many British nurses have moved to other countries, primarily to the US and other Anglophone countries, even though the domestic labour market has offered plenty of opportunities for employment.

The fact that the international migration of nurses has grown in the long term demonstrates that the dynamic that creates the demand for migrant nurses is not a new one, even though it has been strengthened by the institutional changes in the welfare state during recent decades. From the late 1950s, the welfare state projects of many high-income countries boosted the demand for the nursing labour force, but did not satisfactorily cater for the needs of nurses themselves as workers and professionals. The conditions for this workforce were shaped by managerial ideologies that largely reinforce the image of much of nursing as lower-skilled work, the bulk of which can be carried out by a disposable workforce as long as their work is organized by professionals (Davies, 1992; Hallam, 2000; Wrede, 2008a). The elitist strategies of some segments within nursing contribute to this view. For instance, in the UK, the politics of nursing traditionally have been characterized by registered nurses' hostility towards auxiliaries and assistants (Dingwall et al., 1988). There is evidence from the Nordic countries to suggest that the egalitarianism of the social democratic welfare states counteracted such elitist professionalism, even though the basic dynamic of internal competition remained (Henriksson et al., 2006). Nordic women-friendly family policies also helped female professionals. But the situation is changing. Although feminist scholars of the 1980s considered the Finnish welfare state the woman's best friend – 'better than diamonds' – they now argue that this interpretation is no longer warranted in the early 21st century (Julkunen, 2004: 182). At the same time as the Nordic welfare states, such as Finland, redefine the policies that organize nursing work they have also come to rely on an imported nurse workforce (Aiken et al., 2004; Bourgeault and Wrede, 2008).

The impact of the neoliberal reform paradigm on nurse migration and nursing care

As has already been suggested, the international recruitment of nurses started to increase as the governments of affluent countries intensified their efforts to find new pools of flexible, cheap health workers. Indeed, many governments now explicitly seek to redistribute and internationalize care work, including nursing work (Misra et al., 2006). Currently the international migration of nurses is booming and new destination countries are emerging, making the phenomenon even more global. In Europe, Ireland and Finland, both previously source countries, now recruit nurses from other countries (Aiken et al., 2004; Bourgeault and Wrede, 2008; Yeates, 2004). Saudi Arabia and Singapore are other new destination countries, while the former socialist countries in eastern Europe, as well as developing countries such as India and China, constitute new sending regions. Many governments aspire to enter the market of training nurses for export, an activity traditionally dominated by the Philippines, while at the same time their own health sectors are already suffering workforce shortages (Aiken et al., 2004). Indeed, Hawkes and colleagues (Hawkes et al., 2009) calculate that India stands to lose one fifth of its nursing labour force to wealthier countries. A chain dynamic in the migration of skilled healthcare labour powerfully brings to light how social inequalities shape opportunities for nurses. Migrant nurses from first-world countries, even though they are also influenced by push factors such as unemployment, differences in salary levels and the like, are still privileged when compared with migrant nurses from the transition countries of eastern Europe or poor countries outside Europe (Larsen et al., 2005).

The increased managerial pressures on nursing – reflected in the demand for cheap and flexible nurses – are related to the neoliberal welfare state reforms that have become a global movement during the past three decades. Rather than being a unitary programme of specific measures, this movement can be conceptualized as a hegemonic global discourse of 'reform' and 'change' that has travelled 'along national highways' (Kuhlmann, 2006: 7). Commenting on developments in the UK in the 1980s, Davies (1992) argues that neoliberal reforms treated nursing in an archaic way that reinforced the subordination of women's work. Accordingly, when seen from the outside, nursing was understood as a fairly homogeneous activity requiring pairs of hands and qualities such as dedication, sympathy and altruism (Davies, 1992). The trivialization of nursing made possible organizational neglect, and gender was implicated in the style of management applied to nursing in healthcare organizations in that it expressed the devaluation of nurses as a workforce (for contemporary developments, see Chapter 20 by Barry et al.).

International comparison suggests that neoliberal policies have favoured a commercially minded 'market expert professionalism' over the social service professionalism that the earlier welfare state policies often were identified with (Sandall et al., 2009: 548). Such new forms of expert professionalism may even reinforce certain elements of an elitist professionalism. Expert positions – such as, for example, Nurse Practitioners or managerial positions – are only available for some (groups of) nurses. For the majority, the new policies promise to increase direct patient work. Aiming at greater efficiency, the new policies target the health division of labour with the aim of making nursing more efficient, for instance by the tailoring of nursing roles, skill mixes and teamwork to meet the specific needs of organizations (Bourgeault et al., 2008).

Finland provides an example of a country where the impact of the 'efficiency drive' of the 1990s, coinciding with a deep recession, has transformed the conditions for nursing. In a recent representative survey of registered nurses (RNs), nearly 40 per cent of nurses reported that they no longer would choose the occupation and one fifth said they were in doubt as to whether they would. Both groups reported similar reasons: poor salaries, poor working conditions, high responsibilities under considerable pressure and lack of recognition (Santamäki et al., 2009: 33). RNs who graduated during the years 1987–95 are particularly discontented with the occupation (Santamäki et al., 2009: 36). When these nurses were entering the labour market, nursing was being reconfigured along the lines of new management ideals. Research evidence further shows that the 'flexible' work roles that are tailored for auxiliary groups within nursing according to the needs of employing organizations threaten their occupational identity and commitment to the occupation. Auxiliary nurses are seen 'as the flexible workforce that is particularly needed for routine, work-intensive care domains'; thus they are forced to re-negotiate occupational boundaries and give proof of their competencies in different organizational contexts (Wrede, 2008a: 133). It is likely that this reorganization of health-care work contributed to the demand for migrant nurses that first emerged in Finland in the early 2000s (Bourgeault and Wrede, 2008).

Currently, it seems likely that migrant nurses will become a major segment of the nursing workforce in most high-income countries in years to come (OECD, 2008). The increased reliance on migrant nurses occurs in the context of skill-mix reforms that, centring on the notion of skill, suggest a legitimate meritocratic hierarchy in the nursing workforce. As skill is socially constructed, however, it is evident that power differentials and cultural assumptions about gender, 'race', ethnicity and nationality emerge as highly significant cultural ideas affecting the social definition and evaluation of nursing skills (Hallam, 2000; Steinberg, 1990). Accordingly, neoliberal policies can be critiqued for supporting an elitist professional ideology that favours the professional interests of a few segments, such as, for example, Nurse Practitioners, over the shared social interests of all nurses (Henriksson et al., 2006). Indeed, critiques that adopt a global perspective identify social relations of inequality and labour exploitation *among* women as key features in the present re-organization of the global political economy of care (Yeates, 2004). When contemporary globalization processes forge a 'new' global economy of reproduction, governments perceive nurses 'produced' in low-income countries as the future carers, primarily carrying out care-intensive work such as care for the elderly and the long-term sick (Yeates, 2008).

Globalization of nursing

It is too early to claim that nursing is a globalized profession. At present nursing still remains largely organized within distinct national contexts and governed at the national level. Also, in most countries, the proportion of foreign-trained nurses remains below 10 per cent (Aiken et al., 2004). But the situation is rapidly changing as a consequence of the complex configurations of economic, political and cultural globalization. For instance, in the European context, a process of Europeanization of health policy can be identified, occurring primarily as a consequence of the activities of EU institutions outside of the health field (Greer, 2006). An unprecedented restructuring of nursing is taking place globally in national as well as transnational contexts as a result, for instance, of the growing relevance of transnational trade in health services. Trade in health services includes cross-border healthcare delivery, consumption of health services abroad, the commercial presence of transnational companies in national health systems, as well as the managed large-scale movements of healthcare personnel (Chanda, 2001). The scholarship on nurse migration provides evidence of how so-called global cities, such as London, that are hotspots of global markets, also have a high proportion of foreign-trained nurses (see, for example, Aiken et al., 2004). In the USA – the world's main receiving country for foreign-trained nurses – the growing demand has turned the international recruitment of nurses into a lucrative business for recruitment agencies (Brush et al., 2004). As a consequence future scholarship on nursing will have to tackle a complex challenge that goes beyond the traditional scholarship on gender and the professions. Seeing the politics of nursing as limited to national settings perhaps was always too narrow a perspective. But now, more than ever, the literature on nursing needs to engage with the literature on global care chains that attempts to capture the ways the transnational and globalizing dynamics currently transforming nursing are gendered (Yeates, 2004; 2005; 2008).

A transnational perspective on care not only emphasizes the historical legacy of global inequality, but also of institutionalized relationships of subordination (Choy, 2003; Yeates, 2004). From this perspective gendered migration patterns between countries, such as the so-called 'global care chains' (Hochschild, 2000), are understood as transnational processes through which historical relationships between countries give rise to the specific preconditions and conditions for contemporary developments (Yeates, 2004). For instance, it has been argued that, in the case of Filipino nurses migrating to the USA, nursing is not simply a gendered and racialized institution, but an international arena for the conflict and cooperation of predominately women workers worldwide and that from this perspective, migration, colonialism and imperialism are intertwined (Choy, 2003).

This transnational perspective links nurse migration to exploitation and (neo)colonialism rather than simply to the structural forces within the national boundary of the receiving region, such as the 'pull factors' of labour-force shortages or high salaries (Choy, 2003). In her analysis of the migration of nurses from the Philippines to the US, Choy argues that:

> the desire of Filipino nurses to migrate abroad cannot be reduced to an economic logic, but rather reflects [an] individual and collective desire for a unique form of social, cultural and economic success. (2003: 7)

She further states that such success has been seen as 'obtainable only outside the national borders of the Philippines' (2003: 7). In a similar vein, Ishi (1987) stresses the importance of the demands of the service economy in high-income countries. The economic exploitation of low-income countries therefore reinforces the cultural, political and military hegemony of high-income countries.

Those who stand to lose in the new global healthcare labour markets are nurses migrating from poor countries like the Philippines. To be sure, international migration of health workers can be defended with reference to the opportunities that international recruits from poorer countries gain in terms of access to economic mobility by migrating. However, their status also needs to be considered in the context of destination countries. High-income countries continue to have strong capacities to regulate nursing work at national as well as transnational levels and strong nursing trade unions enact protectionist strategies *vis-à-vis* international recruits. These developments may contribute to producing nationality and non-domestic education as sources for new hierarchies of super- and subordination within nursing. Even though nurses are privileged if compared with domestic workers or sex workers, female migrants from low-income countries tend to be particularly vulnerable to the gendered inequalities associated with international migration. Indeed, migrant nurses from low-income countries stand to lose opportunities and encounter exploitation if, for instance, their credentials are not recognized and they end up in assistant roles. For low-income countries this constitutes brain drain, even brain waste, if the nurses they train end up as unrecognized care workers elsewhere. This loss of human capital is most acutely a loss for the populations of the poor countries where the shortage of qualified labour hampers the development of healthcare services.

Conclusion

Kuhlmann (2006) has drawn attention to the similarities of professionalism and citizenship as normative concepts that provide legal solutions for the management of individuals and populations. She further holds that both build on a hegemonic masculinity that denies women and all people labelled as 'others' full access to citizenship and to the professions (Kuhlmann, 2006). Wrede (2008b) suggests that it is helpful to identify the privileged femininities upheld by professional ideologies of female professions as dominant, even hegemonic femininities. The literature cited in this chapter that has critically assessed the ideologies underpinning professional nursing has demonstrated that the hegemonic femininity in nursing is that of white, middle-class women whose activities uphold western interpretations of healthcare work. This professional ideology also dictates the internal social orders that stratify nursing and divide it into segments. Historically, this professional ideology has nevertheless succeeded in producing the disciplining identity for rank-and-file nurses in a persuasive way; that is, by producing an image of nurses as 'angels' who embody specific feminine virtues (Hallam, 2000). This persistent imagery has served to make male nurses and non-white, non-middle-class nurses invisible. This imagery is currently in flux, but in the context of globalized inequality it is likely to persist.

In a context where welfare services become commodities bought and sold in transnational markets, the new professionalizers of nursing steer some segments of nurses towards providing a marketable expertise, while the majority are shaped into flexible workers. Against this background, the concepts of brain drain and brain gain, often used in literature on so-called skilled migrants such as nurses, as well as the notions of push and pull factors, are simplistic if they are not linked to the wider framework of the gendered and racialized injustice embedded in international migration.

The impact of globalization on nursing does not, however, merely come from the emergence of new transnational connections and an internationally diverse workforce. Transformative cultural change also occurs within the national context, when new healthcare cultures emerge. Both non-local reform ideas and migrant nurses are agents in the transformation of nursing, challenging the idea of nursing as a nationally bounded, unitary profession. Traditionally, registered nurses had a strong basis for unity in their professional ideology, while the lower-skilled groups of auxiliaries and assistants were excluded from making claims of being professional. The current emphasis on multi-professional teams, specialization of nurses into specific tasks and the emphasis on separating leadership into a separate function are examples of new, internationally spread ideas that reorder nursing work, challenging traditional professional ideologies and orders. The complex new division of labour boosts new group identities and divides loyalties. Focusing on a high-income-country context in particular, it is evident that some groups and individuals within nursing gain new professional opportunities, while some tasks may disappear from the nursing jurisdiction. Nurses from low-income countries, on the other hand, gain new economic and professional opportunities, but also face a high risk of encountering exploitation and discrimination.

For nursing as a group with a shared professional ideology and imagery, the future is ambiguous. To be sure, the wider politics of expertise and flexibility are increasingly transnational and the problematic legacies of professionalism that helped to construct nursing as an elaborate hierarchy seem to have been revitalized rather than eroded by present developments. As a result, when nursing is globalized along national pathways, the references to professionalism and skill produce new orderings of nurses which reflect the specific dynamics of particular settings. Research into these phenomena requires gender-sensitive analysis that considers the intersections of gendered injustice with other local and global forms of inequality. Furthermore, a critical transnational perspective is needed, paying close attention to how wider, transnational patterns of economy, politics and culture transform the politics of nursing at different levels.

Summary

- Historically, gendered ideology configured professional nursing as a female profession with an internal, class-based hierarchy and an associated internal division of labour. In the context of the nation-state, professional nursing has been articulated in relation to state projects such as imperialism, nationalism and the welfare state.
- Neoliberal economic restructuring has emerged as a global force that has steered nation-states to explicitly create and reinforce the redistribution and internationalization of care work, including nursing; neoliberalism shapes policies in both sending and receiving countries.
- The transnational perspective links nurse migration to exploitation and (neo)colonialism rather than simply to the structural forces within the national boundaries of the receiving region; these include 'pull factors', such as labour force shortages or high salaries.
- When nursing is globalized along national pathways, references to professionalism and skill produce new, complex orderings of nurses within the wider profession. Research into these issues requires gender-sensitive analysis that considers the intersections of gendered injustice with other local and global forms of inequality.

Key reading

Kuhlmann, E. (2006) *Modernising Health Care. Reinventing Professions, the State and the Public* (Bristol: Policy Press).

Mortimer, B. and McGann, S. (eds) (2005) *New Directions in the History of Nursing: International Perspectives* (London: Routledge).

Wrede, S. (2008) 'Unpacking Gendered Professional Power in the Welfare State', *Equal Opportunities International*, 27 (1), 19–33.
Yeates, N. (2008) *Globalizing Care Economies and Migrant Workers* (London: Palgrave Macmillan).

References

Aiken, L., J. Buchan, J. Sochalski, B. Nichols and M. Powell (2004) 'Trends in International Nurse Migration', *Health Affairs*, 23 (4), 69–77.
Allsop, J., I. L. Bourgeault, J. Evetts, K. Jones, T. Le Bianic and S. Wrede (2009) 'Encountering Globalization: Professional Groups in an International Context', *Current Sociology*, 57 (4), 487–510.
Black, L., L. Spetz and C. Harrington (2008) 'Nurses Working outside of Nursing. Societal Trend or Workplace Crisis?', *Policy, Politics, & Nursing Practice*, 9 (3), 143–57.
Bourgeault. I. L., E. Kuhlmann, E. Neiterman and S. Wrede (2008) 'How to Effectively Implement Optimal Skill-Mix and Why', *Policy Brief Series, Health Evidence Network* – WHO Europe, at: www.euro.who.int/document/hsm/8_hsc08_ePB_11.pdf, accessed 20 August 2009.
Bourgeault, I. L. and S. Wrede (2008) 'Caring Beyond Borders: Comparing the Relationship between Work and Migration Patterns in Canada and Finland', *Canadian Journal of Public Health*, 99 (S2), S22–S26.
Brush, B. (1997) 'The Rockefeller Agenda for American/Philippines Nursing Relations', in A. M. Rafferty, J. Robinson and R. Elkan (eds), *Nursing History and the Politics of Welfare* (London: Routledge), 45–63.
Brush, B., J. Sochalski and A. Berger (2004) 'Imported Care: Recruiting Foreign Nurses to U.S. Health Care Facilities', *Health Affairs*, 23 (3), 78–87.
Chanda, R. (2002) 'Trade in Health Services', *Bulletin of the World Health Organization*, 80 (2), 158–63.
Choy, C. C. (2003) *Empire of Care: Nursing and Migration in Filipino-American History* (Durham, NC: Duke University Press).
Davies, C. (1980) 'A Constant Casualty: Nurse Education in Britain and the USA to 1939', in C. Davies (ed.), *Rewriting Nursing History* (London: Croom Helm), 102–22.
Davies, C. (1992) 'Gender, History and Management Style in Nursing: Towards a Theoretical Synthesis', in M. Savage and A. Witz (eds), *Gender and Bureaucracy* (Oxford: Blackwell), 229–52.
Davies, C. (1995) *Gender and the Professional Predicament in Nursing* (Buckingham: Open University Press).
Davies, C. (1996) 'The Sociology of Professions and the Profession of Gender', *Sociology*, 30 (4), 661–78.
Davies, C. (2007) 'Rewriting Nursing History – Again?', *Nursing History Review*, 15, 11–28.
Dingwall, R., A. M. Rafferty and C. Webster (1988) *An Introduction to the Social History of Nursing* (London: Routledge).
Evetts, J. (2003) 'The Sociological Analysis of Professionalism. Occupational Change in the Modern World', *International Sociology*, 18 (2), 395–415.
Folbre, N. (2006) 'Nursebots to the Rescue? Immigration, Automation, and Care', *Globalizations*, 3 (3), 349–60.
Fournier, V. (1999), 'The Appeal to "Professionalism" as a Disciplinary Mechanism', *Sociological Review*, 47 (2), 280–307.

Greer, S. (2006) 'Uninvited Europeanization: Neofunctionalism and the EU in Health Policy', *Journal of European Public Policy*, 13 (1), 134–52.

Hallam, J. (2000) *Nursing the Image: Media, Culture, and Professional Identity* (London: Routledge).

Hardill, I. and S. MacDonald (2000) 'Skilled International Migration: The Experience of Nurses in the UK', *Regional Studies*, 34 (7), 681–92.

Hawkes, M., M. Kolenko, M. Shockness and K. Diwaker (2009) 'Nursing Brain Drain from India', *Human Resources for Health*, 7 (5), at: www.human-resources-health.com/content/7/1/5, accessed 3 August 2009.

Healey, M. (2008) '"Seeds that May Have Been Planted May Take Root": International Aid Nurses and Projects of Professionalism in Post-independence India, 1947–65', *Nursing History Review*, 16, 58–90.

Henriksson, L. (1998) *Naisten terveystyö ja ammatillistumisen politiikka* (Helsinki: Stakes).

Henriksson, L., S. Wrede and V. Burau (2006) 'Understanding Professional Projects in Welfare Service Work: Revival of Old Professionalism?', *Gender, Work and Organization*, 13 (2), 174–92.

Hochschild, A. R. (2000) 'Global Care Chains and Emotional Surplus Value', in W. Hutton and A. Giddens (eds), *On the Edge: Living with Global Capitalism* (London: Jonathan Cape), 130–46.

Ishi, T. (1987) 'Class Conflict, the State, and Linkage: Migration of Nurses from the Philippines', *Berkeley Journal of Sociology*, 37 (1), 281–312.

Julkunen, R. (2004) 'Hyvinvointipalvelujen uusi politiikka', in L. Henriksson and S. Wrede (eds), *Hyvinvointityön ammatit* (Helsinki: Gaudeamus), 168–86.

Kuhlmann, E. (2006) *Modernising Health Care. Reinventing Professions, the State and the Public* (Bristol: Policy Press).

Larsen, J. A., H. T. Allan, K. Bryan and P. Smith (2005) 'Overseas Nurses' Motivations for Working in the UK: Globalization and Life Politics', *Work, Employment & Society*, 19 (2), 349–68.

Misra, J., J. Woodring and S. Merz (2006) 'The Globalization of Care Work: Neoliberal Economic Restructuring and Migration Policy', *Globalizations*, 3 (3), 317–32.

Mortimer, B. (2005) 'Introduction: The History of Nursing Yesterday, Today and Tomorrow', in B. Mortimer and S. McGann (eds), *New Directions in the History of Nursing: International Perspectives* (London: Routledge), 1–21.

Mortimer, B. and S. McGann (eds) (2005) *New Directions in the History of Nursing: International Perspectives* (London: Routledge).

OECD (2008) *The Looming Crisis in the Health Workforce. How Can OECD Countries Respond?* (Paris: OECD Health Policy Studies, OECD).

Rafferty, A. M., J. Robinson and R. Elkan (eds) (1997) *Nursing History and the Politics of Welfare* (London: Routledge).

Sandall, J., C. Benoit, S. Wrede, S. F. Murray, E. R. van Teijlingen and R. Westfall (2009) 'Social Service Professional or Market Expert: Maternity Care Relations under Neoliberal Healthcare Reform', *Current Sociology*, 57 (4), 529–53.

Santamäki, K., T. Kankaanranta, L. Henriksson and P. Rissanen (2009) 'Sairaanhoitaja 2005. Perusraportti', *83/2009 Working Papers*, Yhteiskuntatutkimuksen instituutti & Työelämän tutkimuskeskus, Tampereen yliopisto.

Steinberg, R. (1990) 'Social Construction of Skill. Gender, Power, and Comparable Worth', *Work and Occupations*, 17 (4), 449–82.

Tronto, J. C. (1993) *Moral Boundaries: A Political Argument for an Ethic of Care* (New York: Routledge).

Wildman, S. and A. Hewison (2009) 'Rediscovering a History of Nursing Management: From Nightingale to the Modern Matron', *International Journal of Nursing Studies*, 46 (12), 1650–61.

Witz, A. (1992) *Professions and Patriarchy* (Routledge: London).

Wrede, S. (2001) *Decentering Care for Mothers. The Politics of Midwifery and the Design of Finnish Maternity Services* (Turku: Åbo Akademi University Press).

Wrede, S. (2008a) 'Educating Generalists: The Flexibilisation of Finnish Auxiliary Nursing and the Dilemma of Professional Identity', in E. Kuhlmann and M. Saks (eds), *Rethinking Professional Governance: International Directions in Healthcare* (Bristol: Policy Press), 127–40.

Wrede, S. (2008b) 'Unpacking Gendered Professional Power in the Welfare State', *Equal Opportunities International*, 27 (1), 19–33.

Yeates, N. (2004) 'Global Care Chains. Critical Reflections and Lines of Enquiry', *International Feminist Journal of Politics*, 6 (3), 369–91.

Yeates, N. (2005) 'A Global Political Economy of Care', *Social Policy & Society*, 4 (2), 227–34.

Yeates, N. (2008) *Globalizing Care Economies and Migrant Workers* (Basingstoke: Palgrave Macmillan).

Yrjälä, A. (2005) *Public Health and Rockefeller Wealth. Alliance Strategies in the Early Formation of Finnish Public Health Nursing* (Turku: Åbo Akademi University Press).

29
Complementary and Alternative Medicine: Gender and Marginality

Sarah Cant and Peter Watts

Introduction

It is widely recognized by social scientists that over recent decades the popularity of complementary and alternative medicine (CAM) has increased in the West, and that both users and practitioners are more likely to be women. Despite this, relatively little attention has been paid to explaining the relationship between gender and CAM, an omission this chapter seeks to address. In doing so, we will explore the apparent affinity between CAM, women's health concerns and feminist agendas, and the extent to which CAM has the potential to create spaces for gender-sensitive healthcare. However, in practice this radical potential has been limited by the persistence of gendered power relations embedded within biomedicine, coupled with the position of 'mainstream marginality' (Cant, 2009) that CAM inhabits.

Viewing CAM through the lens of gender also reveals that men comprise a significant cohort of users, particularly in relation to certain illness categories. This implies that the relation between CAM and gender is not a simple matter of binary divisions, but relates to broader questions of gender, 'otherness' and marginality. The chapter also highlights that women's experiences of CAM are context-bound: that there is an intersectionality between gender, ethnicity, class and culture, as revealed by the use of CAM in India, Guatemala and Taiwan, and within different ethnic groups in the UK (Broom et al., 2009; Furth and Shu-yueh, 1992; Green et al., 2006; Michel et al., 2006).

Understanding the relationship between CAM and gender, therefore, invites a nuanced and sophisticated analysis, avoiding any simplistic assumptions about the congruence between CAM and femininity. To this end, in this chapter we review the existing social scientific research on CAM, exploring the demographics of usage and provision. From this we go on to consider whether there is an elective affinity between CAM, femininity and other axes of marginality.

CAM and social science

Complementary and alternative medicine in the West has attracted considerable attention from social scientists, due to its resurgence in popularity, particularly since the 1980s. Key concerns have included its attempts to professionalize; the challenges it poses to biomedicine; the attractiveness to consumers; and possible alignments between CAM and broader social changes, such as the 'postmodern condition' (Cant, 2009). However, any analysis of CAM is complicated by the difficulties involved in defining the terrain to be studied. CAM comprises a wide array of disparate therapeutic modalities. These include: complete medical systems such as homeopathy and acupuncture; diagnostic techniques such as iridology; practical interventions such as reflexology; and spiritual healing activities. CAM modalities also vary significantly in their degree of alignment to conventional medicine, their underlying philosophies, the levels of training required, their popularity, their modes of regulation, and their perceived levels of risk. This diversity is the reason why the most commonly used descriptor is 'complementary and alternative medicine', as this recognizes the reality of various and differential relationships between forms of CAM and biomedicine.

Despite the considerable interest in CAM from social scientists, the research literature is problematic for a number of reasons. Variations in the definitions of CAM used have a significant impact, especially when trying to gauge levels of usage, numbers of practitioners, or when comparing different studies. Nevertheless, reviewing the research literature reveals a number of themes. Sociological and psychological studies have sought to map the socio-demographic characteristics of users and their motivations. Studies of lay practitioners have concentrated on the professionalization of CAM, and this has often necessitated altering practices in order to align them with biomedical knowledge and practice. They have also revealed that CAM has continued to rely on experiential rather than experimental evidence of its efficacy, which has limited the opportunities for state endorsement and funding. There has also been research into the changing disposition of biomedically trained practitioners towards CAM, and the extent to which this has produced integrative healthcare.

These studies reveal that where CAM is integrated into mainstream healthcare, biomedicine nevertheless retains epistemological superiority and practical and professional jurisdiction. As such, CAM has ambiguous status: mainstream in terms of its popularity, but marginal in terms of its status and authority. Such studies have also identified a *prima facie* connection between gender and CAM, in that the majority of both users and practitioners are women.

CAM and femininity: an elective affinity?

Women as users

Most surveys of CAM use in the 'developed' world establish a particular profile of users. They are more likely to be female, middle-aged, middle-class and relatively well educated, with higher levels of self-reported poor health. Research evidence shows that this holds true for the United States (Eisenberg et al., 1998), Canada (Miller, 1997), Australia (Xue et al., 2007), Scandinavia (Hanssen et al., 2005), Switzerland (Wapf and Busato, 2007), Japan (Hori et al., 2008) and the UK (Harris and Rees, 2000). Although such evidence is compelling, it must be remembered that women are also the primary consumers of conventional medicine. As such the general gender differences in the use of healthcare are mirrored and perhaps amplified with respect to CAM.

Considerable research effort has gone into trying to understand why CAM has become more popular since the 1980s. Specifically users are reported as: being sceptical or ambivalent towards science and conventional medicine and having anxieties about side-effects; being drawn towards ideas of holism and harmony with nature; viewing health and healing as a personal responsibility; desiring to take an active role in defining and maintaining their health and healthcare needs, based on collaborative relationships with healthcare providers; seeking to achieve and sustain well-being, and thereby to prevent ill-health. To date, work has tended to focus on exploring the different characteristics of users and non-users, rather than on examining the reasons why women are more likely than men to turn to CAM (Kelner et al., 2003; see also Chapter 14 by Hunt et al.).

Some authors have made an association between CAM and feminist campaigning. Flesch, for instance, contends that the critique of biomedicine emanating from the feminist movement of the 1960s and 1970s is directly implicated in the simultaneous rise of CAM: 'The holistic health movement and the women's health movement are linked in their origins, their concerns, their evolution, and ultimately, their fate' (2007: 169). An alternative approach is taken by Heelas et al. (2005) who locate CAM use within what they describe as the holistic milieu, an array of spiritual rather than religious practices, characterized by a 'subjective turn', and dominated by women, both as practitioners and users.

Sointu (2006) also acknowledges the significance of subjectivity in women's CAM use. She argues that modern selfhood is grounded in being a self-fulfilling, choice-making, reflexive individual. However, traditional gender roles restrict opportunities for women to achieve this ideal. This leads them to develop tactics aimed at redefining dominant cultural messages and practices, and renegotiate life trajectories. In relation to health, these are often expressed in terms of personally assessed notions of well-being, which may be attained through CAM use. It should be noted, though, that Sointu's sample comprised articulate, educated, middle-class women from the UK, and as such her findings may not be generalizable.

What these studies share is the view that CAM affords the opportunity for gender-sensitive healthcare. This contention is supported by the fact that women often use CAM for gender-related disorders. Studies of women with breast cancer, for instance, reveal levels of CAM use that are significantly higher than within the general population. In a review of the research literature, DiGianni and colleagues (2002) found that while 42 per cent of the general population in the United States used CAM, this figure was between 63 to 83 per cent for women with breast cancer, a rate higher than amongst people with other cancers, and increasing over recent years (Eschiti, 2007). Increased use of CAM is also associated with pregnancy (Samuels et al., 2010), menopause (Kang et al., 2002) and enhancing fertility (Rayner et al., 2009).

There is, then, a clear association between increased CAM use and those areas of biomedical intervention about which feminists have historically been most vocal in their critique. Women appear to turn to CAM in the face of health needs which intimately pertain to their sense of femininity, identity and their relation to their own bodies as women. Moreover, pregnancy, fertility and menopause are all domains historically managed by women, but where biomedicine has wrested control. Medicalization of these territories has involved the introduction of invasive practices, dependence on technology, and extensive monitoring, management, manipulation and surveillance (see also Chapter 7 by Bell and Figert, and Chapter 9 by Ettorre and Kingdon).

Whether or not such critiques directly influence women in their decision to use CAM is hard to establish. The studies cited above reveal a number of reasons why women turn to CAM for female-specific conditions. These include: having had negative experiences of conventional medicine and of relationships with biomedical practitioners; the perception that CAM is safer and natural; the desire to boost general health, well-being and quality of life, and prevent illness; the perception that CAM is empowering, affording personal control over health and healthcare; and a desire to maximize the chance of a positive health outcome, when biomedicine cannot guarantee one. Such accounts, though, mirror the reasons for CAM use given more generally in the population and do not in themselves explain the relationship between CAM use and gendered health issues.

Women as practitioners

The possibility of an affinity between CAM and femininity is further evidenced by the fact that the majority of non-medically qualified practitioners of CAM are women, although chiropractic and osteopathy are notable exceptions (Flesch, 2007; Scott, 1998; Taylor, 2010). Flesch (2010) contends that women are drawn to practise CAM because of its caring, nurturing, holistic, person-centred and preventative focus. In contrast, men's motivations to practise CAM are more likely to be derived from reservations about the philosophical roots and practical limitations of biomedicine. Similarly, Taylor (2010) argues that practising CAM affords women the opportunity to escape harmful male-dominated work environments, reinvest work with spirituality, and explore alternative gender subject positions, even if it does not afford much in the way of material rewards.

Scott (1998) made a stronger case, observing a historical congruence between the feminization of homeopathy and feminist health campaigning, such that contemporary homeopathy can be understood as feminist medicine in practice. She argues that feminized homeopathy challenges the ontological dualisms of biomedicine by rebalancing the power relation between practitioner and patient, specifically by giving credence to clients' experiences of their own health and bodies and by sharing the responsibility for healing. She further suggests that homeopathy can provide resources to enable women to maintain well-being in the face of direct male oppression.

It is possible to overstate CAM's radical potential. Cant (2009) argues that as CAM groups have worked to increase their status there has been a tendency to temper their more radical therapeutic claims and forge an alignment with biomedicine (see also Chapter 27 by Cheng et al.). Scott (1998) makes two further observations. Firstly, homeopathy's concern with the subjective experience of the client may extend the possibilities of social control through surveillance. Second, the equal and participative nature of homeopathic consultations does not extend to the organization of homeopathy itself, in which men occupy the positions of highest authority, and take the lead in matters of political mobilization. In fact, more widely, those forms of CAM which have been most successful in establishing themselves as professions (chiropractic and osteopathy) are male-dominated (Taylor, 2010). Overall, the predominance of women in this sector has not been accompanied with status or financial reward and there is evidence of persistent gender hierarchies within CAM, a picture replicated when biomedically qualified practitioners attempt to integrate CAM into their practice.

CAM practice in nursing and midwifery

Since the mid-1980s CAM has had an increasing presence in the female-dominated professions of nursing and midwifery. The attraction of CAM in these contexts has been explained by its supposed affinity to the caring orientations of these occupations and the opportunities such practices may afford for professional development (Shuval, 2006).

In our own study of nurses and midwives working in the British National Health Service (NHS), we found that CAM was attractive to practitioners because it allowed them to develop more personalized relationships with their clients and open new spaces for occupational autonomy, in the face of increasing technological and bureaucratic regulation (Cant et al., 2011). Attempts to integrate CAM into nursing and midwifery practice were most successful when: biomedical interventions were deemed to have limited success (for example, back pain); the practitioners had some existing autonomy from biomedicine (midwife-led units); the risks associated with CAM interventions were considered to be low (normal births); there was a demand from consumers for CAM services; and the medical profession had little interest or did not object to the establishment of CAM services.

In our study, success in integrating CAM into practice and thereby developing a space of professional autonomy was limited. This was partly because the knowledge base underpinning CAM is uncertain in terms of status and efficacy, and therefore did not provide the grounds to assert professional authority. It was also due to the fact that any opportunities for developing occupational jurisdiction were constrained by the existing authority of biomedicine. Specifically: practitioners were only able to develop CAM services in areas already delegated to them by biomedicine; they could only practise forms of CAM which did not challenge biomedical epistemologies; and they were often dependent on referral of patients from medics. All in all CAM allowed for an extension of practice, but not for an enhancement of the practitioners' professional roles (Cant et al., 2011). This can be seen to be a reflection of established power relations between male and female-dominated occupational groups in healthcare, a finding in accordance with Witz and Annandale's (2006) observations about the gendered nature of professionalization projects.

A tension can be seen here. In our study (Cant et al., 2011) nurses and midwives were drawn to CAM because of its potential to reconfigure their practice in two ways – to foster holistic, individualized, caring and arguably *feminized* relations with their clients and to achieve autonomous professional standing. As Flesch observes,

> [. . .] the very qualities of CAM that make it an alternative to conventional medicine are, paradoxically, the same qualities that lock women into caring roles, devalued by society, and by the medical profession, and which render them glorified auxiliaries to their biomedical physician counterparts. (2010: 170)

Theorizing the relation between CAM and femininity

Although a clear empirical association between CAM and women has been established, attempts to explain this in terms of an affinity between CAM and femininity are nascent. Moreover, any attempt to do so must recognize that 'femininity' is a problematic term. However, feminist thinking which draws upon post-structuralism/postmodernism and psychodynamic theory may be insightful here, in that it focuses attention on the underlying rules of thought that inform subjectivity and practice.

Bordo (1986), for example, contends that after Descartes, modern scientific rationality has been characterized by a historical 'flight from the feminine'. Cartesian thought is marked as masculine in that: knowledge is to be gained through the separation of the knower and the known; the relation between the knower and the world is one of objectivity; the approach to gaining knowledge is analytic, privileging *clarity* and *distinctness* as the arbiters of a true idea. It can be seen that the mechanistic instrumental rationalism of biomedicine reflects this approach.

Moreover, Cartesian thinking explicitly denounces other ways of producing knowledge: subjectivity must be abjured, because it blurs the distinction between the self and the world; also forbidden is any notion of *sympathy*, where knowledge of an object is gained through seeking unity with it. Significantly, though, subjectivity and sympathy have historically been understood as feminine epistemological principles. As such, Cartesian rationality masculinizes thought at its root. Furthermore, this flight from femininity was deliberate:

> The founders of modern science consciously and explicitly proclaimed the 'masculinity' of sciences as inaugurating a new era. And they associated that masculinity with a cleaner, purer, more objective and more disciplined epistemological relation to the world. (Bordo, 1986: 358–9)

Masculine science established itself, then, by naming feminine ways of knowing as 'other'. In such a context, contemporary practices which are 'feminine' in that they embrace sympathy and grant 'personal or intuitive response a positive epistemological value, even (perhaps especially) when such response is contradictory or fragmented' (Bordo, 1986: 357) may be read as resistance to the dominance of masculine thought. It can be seen that CAM – whose efficacy is so often determined on the basis of personal, subjective experience – has a fit here: in being characterized by its 'otherness' to masculine scientific thought, it has an alignment to the position of 'otherness' in which femininity has also been placed.

CAM, otherness and marginality

This line of thinking suggests that both masculine and feminine modes of thought are historical social constructs, rather than reflections of any essential male or female nature. As such, it would be wrong to assume a simple binary association between CAM and women on one side, and men and biomedicine on the other. In practice widespread social and developmental asymmetries between women and men mean that women are more likely to associate themselves with such 'othered' approaches to knowing and being. Nevertheless, many men also find themselves in positions of 'otherness' in relation to masculine thought, and more generally in relation to 'hegemonic masculinity' (Connell, 1995). There seems to be some association between such marginalization and use of CAM.

CAM, marginality and men

The dominance of women as users of CAM can mask the nevertheless significant levels of usage by men. In their extensive international review of 110 studies of CAM use, Bishop and Lewith (2008) found that in 63 per cent of the studies women were more likely to use CAM than men, in 36 per cent there was no significant association between gender and use, and in the final one per cent men used CAM more than women. Thomas and Coleman (2004) also found that women and men in the UK used CAM in equal proportions. In the US, Eisenberg and colleagues' (1998) classic study reported that 48.9 per cent of American women used CAM, but it also showed that 38.7 per cent of American men did. Furthermore, McFarland and colleagues (2002) report that 43 per cent of Canadian men use CAM. Levels of usage by men are also considerable in Scandinavia (Hanssen et al., 2005) and Japan (Hori et al., 2008).

The relative focus on women in the research literature means that, beyond generic characteristics of users, little is known about how CAM use and masculinity intersect. Two themes do emerge from the literature. The first of these concerns how men come to see CAM as a practical option: men's engagement with CAM seems to be shaped by wider gendered behaviour regarding illness. For instance, Boudioni and colleagues (2001) found that even though men are as likely to be diagnosed with cancer as women, patterns of health-seeking behaviour varied by gender. Women were found to talk about their problems more openly and to use cancer information services more frequently, and hence be more open to new treatment ideas. Men tended to focus their attention on prognosis and practical issues. Accordingly, they were less likely than women to monitor themselves for signs of disease; to be well informed about gender-specific cancers; to seek online information about treatment options; to seek emotional support; to ask about the side effects of conventional treatment; and to ask about CAM.

This picture is corroborated in a study of male cancer patients which found that men were more likely to be passive recipients than proactive seekers of CAM interventions (Evans et al., 2007). The respondents were relatively unlikely to ask their biomedical practitioners about CAM, or read books or search the internet for information. Instead, CAM use among men resulted from largely female-led lay-referral networks. Especially significant in this regard were wives and daughters who had knowledge or personal experience of CAM.

Second, reviewing the literature suggests that men may be more likely to explore CAM with regard to certain specific health issues such as prostate cancer, impotence and HIV infection. According to Bishop and colleagues (2010) prostate cancer is the most prevalent cancer amongst men in the western hemisphere; and prostate cancer is also associated with CAM use. Studies have identified a number of common motivations for turning to CAM. These include: to treat the disease itself; dissatisfaction with conventional treatment; to increase quality of life and extend life; to give a sense of control and hope; and to boost the immune system and prevent reoccurrence of disease. One of the most frequently mentioned motivations is a desire to counter the side-effects associated with conventional treatment, including impotence, incontinence, and social and psychological impacts associated with these (Bishop et al., 2010; Porter et al., 2008).

CAM use amongst men is also strongly associated with HIV disease. Estimates of levels of usage vary significantly between studies, reflecting different definitions of CAM, but the modal rate is around 70 per cent. This is approximately twice the level of use within the general population, and higher than use amongst people with other chronic, debilitating diseases (Milan et al., 2008). Usage has been shown to increase after diagnosis, to be more likely amongst gay men than straight men, and amongst those who have a negative disposition towards conventional treatment regimens (Hsiao et al., 2003; Sparber et al., 2000). In contrast to prostate cancer, usage is regular and sustained, with rates remaining high despite the widespread availability of effective anti-retroviral medications. Discontinuance of CAM use is associated with financial constraints rather than disaffection with the therapies themselves (Foote-Ardah, 2003). Patterns of use amongst women with HIV are harder to specify, as study samples have tended to be skewed towards male respondents.

Studies identify a number of reasons why people with HIV turn to CAM. These include: to fight both the disease itself, and its attendant symptoms such as weight loss and pain; to mitigate the toxicity of conventional anti-retroviral therapies and their side-effects such as nausea, diarrhoea and fatigue; and to boost immunity and improve general health (Hsiao et al., 2003; Sparber et al., 2000). Studies have also shown that CAM is used to meet wider, holistic needs that are experienced by many people living with HIV. These range from tangible consequences such as insomnia, stress and depression, to general questions of status and identity. Foote-Ardah (2003) found that her respondents used CAM as a means to rebuild a normal, non-diseased sense of self in the face of the impact on self-concept of chronic treatment regimens, and the stigma associated with infection. She writes:

> Many people find CAM attractive because of its healing power to address diverse aspects of not just a person's health, but a person's everyday life. Its use is not only sustained in its perceived ability to contribute to the realisation of desirable ends – managing side-effects, symptom relief, and reducing

anxiety – but in its sense-making capacities to manage stigma, evaluate health status, and increase personal control over the illness experience. (2003: 498)

This trend was even more marked in Pawluch and colleagues' (2000) research, where CAM was seen to afford an opportunity to resist opprobrious biomedical definitions of homosexuality and unsatisfactory or insensitive treatment.

Such studies reveal little about why CAM use should be higher amongst men in precisely those conditions in which masculinity is unsettled. Whilst speculative, useful insights may be drawn from considering this question in relation to 'hegemonic masculinity'. In elaborating this concept, Connell (1995) proposes that masculinity should be understood less as a specific set of characteristics possessed by all men than as a normative set of social structures and practices through which gender is experienced, and which frame and legitimate men's patriarchal conduct in relation to women. As such, hegemonic masculinity is characterized by independence, aggression, rationality and heterosexuality. It is also associated with sexual virility and phallic power. Thus, impotency compromises men's ability to identify with hegemonic masculinity, and hence their ontological security (Segal, 2001). Conditions such as prostate cancer, then, position men in a marginal relation to dominant discourses of masculinity. This marginality may go some way to accounting for the recourse to CAM associated with this condition.

This speculation is strengthened by the review of HIV and CAM use. Hegemonic masculinity exists only in relation to that which it 'others'. This includes both femininities and competing expressions of masculinity, which it is compelled to marginalize and subordinate in order to sustain itself. In this conceptualization, male homosexuality stands as the antithesis of hegemonic masculinity (Connell, 1995). Despite contemporary patterns of infection, there remains in the West a strong cultural association between HIV infection and homosexuality, reflecting how the epidemic developed historically. High levels of infection amongst gay men in the early 1980s coincided with the rise of neoliberal politics, and were exploited in order to restate conservative hegemonic gender ideals. The initial absence of effective biomedical intervention facilitated this, orientating the debate towards the moral regulation of sexual practice. The gay community, however, was already experienced at mobilizing from a position of marginality, and responded robustly, for example through the promotion of safer sex and alternatives to biomedicine, specifically CAM.

CAM was politicised, affording not only the vocabulary but also the practical resources through which to challenge biomedical accounts of HIV disease, the stigma associated with HIV infection and hegemonic heterosexuality in general. In doing so, gay activists were able to reconfigure the terms of the debate such that homosexuality was presented as a positive, responsible, healthy, unrepressed form of sexuality and lifestyle (O'Connor, 1995):

> The use of complementary therapies among gay men cannot be separated from the homophobia and heterosexism that provide the contexts for their lives, nor from the access that some have to organisations that encourage, and support in various ways, a more hopeful and proactive approach to the management of HIV/AIDS. (Pawluch et al., 2000: 262)

In sum, the examples of prostate cancer and HIV infection suggest an association between marginalized gender positions, whether masculine or feminine, and a turn towards CAM use.

CAM, marginality and ethnicity

It is also important to recognize that women's experiences of patriarchy are disparate, such that some will experience greater marginality than others. Sociological studies of CAM have tended to focus on western countries, in which biomedicine is dominant – indeed, it is this focus on western usage that casts non-biomedical practices as 'alternative' or 'complementary'. Furthermore, when considering the intersection between CAM and gender, it is important to acknowledge the historical ethnocentrism of much feminist analysis. First and second wave feminism have been characterized as reflecting the views of privileged women, establishing a white, western, bourgeois, feminist hegemony. As such, the diversity of women's experience was insufficiently recognized. This reflects a fundamental tension within the feminist project: the desire to deny the master-narratives of patriarchy alongside the need to establish alternative totalizing theories for political purposes. Indeed, homogenizing, monocausal theories of patriarchy proved effective at elaborating a critique of biomedicine and can explain to some degree the turn to CAM in the West. They simultaneously marginalize the experiences of many women. This can be seen in the fact that CAM use in the West is dominated by educated, middle-class, high-income white women. It is therefore important to review the use of CAM and traditional medicine by non-white women in the West and in other parts of the world.

The literature reflects the same ethnocentric biases, and research on such women is limited. Existing research suggests that CAM use amongst non-white women is implicated in complex dynamics of gender oppression and resistance. Where CAM has been available to privileged women in the West as a means to resist dominant biomedical definitions, and assert ownership and self-responsibility over their health, this reflects specific cultural and economic hierarchies and is by no means universal. For instance, in India, therapeutic modalities such as Ayurveda, Unani, Siddha and homeopathy are widespread and long-established practices. In this context, Broom and colleagues (2009) found that women with cancer were likely to employ such traditional medicines, because their lack of status and value to the family meant they were denied access to biomedical treatment. Similarly, in Guatemala, Michel and colleagues (2006) found that menopausal women among the Q'eqchi Maya turned to traditional medicine, because access to biomedical healthcare was mediated by gender hierarchies and the authority of the male head of the household. This left many menopausal women not only unable to draw upon biomedical treatments, but also unable to access biomedical accounts of their symptoms.

Strong moral taboos associated with menstruation, pregnancy, childbirth and menopause served to frame women's experiences. This further disadvantaged the women, as menopause was not discussed, leading to anxiety and misinterpretation of the symptoms as indicating cancer or tuberculosis. Moreover, there was a belief among the traditional healers that such ailments could derive from 'the natural aging process, "bad deeds" wished upon them by another community member (witchcraft), or nature's retribution for being disrespectful' (Michel et al., 2006: 738). Amongst family members symptoms were associated with infidelity, which 'has prevented many women from seeking medical attention for gynaecological ailments as their husbands often insisted that their discomforts (specifically vaginal dryness and sexual disinterest) were the result of adultery' (Michel et al., 2006: 737). Overall, then, the examples serve to show CAM use amongst women can be a reflection of gender oppression rather than resistance.

It would be specious to assume a binary division between the nature and effects of western and non-western usage. In some circumstances CAM use amongst non-white women can also be empowering, in ways that reflect specific, complex positions of marginality. For instance, Green and colleagues (2006) found that migrant Chinese women in the UK turned to CAM when their access to biomedicine was blocked due to discrimination or to communication difficulties. However, those women who were able to overcome such communication difficulties would use both CAM and biomedicine in a fluid and flexible way, drawing on whichever practices and explanations better suited their personal understandings of their illnesses.

A similar, syncretic, orientation to CAM use – one which accepts and exploits the inconsistencies and incompatibilities of different healthcare systems – has been observed amongst British South Asian mothers (Reed, 2003). In her study, Reed showed that health choices were informed by rich cultural and social resources, a complex mix of biomedical and non-biomedical approaches. In turn, these choices provided the women the means by which to establish identity and difference. For instance, through casting themselves as mediators of family health and making choices about remedies they were able to assert themselves in their domestic sphere. Choosing traditional remedies also provided the women with the means to assert a strong sense of cultural identity. This finding is not specific to women however: Keval (2009) found both men and women with Type 2 diabetes within Gujarati-speaking South Asians in England drew on traditional medicines to re-negotiate cultural constructions of identity, and resist biomedical constructions of risk. Syncretism here is a powerful resource through which to construct ethnic and gendered identities.

Such syncretism within a context of medical pluralism was also revealed in Furth and Shu-yueh's (1992) research on how Taiwanese women embraced and rejected various aspects of three therapeutic modalities – Buddhist teachings, traditional Chinese medicine, and biomedicine – in order to preserve their dignity when menstruating. All three paradigms present menstruation as something problematic and in need of regulation, but they focus variously on ritual pollution, vulnerability and emotionality. This created a space in which individual women could choose which account to draw upon in any given situation, according to their preference. For instance, biomedical accounts were used to counter popular pollution beliefs, and thereby avoid some of the associated cleansing practices, restrictions on action and emotional restraint. Chinese medicine, however, was used to resist the biological and pharmacological reductionism of biomedicine; in turn, Buddhist beliefs about ritual pollution allowed women to avoid socially embarrassing situations. As such, medical diversity becomes a means to resist patriarchal authority. As Furth and Shu-yueh observe:

> It is certainly possible to read the elaborate behaviour modifications practiced by our respondents as accommodations to a dominant masculinist ideology marking the female as weak and symbolically unclean. [. . .] They might be said to be participating in a specifically female culture of resistance. (1992: 45)

Significantly, within this context it is biomedicine rather than CAM that provides the primary means of unsettling dominant patriarchal constructs of menstrual weakness, which emanate from religious and traditional doctrines.

In sum, then, these examples reveal that the relationship between gender, CAM and empowerment is complex and context-dependent. In some circumstances CAM has been shown to enable white, middle-class, western women to assert an empowered feminine identity, and non-white women to forge a meaningful sense of gendered ethnic identity. In other contexts, however, the turn to CAM is indicative of disempowerment when women are denied access to biomedicine. Finally, CAM can itself be a source of patriarchal oppression, which may be unsettled by biomedicine. These examples also serve as a warning against making simple associations between CAM and femininity and the need to develop theoretical sensitivity.

Conclusion

Interrogating the intersection between CAM and gender reveals a complex picture. On the one hand there is evidence that CAM offers a space for gender-sensitive healthcare, where women's concerns regarding biomedical interventions and their desire for holistic, participatory and empowered healthcare are taken seriously. Moreover, CAM affords some opportunities for feminine forms of therapy to gain legitimacy although with the dominance of biomedicine these are inevitably limited. On the other hand, the appeal of CAM extends beyond women and an affinity with femininity into questions of marginality more generally.

CAM use is also associated with men whose masculinity is non-hegemonic and provides a resource for men and women from some ethnic minority groups to assert and maintain cultural identity. It would be wrong to cast CAM as always empowering though. Studying CAM use across the globe reveals that it is sometimes implicated in relations of male domination when women are denied access to biomedical interventions. Moreover, CAM in the West remains largely in the private sector and as such the opportunities that it affords are stratified by wealth.

Summary

- There is some evidence of an affinity between CAM use and femininity.
- CAM provides some opportunities for female practitioners to extend their professional jurisdiction and develop feminine forms of therapy.
- CAM can be associated more broadly with marginality as shown through the usage patterns by men with HIV and prostate cancer and also by men and women from minority ethnic groups.
- The capacity for CAM to be empowering is always contextual; there are socio-economic and geographical limits to this potential.

Key reading

Broom, A., A. Doron and P. Tovey (2009) 'The Inequalities of Medical Pluralism: Hierarchies of Health, the Politics of Tradition and the Economies of Care in Indian Oncology', *Social Science & Medicine*, 69 (5), 698–706.

Cant, S. (2009) 'Mainstream Marginality. "Non Orthodox" Medicine in an "Orthodox" Health Service', in J. Gabe and M. Calnan (eds), *The New Sociology of the Health Service* (London: Routledge), 177–200.

Pawluch, D., R. Cain and J. Gillett (2000) 'Lay Constructions of HIV and Complementary Therapy Use', *Social Science & Medicine*, 51 (2), 251–64.

Sointu, E. (2006) 'The Search for Wellbeing in Alternative and Complementary Health Practices', *Sociology of Health and Illness*, 28 (3), 330–49.

References

Bishop, F. L. and G. T. Lewith (2008) 'Who Uses CAM? A Narrative Review of Demographic Characteristics and Health Factors Associated with CAM Use', *eCAM*, 7 (1), 11–28.

Bishop, F. L., A. Rea, H. Lewith, Y. K. Chan, J. Saville, P. Prescott, E. von Elm and G. T. Lewith (2010) 'Complementary Medicine Use by Men with Prostate Cancer: A Systematic Review of Prevalence Studies', *Prostate Cancer and Prostatic Diseases*, 14, 1–13.

Bordo, S. (1986) 'The Cartesian Masculinization of Thought and the Seventeenth-century Flight from the Feminine', in L. Cahoone (ed.) (2003), *From Modernism to Postmodernism: An Anthology (Second Edition)* (Oxford: Routledge), 354–69.

Boudioni, M., K. McPherson, C. Moynihan, J. Melia, M. Boulton, G. Leydon and J. Mossman (2001) 'Do We Men with Prostate or Colorectal Cancer Seek Different Information and Support from Women with Cancer?', *British Journal of Cancer*, 85 (5), 641–8.

Broom, A., A. Doron and P. Tovey (2009) 'The Inequalities of Medical Pluralism: Hierarchies of Health, the Politics of Tradition and the Economies of Care in Indian Oncology', *Social Science & Medicine*, 69 (5), 698–706.

Cant, S. (2009) 'Mainstream Marginality. "Non Orthodox" Medicine in an "Orthodox" Health Service', in J. Gabe and M. Calnan (eds), *The New Sociology of the Health Service* (London: Routledge), 177–200.

Cant, S., P. Watts and A. Ruston (2011) 'Negotiating Competency, Professionalism and Risk: The Integration of Complementary and Alternative Medicine by Nurses and Midwives in NHS Hospitals', *Social Science & Medicine*, 72 (4), 529–36.

Connell, R. W. (1995) *Masculinities* (Cambridge: Polity).

DiGianni, J., E. Garber and E. P. Winer (2002) 'Complementary and Alternative Medicine Use among Women with Breast Cancer', *Journal of Clinical Oncology*, 20 (18), 34–8.

Eisenberg, D. M., R. B. Davis, S. A. Ettner, S. Wilkey, M. Rompay and R. Kessler (1998) 'Trends in Alternative Medicine Use in the United States 1990–1997: Results of a Follow-up National Survey', *Journal of the American Medical Association*, 280, 1569–75.

Eschiti, V. S. (2007) 'Lesson from Comparison of CAM Use by Women with Female-specific Cancers to Others: It's Time to Focus on Interaction Risks with CAM Therapies', *Integrated Cancer Therapy*, 6 (4), 313–44.

Evans, M., A. Shaw, E. Thompson, S. Falk, P. Turton, T. Thompson and D. Sharp (2007) 'Decisions to Use Complementary and Alternative Medicine (CAM) by Male Cancer Patients: Information Seeking Roles and Types of Evidence Used', *BMC Complementary and Alternative Medicine*, 7 (25), at: www.ncbi.nlm.nih.gov/pmc/articles/PMC2000907/, accessed 21 January 2011.

Flesch, H. (2007) 'Silent Voices: Women, Complementary Medicine, and the Co-optation of Change', *Complementary Therapies in Clinical Practice*, 13 (3), 166–73.

Flesch, H. (2010) 'Balancing Act: Women and the Study of Complementary and Alternative Medicine', *Complementary Therapies in Clinical Practice*, 16 (1), 20–5.

Foote-Ardah, C. E. (2003) 'The Meaning of Complementary and Alternative Medicine Practices among People with HIV in the United States: Strategies for Managing Everyday Life', *Sociology of Health and Illness*, 25 (5), 481–500.

Furth, C. and C. Shu-yueh (1992) 'Chinese Medicine and the Anthropology of Menstruation in Contemporary Taiwan', *Medical Anthropology Quarterly*, 6 (1), 27–48.

Green, G., H. Bradbury, A. Chan and M. Lee (2006) '"We Are Not Completely Westernised": Dual Medical Systems and Pathways to Health Care among Chinese Migrant Women in England', *Social Science & Medicine*, 62 (6), 1498–509.

Hanssen, B., S. Grimsgaard, L., Launso, V. Fonnebo, T. Falkenberg and N. K. R. Rasmussen (2005) 'Use of Complementary and Alternative Medicine in Scandinavian Countries', *Scandinavian Journal of Primary Health Care*, 23 (1), 57–62.

Harris, P. and R. Rees (2000) 'The Prevalence of Complementary and Alternative Medicine Use amongst the General Population: A Systematic Review of the Literature', *Complementary Therapies in Medicine*, 8 (2), 88–96.

Heelas, P. and L. Woodhead, B. Seel, K. Tusting and B. Szerszynski (2005) *The Spiritual Revolution: Why Religion Is Giving Way to Spirituality* (Oxford: Blackwell).

Hori, S., I. Mihaylov, J. C. Vasconcelos and M. McCoubrie (2008) 'Patterns of Complementary and Alternative Medicine Use amongst Outpatients in Tokyo, Japan', *BMC Complementary and Alternative Medicine*, 8 (14), at: www.biomedcentral.com/1472-6882/8/14, accessed 21 January 2011.

Hsiao, A., M. D. Wong, D. E. Kanouse, R. L. Collins, H. Liu, R. M. Anderson, A. L. Gifford, A. McCutchan, S. A. Bozzette, M. F. Shapiro and N. S. Wenger (2003) 'Complementary and Alternative Medicine Use and Substitution for Conventional Therapy by HIV-infected Patients', *Journal of Acquired Immune Deficiency Syndromes*, 33 (2), 157–65.

Kang, H. J., R. Ansbacher and M. M. Hammoud (2002) 'Use of Alternative and Complementary Medicine in Menopause', *International Journal of Gynecology and Obstetrics*, 79 (3), 105–207.

Kelner M., B. Wellman, B. Pescosolido and M. Saks (eds) (2003) *Complementary and Alternative Medicine: Challenge and Change* (London: Routledge).

Keval, H. (2009) 'Cultural Negotiations in Health and Illness: The Experience of Type 2 Diabetes amongst Gujarati-speaking South Asians in England', *Diversity in Health Care*, 6 (4), 255–65.

McFarland, B., D. Bigelow, B. Zani, J. Newsom and M. Kaplan (2002) 'Complementary and Alternative Medicine Use in Canada and the United States', *American Journal of Public Health*, 92 (10), 1616–18.

Michel, J., G. B. Mahady, M. Veliz, D. D. Soejarto and A. Caceres (2006) 'Symptoms, Attitudes and Treatment Choices Surrounding Menopause among the Q'eqchi Maya of Livingstone, Guatemala', *Social Science & Medicine*, 63 (3), 732–42.

Milan, F. B., J. H. Arnsten, R. S. Klein, E. E. Schoenbaum, G. Moskaleva, D. Buono and M. P. Webber (2008) 'Use of Complementary and Alternative Medicine in Inner-city Persons with or at Risk for HIV Infection', *AIDS Patient Care STDS*, 22 (10), 811–16.

Miller, W. J. (1997) 'Use of Alternative Health Care Practitioners by Canadians', *Canadian Journal of Public Health*, 88, 154–8.

O'Connor, B. (1995) *Healing Traditions: Alternative Medicine and the Health Professions* (Philadelphia: University of Pennsylvania Press).

Pawluch, D., R. Cain and J. Gillett (2000) 'Lay Constructions of HIV and Complementary Therapy Use', *Social Science & Medicine*, 51 (2), 251–64.

Porter, M., E. Kolva, R. Ahl and M. A. Diefenbach (2008) 'Changing Patterns of CAM Use among Prostate Cancer Patients 2 Years after Diagnosis: Reasons for Maintenance or Discontinuation', *Complementary Therapies in Medicine*, 16 (6), 318–24.

Rayner, J., H. L. McLachlan, D. A. Forster and R. Cramer (2009) 'Australian Women's Use of Complementary and Alternative Medicines to Enhance Fertility: Exploring the Experiences of Women and Practitioners', *BMC Complementary and Alternative Medicine*, 9 (52), at: www.biomedcentral.com/1472-6882/9/52, accessed 21 January 2011.

Reed, K. (2003) *Worlds of Health. Exploring the Health Choices of British Asian Mothers* (London: Praeger).

Samuels, N., R. Y. Zisk-Rony, S. R. Singer, M. Dullitzky, D. Mankuta, J. T. Shuval and M. Oberbaum (2010) 'Use of and Attitudes towards Complementary and Alternative Medicine among Nurse-midwives in Israel', *American Journal of Obstetrics and Gynecology*, 203 (341), 1–7.

Scott, A. (1998) 'Homeopathy as a Feminist Form of Medicine', *Sociology of Health and Illness*, 20 (2), 191–214.

Segal, L. (2001) 'The Belly of the Beast: Sex as Male Domination', in S. Whitehead and F. Barrett (eds), *The Masculinities Reader* (Oxford: Polity), 100–11.

Shuval, M (2006) 'Nurses in Alternative Health Care: Integrating Medical Paradigms', *Social Science & Medicine*, 63 (7), 1784–95.

Sointu, E (2006) 'The Search for Wellbeing in Alternative and Complementary Health Practices', *Sociology of Health and Illness*, 28 (3), 330–49.

Sparber, A., J. C. Wootton, L. Bauer, G. Curt, D. Eisenberg, T. Levin and S. M. Steinberg (2000) 'Use of Complementary Medicine by Adult Patients Participating in HIV/AIDS Clinical Trials', *Journal of Alternative and Complementary Medicine*, 6 (5), 415–22.

Taylor, S. (2010) 'Gendering the Holistic Milieu: A Critical Realist Analysis of Homeopathic Work', *Gender, Work and Organization*, 17 (4), 454–74.

Thomas, K. and P. Coleman (2004) 'Use of Complementary or Alternative Medicine in a General Population in Great Britain: Results from the National Omnibus Survey', *Journal of Public Health*, 26 (2), 152–7.

Wapf, V. and A. Busato (2007) 'Patients' Motives for Choosing a Physician: Comparison between Conventional and Complementary Medicine in Swiss Primary Care', *BMC Complementary and Alternative Medicine*, 7 (41), at: www.biomedcentral.com/1472-6882/7/41, accessed 21 January 2011.

Witz, A. and E. Annandale (2006) 'The Challenge of Nursing', in J. Gabe, D. Kelleher and G. Williams (eds), *Challenging Medicine* (London: Routledge), 24–39.

Xue, C. C. L., A. L. Zhang, V. Lin, C. Da Costa and D. F. Story (2007) 'Complementary and Alternative Medicine Use in Australia: A National Population Based Survey', *Journal of Alternative and Complementary Medicine*, 13 (6), 643–50.

Conclusion

Gender and Healthcare: The Future

Ellen Annandale and Ellen Kuhlmann

Introduction

This is an auspicious time for gender and healthcare research. After several decades of dormancy, a range of policy and institutional drivers for change have awakened interest in gender issues. Although presently we are more likely to be disturbed by nightmares of gender-insensitive care than soothed by dreams of care finely and fully attuned to gender, it is now at least possible to visualize a future where health systems are gender-sensitive and the benefits this may bring. The chapters in this Handbook have shown what has been achieved so far and have also identified outstanding concerns and unresolved issues. The purpose of this concluding chapter is to draw matters together and to suggest avenues that need to be travelled in future research and practice.

As shown in the foregoing chapters, despite widescale appreciation that gender sensitivity has the potential to improve healthcare, unfortunately there is no shortage of evidence that health systems and healthcare organizations and professions are stubbornly resistant to the provision of gender-sensitive care even when gender mainstreaming policies have been implemented (Jonsson et al., 2006). Equally, research makes abundantly clear that healthcare practitioners 'do not always deliver the same treatments to male and female patients presenting the same medical condition' (Broom and Doyal, 2004: 21); that this variation is often unjustified; and that it can result in failure to diagnose and treat appropriately (Risberg and Johansson, 2009).

Accumulated illustrations of this kind are important, but they take us only so far. We suggest that two particular problems need to be addressed in order to move forward. The first of these, flagged in the introductory chapter to the Handbook, is the deeply rooted and deceptively simple equation of gender with male/female difference in current research, policy and practice. This fails to appreciate the fundamentally dynamic character of gender in relation to health and healthcare. The second problem is the restricted nature of much research and policy thinking. On the one hand, there is a tendency for research and policy initiatives to drill down to the individual level, concentrating on attitudes and behaviours in isolation from the wider constellation of institutional and other contextual influences upon attitudes and behaviours. On the other hand, research is often slated at the macro-level of health systems and shows limited regard for how policies actually translate into organizational and individual agendas and practices. We therefore suggest that a richer and more complete understanding of the problems that exist and how they might be ameliorated could be achieved by a stronger appreciation of the macro (societal), meso (organizational), and micro (individual practice) levels and by forging stronger connections between them.

Problematizing gender as difference

The concepts of biological sex and social gender have been an unwavering presence in research on gender and healthcare for over 40 years. They are so deeply, and often unproblematically, fixed in the research and policy imagination that they fail to yield to the periodic reflection that is necessary in order to assess their continued relevance and to retain their critical edge. Thus there has been a marked tendency until recently to: 1) use the concepts of sex and gender to divide men and women – and boys and girls – into two distinct groups; and 2) to read social and biological differences off these distinctions. Rather ironically, to an extent this has been exacerbated by the need to collect the gender-disaggregated data necessary to make any inequities transparent. In other words, it is difficult to escape the fixing of binary difference in the research, policy and practice imagination.

Undoubtedly sex or biological differences may sometimes matter, such as in the context of biological or sex-linked diseases (Hølge-Hazelton and Malterud, 2009). Equally, sometimes gender differences may matter, such as when men and women are attached to gendered ways of thinking and acting which influence their health practices and help-seeking, sometimes positively and sometimes negatively. However sex and gender do not *always* matter: there is no one-to-one association between being a man or being a woman and certain health problems, health behaviours or expressions of symptoms. As Risberg and Johansson explain, gender bias

> can arise from assuming sameness and/or equity between women and men when there are genuine differences to consider in biology and disease, as well as in life conditions and experiences. Gender bias can also arise from assuming differences when there are none, when and if dichotomous stereotypes about women and men are understood as valid. (2009: n.p.)

Further complexity is added to the mix when we appreciate that gender often intersects with other factors such as ethnicity, social class, sexuality and age which can also be associated with vulnerability to ill-health, access to care and the quality of care that is provided. Crucially, intersectionality intends to convey that oppressions connected, for example, with gender, class, age, sexuality and race are not simply additive nor do they necessarily act together; rather they often interact in complex ways (Hankivsky and Cormier, 2009). The not inconsiderable challenge, of course, is to identify when sex and gender *do* and when they *do not* matter. Here it is important to appreciate that gender and sex are both sensitive to changes in the societies within which men and women live out their lives. Although we tend to think of social gender as being the most amenable to change, the biological body is not fixed either; 'we *acquire* a body rather than a passive unfolding of some preformed blueprint' (Fausto-Sterling, 2003: 131, emphasis in original). As Krieger and Davey Smith explicate, 'we literally embody the world in which we live, thereby producing population patterns of health, disease, disability and death' (2004: 92). In other words, the circumstances of our social lives get written on our bodies; the social and the biological also intersect. In many societies the everyday lives of men and women are becoming increasingly complex and variable in response to global, national and local changes which impact their lives (Connell, 2012). It is precisely this ongoing process of change that needs to be captured in our understanding of how being a man or being a woman, boy or girl, may matter – or, equally, may not matter – for health and the receipt of healthcare.

This is not easily realized when the meanings of sex and gender are given with an eye to the political influence that can be exerted on policies and practice. As has been pointed out elsewhere in this Handbook, as well as in the wider literature, 'gender and health' used to be more or less synonymous with women's health. From the 1960s, feminist researchers and health activists argued that women's higher prevalence of ill-health resulted from their inferior position in society rather than from their purportedly inferior biology. So, for most researchers, it was social gender rather than biological sex that was the key to understanding women's health. With the social realm to the fore, they sought to understand women's physical and mental health problems from the perspective of what distinguished women from men, such as income differentials and lack of paid work coupled with the demands of work in the home. While this meant drawing attention to male attitudes and behaviours in domains such as work and the family, as is now repeatedly pointed out, from the perspective of men's *own* health, the male body and male health-related practices remained resolutely gender-blind until very recently (see, for example, Broom and Tovey, 2009; Courtenay, 2011).

Many advantages flow from the addition of men's health to the 'gender and health' agenda. It can encourage us to view health through the lens of the social relations of gender that structure the experiences of men and women in complex and variable ways. This in turn prompts us to think about health and illness as at least potentially cross-cutting what are still commonly constructed as fixed divides of biological sex and social gender, although the extent to which they do this will, of course, be highly variable across societies (Annandale, 2009). At a minimum, the more inclusive approach encourages us to question assumptions that particular health problems 'belong' either to men – for example, heart disease, workplace stress – or to women, such as, for example, postnatal depression, anorexia and other weight problems (Lee and Frayn, 2008).

As Wadham (2002) argues, men's health research and policy justifies itself by a strategy of *comparison and equivalence*, that is, by comparing the health of men to the health of women to make the argument that while the resources accorded to each should be equivalent, they are not. It is fairly common, for example, for authors to begin with statistics showing women live longer than men and that men have higher age-specific death rates for heart disease and cancer. A similar case was made several decades before by second-wave feminists who argued that nothing so powerfully demonstrated the damages that patriarchy wrought as harm to women's health (see, for example, Ruzek, 1978). Establishing disadvantage may then be part of legitimating a new field irrespective of the historical time in which it emerges. Comparisons are not necessarily inappropriate in and of themselves; the problem is that they are often made in a zero-sum fashion to advance the needs of men over the health needs of women and invidious comparisons appear, such as rates of prostate cancer 'versus' breast cancer (Wadham, 2002).

These points are of more than theoretical interest. As Coote and Kendall put it some time ago now, over-simplified views of gender not only mean that women and men 'find their opportunities unfairly limited and their quality of life impaired', they also 'distort policy and practice' (2000: 149, 150). Thus, how we approach sex and gender matters because they have become an indispensable part of policy formulation in relation to gender and healthcare.

Although health policy initiatives reflect a gradually growing consciousness of this, they still tend to vacillate between asserting difference – be it on social or biological grounds – and recognizing that gender is about more than simple differences between men and women. Thus, for example, the 2008 Council of Europe Recommendation on the 'inclusion of gender differences in health policy' draws attention to binary difference; remarking that to

> produce both equality, equity, respect for human rights and for the dignity of the individual in the health sector requires that the effects of *gender differences* are taken into account. (Council of Europe, 2008: n.p., our emphasis)

Yet it also acknowledges that 'genders are not homogenous groups and that different social circumstances may all distinctly affect health needs, interests and concerns of each gender and within genders' (Council of Europe, 2008: n.p.). While we can appreciate the value of recognizing these two possibilities, we are still left with an indecisive message as there is little or no sense given of how they might actually *be brought together to* inform policy and practice. These matters need to be borne in mind in light of the next section, which considers macro-level influences upon gender and healthcare.

The macro-level: moving beyond 'difference' and sex-disaggregated data

'Traditionally society has looked to the health sector to deal with its concerns about health and disease' (WHO, 2008: 1). So it is hardly surprising that policy agendas emphasize that, when sufficient and appropriate attention is given to gender issues, healthcare can make a positive difference to the health of men and women. While this makes intuitive sense, 'research on the health effects of gender policy, or the effect of policy on gender differences in health, is rare' (Backens, 2011: 13). Thus, in actuality 'it is difficult to assess what proportion of ... health differences between women and men reflects failures in heath systems as opposed to differences in human and social resources' (Payne, 2009: 6).

Consequently the connection between health status and healthcare is not easily demonstrated. However, it *is* well demonstrated that the root causes of inequities in health are predominantly socio-economic and cultural in form and, consequently, that efforts to tackle them need to begin at that source; namely in the conditions of men's and women's lives (Östlin et al., 2007). Clearly,

> the consequences of and benefits from globalization have been *gender-differentiated* because of the persistence of unequal opportunities faced by women and men throughout all societies, both in the north and the south. (Wamala and Kawachi, 2007: 182, emphasis in original)

This means it is crucial to acknowledge 'the complexities of gender and how roles and identities change over time – and how, in turn, these affect health, its determinants, health care and health policy' (Coote and Kendall, 2000: 160). This is amply demonstrated in the international context where patterns of morbidity and mortality highlight the sensitivity of health to the complex and multifaceted gender-related social changes within and across societies. In many affluent societies of the West recent changes tend to be conceived as 'gender convergence', or as it is more popularly put, 'men becoming more like women and women becoming more like men'. The implication is that, if the lives of men and women are becoming more similar, then their health will follow suit. While life expectancy at birth continues to grow for both males and for females, the gap between them has been reducing and, interestingly, generally is related to larger 'male gains' at all age points (Annandale, 2009).

Much like their counterparts in the West, the women of Eastern Europe also have longer average life expectancies than men. However, in contrast to western countries, the gap in life expectancy between men and women has increased in a number of countries and hence socio-economic changes are associated more with 'gender divergence' and with growing differences in the health of men and women. For example, in the Russian Federation, where this is most marked, the increasing gap is associated with swifter declines in male life expectancy since the mid-1980s; by contrast, female life expectancy has been more stable and relatively high (WHO, 2009). This illustrates that it is often men who have been more vulnerable in these transition countries (Stuckler et al., 2009). This serves as a contrast to the West where, as noted, although men's average life expectancies are still lower than women's, generally they have been gaining more years recently.

Mortality patterns are the ground within which changes in the various life circumstances, attitudes and behaviours associated with gender and the processes connected with biological sex are rooted. But they are a fairly blunt instrument in terms of health planning. Changing patterns of specific major causes of death, such as cancer and heart disease, and so-called health behaviours, such as smoking, can provide more insight. Yet even with regard to major morbidity there is little direct evidence to date that health policy planning is sensitive to gender-related shifts. In the UK, for example, policy strategies and research endeavours are heavily directed towards socio-economic inequalities which rarely get combined with gender (Doyal, 2006; Hunt and Batty, 2009). While healthcare alone cannot alleviate inequalities in health, as many of the Handbook chapters show, in resource-poor settings with reservoirs of unmet need, access to affordable, gender-sensitive care can be essential to survival. Moreover, internationally, health promotional initiatives and interventions extend beyond healthcare in the narrow sense of the provision of immediate treatment and can support the empowerment of disenfranchised groups of men and women which, in its turn, can be a lever for actions to reduce wider gender inequalities (WHO, 2011a).

As Woodward writes, 'in its brief ten-year history as an official United Nations and European Union (EU) policy, the idea of mainstreaming as a means to promote gender equality has gained widespread acceptance' (2008: 289). In the area of gender and health specifically, there is no shortage of high-level recommendations for its continuance from academics and international bodies (see, for example, Council of Europe, 2008; Walby, 2011) or of proposals for how it should be strengthened through reviews of existing practices and mechanisms such as gender budgeting and gender impact assessment (Payne, 2009; WHO, 2011b). By the same token, commentators have drawn attention to limitations in the way that mainstreaming is framed (see, for example, Bates et al., 2009; Sen et al., 2007). Thus, much like the parent concept of 'gender', its offspring 'gender mainstreaming' is very much open to interpretation. For example, it has been pointed out that there are forceful international drivers for the conversion of gender inequality from a 'women's problem' to a 'societal concern' (Kuhlmann, 2009: 146). This risks the political neutralization of gender as it is reduced to a need to attend to differences between men and women, and boys and girls (Braithwaite, 2005). Concurrently, in financially strapped healthcare systems, competing gender interests fight for the political ear within the seemingly more 'neutral space' of mainstreaming. For example, in some western contexts in particular, healthcare is in danger of becoming a battleground for establishing the relative primacy of women's *or* men's health needs. It may be some time before men's health and women's health can peacefully coexist. In such an environment the question that Woodward (2008: 289) poses more generally – 'Can gender survive mainstreaming?' – assumes particular importance for health systems.

As we touched upon in the introduction to the Handbook, initiatives such as mainstreaming can make gender concerns more palatable than they might otherwise be if they were associated with, for example, feminist matters. When reduced to the need to recognize male/female difference, the ostensibly 'neutral space' of mainstreaming can turn into a fertile milieu for new medical approaches which have the potential to damage the provision of gender-sensitive care. For example, so-called 'gender-specific medicine', which rests on the assumption of binary sex difference between males and females, acquires social licence to flourish. As they become normalized, individually tailored health services for men and women seem almost bound to look like a good thing. And yet the reduction of gender to biological difference can actually be quite dangerous. As Epstein remarks, it risks 'improper medical treatment of a patient who doesn't conform to the stereotype of his or her group' (2007: 248). Much 'gender-specific medicine' is hospital-based and high-tech in its approach to care, and is connected with the pharmaceutical industry. The array of social factors that influence health and healthcare, ranging from the social contexts in which men and women live their lives, to the social contexts of care, find little or no place within this highly commercialized and individualized framework (Annandale and Hammarström, 2011).

This discussion of the macro-context has highlighted an array of factors that need to be taken into account when considering the obstacles to gender-appropriate healthcare. This has included conceptual matters such as how gender is conceived as 'specific' to different groups, or as more complex, contextual and changing, and how the choice of approach might inform gender mainstreaming policies. As others have pointed out, 'gender mainstreaming is an essentially contested concept and practice' (Walby, 2005: 321). This means that it is highly malleable. So although, as the term mainstreaming itself implies, the intent is to cascade gender awareness through a systems approach to organizations and their practices, well-intentioned policies can encounter all manner of dams and diversions as they travel from their source. This directs us to the meso-level or organizational context within which policies are implemented. This is especially important at the present time as new health policies and political opportunity structures have expanded from the macro-level of institutional regulation and policies to the meso-level of healthcare providers and service users (see, for example, Kuhlmann et al., 2011).

The meso-level: expanding the scope of gender-sensitive healthcare

As noted in the introductory chapter to the Handbook, gender policies may travel more effectively into the meso-level or organizational level when they are harnessed to business goals and can be seen to contribute to good organizational stewardship of health systems (Payne, 2009; Walby, 2011). This identifies that political opportunity structures for gender-sensitive healthcare are arising not only from women's and men's healthcare activism but also from new – and seemingly gender-neutral – demands for tighter regulation of healthcare providers and an overall changing governance of public sector services (Kuhlmann, 2009). As a result negotiations around gender-sensitive care are becoming more complex, include more decentralized models of governance, and involve a broader range of players than used to be the case.

A fusion of risks and opportunities flows from these new forms of governance. For example, new models of governing and monitoring services, such as target-setting, standardization and evidence-based health policies, can ease the way for the development of gender-sensitive performance indicators and clinical practice guidelines (Kuhlmann, 2009). However, these are not magic potions; practice guidelines can help raise awareness of the relationship between sex and gender factors in healthcare, but they are also in peril of turning into hazardous mechanistic solutions. Just as so-called cultural competence cannot be achieved by learning about the supposed characteristics of various ethnic groups, it is not possible to 'gen up' on gender criteria and simply apply them to practice. There is then a real risk of the routinization and oversimplification that often characterizes top-down approaches to gender mainstreaming at the organizational level.

There is also a danger that gender issues may get lost in the 'jungle' of network-based governance. It has been argued that, to have a chance of being effective, gender mainstreaming needs to be 'owned institutionally' and supported by senior management (WHO, 2008: 148). Although this may be a necessary condition for gender-sensitive care, it is not in itself sufficient. As has been made clear in wider debates, as well as in relation to healthcare specifically, organizational cultures typically are 'thickly encrusted with traditional (usually male dominated) values, relationships, and methods of work which are a challenge to achieving gender equality and equity' (Sen et al., 2007: 149).

Hence cascading gender-sensitive policies and practices through organizations – from senior management to the practitioner dealing directly with patients – is always liable to stumble on the shards of deeply embedded cultural practices. When we add to this the sheer complexity of most healthcare institutions, it is perhaps hardly surprising that gender mainstreaming and associated policies travel slowly and bumpily into the practice of healthcare. Even countries which have had health policy initiatives in place for some time, such as Sweden, have shown only minor improvements in gender equity to date (Jonsson et al., 2006). Given the growing recognition of the central role that middle managers play in the leadership, organization and service performance of health institutions, it is surprising that they have been neglected in recent discussions of gender and healthcare. Thus we know very little about the attitudes that managers below the top management level hold in relation to gender mainstreaming and how it might be achieved (Kuhlmann and Annandale, 2012).

Our existing knowledge of both the gendering of healthcare and implementation of gender-sensitive practice has also been limited to date by the restricted focus of research. Although we should not be too critical given that it is still early days for gender and healthcare research, it is fair to say that the focus has tended to be on particular health conditions, on particular sectors of healthcare and categories of providers, and on particular age groups of patients. Developing a more complete picture of these dimensions of care is important to understanding what works.

As Doyal (2006) remarks with specific reference to the British National Health Service (NHS), health service modernization agendas are beginning to pay attention to the needs of men and women, but most of the strategies proposed are sex-specific; that is, they are concerned with conditions that affect only or mostly men or only or mostly women. She explains that 'there appears too little recognition of the fact that sex and gender issues need to be incorporated into the planning of *all* health services for both women and men' (Doyal, 2006: 155, our emphasis).

Coronary heart disease (CHD) is a prominent exception internationally to the focus on sex-specific health problems. To date CHD has been a – if not *the* – major focus for research on gender and healthcare. The high incidence of CHD amongst both men and women across the globe and related high costs to healthcare providers makes this highly appropriate. Moreover, as is highlighted in several of the Handbook chapters, an array of studies has shown that both biological sex and social gender can be very important to shaping, and understanding, disease, symptoms, diagnosis and treatment. However, we need to keep in mind that insights from CHD are not necessarily transferable to other health conditions or care contexts. With a store of knowledge it is timely to step back and ask: What lessons can be learnt from CHD for other areas of health and healthcare? One such lesson is that when the emphasis is placed on sex and gender as binary difference, as has sometimes happened in gender and CHD, research and practice can be drawn in highly medicalized and specialized directions such as the development of gender-specific – read sex-specific – cardiology which inappropriately pushes gender-related social factors out of frame (see, for example, Michelena et al., 2010).

In the western context, with some exceptions such as mental health (see, for example, WHO, 2004), gender concerns have tended to be associated with acute care and with the activities of particular categories of providers, such as physicians. This no doubt reflects the dominance of hospital-based medicine and the medical profession in the health systems of most resource-rich countries. Even so, the failure to bring a thoroughgoing gender focus to other important areas of care is surprising. For example, women's greater longevity does not seem to have drawn much attention to gender issues in the provision of long-term care or in palliative care. This raises a wider puzzle which concerns age: gender only seems really to matter in infancy (for example, excess female deaths in resource-poor countries), adolescence (for example, sexual health and mental health) and middle age (for example, CHD). There is a relative absence of studies of gender and the healthcare of children beyond infancy and a relative absence of studies of older people. To be sure, attention has been drawn to the role of gender in utilization of services, but there has been minimal attention to the role gender expectations may play in the actual provision of care of various kinds – from minor symptoms to major illness and continuing care – for these age groups. This neglect is notable given the awareness of variations in the self-assessed health of boys and girls (Torsheim et al., 2006) and older men and women (Arber and Cooper, 1999).

The abiding focus on the medical profession – and to a much lesser extent on the nursing profession – has generated a 'black box' in relation to policy and research when it comes to other health professional groups. This is especially surprising in the field of complementary and alternative medicine (CAM) for two reasons. First, CAM therapies are increasingly popular; many healthcare systems across the globe have responded to new demands from service users by including a range of CAM therapies in public sector healthcare and are also improving the regulation of CAM practitioners, thereby furthering professionalization of a wide range of occupational groups (Cant et al., 2011). Second, in western countries, alternative therapies emerged within the context of a medical counter-culture and were especially fuelled by the women's health movement of the 1970s (see Ehrenreich and English, 1979). Thus, CAM seems to be connected to women's demands for more holistic healthcare. In many national contexts women are more likely than men to use most forms of healthcare, something which may be amplified in CAM use where women also make up the majority of service users today (Bishop and Lewith, 2008).

The 'female' image of CAM as highly client-sensitive is complemented by overall high numbers of women on the provider side (Flesch, 2007). It would however be naive to interpret CAM as simply due to a natural female alliance. Although statistical data are limited overall, there is significant variation in both sex ratios and gendered images in the wide range of occupations providing services subsumed under the CAM umbrella. For example, some groups, such as osteopaths and chiropractors, show higher ratios of men than other groups, such as, for instance, herbalists. As well, the provision of CAM therapies is highly dependent on the regulatory architecture of health systems. CAM therapists often do not have a market monopoly since physicians also offer CAM services, such as acupuncture, in many countries. Furthermore, empirical evidence on the impact of the female bias on the quality of care provided by CAM therapists is largely missing.

A further effect of the rather obdurate focus on *particular* professional groups, such as physicians, and to a lesser extent nurses, is that the wider constellation of care can get neglected. Although individuals can make a difference, healthcare is typically a collective endeavour and hence the ways that healthcare providers interact – both within and across professional groups – is vital to the provision of gender-sensitive care. This has become even more important in recent years as healthcare in many settings has become increasingly specialized and complex and in need of effective coordination. Achievements from a pocket of gender-sensitive care in one part of the system can quite easily be neutralized by gender-insensitivity in another. Thus, for example, a primary care provider's appreciation that a young woman might be reluctant to reveal that her health problems are due to intimate partner violence could be effaced by lack of awareness in the acute-care context. Therefore more consideration could to be given to care pathways, to the exchange of information, and to processes of decision-making between different categories of providers in relation to gender. This calls for closer attention to the micro-level of care.

The micro-level: bringing gendered interaction and the patient into healthcare research

It could be said that the very association of 'gender and healthcare' itself originated in micro-level policies and practices. During the 1960s and 1970s, feminist activists and academics threw significant light on the gendered ideologies imported into healthcare to the detriment of women (see, for example, Ruzek,

1978). The dynamics of interaction between the male-dominated medical profession and their female patients became a major focus of academic research
as attention was drawn to the 'medical model' of women which was adjudged
to rest on the tacit belief that men are normal whereas women are abnormal,
which emanates from women's 'natural' reproductive role. An abiding concern
of this time was the casting of the (female) patient in a truly patient or passive
role. For example, studies emerged of sexist assumptions in medical consultation and their impact on information exchange, decision-making and quality
of care (see, for example, Wallen et al., 1979).

We have witnessed a sea change in the conceptualization of the patient in
the intervening years as, with the rise of consumerism, they have been recast
as active negotiators and 'expert patients' in the healthcare encounter. While
this varies internationally, patients are 'active and engaged with others' in
healthcare contexts within which they 'literally create outcomes, new relationships and new structures' (Olesen, 2002: 254). This concerns not only formal
health systems but also the wider healthcare division of labour of which men
and women are a part, such as care in the home and community, something
which can be especially important in resource-poor settings. As Olesen puts it,
patients and potential patients are 'both worker and work object in the interaction with others in the system' (2002: 255).

But we are unlikely to realize this from most research on gender in healthcare,
where patients appear on the stage mainly as supporting characters rather than
active participants. The impression given is that what patients think and do
matters *before* they get into the healthcare setting. Thus we have a growing body
of research on how women and men interpret symptoms, seek help and make
their way into particular care contexts. But there has been relatively little regard
to date for what happens *once they get into care*, since, more often than not, at
this point attention shifts to what *practitioners* think about patients and how this
impacts on their decision-making (see, for example, Foss and Sundby, 2003).

Although organizational life might at first glance appear rule-bound, the
everyday reality is far more precarious. As Strauss and colleagues put it some
time ago,

> hardly anyone knows all the extant rules, much less exactly what they
> apply to, for whom, and with what sanctions ... [Hence] the importance of
> negotiation – the processes of give-and-take, of diplomacy, of bargaining –
> which characterizes organizational life. (Strauss et al., 1963: 148)

If we want to ask how and in what ways gender might get built into this mix,
we cannot find answers the question by reference to healthcare providers alone.
Rather we need to engage the patient's point of view and ask such questions
as: How far are patients themselves attuned to the gendering of care? How, if

at all, do they seek to mobilize gender identities in healthcare encounters to achieve personally desired outcomes? In other words, we need to pay better research attention to the various ways in which the patient's experience of care is impacted by the array of gender matters that suffuse healthcare. One way to achieve this understanding is through context-sensitive observational studies of care 'in action' and, since gender concerns may not be overt and hence readily observable, through interview studies of patient experience.

Conclusion

The objective of this chapter has been to draw connections between the macro, meso and micro dimensions of gender and healthcare in order to facilitate a more complete and forward-thinking analysis of the barriers to and enablers of gender-sensitive care and gender mainstreaming policies. Here we should stress that the connections between levels are context-specific; there is no set formula for how policies and practices travel from the macro to the meso and micro-levels – and potentially back again. Indeed, this process is likely to be highly variable according to the national contexts within which health systems are embedded and the health problem of concern.

A number of other connections have threaded though our discussion of these different levels of policy and practice. First is the connection between biological sex and social gender. We have raised a concern that simplistic binary notions of sex and gender are difficult to get away from. They are easily fixed in the research and practice imagination and lend themselves to naive and potentially risky associations between certain health conditions, attitudes, beliefs and behaviours, and being either a man or a woman, which may work against the delivery of appropriate care. Thus we have suggested that the meanings of sex and gender and the connections between them need to be subject to ongoing reflection so that sterile and ineffective conceptions do not get fixed in practice.

A second kind of connection that has been underscored is the interaction between *all* key stakeholders in health systems, which includes the variety of healthcare providers and managers as well as patients themselves. Finally, as foregrounded in many of the Handbook chapters, there is the awareness that gender never stands alone; in healthcare as elsewhere, its expression will vary as it intersects with the way healthcare generally is governed and with other influential social factors that are also associated with health and healthcare, such as age, ethnicity, sexuality and socio-economic status.

References

Annandale, E. (2009) 'Health and Gender', in W. Cockerham (ed.), *The New Companion to Medical Sociology* (New York: Wiley-Blackwell), 97–112.

Annandale, E. and A. Hammarström (2011) 'Constructing the "Gender-Specific Body": A Critical Discourse Analysis of Publications in the Field of Gender-Specific Medicine', *Health*, 15 (6), 571–87.

Arber, S. and H. Cooper (1999) 'Gender Differences in Health in Later Life: The New Paradox?, *Social Science & Medicine*, 48 (1), 61–76.

Backens, M. (2011) *Gender Policy and Gender Equality in a Public Health Perspective* (Stockholm: Karolinska Institutet).

Bates, L., O. Hankivsky and K. W. Springer (2009) 'Gender and Health Inequities: A Comment on the Final Report of the WHO Commission on Social Determinants of Health', *Social Science & Medicine*, 69 (7), 1002–4.

Bishop, F. L. and G. T. Lewith (2008) 'Who Uses CAM? A Narrative Review of Demographic Characteristics and Health Factors Associated with CAM Use', *Evidence-based Complementary and Alternative Medicine*, 7 (1), 11–28, at: http://ecam.oxford-journals.org/cgi/content/full/nen023v1, accessed 22 November 2009.

Braithwaite, M. (2005) EQUALPOL. *Gender-sensitive and Women-friendly Public Policies: A Comparative Analysis of Their Progress and Impact. Final Report*, EU Research on Social Sciences and Humanities (Brussels: European Commission), at: www.equapol.gr/pdf/HPSE-CT-2002-00136_DEL1_StateOfTheArt.pdf, accessed 22 November 2009.

Broom, D. and L. Doyal (2004) 'Sex and Gender in Health Care and Health Policy', in J. Healy and M. McKee (eds), *Accessing Health Care: Responding to Diversity* (Oxford: Oxford University Press), 19–32.

Broom, A. and P. Tovey (2009) 'Introduction: Men's Health in Context', in A. Broom and P. Tovey (eds), *Men's Health: Body, Identity and Social Context* (London: Wiley-Blackwell), 1–31.

Cant, S., P. Watts and A. Ruston (2011) 'Negotiating Competency, Professionalism and Risk: the Integration of Complementary and Alternative Medicine by Nurses and Midwives in the NHS', *Social Science & Medicine*, 72 (4), 529–36.

Connell, R. (2012) 'Gender, Health and Theory: Conceptualising the Issue, in Local and Global Perspective', *Social Science & Medicine*, at: http://dx.doi.org/10.1016/j.socscimed.2011.06.006, accessed 2 March 2012.

Coote, A. and L. Kendall (2000) 'Well Women and Medicine Men: Gendering the Health Policy Agenda', in A. Coote (ed.), *The New Gender Agenda* (London: Institute for Public Policy Research), 149–61.

Council of Europe (2008) *Recommendation CM/Rec(2008)1 of the Committee of Ministers to Member States on the Inclusion of Gender Differences in Health Policy*, at: www.inmujer.migualdad.es/MUJER/politicas/docs/14_CMRec_2008_1E.pdf, accessed 16 November 2009.

Courtenay, W. (2011) *Dying To Be Men* (London: Routledge).

Doyal, L. (2006) 'Sex, Gender and Medicine: The Case of the NHS', in D. Kelleher, J. Gabe and G. Williams (eds), *Challenging Medicine*, second edition (London: Routledge), 146–61.

Ehrenreich, B. and D. English (1979) *For Her Own Good. 150 Years of Expert Advice to Women* (New York: Anchor Press).

Epstein, S. (2007) *Inclusion. The Politics of Difference in Medical Research* (London: Chicago University Press).

Fausto-Sterling, A. (2003) 'The Problem with Sex/Gender and Nature/Nurture', in S. Williams, L. Birke and G. Bendelow (eds), *Debating Biology* (London: Routledge), 123–32.

Flesch, H. (2007) 'Silent Voices: Women, Complementary Medicine, and the Co-optation of Change', *Complementary Therapies in Clinical Practice*, 13 (3), 166–73.

Foss, C. and K. Sundby (2003) 'The Construction of the Gendered Patient: Hospital Staff's Attitudes to Female and Male Patients', *Patient Education and Counselling*, 49 (1), 45–52.

Hankivsky, O. and R. Cormier (2009) *Intersectionality: Moving Women's Health Research and Policy Forward* (Vancouver: Women's Health Research Network), at: www.whrn.ca, accessed 1 October 2011.

Hølge-Hazelton, B. and K. Malterud (2009) 'Gender in Medicine – Does It Matter?', *Scandinavian Journal of Public Health*, 37 (2), 139–45.

Hunt, K. and D. Batty (2009) 'Gender and Socio-economic Inequalities in Mortality and Health Behaviours: An Overview', in H. Graham (ed.), *Understanding Health Inequalities*, second edition (Maidenhead: Open University Press), 141–61.

Jonsson, P. M., I. Schmidt, V. Sparring and G. Tomson (2006) 'Gender Equity in Health Care in Sweden – Minor Improvements since the 1990s', *Health Policy*, 77 (1), 24–36.

Krieger, N. and G. Davey Smith (2004) '"Bodies Count" and Body Counts: Social Epidemiology and Embodying Inequality', *Epidemiological Reviews*, 26 (1), 92–103.

Kuhlmann, E. (2009) 'From Women's Health to Gender Mainstreaming and Back Again: Linking Feminist Agendas and New Governance in Healthcare'', *Current Sociology*, 57 (2), 135–54.

Kuhlmann, E. and Annandale, E. (2012) 'Mainstreaming Gender into Healthcare: A Scoping Exercise into Policy Transfer in England and Germany', *Current Sociology*, Special Issue, 60 (4).

Kuhlmann, E., V. Burau, C. Larsen, R. Lewandowski, C. Lionis and J. Repullo (2011) 'Medicine and Management in European Healthcare Systems: How Do They Matter in the Control of Clinical Practice?', *International Journal of Clinical Practice*, 65 (7), 722–4.

Lee, E. and E. Frayn (2008) 'The "Feminization" of Health', in D. Wainwright (ed.), *A Sociology of Health* (London: Sage), 115–33.

Michelena, H., B. Powell, P. Brady, P. Friedman and M. Ezekowitz (2010) 'Gender in Atrial Fibrillation: Ten Years Later', *Gender Medicine*, 7 (3), 206–17.

Olesen, V. (2002) 'Resisting "Fatal Unclutteredness"', in G. Bendelow, M. Carpenter, C. Vautier and S. Williams (eds), *Gender, Health and Healing* (London: Routledge), 255–66.

Östlin, P., E. Eckermann, S. M. Udaya, M. Nkowane and E. Wallstam (2007) 'Gender and Health Promotion: A Multisectoral Policy Approach', *Health Promotion International*, 21 (S1), 26–35.

Payne, S. (2009) *How Can Gender Equity Be Addressed through Health Systems?*, Joint Policy Brief 12, World Health Organization, on behalf of the European Observatory on Health Systems and Policies, at: www.euro.who.int/document/E92846.pdf, accessed 11 October 2009.

Risberg, G. and E. Johansson (2009) 'A Theoretical Model for Analysing Gender Bias in Medicine', *International Journal for Equity in Health*, 8, at: www.equityhealthj.com/content/8/1/28/abstract, accessed 22 November 2009.

Robertson, S. (2007) *Understanding Men and Health* (Maidenhead: Open University Press).

Ruzek, S. (1978) *The Women's Health Movement: Feminist Alternatives to Medical Control* (London: Praeger).

Sen, G., P. Östlin and A. George (2007) *Unequal, Unfair, Ineffective and Inefficient. Gender Inequality in Health Care: Why It Exists and How We Can Change It*, Final Report to the WHO Commission on Social Determinants of Health, at: www.eurohealth.ie/pdf/WGEKN_FINAL_REPORT.pdf, accessed 10 October 2009.

Strauss, A., L. Schatzman, D. Ehrlich, R. Bucher and M. Sabshin (1963) 'The Hospital and Its Negotiated Order', in E. Freidson (ed.), *The Hospital in Modern Society* (London: Free Press), 147–69.

Stuckler, D., L. King and M. McKee (2009) 'Mass Privatisation and the Post-communist Mortality Crisis: A Cross-national Analysis', *The Lancet*, 373, 399–407.

Torsheim, T., U. Ravens-Sieberer, J. Hetland, R. Välimaa, M. Danielson and M. Overpeck (2006) 'Cross-national Variation of Gender Differences in Adolescent Subjective Health in Europe and North America', *Social Science & Medicine*, 62 (4), 815–27.

Wadham, B. (2002) 'Global Men's Health and the Crises of Western Masculinity', in B. Pease and K. Pringle (eds), *A Man's World. Changing Men's Practices in a Globalised World* (London: Zed Books), 69–84.

Walby, S. (2005) 'Gender Mainstreaming: Productive Tensions in Theory and Practice', *Social Politics: International Studies in Gender, State and Society*, 12 (3), 321–43.

Walby, S. (2011) *The Future of Feminism* (Cambridge: Polity).

Wallen, J., H. Waitzkin and J. Stoeckle (1979) 'Physician Stereotypes about Female Health and Illness: A Study of Patient's Sex and the Informative Process during Medical Interviews', *Women and Health*, 4 (2), 135–46.

Wamala, S. and I. Kawachi (2007) 'Globalization and Women's Health', in I. Kawachi and S. Wamala (eds), *Globalization and Health* (Oxford: Oxford University Press), 171–84.

WHO (2004) *Gender in Mental Health Research* (Geneva: WHO).

WHO (2008) *Closing the Gap in a Generation. Final Report of the Commission on Social Determinants of Health* (Geneva: WHO).

WHO (2009) *World Health Statistics 2009*. at: www.who.int/whosis/whostat/2009/en/index.html, accessed 1 October 2011.

WHO (2011a) *Human Rights and Gender Equality in Health Sector Strategies: How to Assess Policy Coherence* (Geneva: WHO).

WHO (2011b) *Gender Mainstreaming for Health Managers: A Practical Approach* (Geneva: WHO).

Woodward, A. (2008) 'Too Late for Gender Mainstreaming? Taking Stock in Brussels', *Journal of European Social Policy*, 18 (3), 289–302.

Index

CPSIA information can be obtained
at www.ICGtesting.com
Printed in the USA
LVOW10s1442131217
559594LV00014B/357/P